7th Revised and Extended Edition
1st English Translation
Color Edition

Translated into English by Andrew Schlademan
Cover design by Kristen Albert

ISBN-13: 978-1-948909-00-6
Library of Congress Number: 2018900187

Published by Thirty-Three & 1/ॐ Publishing

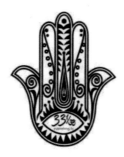

Printed and bound in the United States of America.

Björn Eybl, responsible for content: *"Not being a physician, I am not permitted to practice medicine in Austria. Thus, I hereby point out that I have never done so. Not even with my own method. Only God, Nature and the client himself can heal."*

The Psychic Roots of Disease: 5 Biological Laws of Nature is based on the discoveries of Dr. Ryke Geerd Hammer, M.D.

This extensive desk reference book is designed to share the finds of more than 500 case studies, with Therapists, patients and the curious.

The Psychic Roots of Disease
5 Biological Laws of Nature

Björn Eybl

Table of Contents

INTRODUCTION

Out of the Ancient Medicine 7
Into the New Medicine 8
The Discoverer 8

THE 5 BIOLOGICAL LAWS OF NATURE   9

The 1st Biological Law of Nature 9
The 2nd Biological Law of Nature 13
The 3rd Biological Law of Nature 14
The 4th Biological Law of Nature 18
The 5th Biological Law of Nature 19
Explanations of Important Terms 21

CONDITIONING   24

Conditioning from the Family 24
Conditioning from Past Lives 27
Conditioning from Past Lives 27
Conditioning during procreation/pregnancy 30
Conditioning during birth 31
Conditioning during the first years of life 31
Children are different 32

DIAGNOSIS   34

Getting into the practice 34
Laboratory Values 37
The Initial Consultation - Determining the Conflict 42

THERAPY   46

Possibilities for Conflict Resolution 46
Conflict-active Phase at the brain level/body level 57
Nutrition 57
Repair phase at the psyche level/brain level 60
Repair phase at the body level 61
Medication 62

LEXICON OF "DISORDERS"   64

General Symptoms 65
The Nervous System 71
Eye 81
Ear 104
Hypophysis (Pituitary Gland) 113
Thalamus, Hypothalamus 115
Adrenal glands 116
Thyroid and Parathyroid 118
Heart 123
Blood 133
Blood Vessels 139

Lymphatic System 145
Spleen 149
Nose and Sinuses 151
Larynx 155
Lungs, Bronchi and Trachea 158
Pleura 169
Lips, Mouth and Throat 171
Teeth and Jaw 181
Esophagus 187
Stomach 189
Small Intestine - Duodenum 194
Small Intestine - Jejunum and Ileum 196
Cecum and Appendix 200
Large Intestine - Ascending, Transverse, and Descending 201
Large Intestine - Sigmoid Colon 203
Rectum and Anus 204
Diaphragm 209
Peritoneum, Navel, Gr. Omentum and Abdominal Wall 212
Liver and Gallbladder 216
Pancreas 222
Kidneys and Ureters 228
Bladder and Urethra 235
Ovaries 240
Fallopian Tubes and Uterus 244
External Female Sex Organs (Vulva) 251
Testicles 255
Prostate Gland 258
Penis 261
Breast 265
Skin, Hair and Nails 271
Bones and Joints 286
Muscular System 307
Constellations 313

FINAL REFLECTIONS   **318**

Index 324

LIST OF ABBREVIATIONS

Adeno-Ca . . . . Glandular or mucosal tissue cancer
Ca . . . . Cancer (from the Latin carcinoma) (p. 15ff)
CT . . . . Cerebral CT = Computed tomography (pp. 10, 37)
CM . . . . .Conventional Medicine
EM . . . . Effective Microorganisms (p. 59)
MMS . . . . Miracle Mineral Supplement of Jim Humble–gentle antibiotic (p. 62)
OP . . . . Surgical operation
SBS . . . . Significant Biological Special Program (p 11f)
Syndrome . . . . Active kidney collecting tubules SBS + other SBSs during repair (p 230ff)
Example ➜ . . . . Typical conflict situation
Example • . . . . Real event

The Psychic Roots of Disease

5 Biological Laws of Nature

Acknowledgments

I thank Dr. Hamer for the gift of the New Medicine. This discovery will employ generations of physicians and change much for the better.

I also thank my friends and teachers who have shared their knowledge with me.

Great appreciation goes out to my wife for her moral support and patience during this three-year task.

I thank all of the people who shared their own "case histories" with me; without them, this book would only be half as good.

Thank you, Dr. Wolf Dieter Diersch, for your paternal guidance and legal support. Without you, this book would probably not have been published. I thank Dr. Ruprecht Volz for his thorough editing of both the language and the professional content in the German version.

I also want to express my gratitude towards Wolfgang Kalchmair for graphic direction and typesetting the book and Andreas Meinel for producing the index and looking over the second edition.

I also thank the director of the panel www.gnm-forum.eu, Antje Scherret, who influenced the second edition with her treasury of experiences.

Thanks to Bettina Mayer's team for graphic advice and Mr. Coser Angelo for the graphics processing.

Many thanks go to Carolyn Preissecker and Michael Busboom for the basic English translation.

Andrew Schlademan and Niamh Prior deserve special thanks for this English edition of the book.

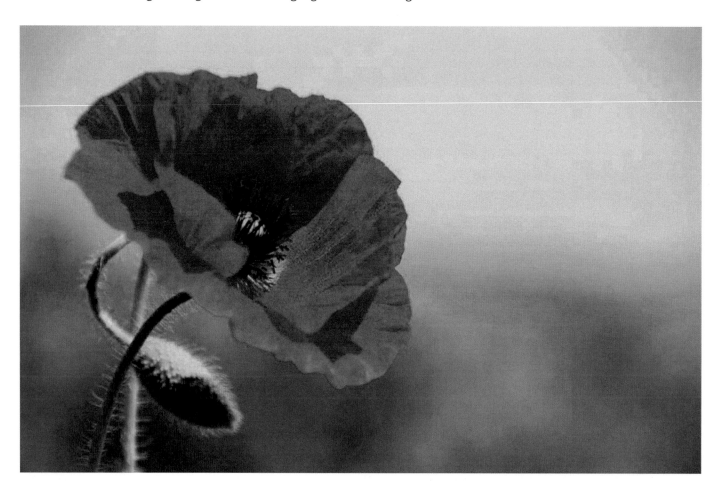

On the Creation of this Book

With this book, I wish to bring the interested layperson closer to the discoveries of Dr. Hamer.

It is not my intention to "adorn myself with borrowed feathers" in order to gain recognition.

The honor and recognition belong to Dr. Hamer alone.

It was he who discovered the 5 Biological Laws of Nature, and found out about all of the rest.

My role is one of a "translator" into the language of the common man who, until now, has hardly had the opportunity to grasp and make use of this medical discipline.

Since this book appeared seven years ago, my scope of knowledge has steadily increased. At the beginning, I strictly kept to Dr. Hamer's conflict and progression descriptions. This seventh edition is also based on his discoveries. However, to be honest, over the course of time the "strictly according to Hamer" perspective became too restrictive for me. And not just for me, but for many others too.

We want to further develop these thoughts, to evolve.

I have asked myself over recent years, how do these conflicts arise in the first place? Which individual preconditions have to exist for this to happen? Which influences lead to which conflicts? What lies in the background behind hereditary diseases?

Dear reader, you are holding in your hands the translated and completely revised seventh edition of this book.

Many new insights from practice and much new knowledge have been incorporated. I hope you will find enjoyment in reading and using this book.

I would like to thank the IBERA publishing house for their fair pricing.

A reasonable retail price was important to me as I did not want to sell an expensive textbook, but rather a "book for everyone" that would be worth its price.

This self-help and reference guide is meant to accompany us into a new era: an era full of uncertainty but one that we can look forward to.

This book presents the current status of my personal knowledge. Some details will perhaps prove to be wrong; *I ask the reader to forgive me for that* — to learn means to err! My guiding principle while writing has been: as simple as possible and as detailed as necessary. I hope that therapists will find it useful and interesting as well.

I often had to hide my enthusiasm behind factual and concise formulation; perhaps it will be sensed from "between the lines."

Out of the Ancient Medicine

For generations, we have become accustomed to receiving medication for every *"illness"* in order to get well.

It's normal that when we go to see a doctor, we come out with a prescription. It gives the patients a comforting feeling. After all, having *"something in their hands"* means having a bit of hope for eliminating the evil from their lives.

These prescriptions confirm our belief that the cause is *"external;"* otherwise, an *"external"* cure could not happen.

It is a satisfying, childishly simple-minded way of dealing with illness. It is a way of handing over responsibility, similar to handing over a broken car to a repair shop.

"The specialists will fix it — why else would they have gone through so much to learn their trade?"

Since we have no idea why we get sick or stay healthy, relinquishing responsibility is the easiest option.

Even if the doctor does not know the cause of the sickness either, they have a system that offers seemingly appropriate support and a therapy that sometimes helps.

The successes in trauma and emergency medicine are so impressive that we feel well cared for in other medical areas of expertise. Of course, over the centuries, the Western medical guild has learned how to credit random successes to their own account.

As a child, I read - with veneration - about the alleged annihilation of smallpox and other contagious diseases by medical giants such as Jenner, Koch, and Pasteur.

At that time, I did not know that when reading history, one must keep the author in mind: either the winner or the loser.

I didn't yet know that - through interest-driven policy - written history is often only a distorted image of reality.

I did not know that the real story is almost always sacrificed on the altar of Mammon. Christianity[1] and medicine have been following the same path for a long time and they share a common concern: keeping the people in line. Has this always been for the good of the people?

Well, it has at least been good for these institutions.

It is well known that the blind let themselves be led without any resistance. Until Christianization, the peoples of Europe believed in reincarnation. The church aristocracy exterminated this primal knowledge with *"fire and sword"* and replaced it with *"heaven and hell."*

For centuries, the fear of eternal damnation was just the thing for keeping people on track. For both clergymen and doctors, it

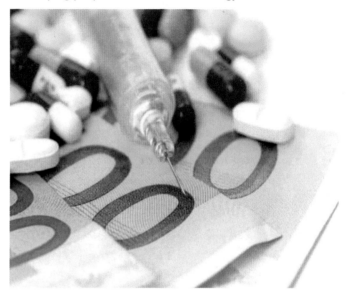

was important to keep the masses ignorant and pretend that they knew everything. For this purpose, the elitist Latin language was ideal: For common people, it was incomprehensible and thus, it provided the perfect protection from criticism.

Would it not have been more honest to say, *"joint inflammation"* instead of *"juvenile idiopathic arthritis?"*

Honestly, yes, but what do you answer if the patient tries to examine the cause of their joint inflammation? Do you have to admit that you don't know?

How am I supposed to justify the chemicals I'm prescribing? Won't the patient ask why he should swallow the stuff if I don't even know why the joint is inflamed? With "juvenile idiopathic arthritis," it's all much easier for me.

If the patient demands, I can answer that this affliction is an "autoimmune disease." If he is not quite convinced, I can then explain the effects of "immune complexes in the reticuloendothelial system."

---

1   With Christianity, I mean the church as an organization and not Jesus' message, which I regard highly

With the knowledge of true biological interrelationships, the doctor no longer needs to hide behind incomprehensible terminology and the patient doesn't have to blindly accept it either. These "fig leaves" (incomprehensible terminologies) are no longer necessary as a cover up, because each patient can know, relatively precisely, about the processes of "his illness." On the other hand, we must be willing to reclaim responsibility for our own health or illness with all its consequences, even the unpleasant ones.

The New Medicine

The basics of the 5 Biological Laws of Nature were discovered by Dr. Hamer in 1981. That is already long time ago when you consider how many millions have died unnecessarily from chemotherapy and radiation, but it's only a short time for a new science. We are at the beginning of a new era in medicine.

The coming years will fundamentally transform medicine.

By means of the "master key," the 5 Biological Laws of Nature, we will see a real paradigm shift and a flood of new findings.

Today, the New Medicine (NM) and conventional medicine (CM) are seemingly irreconcilable with each other. Naturopathy is also struggling with the facts of the 5 Biological Laws of Nature.

It will be a difficult road, but there is no other way around it. For the benefit of their patients, CM and naturopathy will have to be joined with the New Medicine, in order to eventually become a whole.

This book is an attempt to integrate valuable parts of CM and naturopathy into the New Medicine. Integration in the other direction seems nearly impossible to me both professionally and from a functional standpoint.

My first contact with the Germanic New Medicine®

I became aware of "The New Medicine" in 1995 (that's how it was called then and how I continue to call it to this day) through the media when the *"Case: Olivia"* story unfolded in Austria. Like most people, I thought to myself, *"My God, that poor child!– That is absolutely wrong, what the parents and this Dr. Hamer are doing."*

Even after the *"Case: Olivia,"* I kept hearing about Dr. Hamer via the widespread negative headlines, but sometimes also through very positive headlines in various alternative media.

At some point, I wanted to know more and I bought Dr. Hamer's original "Habilitation Thesis."

Although it all seemed Greek to me, I got the feeling that this Dr. Hamer was an honest and conscientious person.

While I was reading the "Habil" a second time, it finally clicked and since then, this subject hasn't let go of me. I attended study circles, lectures, and seminars, and marched in demonstrations in Vienna and Tübingen. I was known for always asking the most questions; this is something I still do today.

The thing that keeps me going is, I got responses that were consistent with my experience as a massage therapist and naturopath. This confirmation of theory in practice and the confirmation I found in diseases I experienced firsthand is what makes this Medicine so valuable to me.

Today, 20 years later, I am ashamed of my quick judgment in the "Case: Olivia." My confidence in the mass media has certainly faltered and I have come to realize that mass media does not inform the masses, but rather reflects the wishes of certain people.

The Discoverer

Dr. Ryke Geerd Hamer was born in 1935 and he studied medicine, physics and theology. In 1972, he became a specialist for internal medicine.

He worked in the Department of Internal Medicine at the University of Tübingen and Heidelberg, where he had to deal with cancer patients on a regular basis.

Even from an early age, he had always been a pioneer and innovator: he invented a scalpel that enabled plastic surgery without bleeding, the so-called Hamer scalpel, a special bone saw and more.

Through income from the patents on these inventions, Dr. Hamer wanted to become financially independent and settle down with his wife, also a doctor, and his four children in Naples, Italy. His plan was to open a surgery clinic for poor people and to work for free, but in 1978 tragedy struck.

During a boat trip to Corsica, his eldest son Dirk was fatally injured by a gunshot from Prince Emmanuel of Savoy and died in the

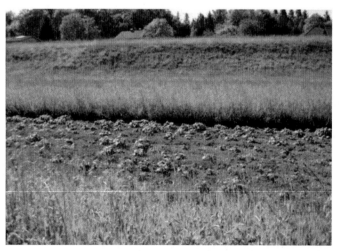
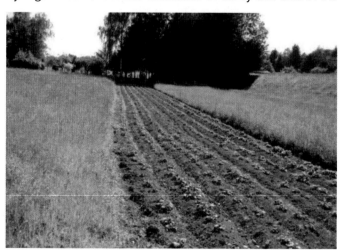

It is sometimes a matter of perspective to recognize the order. In both images, you get to see the same potato plantlets. Dr. Hamer recognized the order in relation to health and disease, because the line of sight agreed psyche-brain-organ.

arms of his father after a four-month struggle.

Three months later, Dr. Hamer unexpectedly fell ill with testicular cancer. It occurred to him that this disease could possibly be related to the loss of his son. After his recovery, he decided to investigate this idea further.

He began to inquire whether his patients in the Munich Cancer Hospital had also experienced tragedy before they got sick. And indeed, his guess was right: Without exception, all patients told of a drastically shocking event. This was the beginning of Dr. Hamer's discoveries. He began to tell his colleagues of this breathtaking correlation, hoping to start a scientific discussion. But this discussion only lasted a short time; he was quickly faced with the choice by the hospital management to leave the hospital or "renounce" his theses.

Fortunately, it was not in Dr. Hamer's nature to give in.

He decided to continue his research, and when he left the Munich clinic, he had formulated the 1st Biological Law of Nature: the "Iron Rule of Cancer".

Until this discovery, Dr. Hamer had an enviable career. He was celebrated as the youngest patent-holding internist in Germany. With his discovery of the psychic correlation to illnesses, the tide turned abruptly: 1986 saw his physician's license revoked for *"not denouncing the Iron Rule of Cancer and not converting back to conventional medicine."* He also experienced two imprisonments and three assassination attempts.[2]

When Dr. Hamer once again presented his findings to the University of Tübingen for review and was again rejected, an in-house counsel whispered to him:

"Our masters have analyzed it hundreds of times behind closed doors; every time they found that everything is correct. If they had found only one case that would not have been correct, they would have invited you for public scrutiny the next day."[3]

On July 2nd 2017, Dr. Hamer died while in exile in Norway. According to his wishes, he was buried in Erlangen, Germany. This is where he met his wife and spent the happiest years of his life.

Why "Germanic"?

Up until 2004, Dr. Hamer published his findings under "New Medicine." Dr. Hamer on the renaming:

"The only reason why I wanted to rename 'New Medicine' is because about 15 other sub-disciplines of alternative therapies also call themselves 'New Medicine' and the name could not be protected. So I had to find a new name, and since this medicine was discovered in Germania, the land of poets and thinkers, musicians, inventors and discoverers, which is also the mother of almost all European languages, I called it the 'New Germanic Medicine®'. Since then, however, sectarianism and even anti-Semitism have been associated with me."[4]

My future vision

We, New Medicine enthusiasts or Germanic health practitioners, practice with respect and appreciation - not only towards each other, but also towards conventional doctors, and therapists.
We shun fanaticism and dogmatism and learn gratitude, love and humility from each other.
We understand that all humans are spiritual beings on their own path of development.
We recognize that the ways of healing are as individual as each person.
The "good" of conventional medicine is combined with the New Medicine.
The New Medicine recognizes that their knowledge is also not a panacea and has expanded their horizons to things like family systems, subtle-energies and spirituality.
Conventional medicine overcomes its crude materialism - the New Medicine overcomes its strict biomechanical-thinking - spiritual seekers take the leap from reading books to implementing their insights in everyday life.

THE 5 BIOLOGICAL LAWS OF NATURE

These laws describe the causes and progression of almost all diseases, but they do not apply to injuries (e.g. accidents), poisoning (e.g. fluorine, mercury) and deficiency diseases (e.g. Coca-Cola-McDonald's diet, the effects of glyphosate (antibiotic pesticide) poisoning).

1st Biological Law of Nature

The Conflict

1st Criterion: Each Significant Biological Special Program (SBS) is formed by a biological conflict, a highly acute, dramatic, and isolative[5] conflict-shock experience on three levels: psyche-brain-organ.

2nd Criterion: The biological conflict is determined at the moment of the conflict: both the localization of the SBS in the brain as a Hamer Focus and the localization in the organ(s) as a cancer or cancer equivalent.

3rd Criterion: The course of the SBS at all three levels (psyche-brain-organ), from conflict to conflict resolution, on to the healing crisis at the height of the healing process and then the return to normalization (normotonia), is synchronous.

Special programs, in my experience, can start without a "highly acute and dramatic" onset: If stress, worries, or concerns of daily life last long enough, they can become solidified as biological conflicts. You hear the typical idioms: *"The straw that*

---

2   Read about it in "Einer gegen Alle" (One Against All) by Dr. Hamer.

3   See German New Medicine Quick Reference, p. 38; Amici di Dirk Publishers, 2008. ISBN: 978-84-96127-31-9, hereinafter cited as "Dr. Hamer, German New Medicine - Brief Information "

4   Dr. Hamer, presentation of the New Medicine, p. 2, see bibliography

5   Isolative means that in this moment, we are left to our own devices.

broke the camel's back!" "That's been torturing me for a long time," "I cannot bear it anymore," and "Yes, it's a burden!"

Simply put: "diseases" begin with events or situations that we haven't "resolved" and are mirrored on the three levels of psyche-brain-organ. *Small disharmonies cause "minor diseases" and great shocks cause "major diseases."*

Example of a slight agitation: A wasp flies under someone's shirt. The fright is transferred into their limbs. A small shock with all the criteria of a biological conflict: unexpected, highly acute-dramatic, isolative. After a few seconds the insect buzzes off again. Since the stress (conflict-active phase) lasted only briefly, there is no visible disease. Although an SBS starts, the time for a physically significant impact is too short (in the jargon: "too little conflict mass"). Small biological shocks are commonplace, as opposed to serious events. These heavier shocks cause "diseases" and this is what this book is all about - the roots of diseases.

Examples of serious conflicts: *Someone is beaten; a woman is raped; a mother loses her child; a man loses his job, upon which he is highly dependent.*

Biological conflicts run *"past understanding,"* meaning our intellect, reason and logic have no impact at this stage - it's about instinctual feeling and sensing. Here, one or more special programs (SBS) may begin, to cope with the "catastrophe" in the best possible way from a biological perspective . Due to the shock, the brain and body ramp up from *"normal mode"* to *"special mode."*

Psychology speaks of "dissociation" in this context: Through not coping with events (traumata), parts of the consciousness can split and can lead to a loss of (conflict) memory, impaired sensory perception and ultimately, disease.

Consider this: a part of the consciousness splits off, "freezes" - in this place, at this time - and is waiting for "redemption." The afflicted is called on to retrieve this frozen portion of their consciousness, in other words, to reintegrate it (conflict resolution). Then, it is once again "complete."

The point in time
The earlier in life conflicts occur, the more formative they are. They determine our character, our personality, and usually elude a resolution of the conflict. The more mature we are, the bet-

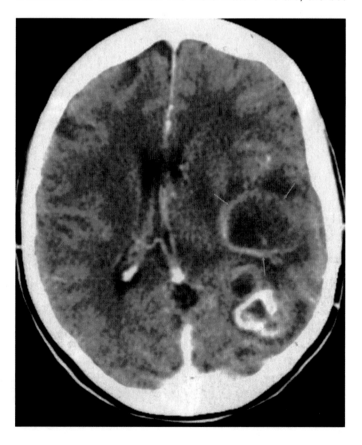

Two sharp-edged (= active) Hamer Foci in the relay for the inner ear. They show that the client has suffered a hearing conflict, which is not yet resolved. "What I've heard cannot be true!" These Hamer Foci can be described as "fingerprints of the soul."
They are living proof that the psyche controls all organs via the brain. To be honest, one has to admit that we are dealing with two, very clear examples here. In principle, they are ususally much less conspicuous.

The arrows point to a Hamer Focus during an intense repair phase (CT with medium contrast). Sharp rings are no longer visible, instead you can see large black areas with embedded cerebrospinal fluid (edema) and a bright connective tissue hem. Affected here is the relay for the coronary arteries, corresponding to a resolved territory-loss conflict in this patient. In the CM, such Hamer Foci in the repair phase are often diagnosed as "brain tumors." In this patient, the CM speaks of a "glioblastoma" ("Very malignant!").

ter we can usually deal with conflicts and allow them to resolve themselves. Most conflicts happen in the first three years of life.

The term Significant Biological Special Program (SBS)

Throughout the book, we will no longer speak of "diseases" per se, but of Significant Biological Special Programs.

Why? Because "disease" implies that something in the body is *"not right,"* *"not functioning,"* *"worn out,"* or *"broken"* (old-fashioned medicine's way of thinking).

By understanding the 5 Biological Laws of Nature, we realize that everything in the body has order and meaning.

What we referred to earlier as a "disease" is, in fact (usually time-shifted), a consequence of an exceptional biological situation - part of nature's survival strategy. If earlier we thought, this or that "does not work," it was because we didn't know how the body works and the natural relationships. Each tissue, every organ has a "normal program" for its standard functioning in "everyday life" and a special program (SBS) for extraordinary situations, for "biological catastrophes."

A technological comparison

Cars with on-demand four-wheel drive (an SBS) have the advantage, for example, to enable someone to drive on snowy mountain roads (exceptional situation).

Undoubtedly, this is a good thing. Who would complain about having 4WD after driving up into the mountains in winter, aside from needing a little more fuel (subsequent disease symptom)? The four-wheel drive is a useful, automobile special program to overcome exceptional situations. Only when we don't understand four-wheel drive would we try to dismantle and remove it from our car.

In terms of time, there is a difference between SBS and "disease:" Each SBS begins with a conflict-shock and lasts until the end of the repair phase. Most "disease" symptoms only occur during the repair phase. (See 2nd Law of Nature.)

Term "Biological Conflict"

For Dr. Hamer, the murder of his son Dirk was the worst event in his life, but it allowed him to discover the 5 Biological Laws of Nature. Each SBS is a shocking event that causes a biological conflict - hereinafter referred to as "conflict."

Instantly, the psyche, brain and organ(s) are changed.

Psyche: Compulsive thinking: thoughts are constantly focused on one thing - the conflict. The person can think of nothing else. Even at night, one cannot stop thinking.

Brain: Sharp-edged Hamer Focus appears in the corresponding brain section (see image below, left).

Organ: Cell growth (tumor) or cell diminishing (tissue shrinkage, ulcer, necrosis) or a respective increase or decrease in function. (See 3rd Law of Nature.)

Term "Hamer Focus"

From the instant the conflict starts, we find a circular target-shaped structure precisely in the area of the brain that corresponds with the content of the conflict - a Hamer Focus. Such foci consist of spherical, compressed brain tissue. In computed tomography (CT scans), Hamer Foci appear as circular discs. They were described by Dr. Hamer's colleagues - derisively - as the "odd

Hamer Foci." Though, the name, "Hamer Focus," finally stuck. The location of the Hamer Focus provides information about what conflict has happened and which organ is affected. Furthermore, one can conclude from the appearance of the Hamer Focus, in which "disease" phase the patient is. A sharp-edged Hamer Focus indicates that the patient has not yet resolved the conflict shock. A blurred, fuzzy Hamer Focus, on the contrary, indicates a solved conflict, which means the patient has overcome the shock and is healing.

Idioms

In the vernacular, there has never been a doubt about the connection between the mind and body:

"I was scared to death." (shock/fear conflict - larynx)

"I was paralyzed with fear." (motor conflict - muscles)

"He spat fire and brimstone." (territory anger conflict - gallbladder ducts)

"I just couldn't swallow it." - Chunk conflict (see p. 15, 16) - throat

"This sits in my stomach." - Chunk conflict (see p. 15, 16) - stomach

"My hands are tied." (powerless/helpless conflict - thyroid excretory ducts)

"The contact is broken." (separation conflict - epidermis)

"I can't endure this anymore." (self-esteem conflict - hip, femoral neck)

"The guy is breathing down my neck." (fear in the neck conflict - retina, vitreous body)

"I lost face." (separation conflict - trigeminal nerve).

Perception

What happened is not the determining factor, but rather how the patient perceives what has happened. What often looks harmless from the outside may have hurt a person deeply, hitting them in their weak spot.

On the other hand, heavy blows by fate are often dealt with easily, but they can look like a biological conflict from the outside. They always depends on the psychic structure, weaknesses and the resonances affecting the individual. So, be careful with remote diagnoses!

Example of varying perceptions

A man learns that his wife was killed in a traffic accident.

- "Normal" would be the sensation of a loss-conflict with SBS of the testicle. The event can also be perceived differently.
- Resistance conflict, when he resists inwardly and refuses to accept the death. *"My wife can't be dead!"* > SBS of pancreatic islet beta cells (diabetes).
- Central self-esteem conflict, when he received all his self-confidence from his wife: *"Without her, I am worthless."* > SBS of the lumbar spine (back pain during the repair phase).
- Loss-of-territory conflict, when he looked at his wife as part of his territory: The alpha-male and his female. > SBS of the coronary arteries (angina pectoris).
- Frontal-fear conflict, if he has the image of the truck, barreling towards his wife in his mind. > SBS of the brachial arches (non-Hodgkin's lymphoma, or branchial duct cyst in the repair phase).
- Only a small conflict and no visible SBS, for example, if he didn't care about his wife anymore.

Biological right or left-handed

Even with the first cell division, the decision is made whether the individual will be right or left-handed. In identical twins, one is always right-handed and the other is left-handed.

The determination of handedness is very important for us, because it follows the simple rule that applies equally to men and women: With right-handers, the left half of the body is the mother/child side. This side is related to your own mother, your own children or the people and animals that evoke these emotions. The right half of a right-handed person's body is the partner side (life or business associates, friends, enemies, partners, pets, colleagues, neighbors, relatives, and all other people).

For left-handed people, it is exactly the opposite.

The cause of a sore right hip in a right-handed person has to do with the partner side. (As for the hip, the conflict is about not being able to endure or prevail at something any longer.)

If a left-handed person has problems with the right knee, we must look for a mother or child self-esteem conflict. (The knees have aspects of an unsportsmanlike self-esteem conflict. In this case, the conflict relates to mother or child.)

A rash on a right-handed person on the left side of the body has to do with mother or child. (Epidermis - separation conflict in regard to mother or child.)

A conflict can also start special programs on both sides of the body simultaneously, e.g., when both knee joints are affected or when the skin rash is over the whole body. These cases involve both partner, mother or child. It is also possible to feel like a mother, a child and a partner to one and the same person (for example, the father in need of care is partially perceived by the daughter "as a child.")

In the SBS belonging to the territorial areas (e.g., coronary arteries, bronchi, or stomach mucosa), the handedness is of particular importance: In these cases, it decides which cerebral hemisphere the conflict "strikes" and which organs react with an SBS. It is only in the brainstem-SBS, the chunk conflicts ("yellow group" - the middle ear, intestine, liver parenchyma and others), that handedness does not play a role (see p. 15 - 17).

The clap test

To determine handedness, have the patient, with their arms not resting on their body, clap their hands.

The leading (active) hand indicates the handedness. If in doubt, they can clap alternately fast and slow. If, when clapping, the right hand is moved towards the left, the person is right-handed.

Usually the leading hand is the one on top. However, be careful, some people clap with the lower hand up into the upper hand. Therefore, always pay attention to "the leading hand." When the clap test is ambiguous, you can use two other tests:

Baby Test: For this test, you actually need a baby. As a baby substitute, you can use a rolled up towel or a cushion. Ask the standing patient to put the baby (the cushion) to their breast. Hand over the baby (the cushion) in a neutral position (vertical) and pay attention to whether the patient places the head of the "baby" on their left or right breast.

If the head is placed on the left breast, the patient is right-handed, if the head is placed on the right breast, the patient is left-handed.

"Bottle Test": Give the patient a bottle with a screw cap and ask him to open it. The guiding hand typically does the unscrewing/screwing. For example, a right-hander turns with his right hand while holding the bottle with his left.

Note: For drummers, people with paralysis or people, who have had injuries to one arm, these tests can bring incorrect results.

In retrained left-handers, (left-handers who were trained/ forced to become right-handers) a reverse training can bring astonishing improvements in various complaints.

Local conflict - regardless of handedness

The location affected by symptoms doesn't always have a parent-child or partner reference. Example: *A right-hander gets a slap on the right cheek. A basal cell carcinoma forms on the right cheek.*

The conflict had nothing to do with mother-child or partner, but simply with the unwanted skin contact. This causes a local conflict - regardless of handedness.

In principle, local conflicts can occur anywhere. Mostly, however, they happen in the epidermis, dermis, connective tissue, joints, muscles, blood and lymph vessels, peritoneum and pleura.

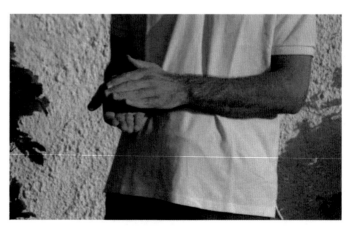

Right hand on top: biologically right-handed

Left hand on top: biologically left-handed

2nd Biological Law of Nature:[6]
The Two-Phased Process

The involuntary or autonomic nervous system consists of two parts: the sympathetic (active nerves) and parasympathetic (resting nerves).

The first regulates our involuntary functions when we are awake (activity, work, sports); the second controls these functions at rest (sleep, relaxation). In the normal state, which means when we are healthy and feel comfortable, these two branches switch

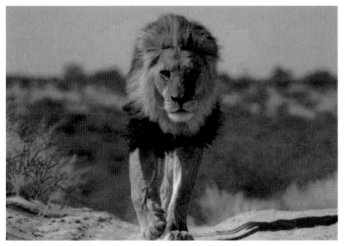

Imagine this lion comes up to you in the wild! Instantly you are in sympatheticotonia!

rhythmically (normotonia, stable circadian rhythm).

Dr. Hamer discovered that after the onset of a conflict, the psyche, brain and organ(s) automatically switch on "constant stress" mode (continuous sympatheticotonia), i.e., the sympathetic nervous system takes over sole command.

Conflict-active phase
We call this stress phase the "conflict-active phase" or simply the "active phase."
Characteristics: tension, thoughts are constantly revolving around the conflict (compulsive thinking), a sharp-edged Hamer Focus in the corresponding brain area, cold hands, increased blood pressure by vascular constriction, faster breathing and heartbeat, poor sleep, feeling "wound up" even at night, no appetite (i.e., weight loss, "cold diseases" such as gastritis, and angina pectoris).

Repair phase
When the individual resolves the conflict (conflict resolution), the conflict-active phase ends and the repair phase begins. Now the parasympathetic nervous system determines what happens. The pendulum swings in the other direction. Permanent stress becomes continuous fatigue (i.e., vagotonia).
Characteristics: relaxation, end of compulsive thinking, emotional relief, warm hands, poor circulation, poor performance, great need for sleep, fatigue - especially during the daytime, large appe-

tite leading to weight gain, headache and fever. The Hamer Focus in the brain shows soft contours due to fluid retention. Most CM "diseases" can be found during the repair phase, including the so-called infectious diseases and other hot diseases.

In the first part of the repair phase, water is deposited in the affected brain section and organ (edema), which can be very distressing for the patient (pain).

If an individual cannot resolve a conflict, he becomes weaker and weaker until he dies of exhaustion (cachexia). Mostly, however, it does not go that far, because instinctively we suppress such con-

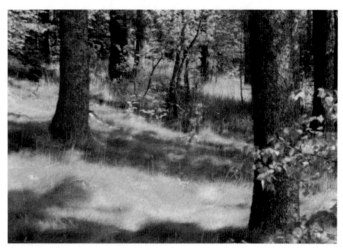

The peace and harmony of the forest promotes relaxation, i.e., parasympathicotonia or vagotonia

flicts from our consciousness or "come to terms" with the matter (downward transformed conflict, see page 22f).

Note: a pure repair phase lasts max. six months. If the repair phase symptoms continue for longer than half a year, there is a reoccurring conflict present.

Repair phase crisis (chills phase, "cold days")
At the mid-point of the repair phase, the moment of truth arrives with the repair crisis (chills phase). With severe diseases, this short, but intense, "sympatheticotonic wave" determines whether we make it "over the hump" or not. Its duration lasts from a few minutes to about three days.

The repair crisis is the most critical phase during the entire SBS. The most prominent healing crises are the heart attack (SBS of the heart) or epileptic seizure (SBS of the skeletal muscle).

Sometimes in these "cold days" of the crisis, one goes through the conflict in slow-motion once again. Through the healing crisis, the rudder is turned around again towards normality.

In the brain and organ(s), the water retention, which has been accumulated in the first part of the repair phase, is eliminated.

The second part of the repair phase, which deals with moving in the direction of normal conditions (normotonia), is characterized by increased water excretion ("pee phase"). This is accompanied by a rapid improvement of the symptoms.

Each SBS has its specific repair crisis, even harmless "illnesses" such as rhinitis (sneezing repair crisis) or laryngitis (repair crisis cough).

6   "Dr. Hamer, German New Medicine®–Brief Information" pp. 14, 15

The course of an illness when the conflict is resolved — our most important graph![8]

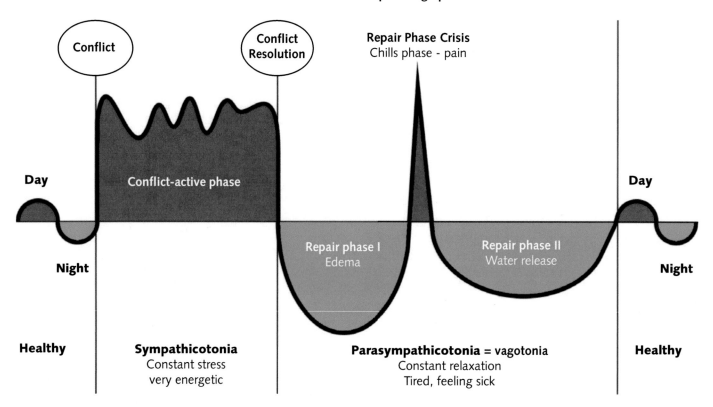

8   Cf. "Dr. Hamer, German New Medicine®–Brief Information " pp. 14, 15

The knowledge of this two-phase process brings order to the "diseases" of CM.

The first phase - the conflict-active phase - has been often overlooked up to this point, since it only accounts for a small number of complaints. During the second phase, the repair phase, "diseases" are diagnosed and treated, but in reality they are just repair phase symptoms.

3rd Biological Law of Nature:[7]
The Ontogenetic System of Diseases or Germ Layer Order

This third natural law states that all bodily processes can be understood and explained through an organism's developmental history (ontogeny).

From embryology, we know that each tissue, each cell in humans and animals is assigned to exactly one of the three germ layers.[8] Dr. Hamer observed the following: On the one hand, there are tumors that grow in the conflict-active phase and "shrink" in

the repair phase. On the other hand, there are cancers that form "holes" (tissue-shrinkage - ulceration, necrosis) during the conflict-active phase, which fill up again in the repair phase. This appeared to be contradictory, seemingly "illogical" behavior.

Through study and comparison of approximately 10,000 patient cases, Dr. Hamer solved this puzzle and discovered a breathtaking order with respect to germ layer, conflict theme and the part of the brain: the ontogenetic germ layer system of nature.

Looking at the four tables on page 15, one can see that the endoderm and old-mesoderm tissues behave the same - this pair works according to the "old brain" model.

The second pair, the new-mesoderm and ectoderm, works according to the "new brain" model; here it functions in exactly the opposite way (see p.15).

To sum up, you can say that with the 3rd Biological Law of Nature, we can understand tissue growth (tumor), tissue breakdown/degradation (ulcer), function reduction (e.g., diabetes) and increased function (e.g., hyperthyroidism). We also know now, which conflict affects which organ and which part of the brain steers the action.

Thus, the idea that cancer "proliferates" uncontrollably until the person is doomed is an out-dated concept. We can recognize, that cancer is not a senseless process carried out by rampaging cells, but one of Mother Nature's perfectly coordinated processes.

7   Dr. Hamer, German New Medicine - Brief Information, p. 19

8   Do not confuse germ cell layers (formed during embryogenesis) with the pathogenic microorganisms commonly known as germs.

* **

Brainstem and midbrain - inner germ layer - endoderm - handedness not relevant

Tissue/organ	Type of conflict	Conflict-active phase	Healing-phase
*Digestive organs, kidney collecting tubules, pulmonary alveoli, uterus mucosa, prostate gland, etc.	Chunk conflicts - Unable to get or get rid of something ("chunk"). (Want to have/ don't want to have conflict)	Increased function, cell division/tumor growth (adenocarcinoma) ⊕	Normalization, cell degradation through fungi or bacteria, night sweat and pain ⊖
**Smooth musculature	Motor chunk conflict	Increased tension	Normalization

Cerebellum - middle germ layer - old-mesoderm - consider handedness

Tissue/organ	Type of conflict	Conflict-active phase	Healing-phase
Inner and outer skins: dermis, pericardium, abdomen, pleura, nerve sheaths, breast glands	Protection and integrity: distortion, attack, defilement, disfigurement, worry or fight conflicts	Increased function, cell division/tumor growth (adenocarcinoma or adenoid tumors) +	Normalization, cell degradation by fungi or bacteria, night sweats and pain ⊖

Cerebral white matter - middle germ layer - new-mesoderm - consider handedness

Tissue/organ	Type of conflict	Conflict-active phase	Healing-phase
Supportive and connective tissue: bones, cartilage, tendons, ligaments Nutrition of the skeletal muscles, usually linked with ectoderm - innervation. Blood and lymph vessels, ovaries, testes, etc.	Self-esteem conflicts, inability conflicts (e.g., relating to occupation, relationship, family, sports, and appearance). One was blamed or demeaned. Something has failed or gone wrong	Functional limitation, Cell degradation (necrosis) ⊖	Function increase, cell growth (mesenchymal tumors, sarcomas) with the help of bacteria + pain +

Cerebral cortex - outer germ layer - ectoderm - consider handedness

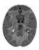

Tissue/organ	Type of conflict	Conflict-active phase	Healing-phase
Sensory organs, epidermis. squamous mucosa: e.g. coronary arteries and veins, bronchial and laryngeal mucosa, tooth enamel	Social conflicts: e.g., separation conflicts, territorial conflicts, bite conflicts	Cell degradation or functional impairment Pain in organs belonging to the so-called gullet-mucosa pattern ⊖	Cell structure or function restoration +
Innervation of skeletal muscles, usually coupled with mesoderm-nutrition	Motor conflict	Functional impairment, (debility, paralysis)	Restoration + healing crisis (convulsions spasms, epilepsy)

Common principle: cell-growth in the conflict-active phase, cell degradation in the healing phase

Brainstem (incl. midbrain) controls the inner germ layer - endoderm.

Nerve conduction from brain to organ not crossed. Handedness doesn't matter!

The digestive tract is arranged in a ring formation in the brainstem - according to Dr. Hamer, following its ontogeny (in my opinion this is an ancient building block of nature): protozoa (e.g., sea anemone), the model state for this, has a single opening for intake of nutrition and excretion.

Right side: The nutrition (chunk) is ingested . Left side: The indigestible (chunk) is excreted.

The same system has been assumed by higher species (including human beings) - but in order to make an elongated, not ring-shaped body possible, the ring was broken apart. The mouth and anus represent the beginning and the end of the former "digestive ring." Conflict theme: archaic "chunk" conflicts; on the right side wanting to ingest/get something and on the left side wanting to get rid of something.

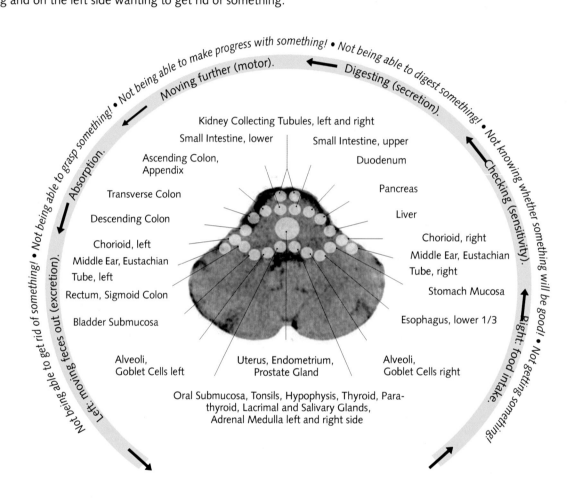

Cerebellum controls one part of the middle germ layer tissue = cerebellum - mesoderm. Nerve conduction from brain to organ are crossed. Consider handedness (right or left). Protection and integrity: Attack, defilement, worry, and fight conflicts.

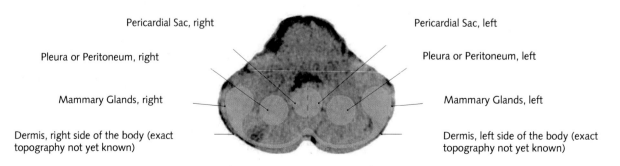

Cerebral White Matter controls the other part of the middle germ layer tissue - new-mesoderm. Nerve conduction from brain to organ crossed (except myocardium). Consider handedness (right or left) or local conflict. Self-worth conflict: one does not feel strong enough. Things did not go well. Something has gone wrong.

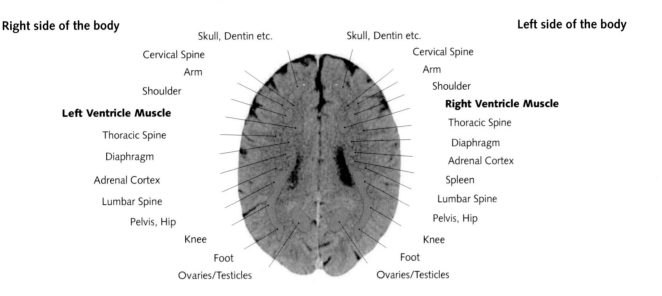

Right side of the body | Left side of the body

Skull, Dentin etc.
Cervical Spine
Arm
Shoulder
Left Ventricle Muscle
Thoracic Spine
Diaphragm
Adrenal Cortex
Lumbar Spine
Pelvis, Hip
Knee
Foot
Ovaries/Testicles

Skull, Dentin etc.
Cervical Spine
Arm
Shoulder
Right Ventricle Muscle
Thoracic Spine
Diaphragm
Adrenal Cortex
Spleen
Lumbar Spine
Pelvis, Hip
Knee
Foot
Ovaries/Testicles

Cerebral cortex controls the outer germ layer called ectoderm. Nerve conduction from brain to organ crossed. Consider handedness (right or left). Social, territorial, separation, or motor conflicts; fear of rear or front attack.

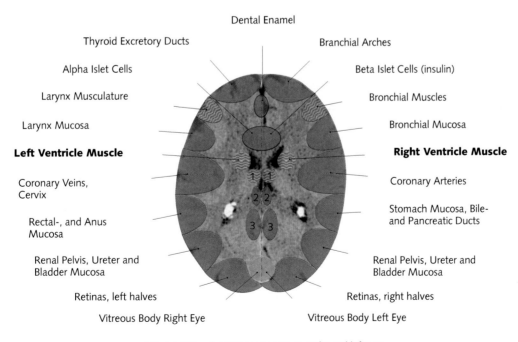

Dental Enamel
Thyroid Excretory Ducts
Alpha Islet Cells
Larynx Musculature
Larynx Mucosa
Left Ventricle Muscle
Coronary Veins, Cervix
Rectal-, and Anus Mucosa
Renal Pelvis, Ureter and Bladder Mucosa
Retinas, left halves
Vitreous Body Right Eye

Branchial Arches
Beta Islet Cells (insulin)
Bronchial Muscles
Bronchial Mucosa
Right Ventricle Muscle
Coronary Arteries
Stomach Mucosa, Bile- and Pancreatic Ducts
Renal Pelvis, Ureter and Bladder Mucosa
Retinas, right halves
Vitreous Body Left Eye

1 Skeletal Muscles (Motor Function), right and left Leg
2 Epidermis, Hair (Sensory), right and left Leg
3 Periosteum (Post-sensory), right and left Leg

Common principle: cell degradation in the conflict-active phase, cell growth in the healing-phase

4th Biological Law of Nature:[9]
The Ontogenetic System of Microbes

This natural law states that fungi, bacteria, and viruses (nucleic acid-protein compounds) are indispensable aids (= symbiotic) and fulfill defined tasks.

We know from CM about the classification of microorganisms into "good/mutualistic" (e.g., coliform bacteria in the gut, mouth flora) and "bad/parasitic" (e.g., tubercle bacteria, streptococci, viruses). The "bad" has been given the blame for various "diseases," namely the "infectious diseases."

This error occurred because coinciding with many "diseases," fungi, bacteria and viruses (nucleic acid protein compounds) are actually found in the body.

What CM likes to conceal is the fact that if you look for them, you can find lots of microbes in healthy people too. If they are found in sick people, they are called "pathogenic" (disease-causing) bacteria - "Here, we've found it! - It's an infection!" They explain why one and the same germ sometimes makes you ill

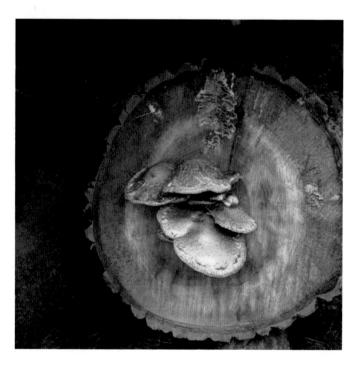

Nothing is where it is accidentally. This is also true for microbes. Here, dead wood is being broken down by fungi.

and at other times doesn't - on the basis of having a good or a bad "immune system."

"Infection experiments" have been repeatedly carried out in secret and have always brought back the same results: germs are partially transferable but the associated diseases are not.

Microbes - The Firefighters

If someone was investigating the cause of building fires, they might come to the following crazy conclusion:

"In all instances of building fires, fire department vehicles and firefighters were present." These vehicles and fire-fighters must be the cause of fires! Right?

Everyone knows that this is nonsense, because the firefighters are actually there to extinguish the fire. Fungi, bacteria, and viruses (nucleic acid-protein compounds) do just the same. They "put out fires" and optimize healing. They are not to blame for the disease.

Faithful Companions

Microbes have been our faithful companion for a long time. Our body is "riddled" with them down to the very last cell (e.g., mitochondria). In nature, nothing is "germ-free." On the contrary, every living thing is full of microbes (such as topsoil/humus). Since the beginning, we've lived in perfect symbiosis with them. Without them, we would fall stone dead on the spot (cellular respiration, digestion).

Dr. Hamer has found out that the three microbial species (fungi, bacteria, viruses) are controlled by different brain regions. From those regions, they receive their orders for targeted "operations." Important: Our little micro-surgeons work exclusively during repair phases!

Fungi and Bacteria

These work at the brainstem's command and clear away excess tissue from the inner germ layer (e.g., candida fungus in the gut and thrush fungus in the mouth). Night sweats means that they are currently at work. The brain-stem gives the command to multiply in the active phase (to produce an appropriate quantity for storage). If they are found in this (asymptomatic) active-phase, CM calls it "non-pathogenic bacteria."

Bacteria

There are many different types of bacteria. Each bacterium has a certain "special field," for example, the gonococcus in the urogenital tract or corynebacteria in the throat. A part of them is controlled by the cerebellum and destroys tissue ("old brain" principle), and another part is controlled by the cerebral white matter and builds tissue ("new brain" principle), e.g., bacteria help during the bone SBS to build up bone substance.

Viruses

To date, there is no direct evidence for viruses being the cause of diseases. "CM's virus evidences" are all indirect tests based on the binding or non-binding of proteins to other proteins. These tests are not calibrated, because to do this, you would first need to isolate the virus. The evidence that viruses cause disease is therefore lacking.

Undeniably, there are a large number of very small nucleic acid protein compounds (globulins) in the blood and other fluids of the body. These globulins can be roughly equated with these so-called viruses. It is possible that the cerebrum works with these proteins to build up missing ectodermal tissue in the repair phase (still unclear).

How do we explain epidemics?

Through collectively perceived conflicts in families (e.g., mom

---

9   Dr. Hamer, German New Medicine® - Brief Information, p. 29

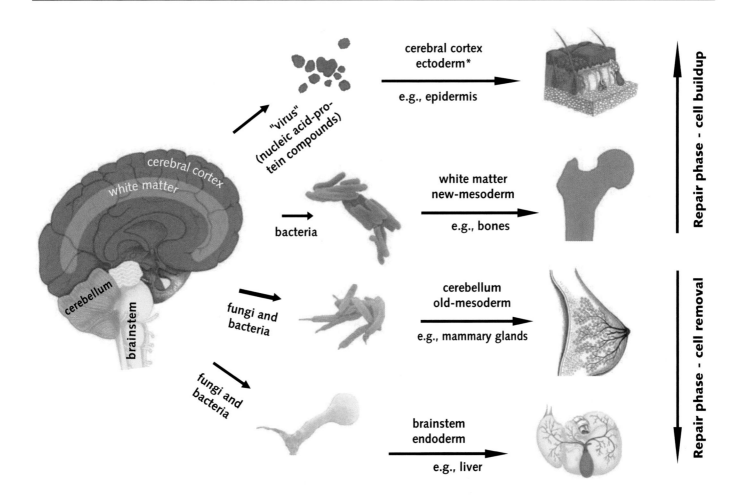

needs to suddenly go to work), school classes (e.g., difficult math test, exam week at the end of the semester), or entire regions (e.g., natural disasters or wars suffered collectively), this is where the group's common field of perception comes into play. Similar stress or negatively experienced emotions lead to similar diseases in the repair phase. See chapters: Vaccination p. 64 and Measles p. 275.

Reservations/open questions

Microbes can only be a problem if they are not part of our "body flora." We come in contact with "unknown" bacteria strains, for example, when traveling overseas. They provide the body with the difficult task of integrating previously unknown bacteria and fungi into the body's microbial pool.

Aside from that, I think that a sick, poisoned environment can also give rise to pathogenic microorganisms. In this context, it is interesting that the medical medium Anthony William (Mediale Medizin, Arkana Verlag 2016) dates the emergence of the Epstein-Barr virus to the beginning of the later industrial revolution (around 1900).

He sees this virus as a cause of very diverse diseases like chronic fatigue, hepatitis and fibromyalgia.

In general, we still know far too little about the precise work of microorganisms, because for over a century, research has only been conducted to study "infection."

5th Biological Law of Nature: The Biological Reason for "Diseases"[10]

Dr. Hamer calls "diseases" "Significant Biological Special Programs (SBS)" with good reason. The name sums it up succinctly: Each "disease" has a significant meaning.

CM assumes that man is a random product of evolution, so the question of "meaning" has never been an issue. According to the CM paradigm, diseases happen by chance or because the "body machine" did not get the right fuel or hasn't been well-maintained, right?

Understanding the meaning of "disease" is probably the best thing about the New Medicine. With this understanding, we can gain insights into the processes of nature. We recognize that everything has evolved to fulfill a purpose. Every SBS has been proven over millions of occurrences. They only start when we are confronted by a certain exceptional situation, when we are caught off guard.

The significance of colon cancer?

"I still can't digest that to this day." - The conflict in colon cancer is "indigestible anger." For example, an employee is looking forward to an upcoming promotion when suddenly someone else is chosen instead. A cell division begins in the large intes-

---

10 see "Dr. Hamer, German New Medicine® - Brief Information" p. 29.

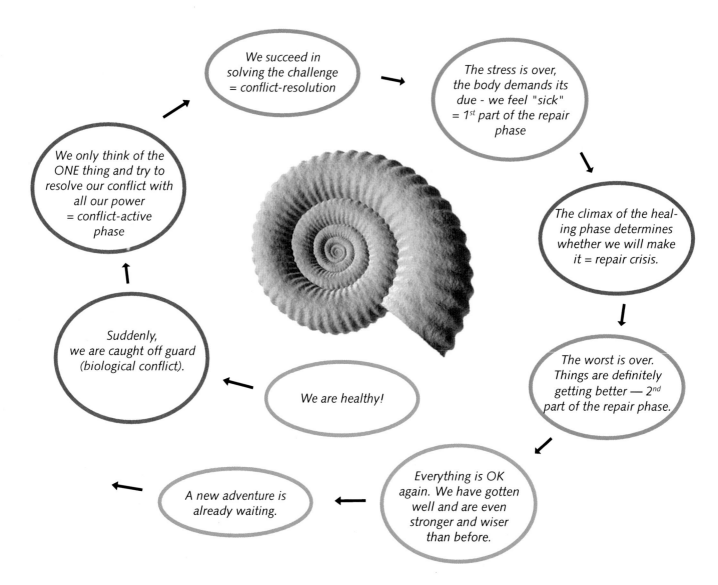

We succeed in solving the challenge = conflict-resolution

The stress is over, the body demands its due - we feel "sick" = 1st part of the repair phase

We only think of the ONE thing and try to resolve our conflict with all our power = conflict-active phase

The climax of the healing phase determines whether we will make it = repair crisis.

Suddenly, we are caught off guard (biological conflict).

We are healthy!

The worst is over. Things are definitely getting better — 2nd part of the repair phase.

A new adventure is already waiting.

Everything is OK again. We have gotten well and are even stronger and wiser than before.

tine. These additional intestinal cells produce additional digestive juice, so that the "anger chunk" can be better digested. The same special program starts in the wolf, when a bone ("chunk") is stuck in the intestines. With additional intestinal cells, nature tries to break down the obstacle. In humans, it is not usually real pieces of food, but "job (chunk)," "house (chunk)" or perhaps even "sports car (chunk)."

The meaning of testicular cancer?

Cell division in the testis occurs after a "loss conflict." *For example: a close relative dies; the beloved cat gets run over or a child makes a permanent move to another city.* Additional testicular cells produce more testosterone (male sex hormone) and more sperm. This hormone acts as a sexual boost, i.e., the reproductive instinct is increased, with the intended result being the quick replenishment of this loss. Nature does not distinguish between the death of a loved one and a beloved cat. Both cases initiate the same SBS to ensure offspring. Women respond to a "loss conflict" with ovarian cancer. Cell growth in the ovaries causes a flood of estrogen. The high levels of estrogen make women very receptive to sex and ready to conceive. Again, nature steps in to insure rapid "replacement." In this case, this is provided by pregnancy.

Musculoskeletal pain

Musculoskeletal pain has the function of bringing a living being to rest so that the affected structure, which has proven to be too weak, can strengthen. Bone, cartilage, tendons, and muscles can only regenerate or rebuild when they are at rest (even cars have to stop if you want to fix them).

When the repair phase (inflammation) is finished, the pain stops and the bone is fully resilient again; what's more, bone becomes stronger than before (luxury group). The associated conflict is the self-esteem conflict.

The purpose of hyperthyroidism?

When an individual suffers a conflict because they perceive themselves as being too slow, cell division begins in the thyroid. For example, a vendor has customers being "snatched away" all the time because he is not fast enough. In this case, Mother Nature makes more thyroid tissue for a higher thyroxine output, which results in an increased level of activity for this living being. The vendor can now act faster. If the conflict is resolved, the thyroid tumor is destroyed by fungal bacteria (thyroiditis).

Note on the 5th Biological Law of Nature
According to my experience, the purpose of symptoms/illnesses sometimes goes beyond biology. The reason often lies in the need to mirror psychic processes in the body so that they can be recognized = Law of Equivalence/Mirroring. E.g., overly active joints (hyper-mobility) show signs of inner instability.

Important Explanation of Terms

"Benign" or "malignant"
This classification is of great importance to CM, but not within the 5 Biological Laws of Nature.
In CM, "benign tumors" are considered harmless and peaceful, while "malignant tumors" are considered to be aggressive and life-threatening. However, what does the biological reality really look like? What makes the "malignant tumor" so "malign?" The decisive factors for CM are size, appearance, growth behavior, and especially the biopsy findings: If in a microscopic examination reveals many enlarged cells with enlarged nuclei, then the diagnosis is "malignant." If uniform cell structures are found, the diagnosis is "benign."

How does cellular growth function?
First, the cell swells to almost twice its original size. The nucleus and the other constituent parts of the cell double themselves. Shortly afterwards, the cell constricts in the middle and divides. One cell becomes two. The "offspring" have - in comparison to the rest of the mass - large nuclei.
Here, CM speaks of "malignant tissue." More correct here would be simply to speak of "growing tissues." This division gets even more absurd when you know that the boundary between "benign" and "malignant" is anything but clear. The same tissue sample often produces divergent findings in different laboratories. The specialists often contradict each other. This happens frequently when the tumor is just beginning to grow or growth has almost come to a standstill.
We used to think tissue growth was a mistake of nature and thus, said it was "malignant."
We now know that tissue does not randomly start to grow. An SBS will only start if there is a biological necessity. If one were to put embryonic or wound-healing tissue under the microscope, according to CM, it would be classified as malignant, "because we see brisk growth."
A similarly absurd diagnosis would be a tissue sample from a healing fracture. The tissue at the break does not differ from the bone cancer tissue, osteosarcoma. We would get the same results from a tissue sample of a pregnant woman's breast. During this phase, mammary cells multiply.
Conclusion: we should quickly forget the classification into "benign" and "malignant" tissues because it has nothing to do with science.

Metastases
"Metastasis is the spread of a cancer from one organ of the body to another... Metastasis is widely accepted to be the result of the tumor cells' migration..." These assumptions can be found in Wikipedia. They are only eluded to as a hypothesis in relation to other hypotheses. Unfortunately, I know of no cancer patient who has had it explained to them as a theory. On the contrary, "metastases" are presented as medical fact by CM.
With this in mind, one true fact remains: no cancer cell was ever detected in a drop of arterial blood.
Blood donations: Why is the blood from blood donors not examined for "metastases"?
Would that not be a medical concern, when you consider that on average, every 4th person falls ill with cancer during their lifetime and "metastases" might be in the blood donor's blood?
Mysterious migrations: How can cells of an intestinal primary tumor "resettle," for example, in the bone ("bone metastases")

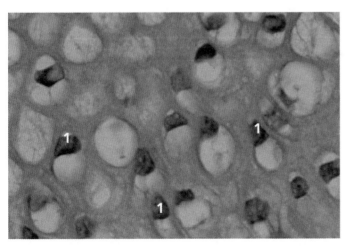

The two images show smears from the cervixes of two different women (400 × magnification).
Above we see almost equally sized cells with normal pale-small cell nuclei (1).
Few are undergoing division = not growing tissues. CM findings: "benign or regular"

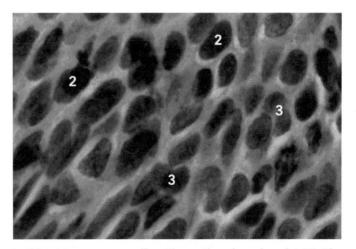

In this picture, we see cells with greatly enlarged nuclei (2). The dark coloration of the preparation shows an increased cell metabolism. Some cells divide (3). All together clear indications of growing tissues. CM findings: "malignant." New Medicine findings: repair phase of a female territory-loss SBS. Source of both images: a hospital laboratory.

and suddenly turn into bone cells? How can specific intestinal cells turn into bone cells? Upon examination, nothing else can be found in the supposed bone metastases.

What then are *"metastases"* if they impossible? They are newly formed cancers (second or third cancers), usually caused by conventional medicine's death-diagnoses and prognosis shocks. *"You have prostate cancer!"* or *"The liver cancer in you is very aggressive. Realistically, you have one more year. Enjoy the time you have left and get all your affairs in order."*

So, if you get information like this without knowing the 5 Biological Laws of Nature, you will suffers a massive conflict. If the patient feels, for example, the fear of death at that moment, a new SBS begins with cellular growth in the alveoli, as it combines the fear of death with *"getting too little air."* After a few weeks and a series of "continuous" check-ups, the so-called pulmonary nodules are found.

It may also happen that a man will suffer a self-esteem conflict along with a prostate cancer diagnosis: *"After the surgery, I'll probably be impotent."*

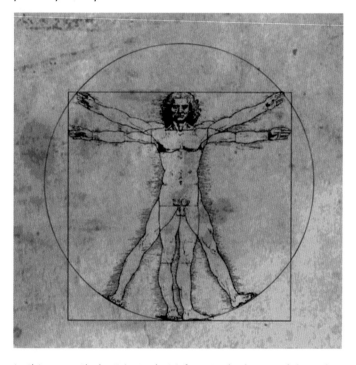

In this case, "holes" (osteolysis) form in the bones of the pelvis or the lumbar spine that CM calls bone cancer.

Why is it that you almost never find *"metastases"* in animals? Fortunately, dogs, cats and parrots do not understand when the doctor tells their owners about the *"malignant cancer,"* which their pet supposedly has. The animal is happy that the visit to the vet is over and it's on its way back home. Another reason why animals are diagnosed with cancer less frequently than humans is because animals are scanned less frequently.

Immune system

We do not use the term immune system because there is no such thing. The fight against hostile invaders (CM's *"antigens"*) does not exist any more than the fight against cancer cells.

What does exist is a kind of *"waste disposal"* system for the body: i.e., scavenger cells (macrophages) break down e.g., dead cells and cell debris. These substances are excreted through the lymphatic system and the blood (= sewer system or drainage system). Also, terms like *"immunoglobulins,"* *"antibodies"* and *"antigens"* are superfluous. It would be better to speak of proteins or globulins.

Recurring conflicts - the multi-phase process
(Diagram top of next page)

Ideally, after the completion of an SBS, the individual returns to health (normotonia). That would be the ideal biphasic course. As it happens, however, multi-phase processes are far more common. Here, after a shorter or longer break, the person is afflicted again by the same or a similar conflict (recurrent), either by a repetition of the conflict or a conflict trigger. The intensity is usually lower in the case of recurrence, because we "already know" the conflict. Nevertheless, we must pass through the entire SBS conflict with its conflict activity, repair phase and repair crisis again. This often happens again and again, like a broken record.

Recurrences and triggers are extremely important in practice, because much of the suffering that confronts us in everyday life is not based on new conflicts, but on the recurrence of old conflicts or conflict triggers. These are complaints that happen again and again without any apparently serious conflict (e.g., repeated stress/frustration at work or constant arguing with your partner). Often, recurrences also happen in the form of memories or dreams.

Persistent conflict activity (central diagram)

If an individual's conflict cannot be solved, it remains constantly in the stress phase and does not make the transition to the repair phase. We speak of persistent conflict activity. A pure, persistent conflict is literally a single-phase process and leads to exhaustion or death. Normally, to keep it from coming to that, we instinctively "adapt" ourselves to the conflict (downward transformed conflict). Statements such as, *"I'll just have to live with it,"* or *"I can't change it, but I suppose it's not so tragic anymore,"* indicate a conflict that has been transformed downward. In practice then, we speak of persistent conflict activity if the activity is interrupted by brief partial solutions, but the active phases predominate (strictly speaking, a multi-phase conflict with an emphasis on conflict-activity).

• *A department manager is demoted. He grapples with his loss-of-territory conflict and this affects his coronary arteries, but he makes the best of it and is now trying to enjoy life more. Nevertheless, at his workplace he is still slightly conflict-active. From this point on, he suffers from persistent angina pectoris (sign of an active coronary artery SBS).*

Persistent repair (lower diagram)

With persistent repair, the situation is reversed. Here, the repair phases predominate the multi-phase progression. Short active phases alternate with longer repair phases. The healing always begins anew, but unfortunately, it is incomplete.

"Hay fever" example: *Just before summer vacation, a student finds himself on the borderline between passing and failing. Despite his best efforts, the teacher gives him a failing grade.*

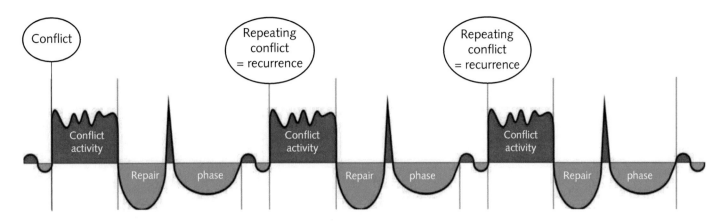

Multi-phase course of events (recurring conflicts) = alternating sympathicotonia and parasympathicotonia

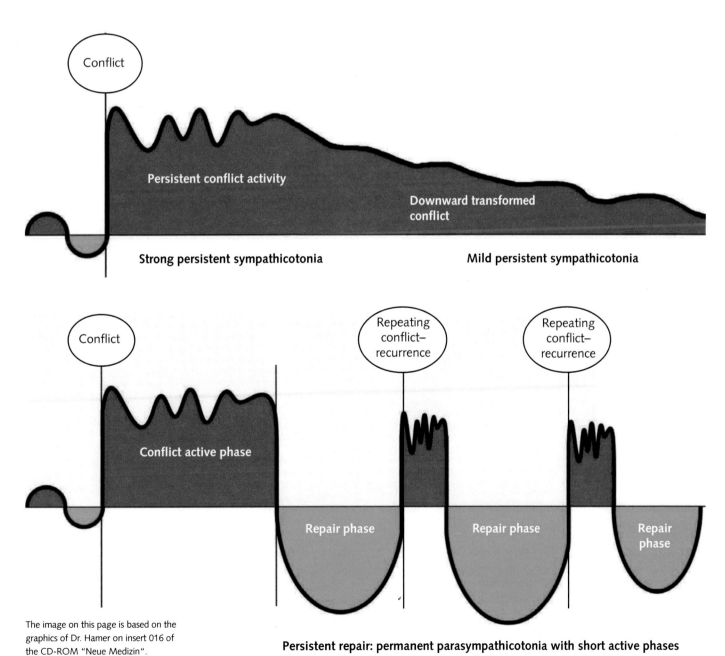

Strong persistent sympathicotonia

Mild persistent sympathicotonia

The image on this page is based on the graphics of Dr. Hamer on insert 016 of the CD-ROM "Neue Medizin".

Persistent repair: permanent parasympathicotonia with short active phases

The student "can't stand it" because now his summer is ruined. Affected organ: nasal mucosa. Trigger: pollen in early summer. From this point onward, he suffers periodically from "hay fever" - persistent healing. (Runny nose is a symptom of the repair phase of a fed up conflict.)

Triggers

At the moment of conflict, the subconscious usually records all of the circumstances accompanying the shock. These accompanying circumstances are stored under the heading "warning signals" and are retrieved on demand from the subconscious database.

Accompanying circumstances are all sensations that are perceived as being connected to the conflict in question: Certain pollen (e.g., birch) or fungal spores in the air, certain scents (e.g., perfumes), wind, drafts, cold, heat, dust, certain types of music (e.g., jazz) or music in general, certain types of noise (e.g., car horns) or any noise, certain voices (e.g., loud male voice) or certain colors. Foods that you eat during a conflict can especially become triggers; however, bodily sensations such as hunger, thirst, a full stomach, cold feet or wet hair can also become triggers.

When a sensory impression matches a "warning signal" from the subconscious database, the brain reacts: "Caution! XY conflict! - Start the SBS immediately!"

By means of the conflict triggers, the subconscious "remembers" the original conflict and starts the SBS. Most of our triggers are "collected" in the time between our conception and adolescence.

Put positively, these early conflicts shape our being, our character.[12] For example, our first contact with water decides if we will feel comfortable in it or whether we'll avoid it for the rest of our lives. If we experience any conflict in or with water, water will become a trigger for that particular conflict.[13]

• A toddler nearly drowns in a swimming pool and suffers a liquid conflict as a result of the accident. It is probable (but not a given) that water will be added to the "warning" database, i.e., it becomes a trigger. Later in life, the person often can't remember the conflict all; however, he notices that his blood pressure is always higher after a bath. (See p. 229.)

Note: A trigger always causes a recurrence and the SBS will start again. If it is possible to resolve the conflict, the trigger becomes irrelevant. Triggers or recurrences are the basis for all allergies.

• Mold allergy: A student lives for a year in a small cottage. It is poorly heated, the walls are partly moldy. One day, a big argument with his best friend takes place in this house. Bad smell conflict: "I can't stand this guy anymore." The mold spores in damp rooms become the trigger here. From this point on, the patient was allergic to mold or damp rooms. (Archive B. Eybl)

• A 40 year-old mother of two has suffered from gastrointestinal issues since she was 23. She experiences a her allergic reactions especially after eating fruit. The following comes to light:

---

12 In psychology, this is called conditioning.

13 Psychology: water is associated with the negative.

When she was 23 and still living at home, she dropped out of college against the will of her parents. At the dinner table, there were constant arguments over this. There was always a large fruit bowl on the table = indigestible anger conflict affecting the intestines. Trigger - fruit. (Archive B. Eybl)

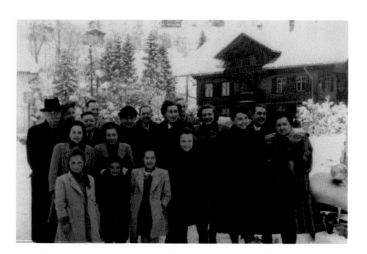

Conditioning from the Family

The 5 Biological Rules of Nature are undoubtably true. They are valid for every living being. However, it would be a bit shortsighted to assume that a person's health is dependent solely on the individual conflicts experienced during their lifetime and how they overcame them.

Earlier, when I proceeded strictly according to the New Medicine, I examined children for personal experiences that they had not coped with yet. However, daily practice showed that often there is nothing to find.

This "shortsightedness" also becomes noticeable when the affected person's complaints don't improve, because you haven't gotten to the crux of the matter.

For this reason, we need to turn to the important questions that lie behind the conflict - how it could even arrive at this point. Which internal, psychological conditions have to exist to give rise to this or the other conflict?

Why do we react so sensitively to one issue when it doesn't seem to matter to others much at all? What makes us into who we are and how we behave?

• A 22 year-old student has suffered from a bladder infection for 10 weeks (= chronic, repeating territory-marking conflict). Her story: For the first two years of her studies, she lived in her own apartment in Vienna, but for financial reasons, she moved into a shared, student apartment 11 weeks ago. After moving in to the apartment, she drove to visit her parents. When she came back, she found her things "pushed to the side" = territory marking conflict ("my territorial borders were not respected"). Despite discussing the situation and "feeling comfortable in the apartment," the conflict persists. Why?

The following conditioning factors came to light: While her mother was pregnant with her, their family lived with her father's parents on a farm. The mother-in-law was constantly violating *her mother's private sphere (territory) and her mother divorced a few years later.*

Just becoming aware of the connections seemed to have a therapeutic effect. For further treatment after that, we made an additional, internal voyage back to the unborn child and her mother at the time. The symptoms disappeared and have not returned. (Archive B. Eybl)

• *A 38 year-old office worker is married and has two children, 7 and 10 years-old. He has an athletic/muscular build even though he isn't very physically active at all.*

He came to my practice because every time he does any physical labor, he <u>always</u> gets terrible back pain for several days afterward. E.g., in the summer, he helped his neighbors with building their garage for a day. The result was three consecutive days of intense back pain. CM diagnosed him with a protruding disc between the 4th and 5th lumbar vertebrae.

Recently, he changed the tires on his car. Again he was in pain the next day! After doing office work, aside from slight tension, he never has any complaints.

In the eyes of the New Medicine, it seemed to be an open and shut case: a self-esteem conflict brought on by physical labor - he knows that he's not the best handyman - repair phase spans the subsequent days.

As his "therapy," I advised him that when he did any physical labor, he had to make sure he told himself, "It's not a big deal," etc. His symptoms, however, didn't get any better. Why? The solution was too shortsighted and the cause lay deeper.

During one of his next appointments, I asked him spontaneously, "What did your father and your grandfather do for a living?" Answer: "My grandfather was a farmer, but came back from Russia with only one leg after the war. He had to give up farming because he couldn't do the work anymore. They took pity on him and gave him a post in the local government. My father had to take over the farm work at an early age because of my grandfather's disability and at the same time he was studying to become an electrician. After a few years, he couldn't do any more physical labor because his back was shot, so he had to switch to an office job."

Now we were getting somewhere: the patient was carrying the

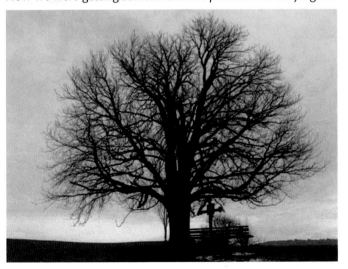

same conflict that his forefathers couldn't resolve. This is why he reacted so sensitively to physical labor. The guiding principle from his grandfather and also his father: "I can't do physical work anymore." Knowing this was the key that this person needed to move forward. It opened up new therapeutic opportunities, namely recognizing the traumata that his direct ancestors experienced, acknowledging it and illuminating it with love. (Raising the patient's awareness - more on that later).

We become increasingly aware of the interdependencies between the family and the individual when we shine a light on the family's history.

For being able to draw on the results of the research into these connections, I owe a debt of gratitude to, among others, Frieda Fromm-Reichmann (neo-Freudianism), Nathan Ackerman (family therapy), Jacob Levy Moreno (psychodrama), Mara Selvini Palazzoli ("Milan systems approach"), Iván Böszörményi-Nagy (multi-generational perspective), Anne Ancelin Schützenberger (psychotherapy, family tree - geno-sociogram), Bert Hellinger (Family Constellation) Dr. Claude Sabah and his student Angela Frauenkron-Hoffmann (biological decoding). The following are some of the most important guiding principles:

Everyone is connected to everyone

This concerns family members in particular. In families, the networking is so strong that we can almost consider it as an independent creature.

We and our children are the last members in a long line of ancestors. As such, we carry all the experiences of our ancestors - the good as well as the bad - in ourselves. A child is, if you will, the result of all of this experience. The experiences that are most important are usually those of the parents and then the grandparents, great-grandparents, etc.

In the family, all events are recorded and the bad/negative wants to be redeemed. In some families, similar tragedies happen again and again. The descendants are confronted with an unhealed issue until it is healed. Even harmless events remain in the family chronicle.

Nothing comes from nothing

Everything proceeds according to psychological or biological habits. Every abnormality, every symptom, every disease in a person has a cause.

<u>These can either be found in the life of the person in question or in the lives of their ancestors.</u>

As with a tree, the leaves (children) get nourishment from the trunk and roots (parents, ancestors). The tree (family as a whole) is dependent on the leaves (children), because this is where the real life is taking place, in the form of photosynthesis. The leaves and bark (the survivors) allow the tree (the family) to grow. The heartwood (of the tree) forms the base and supporting structure. For example, a child may have difficulty learning a foreign language because an ancestor was "opposed" to this language (due to the stress of learning it, by displacement, emigration, hatred of a language group, etc.).

• *An example from the book by Frauenkron-Hoffmann: The 5 year-old Laura can absolutely not stand to be separated* from her mother (i.e., go to kindergarten).

The cause is found in an interview with the mother:

Laura's great-grandmother was an adopted child. At the age of one year, she was given away by her birth mother. Laura has saved the experience of the great-grandmother, although she doesn't know her. She lives in constant fear that she could lose her mother.

Laura was told this story, as part of the "therapy." Her mother also assured her that what had happened to the great-grandmother would never happen to her.

This released the fear pattern in the girl and she suddenly liked to go to kindergarten. (see Frauenkron-Hoffmann, So befreien Sie Ihr Kind, p. 38)

Similar fates within families

show us that the issue that these people are dealing with has not been resolved/healed yet. This is why it appears again.

• The patient - a third-generation hairdresser - comes to an appointment with Mrs. Schützenberger in a neck brace because of a car accident and talks about her family history:

Her grandmother experienced the Armenian genocide first-hand. She saw her mother's and her two sisters' decapitated heads on the ends of lances. "There were so many heads!"

The relationship to the hairdressing occupation over three-generations: The daughter and granddaughter care for and beautify heads.

Mrs. Schützenberger comments: "... as if they could somehow undo the genocide while at the same time needing to remember it and its injustice ..."

Further details: 1. The patient was wearing a neck brace.

2. Her daughter was - almost strangled by the umbilical cord - born handicapped and died young (again the neck). After this, she didn't want to have any more children. 3. The patient's sister, also a hairdresser, had a child that was born with a deformed skull. "Its brain was running out of its head." (see Anne Anceline Schützenberger, Oh meine Ahnen! S. 147ff)

Unspoken and repressed

When unpleasantness within families remains repressed or unspoken, these things have a higher likelihood of coming out "into the open" over the following generations - sometimes in very peculiar ways:

• A 3 year-old girl suppresses her natural bowel movements, sometimes for days. She puts herself through this ordeal the most when she is constantly with her parents, e.g., on vacation. At preschool, the problem isn't so pronounced. Her mother has already tried everything possible, e.g., "poo-poo games" to make it a positive experience, but nothing helps. The little one is even frightened when someone else has to the toilet to go number two.

During her appointment, the mother can't think of any conflict that her daughter might be having. For this reason, I directed my focus on the parents and asked if there is anything that they aren't allowed to or don't want to let out?

"Yes, there is something!" answered the mother. My husband suffers from the so-called Tourette syndrome and that puts a lot

of strain on our relationship. When he's relaxed, he makes arbitrary, animal-like sounds. In everyday life, at work, he always has to pull himself together, but when he relaxed, he lets it all out."

That's it! He wasn't allowed to let his dreadful grunting out. His daughter wasn't letting her stinking feces out. She was mirroring for her father. The family had to come to terms with the situation. Therapy: The parents should speak about it openly and think about why the father isn't allowed to let out his ugly unpleasantness. (The father's family has a history of not discussing anything unpleasant). A few months later, I learned that the little girl was now going to the toilet normally (Archive B. Eybl)

Things left unresolved

Sometimes children act out what parents or ancestors could not translate into action and, in this way, facilitate the healing of the family.

Here's an example from a book by Achleitner-Mairhofer:

A mother is worried about her young son: He belongs to a group of right-wing extremists. He hates foreigners and feels an intense need to protect Austria and his family.

It turns out that the boy is "enmeshed" with his late grandfather: During World War II, while his grandfather was on duty, his family was driven out of their Czechoslovakian homeland. All were able to flee, except the grandfather's sick, old mother, who had to be left behind. Shortly thereafter, she died in a Czech concentration camp. From then on, the grandfather hated the Czechs and he could never forgive himself for not being able to save his mother.

Now to the heart of the matter: The boy in question hardly knows anything about his grandparents, but because he is

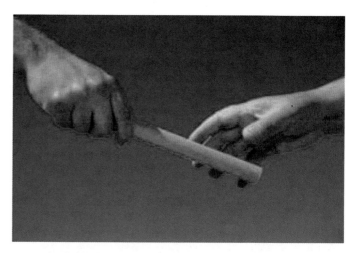

enmeshed with his grandfather, he now feels what his grandparents were feeling. He hates foreigners (and doesn't know why). Since his grandfather couldn't protect his family, the son feels the need to protect his family - the son must basically continue to serve up the hate that his grandfather's unwillingness to forgive left stuck in his throat.

In the course of a family constellation session, the therapist had the son say the following healing words: "Grandpa, I see your helplessness and your grief for your mother." Then she had the grandfather and son bow before the fate of the grandmother and the fate of the Czechs. (see Achleitner-Mairhofer, *Dem Schicksal auf der Spur*)

If we were to concentrate solely on the 5 Biological Laws of Nature, we would diagnose in this young man with a bio-aggressive constellation. (See p. 316)

However, it would remain unclear why the patient, perhaps for almost no reason at all, reacts in this way. Why was he so susceptible to this conflict?

Knowledge of the family history is essential for therapy: In the case of the boy, we can learn the cause of his susceptibility to a territorial-fear conflict - the enmeshment with his grandfather, and resolve it.

Family waltzes

Just like in nature, everything pulsates musically-rhythmically and this is also the case with families. It's easy to trace the duple metre: Here, the connection between the child and its grandmother/father is profound. We see similarities in character, health or in the course of their lives.

The 3 beat rhythm represents the connection me and my great-grandmother/father or between my child and my grandmother/father. You should pay especially close attention to this 3 beat rhythm when it comes to children born with disabilities. In practice, you should keep an eye out for dramas that played out in the lives of their great-grandparents. The key to understanding the disability might lie there.

Nomen est omen

When the same name is repeatedly given within a family, it forms a bond between these people. It can point to a similar fate, similar role/mission/expectation. This means that little "*John*" bears similarities to the old "*John*."

As well intentioned as it may seem, you're not doing your child any favors when you give them the name of one of your ancestors.

Anniversary syndrome

Important events that share the same date (e.g., births, deaths, weddings, accidents) indicate that these events/people share a connection and the issue behind them is waiting to be seen, acknowledged and healed. Also when the birth of one family member and the death of another roughly coincide, it can be that the one will take over the missions/burdens of the other.

• *A 39 year-old man is diagnosed with testicular cancer and after the operation, he declines all further treatments. It turns out that his grandfather died at the age of 39 after being kicked in the testicles by a camel. "Therapy" from Frau Schützenberger: "You can love your grandfather without having to die at the same age as he did!" (see Anne A. Schützenberger, Oh meine Ahnen! S. 138f)*

• *A mother comes to a session because she is worried that her little, firstborn daughter could die of asthma. She reports that for generations in her family, the oldest child always died young. Their family tree goes all the way back to the time of the French Revolution. At the time, the family gave refuge to a priest who was on the run. When the terror ended, the priest came out of hiding and blessed the family with the words, "As thanks, the*

oldest of every generation will watch over you!" For two hundred years, the oldest child from every generation always became a "little angel in heaven" that has watched over the family. Was that a blessing or a curse? Did the new orientation discussion with Mrs. Schützenberger change the situation?

At any rate, the girl regained her health and was still living 10 years later. (see Anne Anceline Schützenberger, Oh meine Ahnen! S. 175ff)

Note: the scientist, Mrs. Schützenberger, doesn't believe in reincarnation or similar phenomena. She documents cases, asks questions about why, but doesn't provide any spiritually-oriented answers.

Birth and death synchronicity

When the birth of one family member roughly coincides with the death of another, it can be that the one will take over the missions/burdens of the other directly.

Comparison: The relay runner hands off the baton (family issue) to the next runner. For the one, the race (life) is over, for the other, it is just beginning.

Conditioning from Past Lives

Even if we are only granted glimpses into past our lives under exceptional circumstances, I am convinced that our previous incarnations have a strong influence on us.

Not all readers of this book will share my belief in reincarnation and I can accept this. I also understand that some think that it's wrong to place science (the 5 Biological Laws of Nature) and religion next to one another, but I am of the opinion that they do belong together.

Schopenhauer called sleep the "brother of death." At night, one dies; in the morning, one is born. At the end of life, one dies and will be born again - if necessary. There is countless evidence, but every one of us, even the most serious, can only accept what we find in our personal world of convictions.

Even the following example isn't evidence, but it is thought provoking: How are we supposed to understand one day in a person's life, without knowledge of the days, months and years that came before this day? How are we supposed to understand their current life situation and mannerisms, if we don't know their history?

• *Bound by an oath: A 55 year-old woman and single mother had a 30 year-old son with a special trait: He feels completely and totally responsible for her. E.g., she planned a trip to Asia. Without even thinking about it, her son said that he would accompany her (although the trip wasn't even interesting to him). He has a girlfriend of 10 years that he wants to move in with, but he stayed true to his mother, staying together with her in their home. At one point the mother went to see a psychic about another matter. The psychic told her that she wasn't here about another matter, but that she was here because of her son. She saw her son next to her and told her that they had already spent many lives together. The last time he was her husband. On his deathbed, he swore that if they should ever be reunited again, he would always take care of her. Today, he doesn't remember this oath, but he is still acting according to it. In a ritual with the*

psychic, the oath was declared to be null and void.
She didn't tell her son anything about it, but soon noticed within a few days that he was behaving differently. He wasn't so courteous and helpful anymore. A few days later he informed her that he was moving in with his girlfriend and they were going to build a house together. (Archive B. Eybl)

According to my experience, in practice, resonance from past lives can be considered similarly to resonance from ancestors. Seen in this way, it will become easier again and provide the same results: "*Recognize yourself as a living being. Develop your character. Make amends with everything that was. This will not only help you, but it will help everyone.*"

You can achieve a great deal by saying prayers that you have formulated yourself when they come from deep within your heart. Example: Through the dissolution of oaths: "*I ask God to help me. Here and now, I release myself from all oaths, vows or promises that I entered into in this or in previous lives. I forgive myself and all involved who I have harmed through these bonds. I am now free. Thank you.*"

Liberation from negative feelings: "*I now let go of all feelings of hate, envy, anger and jealousy that I brought into this world in this life or in any previous lives. I am sorry that in doing so, I have caused others pain or injury. I now let go of these feelings forever.*"

Procreation from a biological perspective

The cycle of sexual reaction in humans and animals is a perfect educational example of how Mother Nature uses the elements of sympathicotonia, parasympathicotonia (vagotonia) and epileptic crisis according to her need. The following describes the male processes in colloquial language:

Normal condition - not aroused: standard day-night rhythm, normotonia, everyday life (1st section).

Sexual distress: "*There she is; I want her. I desire her so much.*

How can I win her over? What will it be like?" = stress, tension, compulsive thought like in the conflict-active phase of an SBS.

Relaxation, intercourse: "*I have her!*" = resolution of the "sexual emergency" > relaxation, vagotonia. Now the penis ring muscles, the bulbospongiosus and ischiocavernosus, contract around the base of the penis and it becomes erect.

(Even at night, men have long erection phases during deep sleep due to the strong vagotonia).

Orgasm: With its involuntary, whole-body contractions, the orgasm constitutes the epileptic crisis (the highest form of sympathicotonia) from natural elements. During these few seconds, both penis ring muscles relax and the penis retractor muscle contracts. This frees the way for the flow of semen. In an SBS, this is where edemata (fluid) is pressed out during the repair phase, here, seminal fluid.

Relaxation, sleep: After the orgasm comes the "sleep,"the second phase of the parasympathicotonia.

In females, everything functions similarly. During the female orgasm, the cervix's exterior orifice opens and the cervix makes peristaltic pumping motions to help transport the sperm cells. Right afterward, the cervix closes again.

Among other realizations that this knowledge gives us, it is clear that sex/procreation can only be successful during a state of relaxation.

Pregnancy from a biological perspective

Knowledge of the two-phase process has important practical consequences for our understanding of pregnancy.

The moon orbits the Earth in 27.3 days. A pregnancy lasts about 273 days.

The first part of the pregnancy - approx. 3 months is sympathicotonic. This causes a boost in growth for the organs controlled by the brain stem and cerebellum (see p. 16) (= sympathicotonic tailwind). The woman is generally nervous, at least not

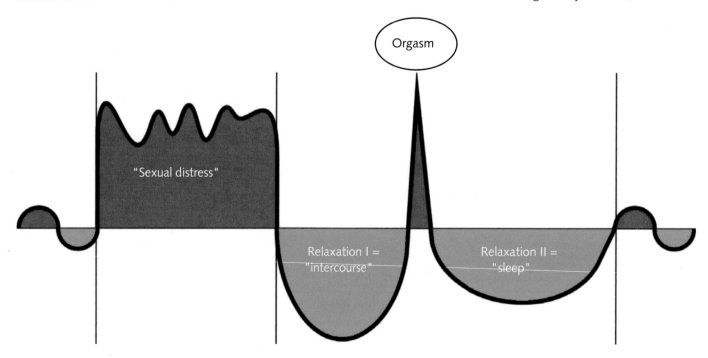

totally relaxed. The cervix is slightly dilated. In these first three months, nature leaves itself the possibility to end the pregnancy through miscarriage. 80% of miscarriages take place within this period. The most common reasons: too much stress, hectic lifestyle ("superwoman"), active conflicts, noise and/or necessities of fate (family energy, karma).

The second part of the pregnancy lasts about six months and is characterized by parasympathicotonia (vagotonia). Now, primarily the organs controlled by the cerebrum are growing (see p. 17). After the first three months are over, the conditions are so good that nature will now want to carry the pregnancy to term. The cervix closes, the woman becomes relaxed and cannot be so easily perturbed anymore. The radiant period! Only severe conflicts can put the mother into such a state of turmoil that the pregnancy would now come to an end.

The birth can be described as an epi-crisis. The first labor pains already count towards the birth. They end the vagotonia, the pendulum now swings in the other direction to strong sympathicotonia.

Our usual method of placing a mother on her back for the entire birth makes the process more difficult: better would be changing positions with squatting and on hands and knees.

The nursing period should last long enough (for the infant) and is again characterized by vagotonia (relaxation). It can be classified as the second part of the "repair phase." Like during an SBS, now liquid in the woman's body is eliminated. The mammary glands are sweat glands that were modified over the course of our developmental history - these now "sweat" the mother's milk out.

If we consider the diagrams below: the red phases are highly intense periods of sympathicotonia in which all events are exactly imprinted in the subconscious. This is where the conditioning happens that we would like to discuss now.

Conditioning during procreation

Procreation represents the (re)entrance into material existence, the beginning of an (re)incarnation, the start of a new life. The thoughts and feelings of the prospective parents, before and during procreation, already have an influence on the child.

It is the difference between whether this procreation was an "accident" or a conscious act. A child that is conceived of pure love - ideally, the mutual wish to create a home for a soul - has the best start in life. It will be able to draw from a large well of primordial force and trust.

Conditioning during pregnancy

Its nest in the mother's body is the cosiest and best place for the child. Day after day during this intimate symbiosis with the mother, the little one collects and registers not only all of the mother's feelings, thoughts and words, but also those of the father, the rest of the family and their environment. This more or less creates the indestructible foundation of feelings and thoughts for its entire later life. It will become the basis for its perception of love, trust, joy and helpfulness, but also for its relationship to God. The foundation is also laid for the way it will deal with difficulties, relatives, authorities, etc. Most significant, though, are those thoughts and words that concern the child itself.

However, even if what's being said isn't about the unborn child, it still feels like it's the one being addressed: I, you, he, she, it, we, they - regardless - the child applies it to itself. If during a fight, the future father says to the mother, *"You don't understand anything!"* Does he know that his unborn child can possibly apply this to itself and later in life (eg., at school) may *"understand little or nothing?"* If the mother often thinks, *"I feel so lonely,"* the child will later often feel *"lonely."* After all, it learned from a very early age to feel that way.

• If the mother or father are worried that they might not have

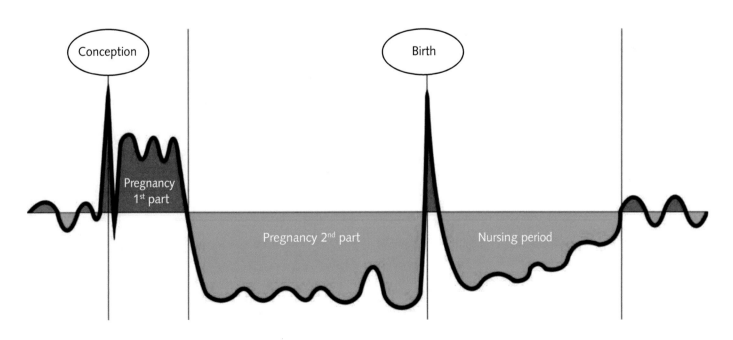

enough money for a (further) child, deficiency conditioning with regard to money could arise. It is probable that later in life, this child could attract this lack of money on itself, because it is already resonates with this condition.

• If the mother, father or both are completely fixated on having a child of a certain sex and are then disappointed, it can turn out that later in life, the child will have problems with their gender identity. Typical example: the girl that tries with all her might to be a boy, gets her hair cut short and plays rough sports with the boys. Example: *The 10 year-old Carl has cognitive problems - he is developmentally delayed and can neither read nor write. The cause: The mother wanted a daughter so badly after her first-born was a son. When the gynecologist offered to let her know the sex of the baby, she said that she didn't want to know. From the corner of her eye, she saw that he entered the male symbol into her record. This shock accompanied her for the rest of the pregnancy. She cried often, trying to convince herself that the doctor made a mistake or that she read it wrong.*

The boy is now living the mother's perception disorder. He cannot (doesn't want to) read and write. He cannot absorb any knowledge and is extremely jealous of his younger sister. However, the causal history goes back even further: The parents of the mother (grandparents of the boy) wished for a boy after two girls. When she - a girl - was born, they were very disappointed. She naturally noticed this and therefore behaved like a boy. She wants to be like a boy. Her parents often say: "You're still our boy..."

As therapy, the mother should talk with her parents about this matter and meditate to heal her own gender-rejection. Every night at bedtime, she should say to her son Carl, "We are delighted that you're a boy. We are delighted that you are here with us." (Archive B. Eybl).

• Unwanted child: If the mother or father consider an abortion, it is a tragedy for the child, because firstly, its trust in the father or mother is gone and also its joyful anticipation of life. It will be at the mercy of this dominant feeling. Later in life, this can be expressed by mistrust toward the parents or all people, an inability to make emotional commitments or by low self-confidence (one always remains unnoticed).

• When the mother is a fearful person, she passes these fears on to her child. It will be just as overcautious as its mother. Most will even transfer the details: e.g., fear of losing their partner, of certain animals, of heights, etc. As the case may be, if the father behaves differently, this conditioning may be balanced (like always, it depends on who the child primarily takes after).

• If the mother or father are afraid that the child could be sick or handicapped, a special fear seed is sewn: mistrust in one's own health. In the later life of the child, this usually leads to medical bondage (hypochondria) or frequent visits to the doctor. This parental fear is normally masked by solicitude: "*We don't want to take any risks with our child, that's why we naturally take advantage of all of the recommended precautions.*" (Ultrasound, amniocentesis, etc.) The pediatrician will praise the parents for their "responsible" behavior and the media sounds the same

trumpet. What we forget is that every preventative examination is done out of mistrust - and the child can sense it. Note: Examinations carried out for a distinct symptom are okay of course.

• When the parents fight frequently, the child naturally picks up on this. The programming reads: "*Fighting is normal and is a part of life.*" According to the law of resonance, it will attract conflict, even though it might possibly be longing for harmony. Certain conflicts can produce special impressions:

A 4 year-old preschooler refuses to sing and dance with the others, but alone at home she always sings with her dolls while she's playing. The cause: The father is a trucker and always likes to sing along with the radio while he's driving. During the pregnancy, whenever he sang along with the radio at home it got on the mother's nerves and she would say to him, "Why don't you just shut up! You're ruining the whole song!" After this programming was explained to the little one, she always sings along enthusiastically with the other children. (See Frauenkron-Hoffmann, So befreien Sie Ihr Kind, p. 24f)

• Some of us (about 10 – 20 %) were not alone in the womb during the first weeks after conception, but rather, we had a twin. Nature/fate wanted us to be born, while our little sister or brother died off (and was reabsorbed). Most of those affected don't have any idea that this happened, but are sensitized to separation, departure, loss or death due to this early conditioning. > If someone has an inexplicable, heypersensitive reaction to these topics, a "lost twin" should be taken into consideration.

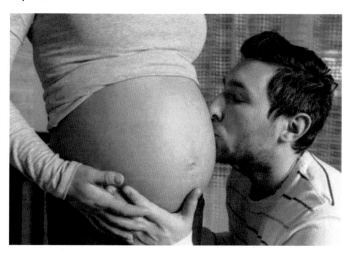

Up until now, I have just sketched out some prenatal conditioning - trailblazers for later conflicts. Conditioning has limits - and conflict is blurry. What follows are the most common, concrete conflict situations that occur during pregnancy:

• Noise of all types (domestic, traffic, construction, motorcycles, aircraft, fireworks, aggressive music, pop concerts).

• Conflict: 1. noise components, 2. emotional components.

• Danger or fear of all types.

• Ultrasound examinations: The No. 1 preventative examination. The sound waves mean enormous noise stress for the child. Some can tolerate it, others can't and suffer hearing, territory or separation conflicts that manifest as corresponding diseases after birth.

What's the use of the ultrasound? What's the use of knowing the length of the femur or the size of the head?

• The amniocentesis is even more dangerous and prone to conflict. I wonder: Why take this risk? Would I abort a child who is possibly handicapped? Here is something on the subject from Werner Hanne's brochure "The Development of the Child - What's Going on There?" (Die Entwicklung des Kindes - was spielt sich da ab?): Is it not possible that a soul would like to incarnate in a body that doesn't conform to our expected norms in order to introduce the parents to a very important, albeit wholly extraordinary, learning experience?

Conclusion: "*Expecting mothers, step back from your daily lives and be happy about your child. Leave of all your worries and fears behind you and go forth in confidence!*"

Conditioning during birth

According to Frauenkron-Hoffmann's observations, labor and delivery determine the child's approach to work and life's ordeals. The way the mother prepares herself to give birth can also be an indication of how the child (later as an adult) will cope with ordeals. Midwives or doctors should help the child to get through (through the birth canal). Later, teachers should help the child get through ordeals (tests). For the child, the teacher has a similar status to those who helped with their birth (positive or negative association).

The birth is the first great challenge in life. The mother's anxiety before birth can later express itself as test anxiety in the child.

A Cesarian section can condition the child insofar as that it now believes that it can't get anything done without external help. (Parents have to help extensively with school work, a need for tutoring; later in life, always trusting experts instead of one's own common sense).

A normal birth - even if it was difficult - confirms to the child that it can do it, if it puts in the effort. Also, trust and confidence between the mother and child is strengthened.

Children delivered by Cesarian section suffer more often from depression, respiratory illnesses and much more. This is probably also because oxytocin, a social-sexual hormone, is only sufficiently produced during a natural birth.

Deciding the time of the birth normally affects the child as well: The release of cortisone from the adrenal cortex initiates the contractions. If the birth is artificially induced (usually for reasons of hospital organization), it could be that later in life, the child has difficulties making their own decisions.

Some behaviors can be explained and thus resolved by understanding special circumstances at birth:

• *A 10 year-old regularly makes a "terrible mess" at the dinner table. Cause: During the delivery, a Cesarian section had to be performed because of a placenta praevia (placenta located in the lower uterine segment). The whole procedure culminates in a "terrible mess." The delivery theater was full of blood. For the boy, the mess was basically a prerequisite for survival. The mother explained the connection to him and told him that as of now, he can eat like a normal person, neatly, just like she does. Since then, the boy has acted normally. (see Frauenkron-Hoff-*

mann, So befreien Sie Ihr Kind, p. 59f)

Summary: "*Expecting mothers, find yourself a good midwife and a good place for your delivery. Accept all help and devote yourself to love.*"

Conditioning during the first years of life

Conditioning can be generated throughout our whole lives - just think of how adults return after being at war. For the most part though, it is the "formative" years that make us who we are. This decreases as time goes on. Mind you, all of this unfolds according to the blueprint left for us by our previous lives, ancestors, pregnancy and birth.

Survival after birth is not something that is self-evident, because without love, in the form of attention, warmth and nutrition (mother's milk), we die.

Strategies to receive love - to be loved - arise from our will to survive. These accompany us later, mostly unconsciously, through the rest of our lives.

A baby learns: "*When I scream, somebody comes. When I scream even more, mommy comes. Then everything's how it should be.*"

"*At nursery school, mommy isn't there. When I scream, auntie comes. That's okay. Once, I fell down and got a bloody nose. Then, mommy came right away. We went to the doctor and then home. Mommy loved me more for those few days than she had in a while.*"

"*That always works and I've learned: To be loved, something bad has to happen to me first, but it doesn't matter, because love is more important to me.*"

Result: Suffering, sick, acts needy for love.

Another child learns: "*When I laugh, everyone comes and hugs me, even mommy comes and is happy.*"

Result: friendly, perhaps even over-friendly.

Or it learns: "*When I do my homework, everyone praises me. That is nice.*"

Result: hard working and conscientious for love.

Or it learns: "*When I can't do my homework, daddy comes and helps me. I have to do poorly in school, because then daddy will come. He gets angry a lot, but still, I have him with me.*"

Result: A failure for love.

I, myself, grew up in a home where efficiency was the most important value. I received my father's recognition when I performed, when I proved myself in life. At school, I was mediocre, but I was good at sports and this brought me my father's recognition. Even though my father passed away 20 years ago, I still try to be as efficient as possible..."

The intellectual calls love recognition, but love is what we're all striving for - the small child, the adult, the elderly.

The following example should show what a large effect a small event can have when it harmonizes with an important resonance:

• *A 50 year-old mother of 4 came into the practice, because right after ending a telephone call, she was hit with a sudden bout of brachial neuralgia that she had been suffering with for a week ("only birth was worse," pain killers didn't help).*

Her girlfriend had asked her over the phone if there was anything she could do to help her get her apartment in order now that her partner had died. Could this trifle have had such an effect? The following came to light:

While she was still an infant, her oldest brother had died while he was still a small child. When she was two and a half, her second brother died. Finally, 4 years ago, her third brother died as an adult. After this last death, her parents forced her to immediately liquidate her brother's apartment, but she felt she still needed time to grieve.

I sensed that for her healing, we had to go back to the little, two and a half year-old girl: We spoke to her and explained to her that she also is loved. "You are not alone. You are loved. Your mother loves you too, but she is grieving for her son." Then, we hugged her in our thoughts and sent her a portion of love from the present time.

Immediately after the meditation, she reported that her pain had subsided by about 70%. The patient told me a week later that she now felt lighter than she had felt in a long time. (Archive B. Eybl)

Children are different

When we are looking for the cause of diseases in children (this also applies to house pets), we have to take two possibilities into consideration:

1. The child has suffered their own individual conflicts. Here, the 5 Biological Laws of Nature apply (see section).

2. The child is bearing something for its parents, ancestors or loved ones. In this chapter, we would like to delve into this aspect and thus, go beyond the 5 Biological Rules of Nature. Family-centered thinking is needed here.

The essentials: Children do not yet carry any responsibility. This lies with their parents or ancestors respectively. The child can do nothing about its bad habits, weaknesses or misbehavior. In principle, it has no other choice. Indeed, it has a resonance with the issue. Through their behavior or their illnesses, children reveal the issues in their family or their surroundings that urgently need to be resolved or healed. This, or their behavior is part of a special survival strategy (this is most prominent with hyperactivity, see below). Finding the cause frees the way for healing.

• A 3 year-old girl has recurring nightmares that wake her up because she feels like she's suffocating. Mrs. Schützenberger's research into the cause reveals that during WWI, the girl's great-uncle fell to poison gas at Ypres and her great-grandfather was wounded at Verdun. After the issue was discussed as a family, the nightmares and complaints came to an end. The girl was born on April 26th 1991, Ypres witnessed the first major gas attacks of the war over April 26th 1915 (see. Anne Anceline Schützenberger, Oh meine Ahnen! p. 219f)

Also, in the next two case examples, we may recognize that our little patients are not actually the real patients:

• The 7 year-old Peter, an intelligent, right-handed boy, had been suffering for two years from epileptic seizures. It always started like this: First, his right eye twitches, then he pulls his arm up involuntarily and covers the affected eye with his hand, as if to protect it.

CM diagnosed a "frontal lobe epilepsy" and treated it with anti-epileptic drugs (unfortunately without success). When I asked about the family history, the cause was clear: Peter's father fell ill two years ago with a disease in his right eye. After surgery, it was better in the short-term, but eventually he became blind in one eye. The whole family had been worried ever since, the relationship between the parents and the financial situation was still tenser than before. Explanation: Due to his father's illness, Peter suffered a motor conflict. Now, he wants to actively protect his father's eye for him. He does not want his father to suffer. He does not want the family to break up. Therefore, during the seizure, he puts

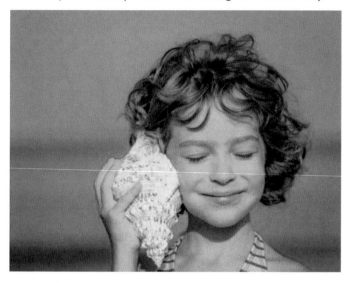

his hand over his right, "daddy-eye." The conflict "persists" because of the continuing bad familial situation. Epileptic seizures are the healing crises of a motor conflict. The attacks will stop when the conflict is permanently resolved.

Note: Children can usually cope well with parental disabilities. That said, suffering or quarreling parents have more potential to cause conflict in children.

The main treatment for Peter would be harmony and joy being restored in his family. The father should tell him often that he is doing fine with only one eye and that everything is okay now. Healing sentence: "Thank you for taking that on for me, but now you don't have to do it anymore, because I'm okay." (Archive B. Eybl)

• Aortic valve stenosis: A 4 year-old boy was diagnosed with an aortic valve stenosis = persistent self-esteem conflict affecting the heart. History: When his mother was pregnant with him, his great-grandmother on his mother's side's was in critical condition with arterial sclerosis of the coronary arteries (her bypass OP was unsuccessful). Her only wish was to see her great-grandchild. She waited until after the birth and then died two weeks later. At the same time, the mother's mother, with whom she had a very close relationship, was diagnosed with restrictive heart valves. So, two close relatives had heart problems. The 4 year-old bore it with them (here, Hellinger speaks of "familial solidarity"). As the "therapy," I suggested that the grandmother and mother completely make their peace with the death and the heart problems respectively. The mother should say the healing phrase to her son: "People come and people go. Your great-grandmother is doing well on the other side. We, the living, can accept that and we're also doing well. Thank you, but you don't have carry this weight for us any longer." (Archive B. Eybl)

The following are, for the most part, derived from a book I recommend by Angela Frauenkron-Hoffmann, "Biologisches Dekodierung: So befreien Sie Ihr Kind" (Biological Decoding: How to Free Your Child):

Aggressiveness, destructive anger

The child mirrors the anger that the mother and/or the father (or ancestors) keep bottled up inside (pregnancy) or express (presently).

Therapy: Determine the anger-causing situation, evaluate it, acknowledge it, speak about it and resolve it. Explain to the child that it doesn't have to act it out anymore and thank them for pointing out the problem.

Hyperactivity

Children with Ants-in-the-Pants syndrome don't fidget for fun, but they do it because they have to. For them, constant movement is a part of their survival strategy.

• A common situation: The mother has experienced a past miscarriage. She morns and thinks to herself, "The next time, I will pay very close attention to the child inside me and its movements. Then I'll be sure that it's alive." Now she is pregnant again and focused on her child's movements. For the child, the programming reads: "I have to move, otherwise I am (or will be considered) dead!"

• An example from the book by Frauenkron-Hoffmann: The

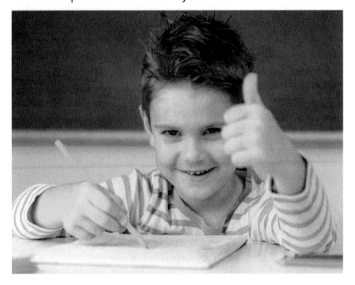

4-year-old Anton is hyperactive. His parents are nervous wrecks. The history: Anton's mother lost her baby in a previous pregnancy in the eighth month. She suddenly felt no fetal movement. Shortly thereafter, when she is pregnant with Anton, she directed all of her attention toward signs of life from her unborn baby. Once, she did not feel any movement, so she pushed against her stomach with her fist to induce fetal movements.

The child receives the message: "I have to move, otherwise I'm considered dead!"

This principle follows Anton in later life: "If I move, every body know that I'm alive." His motto: "Always move!"

Therapy: Find the cause and explain to the child that the matter is now settled.

Attention Deficit Syndrome (ADS)

It comes to this when the mother or father want to "tune out" during the pregnancy but can't.

• A pregnant woman has to listen to her mother-in-law and all of her endless stories the whole time.

• After giving birth, a woman is visited by a flood of well-wishers who are constantly talking. She needs rest and tries to ignore them, because she is too polite to send them away. Another common situation according to Frauenkron-Hoffmann is: A woman accidentally becomes pregnant and doesn't want to accept the reality of her situation. The child learns from this: "It is better just to tune out when someone wants to tell me something," (teachers, parents).

Reading problems

can be an issue if the mother, father or ancestors have experienced stress while reading at decisive moments (especially during the pregnancy). The details of the problems provide a guidepost to the cause. A very slow reading tempo indicates, e.g., that someone was too slow (there wasn't enough time) or too fast (something important was missed).

• A 6 year-old boy was far behind with his reading and was scheduled to repeat the school year again. During dictation though, he always did very well.

History: The mother had prepared a prayer for the birth that she wanted to read when the contractions started. When the time came, the mother tried to read the lines, but she couldn't because of the stress. The boy was thus blocked. "I see letters, but I can't read them because of the stress."

Whenever he has to read something, his brain remembers that = trigger. If the mother hadn't tried to force herself to read, this program wouldn't have been created. When he understood why he couldn't read, he quit having the problem, because it didn't make any sense anymore. (See Frauenkron-Hoffmann, So befreien Sie Ihr Kind, p. 23f)

This boy was able to do it, otherwise his skills would have also been weak during dictation. He took up his mother's stress and carried it on; he was basically mimicking her.

Grammar problems

are, according to Frauenkron-Hoffmann, linked with the father, authority, order, law, police, etc. When a child can't follow the rules of grammar ("law and order") you should examine these issues among its forefathers. Conflict search: more often with the father or male ancestors than with the mother. Also, situations during pregnancy or birth in which there was real stress. Therapy: Find the cause, examine it, acknowledge it and discuss it. Explain to the child that the issue is now resolved and thank them for pointing out the problem. They may now write according to the rules.

Word or spelling problems

Grammar orders the words in their proper places and defines their relationship to one another. Words stand for people, sentences for families. A child having problems with words or putting letters in the right place is not aware of their rank or their place in the family. E.g., friendly relationship between the parents and child (as opposed to a parental relationship) or true family relationships are actually being kept secret from the child. It is also possible that ancestors got into trouble because of family relationships that weren't clear. Therapy: see above.

Foreign language problems

indicate that the mother, father or ancestors are having or had stress with this language or the speakers/nation of the language. When the mother or father regularly criticizes a language group during the pregnancy, it is likely that this language group will be blocked for the child. It will be harder for them to learn it later. When one parent is bilingual, the partner should truly appreciate the second language and thus also participate in the "programming."

• *My mother is an absolute Francophile. She loved this language. My father acknowledged her enthusiasm. This is the reason that French in school was a walk in the park for me. I hardly had to study because I knew the grammar and vocabulary "just like that." Everything about the language simply made sense.*

Math problems

Problems with division (common) can indicate that the child is afraid of "being divided apart." Standard situation: The parents fight - the child fears a "division" (divorce) or it fears a separation from its school class due to changing schools (class will be divided). Ancestral trauma of this sort can also be a reason.

Problems with multiplication (rare) can mean that the family is getting into trouble because of "multiplication" (too many children).

Problems with calculating percentages indicate that someone in the family had stress with percentages.

• *A 10 year-old girl couldn't calculate percentages. Cause: The parents were renovating their house during the pregnancy. The father was counting on a tax of 6%, but suddenly he realized that in their case, they would have to pay a 21% tax. He wasn't counting on that. (See Frauenkron-Hoffmann, So befreien Sie Ihr Kind, p. 105f)*

Therapy: Find out the cause, examine, acknowledge and discuss. Explain to the child that the situation is resolved and thank them for having pointed out the problem.

Getting into the practice

Remain realistic

Without a doubt, the strength of the New Medicine and the 5 Biological Laws of Nature is that we can now understand and explain the body's processes. Cell growth and cell diminishing processes, inflammation and pain become comprehensible. This makes the New Medicine (in contrast to today's conventional medicine) a science. This leap in understanding is so great, it gives rise to extreme expectations: *"If the New Medicine can explain almost everything, then it can certainly heal almost anything."*

This describes my experience and it is similar to almost everyone's reaction when they encounter the 5 Biological Laws of Nature for the first time. However, this is misleading.

The fact of the matter remains, in spite of this knowledge, we can often do very little. This means that we have less influence on diseases processes - particularly with advanced cancers and psychosis - than we would like to have.

This is not because the New Medicine is not correct; it is because we humans seem to be unable to cope with difficult situations and many continue to drag the same heavy baggage along with them for years. We are at the mercy of a culture of fear - pure poison for our bodies and souls.

This is sobering and disappointing, but that's the way it is.

Dr. Hamer raised enormous expectations in his publications. The 98% survival rates in the New Medicine, which he continued to claim, are nonsense. This number, which is hypothetical at best, could only apply to a time in the future when the New Medicine is used by all physicians in all clinics and in an era free from the fear of cancer.

In the lexicon, starting on page 64, I describe all known SBSs and their ideal course: as a special, temporary natural/biological aid for optimally overcoming exceptional situations (conflicts).

Nature anticipates that conflicts will be resolved in a relatively short time (a couple of days or a few weeks).

This is how it is has evolved and how it should be. When this is the case, the SBSs run as described and they are actually beneficial. On the other hand, when conflicts last longer and are repeated over and over, vicious circles arise. Unfortunately this is often the reality we find ourselves in and this is when things can get ugly: tumors that enlarge, tumors that don't break down, pain that doesn't stop or always comes back. Nature and the New Medicine cannot be blamed for this.

With this in mind, I ask the therapists who are reading this to be **realistic and humble** despite your enthusiasm.

Case Example: Osteoporosis

Osteoporosis is a disease that mostly affects older women. It is a progressive loss of bone mass. As a result, the bones become weak and susceptible to fractures (e.g., hip fractures). Conflict: self-esteem conflict.

During an extended conflict-active phase, cells in the bone break down. In the short time between regeneration phases (cell development) pain may occur. These are times when self-worth receives a boost, for example, through a beautiful event. (See also p. 289).

The woman, now 61 years-old, is right-handed, a gymnastics and mathematics teacher and a single mother of one daughter, now an adult. She lives for sports: running, tennis, hiking, skiing, gymnastics, etc., usually in the company of friends. No one would have ever thought that such a physically fit, non-smoker with a healthy diet could be diagnosed with osteoporosis at age 47.

During a checkup in August 1999, a "manifest osteoporosis" was discovered in a quantitative CT scan. By September 2002, the values had deteriorated. In the left thigh, a density of 0.576 g/m³ was measured. She takes her doctor prescribed osteoporosis drug (bisphosphonate) on a regular basis.

Conflict history

The patient had been unhappy teaching over the last two years. Things were not going well in school - it wasn't just the school director that was getting on her nerves. However, this was only the "background music."

The main conflict is her daughter - her pride and joy. She has become independent and has moved out. Yes, it gets even worse. She is going to go to Australia, where she has received an in interesting job offer. In the fall of 2002, the patient is sitting at home alone, with an autumn mist hanging in the air and she doesn't know what she's going to do with her life anymore. Suddenly, she has an idea: "I will go and visit my daughter in Australia. The school will be begging for me to come back after this!" Note: in Austria, teachers can take a year sabbatical without fear of losing their teaching position.

After tying up loose ends at school, the patient took the trip to Australia in January 2003. Since the osteoporosis drug did not help anyway, she leaves it at home. From January 2003 up to June 2004, she spent a fabulous year with her daughter under the Australian sun, "the best time of their lives:" swimming, the beach, tennis, trips and so much more. She recalls that she did not have any back pain at all in Australia, but before that, it was troubling her continuously. (Constant back pain is an indication of a chronic, persistent self-esteem conflict).

After her return in June 2004, she arranged to have her bone density checked again. And lo and behold, with 0.590 (p. 36, color graphic, no. 3 on the x-axis) she was once again above the osteoporosis threshold, which means she was healthy again. The cure "happened" in Australia without any medication.

When measured in August 2000, the bone density on the right femoral neck had 0.599 g/cm³, and the left had 0.554 g/cm³. Here, the right-left correlation shows clearly that the self-esteem conflict is mainly concerned with her daughter, because the patient is right-handed, i.e., the left half of the body is her mother-child side. In September 2004, the teacher started getting back into her daily life. After the glorious year in Australia, she swings into the "worst school year." Since leaving her daughter, she misses her worse than ever and the foggy autumn weather is depressing = conflict recurrence.

The results of the density measurement in 2005 at the left femoral neck has a value of 0.522. Again, the osteoporosis is back with a vengeance! The values are reflecting the swings in her psychological condition. In the winter of 2005, the tide turns. Her daughter returns from Australia and the patient also feels better at school. Basically, she now sees everything in a much more positive light. It was during this time that she encountered the New Medicine.

With her new lease on life, she endured even the dark winters over the subsequent years too (p. 36, Nr. 5, 6, 7, 8, 9). Her bone density improved steadily. This is no medical miracle; this is because her daughter moved back to their hometown again and bones <u>can</u> regenerate (heal themselves - like we're all sure they will after a break).

Another case example/true story

An 84 year-old female retiree with chronic diarrhea was admitted for a colonoscopy at a hospital in Upper Austria. After the procedure, the patient was administered an infusion. Still hanging on the drip, she asked what the drip was for. The answer: "It's against osteoporosis, which everyone has at your age."

The patient is surprised, because three months before she had her bone density measured in another hospital and the result was: "Everything is OK." The current visit was entirely about to her intestines. Nobody even examined her bone density.

Shortly after the first osteoporosis infusion, she was administered two further infusions. She asked, "What's happening now?" Answer: "These are painkillers that we administer to control the pain caused by osteoporosis."

In the patient, discontent was spreading and indeed, she felt a lot of pain - pain that she didn't have prior to getting the infusions. Now to the point: That evening in her hospital room, she was watching TV. Coincidentally, the program included a report on the clinic where she was staying: "…the largest osteoporosis center in Austria and the one with the most patients…" It took a few weeks before the woman was able to recover from this hospitalization.

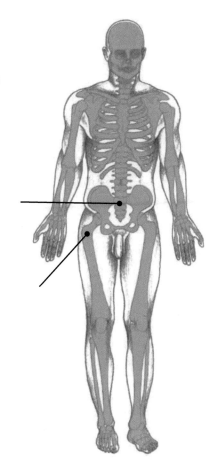

Bone in general
self-worth conflicts

Lumbar spine
**central
self-worth
conflict.
"I am totally
worthless."**

Hip and
femoral neck
**self-worth
conflict,
something can't
be overcome.
"I cannot
do that."**

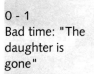

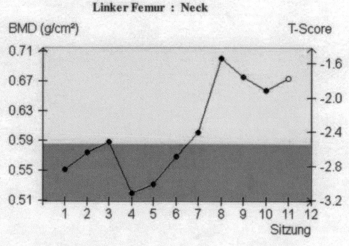

0 - 1
Bad time: "The daughter is gone"

2 - 3
Beautiful Australia-year

3 - 4
"Worst School year"

5 - 7
"The daughter comes back"

8 - 11
Good Time: "The daughter is back home"

	Linker Femur
Durchschnitt (g/cm²)	0.606
SD (Standard Deviation)	0.063
Variations Koeffizient (%)	10.39

Untersuchungsdatum	Alter	BMD (g/cm²)	Anwender
24/08/2000 08:44:00	46	0.554	
02/09/2002 09:47:00	48	0.576 (4.05% / 4.05%)	
16/06/2004 09:38:00	49	0.590 (6.63% / 2.48%)	
21/11/2005 11:08:00	51	0.522 (-5.66% / -11.53%)	
04/12/2006 08:19:38	52	0.534 (-3.56% / 2.23%)	
10/04/2008 11:21:06	53	0.571 (3.10% / 6.90%)	
15/06/2009 10:58:30	54	0.603 (8.88% / 5.61%)	
19/04/2010 10:03:07	55	0.703 (26.97% / 16.62%)	L
04/04/2011 10:12:58	56	0.678 (22.43% / -3.58%)	K
06/06/2012 09:39:55	57	0.659 (19.11% / -2.71%)	L
12/06/2013 09:49:28	58	0.676 (22.09% / 2.50%)	M

* = nicht berücksichtigte Daten   Variation (Ref / Vorherige)

Knochendichte - Befund

Es wurde folgender Befund erhoben:

Messort	BMD (g/cm2)	T-Score
LWS (L1 - L4)	0,873	-1,6
Re. Schenkelhals	0,584	-2,4
Li. Schenkelhals	0,633	-1,9

Gerätetyp: Hologic QDR-4500

Beurteilung: Oteoporosis is no longer detectable
In der LWS und im Schenkelhals beidseits finden sich - bezogen auf den T-Score - im unteren Normbereich gelegene Knochendichtewerte, gegenüber der Voruntersuchung vom April 2008 zeigt sich in der LWS ein Anstieg des Knochenmineralgehalts um knapp 5%, im Bereich des Schenkelhalses im Mittel um knapp 6%. Es zeigt sich somit eine Befundbesserung gegenüber den Voruntersuchungen, der Befund spricht nun für eine **Osteopenie**, eine Osteoporose ist nicht mehr nachweisbar.

Kommentar:

Making a Diagnosis

When we make a diagnosis, we are not only dependent on physical aspects like in CM, but we have three levels available: psyche - brain - organ.

Example: An ovarian cyst always means there is simultaneously a Hamer Focus in the repair phase (soft-contoured) in the corresponding brain location (in this example, the ovarian relay in the cerebral white matter) and a psychic cause, a resolved loss-conflict.

Each finding on one level must agree with the other levels. As a result, errors in diagnosis can largely be avoided. The old saying, "As many diagnoses as there are doctors," should now be a thing of the past.

The Diagnosis of the Brain

The brain level of the diagnosis has enormous scientific value, because it proves the interrelationship between the psyche and the physical body.

In practice though, reading the CT scan has little actual meaning. A CT scan of the head can possibly help when the disease patterns are unclear, but as a rule, we do NOT need it. Why?
1. Because it has a high potential for causing diagnosis shocks.
2. Because a cranial CT scan can't usually be interpreted with 100% accuracy (it isn't easy to find Foci and to match them properly).
3. Learning to read CT scans takes a long time. It takes experience with hundreds of scans before someone can make even partially reliable claims. There are hardly any therapists that can do this. Fortunately, you can work with the 5 Biological Laws of Nature without a CT reading, because we still have two levels (psyche and body) to cross-check.

If you still decide on a CT, it must meet the following criteria:

- CT (brain area), note: MRIs are unusable.
- Parallel to the base of the skull.
- Without contrast material ("native").
- Digital images (CD-ROM), (paper printouts are useless).

The evaluation of CTs is not the subject of this book. CT reading is difficult and requires profound study. For those interested, the corresponding relays are shown in mini-brain images in the lexicon.

Note: CM now calls Hamer Foci "ring artefacts," which also happen and are an effect of CT's radial motion. Obviously, when there are multiple, non-concentric Foci or the Focus does not correspond with the radial axis of the CT scan, it cannot be a ring artefact. New generations of CT machines are being designed to eliminate ring artefacts.

Diagnoses on the Psychological and Physical Levels

CM diagnoses:
It is good when we have all CM diagnoses on hand. However, note this: only about 60% of all CM diagnoses are correct, i.e., 40% are incorrect. Also, X-ray images are often misinterpreted. Even large cysts are often assigned to the wrong organ. These errors can happen because CM works without cross-checking the psyche and brain.

Laboratory Values

are an important pillar of diagnostic assessment for monitoring progress.

With the knowledge of the 5 Biological Laws of Nature, some values will take on a new and different meaning, while others will remain consistent with CM. Some values, such as the pancreatic enzymes lipase and amylase, are highly variable and are only meaningful when they are compared with previous values in the same patient.

Laboratory testing comes with the great danger that the results themselves are deemed to be so important, the data itself creates a conflict for some patients. People prone to hypochondria often run from one examination to the next until the trap they have built for themselves ("abnormal results") eventually snaps shut.

Thyroid laboratory values
Triiodothyronine (T3) and thyroxine (T4)
The majority of these two types of thyroid hormones are bound to proteins in the blood. Only a small portion is provided in the form of free thyroxine (FT4) or free triiodothyronine (FT3).
CM-normal values (serum):[14]
T3 67–163 ng/dl, free T3 2.6–5.1 qg/ml, T4 5.1–12-6 µg/dl, FT4 1.0–1.8 ng/dl.
<u>Elevated</u>
- Conflict-active phase of a thyroid gland chunk conflict.
- Slightly increased in conflict-active phase of a powerless conflict (thyroid excretory ducts).

<u>Reduced</u>
- Persistent-repair or the condition after a thyroid gland chunk conflict.

Increased or decreased TSH levels are an indication of an SBS of the thyroid excretory ducts (p. 121).

Blood laboratory values (See also p. 133ff.)
Erythrocytes (red-blood cells)
CM normal value:[15] women 4.0–5.2 million/ml,
men 4.2–5.9 million/ml
<u>Reduced</u> (anemia)
- Active-phase of a self-esteem conflict: bone SBS. Whether the bone SBS is noticeable in the blood count depends on how many and which bones are involved, because blood formation (hematopoiesis) takes place mainly in the flat bones (e.g., sternum, vertebrae). SBSs in the tubular bones are hardly reflected in the blood count.

<u>Elevated</u> (high red blood cell count)
- Repair-phase of a bone SBS. At the beginning of the repair-phase, the erythrocyte count falls even further, but only in appearance, because the blood is thinned by vagotonic blood vessel dilation with additional serum (lower hematocrit value). The erythrocyte production is running at fully capacity at this time, so the actual amount is already increasing.
- In endurance athletes or with very good physical fitness.

---

14   see http://www.netdoktor.at/laborwerte/fakten/schilddrüse/t3_t4/htm

15   see Böcker/Denk/Heitz, Pathologie, Urban & Fischer, 3rd ed. 2004, Spickzettel Pathologe, hereinafter cited as B/D/H - Pathology

Leukocytes (white-blood cells)
CM normal Value:[16] leukocytes (Adults) 4–10t /mcL (4–10 G/l)
Reduced (leukopenia)
• Conflict-active phase - self-worth conflict (bone).
• Spleen SBS (rare).
Elevated (leukemia)
• Inflammation (repair-phase) somewhere in the body (the leukocytes have the function of "garbage collection" in the body).
• Self-esteem conflict in repair-phase.

Hemoglobin (red blood cell pigment) along with the red blood cell count (RBC) is an important parameter for anemia.
CM normal values:[16] women 12–16 g/dl, men 14–18 g/dl
Reduced
• In the active-phase of a self-esteem conflict - anemia.
• In the repair-phase (vagotonia) of other conflicts due to dilated blood vessels.
• In the second (vagotonic) part of pregnancy due to dilated blood vessels.
• If bleeding (injuries, internal bleeding, heavy menstrual bleeding).
Elevated
• In the repair-phase of a self-esteem conflict (bone). At the beginning of the repair-phase, the hemoglobin and the RBC fall further, but only because the blood is "thinned" by the vagotonic blood vessel dilation with additional serum.
• In the conflict-active phase of other conflicts. Blood vessel constriction increases the vascular blood cell concentration.
• In endurance athletes or with very good physical fitness.

Hematocrit (proportion of the cellular portion of the blood's volume). This value indicates how thin or thick the blood is, i.e., the concentration in which blood cells occur (viscosity).
CM normal values:[16] Women 37–46%, Men 41–50%.
Reduced
• Conflict-active phase of a self-esteem conflict (bone) by reduced production of blood cells. Even lower values at the beginning of the repair phase.
• Conflict-active phase of a refugee conflict (kidney collecting tubules SBS). Fluid retention in the blood also. The blood is thinner, even though the blood cell count hasn't changed.
• In the repair-phase of other conflicts (vagotonia - blood vessel dilation).
• In the second (vagotonic) part of pregnancy, hematocrit is lowered due to dilated blood vessels. (Absorption of fluid into the vascular system) infusions briefly reduce hematocrit due to dilution.
Elevated
• In conflict-active phase other than the conflicts described above. With constriction of the blood vessels, the blood cell concentration increases.
• In athletes, especially after altitude training through increased production of red blood cells. The blood thickens, the ability of the blood to transport oxygen increases.
• By loss of fluids or dehydration (sweating, thirst).

[16] see B/D/H–Pathology

Erythrocyte sedimentation rate (ESR)
One of the oldest and simplest blood test methods:
In a glass tube, the amount of blood cells that have settled to the bottom is measured after one or two hours.
According to CM, an elevated erythrocyte sedimentation is an indication that inflammations are underway in the body.
Normal values:[16] 1h : women 6–11 mm, men 3–8 mm. 2hr: women 6–20 mm, men 5–18 mm.
Elevated
• Repair-phase (inflammation), somewhere in the body.

C-reactive protein (CRP)
This is one of the so-called "acute-phase proteins." When an inflammation is taking place anywhere in the body, CRP rises the fastest of all values.
Normal Value:[16] 10 mg/l
Elevated
• Acute repair-phase of any organ.
• After surgery, injury, accidents, after a heart attack (also repair phases).

Cholesterol
In CM, cholesterol is not determined in order to detect certain disorders, but rather to estimate the risk for vascular disease. It is considered a "risk factor" for heart attack, stroke and other diseases. LDL (low density lipoprotein) is believed to be responsible for vascular damage and is considered "bad," while the "good" HDL (high density lipoprotein) is attributed a vascular protective effect, as far as the CM opinion goes.
In fact, cholesterol - HDL and LDL - is absolutely vital and is produced for the most part by the body itself.
We can assume that Mother Nature produces nothing that is nonsensical or bad.
Cholesterol cannot be transported in the blood because it's not - as fat compounds (lipids) - soluble in water. It is transported by binding to HDL and LDL. We therefore speak of a HDL and LDL lipoprotein-cholesterol complex.
HDL lipoprotein receives the cholesterol absorbed by food and transports it to the liver for processing into bile acids and free cholesterol.
LDL lipoprotein receives the cholesterol made by the liver and leads it to the body's cells.
The cholesterol transported through LDL is the basic substance of steroid hormones (sex hormones, cortisol, etc.), vitamin D3, bile acids, etc. It also takes care of the sealing of arteries and membranes.
To depict LDL as harmful is absurd.
Since 80% of the cholesterol is formed by the liver itself, diet can have little influence on cholesterol levels. Thus, the value can be reduced at most by 5%, and only for a period of 24-48 hours, as the liver otherwise engages to increase its own production. To win about half the population as "patients," the cholesterol "limit" was arbitrarily set to 200 by the pharmaceutical industry. Since then, patients have been "treated," at the cost of the severe side effects associated with lipid-lowering medications.
"Cholesterol appears to be involved as a repair or putty substance

in the restoration of vascular damage."[17]

The fact is, the so-called plaques consist mainly of connective tissue, in which cholesterol can only be found only in minimal amounts (about 1%).

Cholesterol is an important part of the body's outer sheath of cells. It increases the stability of the membranes.

Total cholesterol
CM normal value:[16] 120–200 mg / dL (3.1 - 5.2 mmol / l).

LDL-cholesterol
CM normal value:[16] <150 mg / dl (<3.87 mmol / l)

HDL cholesterol
CM normal value: > 50 mg / dL (> 1.3 mmol / l)
We can probably derive only little from high or low cholesterol

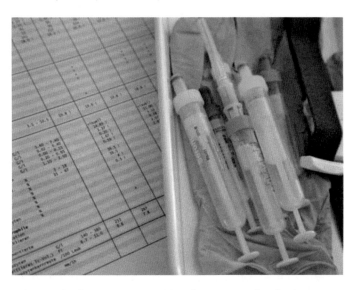

values (whether LDL or HDL) (it often runs in families).

If the value changes suddenly (it rarely does), you can possibly give it some thought:
Elevated
• Lack of exercise, obesity (overweight), alcohol.
• Medication side effects (cortisone, beta blockers, etc.)
• In general, a sign of increased stress.
• Especially to be considered: thyroid, kidney collecting tubules, adrenal, liver and pancreas SBSs.

Liver laboratory values
Gamma-GT
The liver enzyme gamma-GT is the most important parameter with respect to an SBS of the gallbladder ducts.
CM normal values for the new unit: women up to 36 U/l, men to 64 U/l.
Elevated
• Repair-phase of a territory-anger or identity conflict (gallbladder ducts). The critical phase (repair-crisis) begins when the gamma-GT value starts to drop. For values up to 400, the repair-crisis usually proceeds without complications. At values of 400–800 it

is critical, at values above 800 it is very critical (new unit).

GOT (glutamate oxaloacetate transaminase)
According to CM, GOT is elevated in cases of liver, heart and muscular diseases.
CM normal value (new unit):[18] adults 34 U/l
Elevated • Probably like gamma-GT: Territory-anger or identity conflict (gallbladder ducts) - repair phase

GPT (glutamate pyruvate transaminase)
An enzyme whose highest concentration occurs in the liver, and at lower levels in skeletal and cardiac muscles.
CM normal value for new unit:[18] Adults 55 U/l.
Elevated
• Territory-anger conflict (gallbladder ducts) - repair-phase.

AP (alkaline phosphatase) will indicate if a bile duct or bone SBS is in progress.
Normal Value:[18] 40 - 150 U/l (age 60–170 U/l)
Elevated
• Territory-anger conflict (gallbladder ducts) - repair-phase.
• Self-worth conflict (bone) - repair-phase.
• Following bone fractures.

Bilirubin
Bilirubin is a liver value. The amount of bilirubin is determined in order to detect and control the course of jaundice. Bilirubin is a waste product of hemoglobin and is normally excreted via the bile ducts. If it is backing up, bilirubin increases in the bloodstream.
CM normal value:[16] Bilirubin, saturation — adults 0.2–1.1 mg/dL (3.4–18.8 micro-mol).
Elevated
• Territory-anger or identity conflict (gallbladder ducts) - repair-phase. Repair swelling of the bile ducts with temporary closure of the outflow.
• Accelerated breakdown of red-blood cells (hemolysis) by blood, poisons or medicines, large bruises (blunt injuries), malaria.
• Even though rare, bilirubin levels can increase because of a liver parenchyma SBS (starvation or existence conflict), if a major bile duct within the liver (intrahepatic) is closed off due to lack of space.

Cholinesterase
In CM, the cholinesterase value is assessed for the detection of liver damage and poisoning. Because of its strong individual variations, it is better suited to monitor progress than to diagnose.
CM normal value:[16] adults from 3000–8000 U/l.
Elevated
• Starvation-existence conflict - active-phase (liver parenchyma). Increase due to increased metabolic function of the liver.

Pancreas laboratory values
Blood sugar
The blood sugar value indicates the concentration of dextrose (glucose) in the blood. It is controlled by the pancreatic hormones insulin and glucagon.

---

17 http://www.westonaprice.org/knowyourfats/skinny_de.html

16 see B/D/H–Pathology

18 see http://www.netdoktor.at/laborwerte/fakten/leber/ap.htm

16 see B/D/H–Pathology

CM normal value:[16] adults 70 - 100 mg/dl (3.89 - 5.55 m-mol/l).
Reduced (hypoglycemia)
- Fear-disgust or resistance conflict SBS of the alpha-islet or beta-islet cells of the pancreas (see p. 222ff).
Elevated (hyperglycemia)
- Resistance, or fear-disgust conflict SBS of the beta-islet or alpha-islet cells of the pancreas (see p. 222ff).

Amylase (Alpha-amylase)
The enzyme alpha-amylase is produced by the pancreas and is used for carbohydrate digestion. In CM, it is determined in cases of suspected pancreatitis.
Amylase may be measured in the blood (serum) or urine.
CM normal value (serum):[16] adults 70–300mm U/l.
Elevated
- Territory-anger or identity conflict - repair-phase. Pancreatic inflammation (pancreatitis). Repair swelling of the bile ducts with temporary closure of the outflow. Increase of pancreatic enzymes amylase and lipase.

Lipase (phospholipase)
Lipase is the generic term for a group of digestive enzymes (esterases). Their task is to break down fats. Lipase is the most sensitive parameter with respect to the pancreas.
CM normal value:[16] adults 30–180 U/L.
Elevated
- Territory-anger or identity conflict - repair-phase (pancreatic ducts). Repair phase swelling of the bile ducts with temporary closure of the outflow. Pancreatitis, increased pancreatic enzymes amylase and lipase.

Kidney laboratory values
Creatinine
In the view of CM and also in NM, creatinine is the most important kidney value, but it is interpreted quite differently. Creatinine is a metabolic end product of the muscles, so the value is "muscle-dependent." We are mainly interested in the serum (blood) value and not the amount of urinary excretion of creatinine, the so-called creatinine clearance.
CM normal value (serum):[16] 0.5–1.2 mg/dl (44–106 micro-mol)
Elevated
- In the conflict-active phase of a refugee conflict (kidney collecting tubules SBS). This "energy saving program" stores liquid and recycles nutrients. Creatinine, urea and uric acid are kept in the blood system in order to store more energy for use in times of need (CM: "uremia"). This recycling process is called the nitrogen cycle. In CM, dialysis is performed from about 4 mg/dl. With the understanding of the 5 Biological Laws of Nature, dialysis only comes into consideration from 12 — 14 mg/dl.
- In very muscular people, after muscle strain and meat consumption.

Urea
CM-normal value (serum):[16] 10–50 mg /dL (1.64–8.18 mmol).
Elevated
- Refugee conflict (kidney collecting tubules SBS) - active-phase. In the so-called nitrogen cycle, protein is "recycled" from urea.

- After diarrhea, vomiting, fasting, excessive sweating, burns, dehydration.
- After injury, accidents, transfusions (protein breakdown).

Uric acid
In CM, this is the parameter for diagnosing "gout."
For us, the diagnosis of "gout" means that an active refugee conflict combined with any self-worth conflict is present in its repair-phase. (= "Syndrome," see p. 230ff)
Uric acid is the end product of purine metabolism. It is produced during the digestion of meat. So the value is also dependant on nutrition or toxins. In an active refugee conflict, the body tries to obtain excess energy from the uric acid by leaving it in the blood, rather than excreting it.
CM-normal value (Serum):[16] women <5.7 mg/dl, men <7 mg / dl.
Elevated
- Refugee conflict active-phase (kidney collecting tubules), - analogous to creatinine and urea.
- Due to increased purine intake through food (meat, offal, etc.).
- Due to increased purine formation: cell death by drugs - e.g., chemo, blood thinners, blood pressure medication and many more.

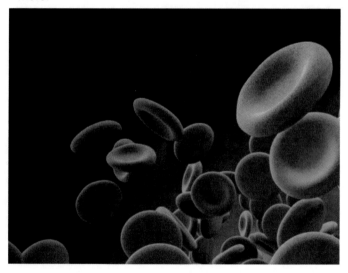

Protein (albumin, microglobulin) **in urine** (= proteinuria)
Alarming sign for CM: Indication of poor renal filtration performance ("nephrotic syndrome"). However, the protein does not pass, as CM believes, from the blood into the urine, but comes from the kidney collecting tubules during repair, thus, from the kidneys themselves (kidney tuberculosis) = breakdown of tumor tissue (see p. 230ff)
Positive test (detection of protein)
- Repair-phase of a refugee conflict (kidney collecting tubules SBS). Breakdown of the tumor > the broken-down tissue is excreted in the urine > protein in the urine.
- Repair phase of a sexual conflict (prostate), or the repair phase of a barely-digestible, unpleasant-situation conflict (bladder

---

16 see B/D/H–Pathology

submucosa) - bladder tuberculosis.
In both cases of tubercular breakdown of tumor tissue > washing out through the urine. > Protein in the urine, accompanied by night sweats.

Blood in urine (hematuria and hemoglobinuria)
If, with the naked eye, red coloration of the urine is visible, it is called "hematuria," as opposed to "microscopic hematuria," which is detecting traces of blood only in the laboratory.
Test positive (detection of blood)
• Territory-marking conflict - repair phase (renal pelvis, ureter, bladder or urethral mucosa). Reconstruction of the transitional epithelium (urothelium). Blood in the urine indicates an inflammation of any of these structures.
• Refugee conflict (kidney collecting tubules) - repair phase. Breakdown of a kidney collecting tubules tumor with the washing out of protein and blood. (Here additional night sweats).
• Barely digestible, unpleasant situation conflict - repair phase (bladder submucosa).

Prostate laboratory values
Prostate-specific antigen (PSA)
The enzyme PSA is produced in the prostate gland and is, according to CM, a parameter for the size of the prostate gland or tumor. That this relation is uncertain is also widely known by conventional medicine, because PSA is also produced in the liver and in part in the pancreas.
CM-normal value:[16] 0–4.5 ng/ml
Elevated
• Sexual conflict, conflict-active or repair-phase (prostate).
• In cyclists and horseback riders.
• After sexual intercourse, after prostate sampling and analysis, among others.
• In women after menopause.
• During a liver SBS.
The fact is, the more often the PSA level is tested, the more often (practically healthy) people die from prostate cancer. From the perspective of the 5 Biological Laws of Nature, even values far above the norm are no cause for excitement. Due to the risk that learning of a raised value can trigger a conflict (with the danger of a vicious circle), it is recommended that the PSA value shouldn't be tested.

Intestinal laboratory values
Blood in the stool
This can be seen with the naked eye. With a stool sample, however, we can look for "hidden" (occult) stool blood in the laboratory.
Positive findings (blood in the stool)
• Repair-phase in a section of the digestive tube (esophagus to rectum). The darker (older) the blood, the farther "upstream" the source of bleeding is to be found.

Rheumatism laboratory values
Rheumatoid factors, antinuclear antibodies (ANA)
Among rheumatoid factors, CM understands "antibodies" that are directed against endogenous structures or proteins that fight

against their own body.
To determine the "rheumatoid factor," the reaction of the blood serum is observed with other proteins in the test tube or on a testing surface. For this, CM has various tests such as the so-called Waaler-Rose test or the ELISA assay.
From the perspective of the 5 Biological Laws of Nature, the rheumatic hypothesis is false and determining the "rheumatoid factor" is meaningless.

Immunoglobulins (Ig) M, G, A, E, D, among others.
The terms "immunoglobulin," "antibodies" and "antigens" can be disregarded. It would be correct to just speak of globulins.
Globulins are the smallest of the body's own protein compounds, which play an important role in the growth of tissues and for sealing off injured cells.
Globulins are found in the blood in higher quantities after poisoning (vaccinations, drugs, alcohol, etc.), injuries (bruising, sprains, etc.) or during repair-phases.
Using electrochemical procedures (electrophoresis), globulins can be classified according to size. The determination of "immunoglobulins" has no meaning for us.

"Infection" laboratory values
AIDS-Tests
AIDS tests such as the ELISA assay and the Western Blot test are not able to identify the HI-Virus. Scientific evidence for the virus has still not been produced to this day. These tests are indirect, non-calibrated detection methods, which do not work.

"For today's so-called anti-HIV antibody tests, there is no international standard. The test result "HIV positive" or "HIV negative," i.e., test scores above or below the specified measurement thresholds in the same person, vary from continent to continent, from country to country, from city to city and even from laboratory to laboratory. In the African test sets, for cost reasons, often only 2 different test proteins are included. When "HIV-positive" people from Africa are retested in Europe, they are often called "HIV-negative," in other words they are no longer "HIV-infected."[19]

The HIV test is not standardized. The test result must be interpreted; the criteria for this interpretation does not only vary from lab to lab, but from month to month.[20]
On the package of the AIDS testing kit (Roche Manufacturing), you can find the following admission: "A negative test result does not exclude the possibility of HIV infection."
Factors that are known to cause false-positive test results are:[21]
• Flu
• Infections of the upper respiratory tract
• Hemophilia
• Herpes simplex
• Cancers
• Swollen lymph nodes

---

16   see B/D/H–Pathology

19   see Dr. med. Krämer, Die stille Revolution der Krebs- und AIDS-Medizin

20   New England Journal of Medicine, Ausg. 317

21   Cf. Michael Leitner "Mythos HIV", Videel publishings

- Renal insufficiency, "blood cleansing" in renal failure
- Currently existing "viral infections" such as hepatitis
- Naturally occurring antibodies
- Antibodies in forms of rheumatoid arthritis
- Blood transfusions
- Tetanus, influenza, hepatitis B vaccinations
- Organ transplants
- Administration of immune globulins
- Receiving anal intercourse

Borrelia Antibodies

Lyme disease is, according to CM, an "infectious disease" caused by the bacterium Borrelia burgdorferi and transmitted by insect bites. (See also p. 69.)

From the perspective of the 5 Biological Laws of Nature, Lyme disease is a separation conflict in the repair phase - with or without insect bite or tick. The Borrelia laboratory test (IgM and IgG "antibody" test) is certainly useless. Even in CM, it is not considered to be very meaningful.

The result is not yes or no, but it is either lower or higher than a certain threshold. If the so-called "tilter" is located above this arbitrarily fixed threshold, Borrelia is regarded as proven (= indirect test).

Chlamydia, campylobacter, streptococcal antibodies

These tests are analogous to the AIDS and Lyme antibody tests.
> Indirect limit value tests without a biological basis.

Tumor markers

Carcinoembryonic antigen (CEA)

In CM, this is the most important tumor marker, especially in relation to colon, lung, and breast cancer.

The name alone is an indication of CM's tumor medicine dilemma: This protein appears to be an indicator of cell division, but cell division is high in both embryonic as well as in tumor growth.

Normal Value:[16] 2.5–10 µg/l
Elevated
- Conflict-active or repair-phase of an SBS.
  Probably old-brain organs in the active-phase or cerebral organs in the repair-phase.
- In smokers (poisoning-repair-metabolism).

Carbohydrate antigen 19/9 (19/9 CA)

is a part of the human blood groups' characteristics.
Used in CM as a marker for pancreatic, liver and gastrointestinal tumors.
Normal Value:[22] <37.5 U/ml
Elevated
- Conflict-active phase or repair phase of the related SBS.

Alpha-fetoprotein (AFP)

Much like CEA, AFP is produced in embryonic tissues and in various tumors. In pregnant women and in infants, the value is

also increased. In both cases, high mitotic rate like in tumors. CM marker for liver, germ cell, bronchial and gastric tumors.
Normal Value:[23] <20 ng/ml
Elevated
- Conflict-active or repair-phase of the related SBS.

Tumor marker pregnancy-specific beta 1-glycoprotein (SP-1), human chorionic gonadotropin (HCG)

Again, you can see how tumor growth is related to pregnancy from a biological perspective. Both SP1 and HCG levels are elevated during pregnancy. For non-pregnant women, they serve as tumor indicators. According to CM, cell division in pregnancy is normal and "benign;" later in life, cell division is considered as abnormal and "malignant."

INITIAL CONSULTATION - DETERMINING THE CONFLICT

As therapists, we try to understand a person as a whole in order to determine their conflict and the previous conditioning associated with it. First, it makes sense to concentrate on the patient's most important symptoms or main manifestations of distress.
I proceed as follows:
1. I try to correlate the symptom with the right special program (SBS). (See lexicon).
2. I determine the phase (conflict-active, repair phase or recurring) that the patient is experiencing.
3. I/we look for the cause of the conflict.
4. I/we look for the underlying conditioning.
5. We plan the path to recovery: through changes in their emotional life/their attitude and through changes in the external situation if this is possible.

If the patient is not yet familiar with the 5 Biological Laws of Nature, the basics should be explained first. Just getting to know the biological connections can have a healing effect because the patient is relieved and fear loosens its grip.

The amount of time required for the initial consultation depends on various factors: the patient's familiarity with the 5 Biological Laws of Nature, their cooperation and the complexity of their medical history.
Many therapists schedule three hours for the first session.

The therapist - patient relationship

For reasons of simplicity, I speak of the "therapist" and the "patient," but this traditional relationship - on this side, the knowing therapist and on the other side, the needy patient - isn't a good basis for a relationship. The reason is that this type of relationship is based on a disparity and creates a dependence (like a child to its parent).

A good therapist knows that whether the patient will recover or not does not lie within their power. They hand over all therapeutic decisions to the patient. They help humbly, because they know that there are greater forces are in play. They see the family in the background and the divine core within the person seek-

---

16 see B/D/H–Pathology

22 see http://www.laborlexikon.de/Lexikon/Infoframe/a/Alpha-1-Fetoprotein_als_ Tumormarker.htm

23 New Eng land Journal of Medicine, # 317

ing assistance. When a patient complains about their parents or others, they are giving these people a place next to themselves in their soul and not condemning them.

Now it comes down to asking the right questions, being a good listener and being able to sense what is resonating behind the words of the patient.

Questions about the conflict

Cold or warm hands?

The first handshake when we meet the patient tells us whether they have warm or cold hands. Cold hands indicate conflict activity. It could be that the patient is conflict-active because they are nervous at the beginning of the session, because of their "disease" or simply because the weather is cold. Be careful not to judge too quickly!

Biologically right-handed or left-handed?

Carry out the clap test and determine which hand leads (see p. 12).

Familial status, occupation, age?

We are interested in their age so we can estimate their possibility

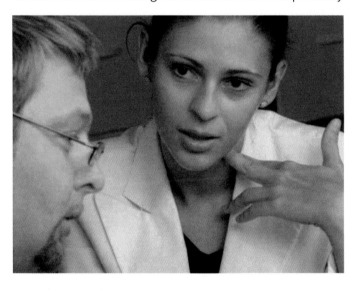

for regeneration, but also with regard to the state of their hormones (first menstrual cycle, menopause, etc.).

Caused by a conflict - yes or no?

Some disorders - usually smaller ones - are not caused by conflicts:
• *Example: An athletic young man has been suffering for a week from mild pain in both Achilles tendons. The tendons and both ankle joints are reddened and lightly swollen. He especially feels pain with the first couple of steps when he gets up in the morning. - It turns out that, following a half a year of not working out, he has started again with strength training in his legs = strengthening of the Achilles tendons, and the symptoms are the same as sore muscles after unusual muscle use - adaptive reaction, training effect, probably not caused by a conflict (= "organ conflict").*
• E.g.: Reddening of the skin due to sunburn. Increase in the pigment cell layer - adaptive reaction to UV radiation.
• E.g.: Digestive problems after gluttonous behavior - poisoning by "overdoing it" or an unwise combination of foods.
• E.g.: Corns caused by ill-fitting shoes.

Deciding whether a conflict is the cause or not isn't always self-evident. Purely adaptive reactions usually pass quickly. During the training pause, for example, our young man could have suffered a local self-esteem conflict with regard to his physical fitness. *("I probably can't run as fast as I used to.")* > Through a good period of training, he could come into a repair phase and experience > pain.

Repair-phase, conflict-active phase or recurring conflict?

When the patient explains their woes, they either describe symptoms of repair or conflict-activity or both of them alternately. For example, constrictive chest pains (angina pectoris), a painful stomach ulcer (gastritis) or diabetes are signs of an active conflict, whereas a slipped disc or pneumonia are signs of a resolved conflict.

Our task is to classify the symptoms correctly. To do this, we need to know the individual SBS.

If the patient describes conflict-active symptoms, we know that the patient carries around a conflict within themselves that they (we) need to identify and resolve as necessary.

If the symptoms are repair phase symptoms, we know that the patient has resolved the corresponding conflict or conflict trigger already, namely just before the complaints started.

General conflict-active symptoms: thoughts revolve around the conflict (compulsive thinking), stress, insomnia, poor appetite (possible weight loss), cold hands and feet or sensitivity to cold.

General repair phase symptoms: psychologically relieved and more easy-going, but physically "sick and tired," fever, sweating, fatigue - especially during daytime hours, healthy appetite (possible weight gain), warm hands and feet.

Symptoms - since when?

The most important question - the clue to the conflict.

Most complaints are repair-phase symptoms. The conflict must have been resolved just before the symptoms appeared for the first time (i.e., something good must have happened). After identifying the event that brought the conflict to an end (e.g., "mom is back," the beginning of the holidays, starting retirement, new love, passed the exam, a clarifying or conciliatory conversation or recognition from their partner or boss) - it is usually easy to get to the conflict. Sudden conflict resolution > sudden onset of symptoms (usually in the evening or at night).

Symptoms that we can attribute to conflict activity or the conflict-active phase must have started with a negative event (conflict) (e.g., dispute, loss, anger, separation).

Please remember: Most important is not the external event itself (this could even appear trivial), but rather the internal perception of the event.

New conflict or recurrence?

Most complaints are not based on new conflicts, but on recurrent conflicts or triggers. In order to clarify this, you should ask the following question: *Are you experiencing these complaints for the first time in your life or have they happened before?* If yes: > new conflict.

If no: > conflict recurrence or trigger. > Next question: *When did that happen? What happened at that time? After or during* which events did your symptoms appear? > Find the original conflict. Assuming you can find it, you will usually find the cause of the present recurrence.

Recurrent dreams?

Does the patient describe dream imagery that appears regularly? Have their dreams changed since experiencing one particular event or another?

During the night, the subconscious mind processes what has happened during the day and in the past. Some dreams, but not all, are conflict related. Recurring dreams often give us a distinct indication of what the conflict is about. Dreams can also have the effect of keeping conflicts active.

• A schoolboy's uncle dies. The two of them had a very close relationship. The boy suffers a loss conflict (testicles) and a general self-esteem conflict (anemia, leukemia). Regularly, he dreams of his uncle's death, in this case the conflict is protracted (persistent-active conflict). Once the conflict has been found, a decision is made to proceed as follows: The anniversary of the uncle's death is approaching. The boy is taken along to the requiem mass and people talk freely to him about his uncle. At last the boy gets warm hands again (repair phase). The boy needs blood transfusions for a period of time and then everything is fine. In CM, the repair phase is diagnosed as "aleukemic leukemia." (Cf. Dr. Hamer, Goldenes Buch (Golden Book), vol. 1, p. 573).

• Muhammad Ali reported that he regularly dreamed of his match with Joe Frazier in March 1971. This fight resulted in his first and certainly the most painful defeat of his boxing career. As a result, he suffered from the following conflicts: not being able to cover oneself > trembling hands. Fear-fright conflict > speech impediments. Not being able to flee from the ring > walking difficulties. With every dream, he briefly enters into conflict-activity. The Parkinson's disease (trembling) represents the repair phase or more precisely, the repair phase crisis, which never ends (= persistent repair).

Unsuccessful conflict searches

Some people think that terms like "identity conflict" or "chunk conflict" (see explanations p. 15, 16) don't apply to them because they try to understand these expressions literally. In this case, it is often helpful to simplify the questions:

What was the worst thing that happened to you at the time? What causes you the most stress when you think of the near future? What thoughts keep going around and around in your mind? What would you like to change in your life? What are you most afraid of? What is your happiness most dependent on? How were your school days?

Also, try remember or get information about prenatal or early conflict: What was the pregnancy and birth like (complications, Cesarian)? Were you breast-fed? How was your childhood?

It's not uncommon for a conflict to lie so far back in the past that it can't be identified anymore. In cases like this, we can only find out what events reactivate/trigger the conflict (= recurrent). Fortunately there are methods like total forgiveness (p. 49f), music therapy (p. 53) or ho'oponopono (p. 56) that enable us to move forward, even in situations like this.

Questions about conditioning

Family

Is there a family history of similar illnesses - mother, father, ancestors? If yes: There must also be psychological parallels here or common patterns (often down the whole family line). For clarification: Did the mother, father or ancestors have similar difficulties, behavior patterns, familial situations?

What secrets did/does the family have (skeletons in the closet)?
What topics are/were taboo?
Early or dramatic deaths of ancestors? Causes?
Was there a tragedy in the family?
Are there heroes or black sheep?
Has anyone been rejected/excluded from the family? Why?
Does the family have a typical feature or a creed?
What were the worst experiences in the mother's life?
What were the worst experiences in the father's life?
What was the financial situation like?
Was the mother's pregnancy planned?
Was there anything out of the ordinary/problematic about the patient's conception?
Were there miscarriages or abortions before/after the patient was conceived?

Birth (mother questions)

How was it?
Was the patient allowed to be with their mother immediately after the birth?
What was the mother's reaction after the birth?
Was the patient breast-fed? How long?
Did the mother fear giving birth?
Premature birth, episiotomy, Cesarian, breech birth?
How was the relationship to the midwife, obstetricians?

Pregnancy (mother/parents questions)

How was it? (Ask about the details: conditions, situations, accidents, deaths (of family/friends) etc.).
Was the pregnancy criticized by anyone?
What was the relationship like between the mother and the father during and after the pregnancy?

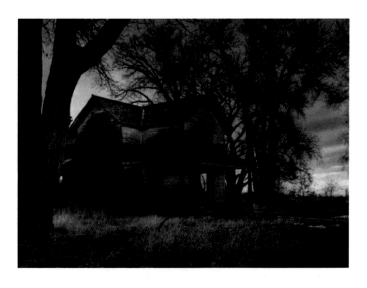

Were there fears about the health of the child or the mother during the pregnancy?
Was the weight gain okay for the mother?
Did the sex of the child make a difference?
Do any ancestors have the same name?

Childhood

Was there anything that characterized the first years of life? (mother questions)
What problems did the parents have?
Were there operations or stays in the hospital?
Was one of the children the favorite/given preferential treatment?
How was school life?
What difficulties were there?
What would the patient criticize about their parents?
The first love?
The first partner?
What is the decisive conditioning with regard to my main problem? > Work it out and formulate it.
Which religious beliefs/convictions were inherited/formed?

Q & A examples for determining conflict

Knee joint pain

A right-handed, 69 year-old woman has been complaining about intense pain in the left knee since the end of the previous week.
Deduction: last week a non-athletic, self-esteem conflict with regard to mother or child must have been resolved (healing symptoms). Now we have to ask about the family situation.
Q: *"Do you have children? How old are the children? What do the children do? Do you have pets ("pet-child" or "pet-partner")? Is your mother still alive? How old is she? Does your mother live with you?"*
A: *"Two grown daughters, the mother died many years ago."*
Deduction: Mother - conflict is unlikely, it probably has to do with the daughters. Now, we need to clarify whether it is a recurrence or a trigger or if the complaints are the result of a new conflict.
Q: *"Have you had pain in your left knee before?"*
A: *"No."*
Deduction: Now I know the complaints are the result of a new conflict. At this point, I don't know when this happened. If the patient had said yes, she had previously suffered pain in the left knee, the symptoms could be the result of a trigger. Next, I try to zero-in on the conflict from the direction of repair phase symptoms.
Q: *"When does your knee hurt the most?"*
A: *"At night, when I turn over."*
Deduction: Clearly the repair phase due to night-time vagotonia. Definite inflammation and energy abundance.
Q: *"Did the pain come suddenly from one day to the next or did it start gradually?"*
A: *"The pain started suddenly."*
Deduction: Sudden pain indicates sudden conflict resolution. Therefore, a clear, positive conflict-resolving incident must have occurred. (With gradual conflict resolution, e.g., pain that increases slowly over several weeks, they usually don't undergo a sudden healing experience, but rather a slow, often hardly noticeable improvement of the conflict situation).

Q: *"What kind of positive experience did you have at the end of last week? Did you have a nice experience with one of your daughters? Did you receive good news?"*
A: *"How did you know that? Yes, I spoke with my daughter on the phone. She told me that she received a job offer."* Note: the daughter lives abroad and has just completed a time-consuming, rather doubtful (for the mother) job-training program with few job opportunities. (Her financial situation is rather precarious due to her three sons).
Deduction: That's it! Non-athletic self-worth conflict due to unsatisfied ambitions regarding her daughter. The conflict had been active for years and thanks to the positive news, now (partly) resolved. If the daughter really gets the job we should anticipate that there will be no further aggravation of the knee symptoms. (Archive B. Eybl)

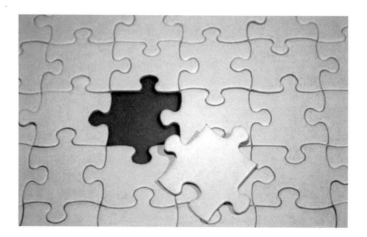

Pain at the back of the head

A 48 year-old, right-handed, unmarried, slender patient works in an office and has no children. Exactly one year ago, on Good Friday, sudden pains began radiating from the back of her head to her jaw and face. In CM, nothing was found. Countless examinations were made and a tooth was needlessly pulled out. The skin was and is not sensitive or reddened or otherwise conspicuous.
Deduction: not a skin SBS.
The facial muscles (facial expression) are OK; there are no signs of paralysis or nervous twitches.
Deduction: no facial motor impairment (being made a fool of conflict).
At this point, I draw a false conclusion: bone SBS, intellectual self-worth conflict.
Q: *"What positive event happened on that Good Friday or in the days before?"*
A: *"Nothing - on the contrary, I can remember exactly how badly things were going for me on that day. I felt miserable, extremely cut off from everything, especially from my partner."*
Deduction: I was wrong. Not a self-worth conflict. The pains are occurring in an active phase. It could only be a periosteal ("bone skin") SBS.
Q: *"Do you suffer from cold feet?"*
A: *"Yes."*
Q: *"Do painkillers help?"*

A: *"No, not at all."*

Deduction: Cold feet = sign that it's periosteal, painkiller ineffectiveness as well.

Q: *"Do you feel the pain more intensely during relaxation or in stress situations?"*

A: *"In stress situations and during the day I feel the pain. At night, it is gone. On the weekend it feels better too."*

Deduction: Clearly pain during sympathicotonia - bone SBS can be ruled out as a cause of the pain.

In further consultation, it turns out that the patient had a very painful separation from her partner. On that evening two years later, she felt the pain of the separation intensely. Everything came back up, especially since she has still not found a new partner and things are not going very well at work either (intense separation conflict affecting the periosteum at the back of the skull). Has been active for exactly one year. (Archive B. Eybl)

Atopic dermatitis/eczema

A 4 year-old girl has atopic dermatitis all over her body. The mother wants her to undergo rigorous treatment. I suggest looking for the cause first.

Deduction: Atopic dermatitis indicates the repair phase of a separation conflict.

Q (for the mother): *"When was the first time you noticed the rash?"*

A (mother): *"A week after birth by Caesarean section we noticed red spots on her face."*

Deduction: Delivery by C-section or the circumstances thereafter was already the reason for the original conflict. One week after birth, the baby entered the repair phase for the first time.

Q: *"On which side of her body did the rash appear most?"*

A: *"On the whole body, everywhere."*

Deduction: A generalized separation conflict. The child suffers from the separation from father and mother. She is lacking skin contact in general.

Q: *"When did the rash appear the worst so far?"*
64full force."

Deduction: The first few days of vacation - strong repair phase, because the whole family was there. She could "cuddle" whenever she wanted. Before the vacation was over, the healing was completed.

After the vacation, the child was conflict-active again and remained in a conflict-active state until Christmas.

During Christmas vacation, she went into healing.

The mother says that after the first half year of her maternity leave she went back to work. The work is only part-time, but the child must nevertheless spend two and a half days a week at her grandmother's. The separation at birth was the initial conflict. The separation from the mother, due to the part-time job initiates a recurrence of the conflict. > "Atopic dermatitis breakouts" in the repair phase (Archive B. Eybl).

THERAPY

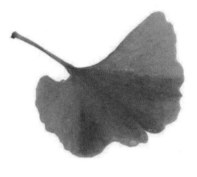

Since we were little children we have been administered various medications whenever we were ill. Although we were usually given our "therapy" during repair phases, the medication was still a comfort, a companion and it gave us hope.

Now, I think we must take our time and organize the existing therapies according to the criteria of the 5 Biological Laws of Nature. This cannot be done by simply waving a wand. On the contrary, it requires the cooperation of medical specialists who have first become acquainted with and then studied the 5 Biological Laws of Nature.

Again and again I experience people diving into the subject matter enthusiastically and then resurfacing to ask, *"Yes, that's great and all, but what now? Where is the therapy?"* To simply do "nothing" is inconceivable for the vast majority of us. We are too deeply conditioned by our previous medical experiences for that. In this book, I attempt to give therapy its rightful place. What I mean is: everything that helps is welcome.

Of course, understanding the biological interrelationships of the New Medicine is important, at least until the time comes when all doctors employ it.

Even then, there will still be people who find it too inconvenient to have to think for themselves and will still just want to "believe" their doctor. We have to accept this.

Regardless, knowing what's going on frees patients from torturing fear and uncertainty. When someone knows, for example, that pain in their musculoskeletal system is part of the repair phase, they can tolerate it and even welcome it. Deducing the causes can even become a hobby.

In the following, we will take a look at what we can do in relation to the phases on the individual levels - psyche, brain and body. In the lexicon, you will also find special treatment suggestions for every "disorder."

Treatment - conflict-active phase psyche level
Possibilities for conflict resolution

The purpose of every SBS (Significant Biological Special Program) is to overcome a certain "catastrophic situation" (biological conflict). Nature places this "tool" in our toolkit for our survival. In making use of it, however, we cannot allow ourselves an endless amount of time. We are talking about a limited special program here, which puts an inordinate amount of strain on our psyche-brain-body system and would exhaust it over the long run. The consequence of constant stress: emaciation or repair phases that can hardly be endured. All SBSs have their origin in the "soul" or psyche, and here lies the key to healing.

When the conflict, triggers and conditioning have been discovered, we can start to think about how to resolve the situation.

Just as every person and every fate is individual, so is are the possibilities for resolution.

Our guiding principles: 1. Determine the conflict and the conditioning. 2. Actively and, if possible, tangibly bring about the solution.

Examples:

• *In preschool, a child is put under pressure to always eat all the food on his plate, even if it doesn't taste good (= conflict, not wanting to swallow the food). Since he started going to preschool, he has regularly suffered throat infections. Tangible conflict resolution: the mother agrees with the preschool teacher that the child only has to eat what it really wants to. = Tangible solution by action. The child has no throat infections any more, since it has been allowed to eat "voluntarily." (Archive B. Eybl)*

• *A left-handed man always experiences a territorial fear trigger (larynx mucosa) whenever his free time gets "filled up" with too many appointments.*

Tangible conflict resolution: the patient holds true to his rule of not scheduling fixed appointments in his free time any more. Since that time, he no longer has had laryngitis, just some "light touches." (Archive B. Eybl)

Unfortunately, there are also difficult cases in which a tangible solution is not that simple:

• *Following a divorce, a young woman is left with a mountain of debt (= existential conflict - water retention, weight gain, headache). A practical solution would be a big box full of money for the patient, but more realistic would be moving back in with her mother to save money or to file for bankruptcy. For the patient, however, neither option is acceptable. (Archive B. Eybl)*

In such cases, we have to try to come up with an alternative, a "plan B."

The subconscious mind - the decisive factor

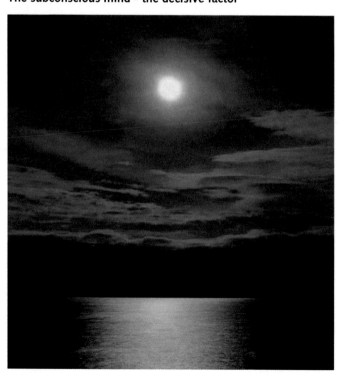

Wanting to try and resolve the conflict with the conscious mind is good, but it's not that simple. This is because the levels of perception at which the biological conflicts have settled have little to do with the intellect and the conscious mind.

Therefore, the key to success is getting the subconscious involved. The subconscious mind represents an essential, indeed the larger part of our psyche. It holds an unbelievable treasure of experiences, including all of the so-called triggers. In order to "delete" triggers, we must reach the subconscious. When compared to the subconscious, our everyday consciousness is of little significance. Comparing it to a car, one could say that the subconscious is the drive chain and the chassis while consciousness merely represents the steering wheel. Nevertheless, our consciousness has a decisive, defining influence on the subconscious.

The following citation is from the 1990s:
Mind your thoughts, for they will become your words.
Mind your words, for they will become your actions.
Mind your actions, for they will become your habits.
Mind your habits, for they will become your character.
Mind your character, for it will become your fate.

Or, as Marcus Aurelius said nearly 2,000 years ago:
"The things you think about determine the quality of your mind. Your soul takes on the color of your thoughts."

If the subconscious does not cooperate with the chosen therapy, no amount of effort will help. Understanding alone is not enough. So how do we bring the subconscious *"on board?"* Involve as many senses as possible. The more senses that are involved, the more likely it is that the subconscious will get involved.

Over the years and decades, our conditioning and the triggers we respond to have worn deep ruts in our souls. They have become an integral part of us. Powerful impulses are necessary in order to get out of these ruts and replace them with new patterns.

The Russian doctor Mirsakarim Norbekov ("The Experience of a fool who had an epiphany about how to get rid of his glasses") gives us guidance on how to reprogram the subconscious: He calls the power that is to be applied and activated by therapists, "the Octave." The "Octave" is the most beautiful feeling we can imagine or that we have experienced in our lives. For example: a great success which gave us the feeling of being in "seventh heaven," a wonderful sunset shared with a loved one, the moment we were able to take a small child in our arms or the unforgettable beauty of a river. "The Octave" is the coming together of conviction, determination, power, strength and firmness with tenderness, love and goodness and with the feeling of weightlessness and joy. "It is the relaxed, quiet, confident feeling that something will be as you wish it to be. At the same time, the Octave is the driving force toward achieving our goals. The Octave is the art of steering your own body, commanding and forcing it, step-by-step, both outwardly and inwardly, into transforming into the picture we wish to see."

The inner effort must be very strong. It is a kind of inner attitude that says:
"I am the will
I am the power
I am the love

I am the forgiveness
I am the youth
I am the health
I am the wisdom
I am the joy of living
I am everything beautiful
Everything depends on me
Everything lies in my hands. "

Practicing, performing rituals or providing therapy with this inner attitude can change the subconscious. It cannot withstand this powerful impulse. With this mind set, we can heal ourselves of chronic suffering. With this mind set, we are no longer the little, insignificant people, who are "steamrolled" by one conflict after another anymore; instead, we elevate ourselves to become the masters of our own destiny.

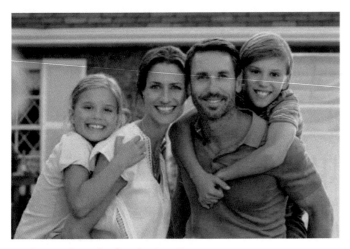

Understanding the family situation

Whoever is familiar with the hidden ordering in families as discovered by Bert Hellinger will be able to find resolutions to conflicts more easily. The clarification of the family situation is part and parcel of my work. Next to the awareness of early conditioning, it is the most important instrument for progress/healing. You aren't required to work out the family constellation - that's not everyone's cup of tea. You can explore the family dynamics in other ways - e.g., through a conversation. Here, the most important few: (book recommendation - Bert Hellinger, "Love's Hidden Symmetry," Zeig, Tucker & Co.).

• We are bound to the family/clan that we are born into. Our (clean/guilty) conscience is part of the family's conscience. Total freedom is an illusion.
> *"I am the continuation of my parents and my ancestors. "*

• If someone in the family has committed an injustice (or the family as a whole) and has not atoned for this, a descendant will later feel responsible for this (unconsciously) and will want to make up for this in their own way (usually to their detriment).
> *"Whatever you did, I'll leave you with the blame. I don't have to shoulder it. I am only a child. "*

• The hierarchy is ordained. Whoever is there first has a higher rank than those who come afterward. This mean the parents come first and then the children in their order. The first partner

(and their common children) come before the next, even when they are divorced. Also, the parents have mothers and fathers and they come before the parents. From this, we get an endless row of ancestors with a natural order. This hierarchy also applies to groups like cliques, organizations, etc.
> *I insert myself into this hierarchy - freedom grows from it.*

• Even the outcasts belong to the family (e.g., a handicapped member living in an institution), the deceased (the premature or stillborn, abortions) and ones who moved away. If these aren't given their place, disharmony/illness arises in the family system.
> *I give them all a welcome place in my heart!*

• The children should accept their parents just as they are. There are none better (even when they were/are bad). Whoever only takes what they want from their parents (like from a buffet), is not taking them as a whole. Whoever despises their parents is cutting themselves off from the power completely. Then again, whoever says "Yes" to their parents wholeheartedly is in agreement with their life and their destiny. (This doesn't mean that you can't be of another opinion and travel down a completely different road than your parents.) Hate and contempt are chains of bondage. Love makes you free.
> *"Thanks mom, I accept everything from you. I keep you in my heart. Thanks dad, I also accept everything from you and I honor you. I follow my own path with strength. "*

• If a boy or a man can't accept his father, the "masculine energy" can't flow to him. His masculinity is restricted, he tends toward depression.
> *"You are my only father and the best one for me. Thank you. "*

• When a girl or a woman can't accept her mother, she can't be/ become a complete woman.
> *"You are my only mother and the best one for me. Thank you. "*

• When it comes to their relationship, parents should not confide in their children. When parents say something to their children that is none of their business, children should ignore it.
"Don't say anymore, I'm only your child. "
Children have just as little right to get involved in their parents' relationship(s). E.g., an affair, divorce or abortion is the parents' exclusive business.
> *"That's none of your concern my child. "*
It's not appropriate when children act as a substitute partner. The child often feels flattered, but the rank is not suitable.
> *"I am only your child. "* (Also with adult children.)

• When it comes to parenting, children should know who's in control. Children need loving AND strong parents. Children develop by obeying and also breaking the rules. Both are important. This is why rules are necessary.
However, the essentials of parenting happen in the way the parents model behavior. Children mimic them automatically.
If the parents disagree on questions of parenting and the father stands down (often), the child will unconsciously show solidarity with him, because it will want please both parents. Eventually, it will become just like the father. This will be even more pronounced the more the mother tries to shut out the father (e.g., alcoholic, failure).
> *"You are allowed to become like daddy or like me. "*

• Children often forgo their own happiness and take on the unresolved/difficult/hushed-up/guilt-ridden issues of their ancestors (usually parents). Often, this is where you can find the deep roots of addiction, illness or problematic character traits according to the motto: "I should suffer too" or "I'll follow in your footsteps."

• The end of the couple's relationship doesn't mean the end of the parental relationship. The mother will always remain the mother and the father always the father. (Always remember to tell this to the child!)
> "We have separated from one another - that doesn't have anything to do with you. We are still your parents."

• After a divorce, children should go to the parent that holds the other in the highest regard. The reason: The other parent has a greater presence there. A child should not be entrusted with this decision (they will be left with feelings of guilt).

• Adoption motivated by, "We want a child," is inauspicious. Temporary foster care is okay.

• In relationships, giving and taking must be balanced. Whoever is constantly giving and never takes always become more powerful, will want to maintain their superiority and this endangers the relationship. Whoever constantly takes and doesn't give anything destroys it as well.
Parents give children so much (life) that the possibility of achieving balance is only limited: when the parents get old.

• "I'm sorry" is better in a relationship than "please forgive me." Through the former, you're more likely to find equal footing than with magnanimous forgiveness. Making amends can also bring things back into balance.

• Hellinger's great guiding principle: "You always have to search for the love - that is where you will find the solution."

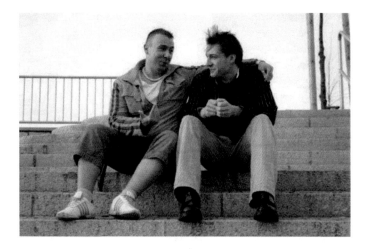

Talk about the conflict and your conditioning

Men find it harder to talk about their feelings - this is probably one of the reasons why women live longer.
The earlier and more we talk about a conflict we've experienced, the faster we come out of the conflict-active phase. If it was deeply hurtful or embarrassing, this is not easy. However, we should move outside of our comfort zone and talk about the experience "from the heart."

It is possible that the person we are talking to has experienced something similar or knows somebody who has experienced something similar. Knowing that you are not the only one with the conflict makes it less dramatic.
Through talking, the "thinking in circles" comes to an end. Afterwards, we see more clearly, can put things into some sort of order and perhaps even find a solution. The important thing is that we talk to someone, whether it is a friend, a partner, a colleague at work or someone else. What's decisive is putting an end to the psychological isolation.
If there is no one we can talk to, we can tell our story - our suffering - to an animal. Pets are excellent listeners. They have certain disadvantages, but also advantages: They do not interrupt, judge, or gossip about us afterwards.
Obviously, the ideal person would be someone who is familiar with the 5 Biological Laws of Nature and someone we trust.
"Professional help" from psychotherapists or psychologists makes sense if they are also familiar with the 5 Biological Laws of Nature and the effects of family conditioning.

Write about the conflict

It is also possible to write about the conflict "from the heart." Through writing, we often get to the point better because we have time to consider everything. Writing clarifies things. Writing can also help us come to conclusions. In light of the 5 Biological Laws of Nature, keeping a diary is valuable for many reasons: for diagnosis, for keeping a record of events as they play out over time and for therapy, because through writing about it, we have already "worked through" the conflict.
With some (interpersonal) conflicts, writing an honest letter often helps you to get things off your chest. You can then consider if you really want to mail the letter (caution: you probably don't) or only mail it symbolically by means of a small ritual. It doesn't matter if the recipient is alive or has already died. An example ritual could be: after writing the letter, take it to the bank of a river, ceremonially burn it and then commend the ashes to the flowing waters.

Forgiving - reconciling

Most conflicts happen in relation to other people. Many recurring conflicts are "kept alive" by holding a grudge against someone. In this case, forgiveness is a simple recipe. Sometimes we don't even need to forgive, but only to put ourselves in the other person's shoes and try to understand their words and actions. Every action a person performs is based on their own individual history and personal conditioning. If we have had the same history, we would have acted likewise. Sometimes we drive ourselves to madness by thinking that somebody wants to hurt us, to rob us, to ruin our reputation, etc.
There is also a deeper aspect of forgiveness:
We have caused everything that happens in our lives ourselves - in this life or in a previous one. Our environment, our fellow human beings are just holding up the mirror for us. Everything we emit from ourselves (thoughts, words, and deeds) comes back to us -

the effect of the "law of attraction." This law works, whether we believe in it or not, and it works as precisely as a clock.

I recommend the book on this topic by the practicing naturopath Marion Kohn (see source list). Using case examples, she shows that conflicts do not just "fall from the sky," but they appear according to plan. She links the 5 Biological Laws of Nature with the spiritual realm. In this way, forgiving becomes easier, because we realize that greater forces are at work behind the biology.

There's no doubt about it, it's easier to feel like the poor victim than to take personal responsibility for our own lives and accept the strokes of fate with gratitude.

The truth is: we are always the victim of our own deeds. Once we understand this completely, there is no reason to be angry with anyone. - Why should we be angry with someone who brings back a part of our self to us? Consequently, when we see the world in this way, there is then also no need to forgive anymore. All that remains is gratitude and amazement at the wonderful order in which all of our lives are embedded. Personally, I find the easiest way to forgive someone is if I remind myself: What was acting here was this person's *"little ego"* and not their divine core.

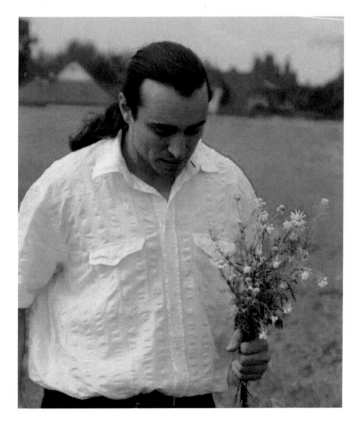

With this in mind, I can't possibly be angry with this *"little ego."* A prerequisite for forgiveness is mental maturity or religiousness in the sense of a connection to a spiritual world.

Forgiving does not mean "backing down." It is not a contradiction when you turn away from someone and also forgive them at the same time. You can even fight with someone and at the same time still forgive them and understand why they don't act in another way.

When we forgive a person, it's best to let them know, because your forgiveness can also be a healing factor for that person.

The act of forgiving someone registers directly in the subconscious when we make a small, ceremonial ritual out of it (e.g., a handshake, a hug, a present, or an invitation). If forgiveness doesn't come from our hearts, but only from our minds, the conflict resolution usually doesn't work.

Playing out conflicts and solutions
("Theater therapy," psychodrama acc. to Moreno)

Theater is as old as mankind itself. Only on the surface do we perceive theater as entertainment. However, the deep meaning of theater is healing. Healing of the audience and society respectively and the healing of the actors.

The ancient Greek tragedies, like many classical works of music, are constructed in two phases and were intended as *"healing exercises"* for the audience.

Theater attempted to show individual or collective conflicts and increase awareness. In the protective atmosphere of the theater, the conflict can be felt again. The renewed experience of distress motivates the individual to a solution (which can then be played out).

If a person was denied his freedom because of a conflicting event in real life, theater reopened the door to freedom. Theater touches all of our senses and, thus, reaches our innermost being.

The subconsciousness can be programmed anew by reenacting the conflict and "playing out a solution." If one day, the knowledge of the 5 Biological Laws of Nature is integrated into so-called theater therapy, we will be able to expect quite a lot.

What is presented to us today as "modern theater" is practically meaningless. It lacks connections to nature and to spirituality and the responsibility for healing is missing. For our purposes, we don't necessarily need a stage and the fancy term "theater therapy." We can act out, alone or with others, a certain scene that we cannot come to terms with in real life - one which *"won't let go"* of us, in the form of triggers, and is making us ill over the long run. We relive the conflict and *"let off its steam"* reduce its significance, rearrange it, and evaluate it in a new way. The old programming, with all of its triggers, is wiped clean and new, positive programming is anchored firmly in its place!

• *The story takes place in France: A four-year-old boy is often naughty, so the parents hire a Santa Claus (Papa Noel), who should "read the riot act" to the child. When the doorbell rings, the father tells him, "That is Papa Noel, so you'd better pay attention."*

For 10 minutes, there is thumping, scraping and scratching on the door - a horrifying eternity for the boy. Afterwards, it seems as if he had been struck by lightning (a motor conflict of not being able to flee and a separation conflict from the fear of being taken away). He dreams about the scene every night (= recurrent). Up until the age of 26, the boy suffers from epilepsy. The conflict was successfully resolved thanks to Dr. Hamer, who reenacted the scene. Again, a stunt Santa was hired and a corresponding set was constructed. Again, there was thumping and scratching, but when "Papa Noel" finally entered the room, the tables were turned. This time, Santa Claus was given a proper thrashing. Since then, the patient was healed. (Cf. Dr. med. Mag. Theol. Ryke Geerd Hamer, Vermächtnis einer Neuen Medizin, Teil 1, Amici di Dirk Verlag, 7. Auflage 1999, ISBN: 84930091-0-5. Hereinafter cited as "Goldenes Buch vol. 1" p. 143)

• At the age of six months, an infant is operated on for an anal fistula. In order to clean the wound, both of the child's parents have to hold the child's arms and legs. The poor baby screams painfully (motor conflict of not being able to escape). In the following months, the boy shows a marked slowdown in his motor development. The parents, who are familiar with the 5 Biological Laws of Nature, discover the conflict six months later and release him by replaying the scene.

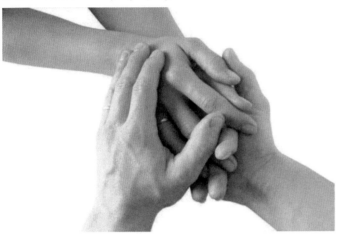

The father's story: "So we laid him down on a table again. I held his legs and my wife pressed around on his bottom, so that he would be reminded of the situation. As soon as I took hold of his legs, the joy and smile disappeared from his face. His eyes opened wide with fright in anticipation of the pain! It was so clear! My wife pressed a little bit on his bottom exactly on the same spot, so he could remember. He was absolutely tense, in panic, about to start screaming. I loosened my grip so that my hands were barely touching him. Actually, I was expecting him to start kicking, but he lay completely still. I waited. Then I felt a little bit of movement in his legs. I overreacted and acted as if he had pushed away my hands, raised my hands and arms and took a step backward. He just looked at me. Again I went close to him and took hold of his legs, but not as tightly as before. My wife pressed on the spot of the already-healed wound on his bottom again. Following a more noticeable movement of his legs, I let him push me away again. His eyes were fixed on me. We went through this routine about 10 or 15 times and each time the movement of his legs became a little stronger and slowly the fear and panic disappeared. In the end, he even liked it and laughed.

As I am writing this story, I have to think of Dr. Hamer's words: "A conflict is then resolved when the person can laugh about it." How true! Now he had a big smile on his face. While I held him, he stretched out his legs and I let myself fall on my back. It was so good to see how he be-came "free." His little legs had no strength, but he made the flexed them to push me away. It

was wonderful to see how he had changed.

It was late afternoon and bedtime soon, so we decided to repeat the play the next day. The next morning we were surprised: he had slept through the whole night - the first time in months! During the day, we also found that his hands were warmer and that he was much more even-tempered and whined less. We played the game again and again. No more panic was seen in his eyes - he wanted to start the game right away and "knock me over." Two days later, we stopped playing the game; we did not want to do it too often. The following nights, he continued to sleep through. So it all hadn't been by chance. His ability to crawl slowly improved about two weeks after the resolution of the conflict. We could clearly see how he was getting more and more active as he turned, crawled, stood up and even walked. Six or seven weeks after resolving the conflict, he took his first steps holding onto a little play buggy. Soon he was walking alone, rarely falling. Now he is two and a half years old and has completely caught up. The examinations show that he is developing normally." (see www.germanische-heilkunde.at)

Performing rituals

Rituals are symbolic actions for sealing intentions or decisions. They are not relics of the past, but powerful therapeutic tools we can apply specifically with our knowledge of the 5 Biological Laws of Nature.

Our goal is to inform the subconscious and to reprogram it. If, for instance, we cannot get over the separation from our partner (= separation conflict), we can perform a farewell ritual where we make a clean break and cut the cord that still binds us to the relationship.

Examples:

• I revisit a place where I had spent happy hours with my partner. I light a candle, thank fate for the time we spent together, say goodbye in my thoughts before blowing out the candle

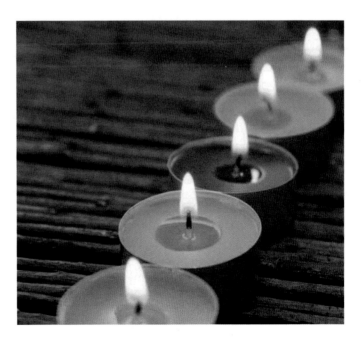

and leaving the past permanently behind me.
- I fumigate the apartment with incense, light a scented candle.
- I build a campfire, throw the partner's letters into the fire and say goodbye in my thoughts.
- I meet with the partner for a last time and say good-bye in a deliberate and formal way.

In the case of a persistent fear-of-rear-attack conflict, we can consider a protection ritual.

We can end a persistent territorial-marking conflict by clearly marking our territorial borders.

The most important thing is that we "get to the point" and experience it with our whole heart. The more feeling we put into the ritual, the more effective it will be. The best rituals are the ones that occur to us spontaneously.

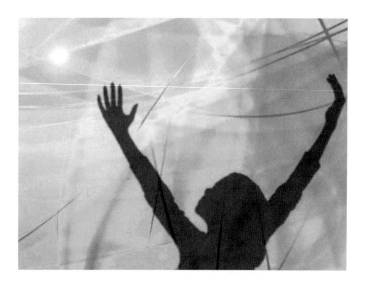

Religiousness, praying, and meditation

Through prayer and meditation we try - based on our attitude and orientation - to come in contact with a higher power, be it God or the Gods, angels or our guardian angel.

The motives for prayer are various and everyone should pray in their own way.

The connection to "above" is immensely important, at least as important as being grounded, in other words, standing with both feet firmly on the ground.

Someone who is connected to a spiritual world does not suffer from every "trivial" conflict they experience. A person who knows that life is just a brief intermezzo in a long journey, can't be thrown off balance easily, since their foundation is of a spiritual nature and therefore indestructible.

When we pray and meditate with regard to conflicts, we shouldn't make the same mistake as the young woman on page 56f.

Praying can also be a request - asking for help. It is okay to ask for help if we find ourselves at a dead end or if a conflict situation appears to be hopeless.

The possibilities for receiving help from the spiritual world are enormous. Every one of us has a protective spirit who is happy to help us if they are allowed to intervene, that is, if the inter-

vention conforms with our life's plan.

As a therapist, I have become used to silently asking for the recovery of everyone seeking help. The act of asking brings a certain comforting humility. I think that every patient should also sincerely ask for healing. Regardless of the phase, we will be helped!

Making amends

Many conflicts remain active because we cannot forgive ourselves, usually for thoughtless words or deeds that hurt someone or caused damage.

I.e.: *We have committed, in effect, a hit and run.*

E.g.: A man cheats on his wife one single time and is plagued with guilt for many years afterward until he finally "confesses" the fling to his wife. (Archive B.Eybl)

"*A guilty conscience*" usually begins a shoulder SBS. But it can also turn into a trigger for some other conflict.

Please note: This is not about being right or wrong in a moral or legal sense, but rather, it's about someone's personal feeling of having done something wrong.

An violent criminal who feels no remorse for what they have done will also have no conflict, no SBS will begin. - That at some point fate will make them pay the bill in full - well, that's another matter. People are only tormented by lingering guilt when they don't acknowledge it and they try to suppress it instead. When guilt is faced and fully acknowledged, the guilty feelings mysteriously disappear.

Even if it takes great effort, we should resolve conflicts whenever possible by making amends or even by turning ourselves in (if you believe in the judicial system). "*I am sorry,*" often works wonders.

Leaving the conflict behind you ("Toilet Bowl Therapy")

Each of us knows what needs to be done on the toilet: leave a little pile, wipe, flush and you're finished. A simple procedure

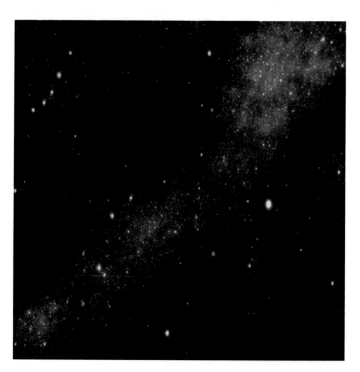

that we've done thousands of times.

Now let's just imagine the following: A person leaves his little pile. But instead of flushing, they use the toilet brush to spread out their faeces - insane? Of course, but this is what many of us are doing over and over.

Instead of flushing conflicts (= toilet bowl contents) away and forgetting about them, we carry them around for days, weeks, years, and even our whole lives (persistent conflicts).

Grumbling and brooding, more or less thinking in circles, we block our life energy. Always thinking about old burdens from the past, we stagger into the next ditch fate puts in front of us, because we are not living in the present.

Enough of that. Get rid of the old baggage. Learn your lesson from the past, but then leave the ballast behind. Let's begin every day fresh.

Putting the conflict in perspective
(Example: the Milky Way therapy)

Consider the Milky Way: estimated at over 200 billion suns and their planets. The Earth is a small planet near the edge of the galaxy - one of hundreds of billions of others.

On this earth alone, we live as one of over 7 billion people. Each of us considers him or herself to be the most important of all - the center of the world, every man for himself. But be honest: From a cosmic perspective, are we not incredibly insignificant? Dust particles of the cosmos, tiny cells in a giant organism.

Why do we think we're so important? How meaningless, how trivial are our little human "mini-problems?" Let's broaden our horizons and put things in perspective.

> *"Above the clouds, the freedom must be boundless.*
> *All fears, all worries, they say,*
> *remain hidden down below and then,*
> *what seems grand and important to us,*
> *would suddenly seem be trivial and small..."*
> (Chorus of "Über den Wolken," a song by the German singer-songwriter Reinhard Mey)

Music therapy, singing — dancing

Experiments with plants and animals show that music has a positive effect on their health. First and foremost, music doesn't heal the physical body of the plant, animal or human; it first heals their souls and only then the body.

Music opens our hearts - actively making music as well as listening to music.

I think that basically any music you like heals, at least a little. Although, you probably can only speak of healing music when it is naturally balanced and harmonizes (resonates) with the good, the beautiful and the divine that is in all of us.

Ideally, this kind of music can evoke our conflict (with its disharmonic aspects) and then heal or carry it away on its their harmonic waves.

True healing music is inspired and comes from the spiritual realms. It reflects the divine cosmic order, as well as sacred geometry (Melchizedek), mathematics (Plichta), physics (Schauberger), biology, chemistry (Russell) and indeed the whole of nature.

Through the knowledge of the 5 Biological Laws of Nature, the therapeutic use of making and listening to music and dancing and singing will certainly receive increased recognition. Dr. Hamer recommends his song: *"Mein Studentenmädchen"* (can be heard on YouTube).

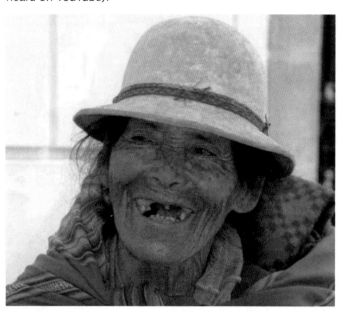

Laughter

Laughter is the best medicine. - We can learn this from the Mediterranean cultures. It is not just the olive oil and tomatoes that allow them to live longer, but their lightheartedness and cheerful outlook as well.

With humor, we can overcome conflicts and crises better. We should not take ourselves and our life, the "game of life," too seriously. We won't get anywhere in life when we only have a doggedly rigid attitude - and certainly not when it comes to resolving conflicts. When the rigidity gives way to laughter, we're already winners.

Imagine health - imagine the solution
(Visualization)

Our thoughts and the images we see are forces which will manifest themselves sooner or later. Negative thoughts and horrible imagery manifest themselves just the same as positive thoughts and happy visions do.

Even if the conflict cannot be solved in real terms, we shouldn't constantly linger in a haze of conflict and "sickness." We have to look forward. By imagining health or the solution to our conflict in intensive imagery, we set powerful forces in motion. Today's dream is tomorrow's reality. The most effective visualizations are those in the state between being awake and dreaming. In this relaxed state of awareness, our brain oscillates at a frequency of around 10 Hz (= alpha waves). This is the point where dreaming starts and the inner imagery appears by itself.

If we decide in favor of visualization exercises, we need to set up a certain time in our daily routine, e.g., before getting up in the morning or before going to bed at night.

Example: Someone has been suffering from pain in their lower back for a long time, because when they were a child they had the feeling that they were not worth anything (persistent conflict). Possible visualization: e.g., being in a beautiful field of flowers, running around and dancing in a completely healthy body. My spine feels light and free. I acknowledge the dark chapter in my childhood and leave it behind. I look forward to a new feeling of being alive.

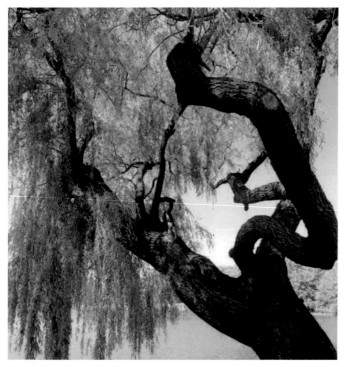

Bach Flower Remedies

During the course of his life (1886–1936), the English physician Dr. Edward Bach came to realize that all physical ailments have a psychic or spiritual origin. During the last years of his life, he fully devoted himself to looking for natural healing methods, which showed no side effects. With his innate sensitivity, he wandered through the woods of Wales and sensed the characteristics of various plants. By the time of his death in 1936, he had developed a system of 38 flower concentrations, produced from the blossoms of wild plants, trees, and shrubs.

According to Dr. Bach, illness is the reaction of the body to psychological disturbances (conflicts). Using Bach flowers, negative feelings are not suppressed, but rather transformed into positive attitudes. E.g., through its unique nature, the yellow willow can help us to forgive past injustices and let them go. Careworn people, blocked by self-pity and bitterness, can recover with the help of this plant.

Dr. Bach always advised chronically sick people not to pay attention to their physical symptoms, but rather to work on the continued development of their soul. When harmony is restored on the spiritual level, the complaints will improve automatically. In practice, Bach flower remedies can hardly be used symptomatically, because in the Bach flower system there are no correlations between conflicts and organs.

Bach flower therapy is especially suited for the conflict-active phase, but also for providing moral support during the healing-phase. The choice of flowers can be rational, intuitive, or made by the patient themselves. The patient, for example, is allowed to pick his own essences. - When you are making your selection, ask for guidance from "above."

Painting therapy

"When put onto paper, inner visions (imaginations) can represent unconscious needs or conflicts in the form of deep psychological symbols. In the act of doing so, conflicts are expressed and experienced.

With the support of therapists, flashbacks to traumatic scenes are made possible in a protected environment. Feelings and conflict tensions are registered. By viewing the image with its symbolism from a different perspective and with a certain distance, internal relationships can be recognized. This new perception makes it easier to find creative solutions to the problem - at first on paper and then in real life." (www.maltherapie-zentrum.at)

Painting therapy seems to be especially well-suited for people, who cannot be reached intellectually (through conversation), whether this is because they are too young, or they have a mental disability or a communication disturbance disorder (such as autism). It could also be the right thing for people, with old, deep-rooted conflicts and for people, who are drawn to painting. The language of animals is images. - If you want to communicate with them, you have to send them pictures.

Telepathic messages are inner images. Inner images are telepathic messages. Images are "in-FORM-ation." Images form matter. In other words, images shape our future, consciously or unconsciously.

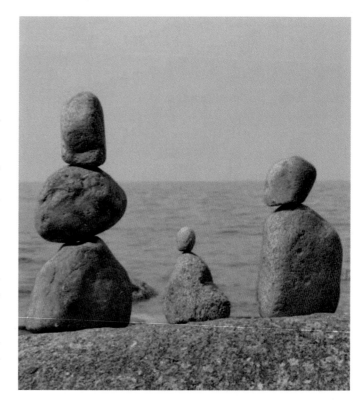

Psychotherapy

Since psychotherapy has always been concerned with the healing of the soul, we can not ignore it.

The last decades have brought about countless psychotherapeutic techniques. This makes the field so vast that it is hardly manageable, even for "insiders."

One valid guiding principle in this jungle of methods is the saying, "*The healer is right!*" Those methods that helps us out of conflict-activity, "are right" and are "the right methods." (On a physical symptom level, the saying has only limited validity.)

However, two things are crucial:

First, the psychotherapist should try to help the patient find a real resolution to their conflict. Real conflict resolution means a biological solution of the conflict that overshadows all "tricks" by its effectiveness.

The psychotherapist should work on the basis of the 5 Biological Laws of Nature.

The best psychotherapist is a physician and the best physician is also a psychotherapist.

We need to breathe new life into the methods of psychotherapy by applying the 5 Biological Laws of Nature.

This work must be carried out by specialists of the relevant medical fields.

Matrix Reimprinting

This very effective treatment is a further development of the, fairly well-known EFT (Emotional Freedom Techniques).

The founder Carl Dawson assumes that in a conflict shock, a part of our psyche splits off and, in doing so, "freezes."

One now gets in touch with this "partial-I" to convince it that the act of splitting off was well-meant, but it is no longer necessary. Through this process, the release of conflict mass and reintegration of the partial-I happens instantly. Carl Dawson is familiar with the 5 Biological Laws of Nature.

Regression therapy, reincarnation therapy

A regression therapy, whether under the guidance of a therapist or alone (in meditation), makes sense if the conflict arose a very long time ago or if it has been forgotten. Regression is finding the conflict first and then conflict resolution by "bringing up" the conflict and experiencing it again.

• *The author Christopher Ray describes in his book: 100 Days Heart Attack,[24] how he resolves a territorial loss conflict, which he suffered in the womb, through a regression that he carried out himself.*

He found himself with his little sibling (twin) in his mother's womb when she decided to have an abortion. This was only partially successful, meaning his sister died and left the womb. = Loss-of-territory conflict (he felt that is sister was part of his territory).

He was then born, but because of the unconscious memory of his sister, he had massive heart problems his entire life. After 6 decades of activity, the conflict resolved itself through the

regression. As a consequence, he suffered a series of heart attacks over a period of 100 days, which he fortunately survived. After that, the chronic angina pectoris that plagued him before the regression disappeared.

As we can see, regressions are somewhat risky, even the ones that are carried out with guidance. It can be dangerous to cut through the veil of forgetting, for we do not forget in vain. Forgetting is a sensible form of protection.

This also corresponds with the findings of Dr. Hamer. Old conflicts, especially the so-called territorial conflicts, should not be resolved after the passage of so much time. Consider the boss at a company, who carried a job-related territorial conflict around with him his whole life, and then, a few weeks after retiring, dies of a heart attack during his repair phase crisis.

There are very specific instructions for conducting regressions in the book, "The Journey"[25] by the American author Brandon Bays. Her methods are well-suited for our purpose.

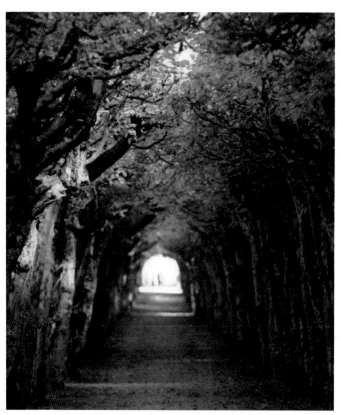

In the reincarnation theory, one tries to return to a previous lifetime and find the cause of the problem(s). There is no doubt that existing therapy successes speak for these methods.

The "overview" over many incarnations and the parallels to today's problems in life may have a healing effect. This also goes for an understanding of certain weaknesses and preferences that one may have had in previous lives.

On the other hand, I think that there's a reason that nature put a barrier between lives. Obviously it is best, with a few

---

24 Monika Berger-Lenz & Christopher Ray, Neue Medizin 8, 100 Tage Herzinfarkt, Faktuell Verlag, Görlitz 2009

25 Brandon Bays, The Journey: A Practical Guide to Healing Yourself and Setting Yourself Free, Atria Books, Reissue edition, 2012

exceptions, that we concentrate on this life rather than poke around in the past. How does it help us to know who we were and where we lived, whether we were rich or poor or what occupation we had? Maybe it's interesting to know all that, but it doesn't help bring us any further.

What does help is treating our neighbors as we would like to be treated ourselves. To recognize and solve our life's tasks (main conflicts) - in the here and now - that's what helps us further. This should give us - every one of us - enough to do for the rest of our lives.

I am perhaps cautious when it comes to reincarnation therapy, but the knowledge that we are repeatedly born again with the sole purpose of furthering our spiritual and emotional development is, in my opinion, the basis for a meaningful life free of fear.

Healing by assuming full responsibility (Ho'oponopono)

This wonderful, unbelievably appealing method gained worldwide recognition through the success of Dr. Ihaleakala Hew Len in Hawaii. To put it briefly, we can heal sick people, ourselves and Mother Earth in the following way:

- I see the sick person and recognize the illness with all of its burdens and weight.
- I recognize that all of it has something to do with me, for the external world is just a mirror of my inner self.
- This is why I assume full responsibility, for I am in some way partially responsible for the situation.
- Now I want to make amends and say, *"I am sorry that I was part of the cause.*
- *Please forgive me, Creator! And I forgive myself too!"*
- *"Thank you, for now I have the chance to heal it!"*
- *"I love you!"*
- Ho'oponopono short form: *"I'm sorry, please forgive me, thank you, I love you."*

How I proceed in my practice

1. Beforehand, I ask the patient to bring the results of all of their medical examinations (blood work, x-rays, etc.). At the beginning of our conversation, they can describe their complaints/symptoms.
2. I try to assign the symptoms to the right SBS and the right phase.
3. After that, I ask targeted questions to find the corresponding conflict. E.g.: "In terms of the New Medicine, this appears to be a persistent separation conflict. Did you experience something of the sort five years ago?..."
4. We work together to find out what conditioning underlies the conflict. This is where we will find the actual cause. At this point, the patient can decide for themselves if they would like to proceed with this information alone or if we should proceed together.
5. An appropriate therapeutic massage to facilitate relaxation.
6. Following that, a meditation in this prone position:

Step 1. Prayer
Silently (or aloud), ask for spiritual help in resolving the conflict or for helping the patient. Make the connection to God.
Step 2. Naming, declaring the intention
I name the conflict/conditioning again briefly and ask the patient if they are now ready to resolve it.
Step 3. Reliving

The patient should place themselves in the situation or conditioning once again (e.g., Mommy wasn't there...).
Step 4. Appreciation
Ask the patient to express their appreciation for the conflict situation. In other words, they should say, *"Thank you that I was able to experience this situation, so I could learn from it."*
Step 5. New conditioning
Based on the conflict situation, we imagine a good situation. *E.g., Mommy comes back and gives me a big hug and says that she's always there for me."*
Step 6. Enjoyment
The patient should "bathe" in this new feeling with pleasure. This energy should fill their whole body.
Step 7. Giving thanks
We thank the spiritual world for its help.
Homework: Every evening for three weeks, the patient should relive/feel the healing thoughts/imagery as intensely as they possibly can. In their daily lives, they patient should consciously deal with matter they identified in a new/different way.

The method that I have just outlined is just one of many possible ways of proceeding. There are *"many roads that lead to Rome."* This is confirmed by the many letters I received following the first edition of this book. Successes in resolving conflicts were also reported by using neuro-linguistic programming (NLP), the Chinese Quantum Method (CQM), quantum healing, matrix energy, two point methods, and many others.

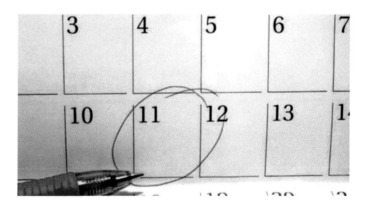

Set a time limit for the therapy

In naturopathy, we know the basic rule of therapy that states: a certain remedy should only be taken for a certain period of time (e.g., drinking a tea mixture for three weeks). Taking it for any longer doesn't make any sense. This rule also applies to psychic healing as well.

A good therapy first brings up the conflict on the conscious level and makes us briefly conflict-active. In the second step, we try to resolve the conflict somehow. If the resolution is not successful within a certain period of time, we should stop the therapy. This is because there is a certain danger of keeping the conflict alive artificially. This result would be counterproductive - well-intentioned, but off-target nonetheless.

- *Example: A young woman is suffering from a loss-conflict because her mother has died. She makes it a habit to pray for her mother every day. Years later, after she finally stops doing it, an ovarian cyst grows, which is diagnosed four months later. Note: Rather than to conclude with the event and starting new again, she keeps the conflict alive for years with her daily prayers. The unusually-long conflict period results in an unusually large conflict-mass. Instead of a small cyst, a large cyst grows in the repair phase. (Archive B. Eybl)*

Excursus: The Phenomenon of First Worsening

In natural healing, the "first worsening," in Chinese medicine and homeopathy also often referred to as a "healing crisis," is when the symptoms get worse at the beginning of the therapy. The "first worsening" is - for homeopaths and natural healers - a welcome sign, because it shows that the therapy has taken hold and is starting to work. How can this phenomenon be explained?

Many years ago, when I first took an intense interest in the findings of Dr. Hamer, I plowed through all the different illnesses with their various conflict origins and compared them to my own illnesses. Soon, I became sicker than I ever had before. What had happened? I had "dug up" my old, unresolved conflicts and by understanding how things were interrelated, I had resolved them through this process of reevaluation.

Chronic processes have to be taken back to the acute stage if they are to be healed. This is true for the body level as well as for the level of the psyche.

Abscesses (encapsulated pus) can be caused "erupt" (e.g., with heat treatments. - A first worsening (pain and even more swelling) is unavoidable.

How do natural healing and homeopathy "kick-off" the healing (= first worsening)? Could it be that in this process we're dealing with a resonance phenomenon?

Nobody doubts that every person has a certain character - certain psychological traits. This is also true of animals and plants; something that is now recognized by science as well. Shouldn't we also attribute a certain character to "dead materials," such as stones, minerals, metals, salts, and so forth? After all, all materials are of a spiritual origin and therefore also have specific spiritual-psychic characteristics. Isn't it possible that, e.g., the specific character of a pasque flower (*Pulsatilla vulgaris*) could come into resonance with the specific conflict-active spirt of a person and heals them in this way?

On the organic level, these means strengthen the vagotonia, so that after the first worsening, a thorough healing can follow.

What can stand in the way of healing

1. Advantages through the illness: Many people are lacking attention. As a child or an adult, they may have experienced that they receive love and attention when they're sick. From this, a program is created: "*I may be sick, but that's not so bad, because now I am loved.*" Unconsciously through this, they will cling to their suffering. Also, consider the advantages of early retirement, disability, care allowances, and other "benefits."

2. Some people identify themselves as a victim (e.g., of a bad partner, an unloving mother). With an illness, they can get revenge by giving the "oppressor" a guilty conscience: "*Look*

how sick I am (silently: *because of you*)."

3. Healing requires change. Some people don't want to change themselves (mostly due to laziness or fear).

> *I'll check and see if these patterns are right and then forget about them!*"

Therapy - conflict-active phase at the brain level

I am not aware of anything that can be done during conflict activity at the brain level.

What's decisive is approaching conflict resolution at the psychological level (see previous pages).

Therapy - conflict-active phase at the body level

Most SBSs do not cause physical symptoms in the conflict-active phase; this is because we do not feel "ill."

In fact, the body usually functions especially well during this phase. It is more or less in a state of "doping" by the sympathetic nervous system. - A natural overdrive for overcoming the conflict. We pay for that later in the repair phase in form of a "healing hangover" (= vagotonic repair phase). Even if we know that a conflict has just taken place on the body level, unlike with the psychic level, there is not much we can or should do.

As the "executive body," the body carries out the appropriate special program. When it comes to starting (psyche) and steering (brain) them, the body only has influence within the framework of its own "feedback"

For example, if an intestinal tumor develops because of indigestible anger (= conflict-active phase), we have to try to deal with the conflict on the psychic level. At the body level, we can or must intervene, e.g., if the conflict lasts too long and there is a risk of a bowel obstruction (ileus). In such cases, we are happy and thankful for modern surgical interventions and certain medications.

Nutrition

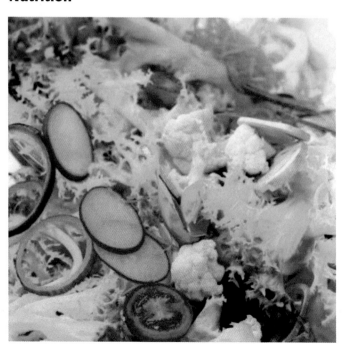

During the conflict-active phase, repair-phase and also when we are experiencing no phase at all (normotonia), healthy, organically pure, genetically unmodified and balanced nutrition is important. During conflict-activity we tend to eat less. At the same time, the body is running at "full speed," meaning it is willing and able to perform.

Logically, fasting or a reduced diet is the wrong thing at such a time, especially for thin people.

The few things that appeal to us should be nourishing and biologically valuable. Overweight people might want to take advantage of such a situation and lose some weight - this is especially easy during this phase (except in the case of an active refugee conflict (kidney collecting tubules).

I have found out that in a conflict-active (stressful) phase, I tend to reach for less valuable foods (sweets, white flour, etc.) more than I do in good times. The biological explanation for this is that

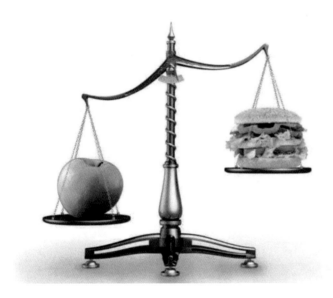

short-chain (simple) carbohydrates give you more energy quickly and easily cover your energy needs during conflict-activity.

Let's be honest: just about every one of us knows what good nutrition is. We all know exactly what is good for us - organic, natural, full-value, balanced foods in reasonable amounts. We all know it and nevertheless, few of us are strong enough to follow through with it, actually "do the right thing." At first, let's try to stop making our worst dietary mistakes by overcoming our "weaker selves." In the following, I limit myself to the basic interrelationships.

Nutrition and cancer

Along with inner balance, good nutrition is the second most important pillar for stable health. An undernourished, "run-down" living being is prone to attract conflict upon themselves. E.g., self-esteem conflicts because they feel inferior, territory conflicts because they are too weak to defend their territory, anger conflicts because they have lost the fight for the "chunk." So saying that poor nutrition predisposes someone to cancer is correct in this sense.

I am also of the opinion that continuous poisoning (fast food diet,

residual pesticides, electromagnetic pollution, chemtrails, pharmaceuticals, immunizations, and much more) can cause feedback effects via the brain that eventually do lead to cancer. It's not only bad nutrition that can undermine our vitality, but also active or passive smoking, drugs/alcohol, too little, too much or too monotonous physical activity, improper breathing and bad posture. A well-fed individual - because of their vitality - can deal with a repair phase crisis better than an individual who has been weakened by the consumption of poisons.

There is no doubt that having a healthy diet increases the quality and quantity of life.

The medical medium, Anthony William has been able to heal thousands of people through his nutritional recommendations alone. His credo: fruit, vegetables and herbs above everything (don't be afraid of fructose).

His favorites: apples, pears, lemons, oranges, blueberries, apricots, melons, mangoes, papayas, salad, asparagus, beans, celery, red beets, radishes, garlic, onions, spinach, avocados, sprouts, nuts, dates, honey, parsley, spirulina, barley grass powder, thyme, sage, tumeric, stinging nettles (an amazing plant that is almost completely overlooked) and lemon balm.

To be avoided according to William: meat, animal fat, milk products, marine fish, mussels, etc. (due to mercury).

The atmosphere at mealtime

Eating in a positive atmosphere, enjoyed with pleasure and due concentration, also promotes one's health.

Eating and drinking makes us ill when we are angry, afraid, or worried. It can cause triggers to be set that can reactivate throughout our whole lives (food allergies). To eat while driving is also dangerous, because conflicts can happen at any moment while driving.

The acid-base balance

In natural healing circles, over-acidity is heard quite often and has become something of a "knockout argument." Over-acidity has been made the culprit for nearly every illness imaginable. From the point of view of the 5 Biological Laws of Nature, over-acidity means basically the same thing as conflict activity.

Stress, negative thoughts and feelings, all increase the acid milieu in the body. When something doesn't suit us, we become "sour" - psychologically and physically.

Vagotonia is alkaline. Positive feelings and thoughts lead to an alkaline milieu in the body.

It is interesting that in the body, poor nutrition, in terms of the acid-alkaline balance, is hardly more noticeable than stress. You can prove this for yourself by means of a test that measures the urine's pH value.[26] A good mood, the joy of living and positive experiences cause the urine's pH to be higher than 7, even when eating a less than optimal diet.

Similar values, but with not quite as high a pH, can be obtained from alkaline meals (e.g., raw vegetables, bitter herbs, etc.).

Conflictive events, stress, bad moods and so on, lead to low pH values in the urine (acidic). A person can eat as many

---

26 I use the "indicator paper Uralyt-U ph 5.2–7.4" from the company Madaus.

carrots and vegetable as he wants; in such a psychological state, the pH value will not go up appreciably.

Taking alkaline powders is a chemical-mineral means for "fighting" the level of acidity. This is fine in the case of heartburn, but using them over a longer period to lower the bodily milieu, is not good (in my opinion). To lower the level of acidity, we have to change our inner lives, the habits of our everyday lives and our nutritional habits.

Organically-bound bases in our daily fruits and vegetables (sprouts, bitter herbs, etc.) can be absorbed by the body far better than non-organic alkaline powders.

Edgar Cayce, the "sleeping prophet," recommended that we should consume 80% alkaline and only 20% acidic foods. Translated onto the level of the psyche, this means in order to stay healthy, we should be relaxed and happy for 80% of the day and only be under stress 20% of the time.

The strongest providers of alkalis are medicinal herbs that grow in the wild, such as dandelion, common centaury (Centaurium erythraea), bear's garlic (Allium ursinum), sage, peppermint, daisies (Bellis perennis), stinging nettles, Melissa, buckhorn (Plantago lanceolata) and many more. The ingredients from "God's pharmacy" are free for the taking and, for healing, are a thousand times better than all of the expensively packaged products in the stores. Pick them as you take a relaxing nature walk. When finely chopped, they can give a variety of dishes an organic upgrade.

Wild herb base drink (alkaline tonic):

Mince a handful of wild herbs according to your preference or a specific organ's need. Place them in a container and cover them with about one cup of cold water. Puree with a hand blender and pour through a sieve or strain. That's all there is to it - drink the green juice. In spring this is recommended as an alkaline tonic - a drink full of vitality!

The amount of protein

According to the World Health Organization (WHO), a clinically relevant protein deficiency begins at about 30–35 g or less per day. The Dutch Professor Oomen followed up on this assertion and found a tribe of natives in New Guinea who live exclusively from sweet potatoes. They eat practically no meat. According to CM,

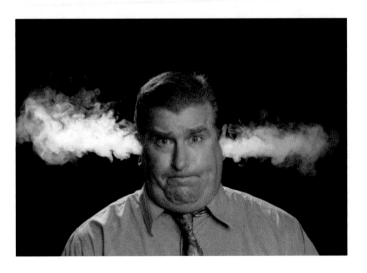

with their 9-24 grams of protein per day, this tribe should suffer from chronic protein deficiency. The people should also suffer from emaciated muscles, anemia or hunger swelling - but the opposite is the case. They are very energetic and downright muscular. He wanted to look into this discrepancy and discovered that anaerobic bacteria (clostridium) in these people's intestines produced proteins from carbohydrates with the help of ambient nitrogen. Vitamin B12, mainly found in animal food, is also produced by intestinal bacteria.[27]

Studies show that many people in our affluent Western society are *"eating themselves to death"* by consuming an excess of meat. Too much animal protein is an unnecessarily burden on the body and over-acidifies it. This is particularly true in the case of pork from factory farming.

Putting an end to our Western overconsumption of meat and protein would not only be good for all human beings, it would also be good for "Mother Nature." Raising livestock causes untold suffering, and besides, three-quarters of the original nutritional energy is lost during its detour through animals' digestive systems, which we euphemistically call a "refining process."

We could easily give back the tremendous portion of the earth's surface which is now used for keeping and producing feed for livestock, if we could just give up eating so much meat.

The amount of food

In laboratory feeding tests with rats, it was determined that the ones who were always being fed sooner put on weight sooner, grew older faster and died earlier.

When the rats always had a full food dish, they lived an average of 600 days. With fewer feedings, the rats were always a little hungry, but they lived an average of 900 days. These rats were a little smaller, but quicker, more intelligent, more curious, and more active than their well-fed contemporaries.[28]

The most vital people in the world are not those in the well-fed, rich Western countries, but those in the poor mountain areas of Asia.

In any case, a simple lifestyle and meager diet doesn't appear to be harmful. The habits that are a necessity for these people can also be a virtue for us as well - and one that would increase our life expectancy.

Effective Microorganisms (EM)

EM were discovered by the Japanese agronomist and university professor Dr. Teruo Higa.

EM are a mixture of lactic acid and photosynthesis bacteria, yeasts, and fungi.

EM are used worldwide in agriculture and in the fields of the environment, industry, and health. Although ordinary EM are not permitted in foods and medications, they may be used internally as well. I personally use them for the regular freshening up of my bacteria and fungi reserves. When I do this, I take a regimen of

---

27 See Dr. Ralph Bircher, Geheimarchive der Ernährungslehre, p. 40–44, Bircher-Benner Verlag, Bad Homburg, 11th edition, 2007

28 See Dr. Ralph Bircher, Geheimarchive der Ernährungslehre, p. 40–44, Bircher-Benner Verlag, Bad Homburg, 11th edition, 2007

one teaspoon of EM1 in a glass of water every day for a week.

Homeopathy

Classic homeopathy is a gentle method that can be used to support patients through all the phases of an SBS.

It's best when the therapist is skilled in both the 5 Biological Laws of Nature and the basics of homeopathy.

I cannot recommend individual medications here, as my knowledge is not extensive enough and because they have to be exactly and individually matched to the phase and the condition of

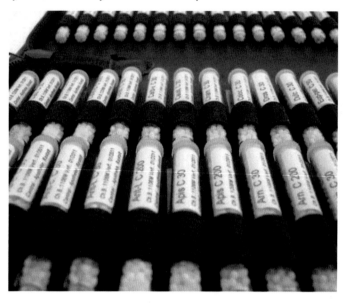

the patient.

Massage

may help in the conflict-active phase and in the repair phase:

- Lymph drainage is a good method to use in the repair phase, especially when there is fluid retention (syndrome).
- Classic massage, segmental massage, as well as foot and ear reflex-zones and acupuncture massages are suitable for both phases.
- According to Chinese energetics, the corresponding meridian area shows a shortage of energy in the conflict-active phase. A shortage of energy demands an influx of energy.
- Osteopathy: There are many different manual techniques associated with this term. The idea is to ease problems in the musculoskeletal system with various pressure, stretching, and movement stimulations - useful in the active and repair phases.
- In classic and segmental massage, energy is applied in a pleasant way. Stroking, pressing, and dispersing, improve the body's metabolism and energy flow. Inner organs, which have been affected by an SBS, can be reached therapeutically by means of skin and muscle stimulations (cutivisceral reflex arcs) in the back.
- With foot and ear reflex-zone treatments, we can supply the inner organs with energy and harmony.

Massages do not affect the person's conflict on the psychic level directly, but the relaxation, being indulged, being touched, and gaining trust can bring about a change in attitude - a good

basis for healing.

Therapy - repair phase at the psyche level

Dr. Hamer rightly criticized that therapy need not be carried out during the repair phase. Repair phases are times when the body repairs and regenerates itself. To view repair phases as "illness" and to try to treat it is a good indication of ignorance, a lack of knowledge of biological interrelationships = old medical paradigm.

- What does make sense, however, is attending to the healing-phases - easing the symptoms, making the suffering bearable.
- Provide courage and confidence.
- Make clear to the patient that the conflict will be resolved and everything will be all right again.
- Provide a "protective atmosphere" for the patient. In other words, protect them from the negative. Keep them away from new conflicts and avoid recurrences.
- Guiding thoughts: *"I am going to be completely well again!" "I am at peace with everyone and everything." "I am looking forward to a new beginning."*

Therapy - repair phase at the brain level

A Hamer Focus in the brain during the repair phase causes fluid retention. The Hamer Focus expands and displaces the surrounding areas of the brain. The brain itself has no receptors for pain; however, the cerebral membrane (meninges) does. > Headaches are caused by the pressure on the meninges. In severe cases, it is advisable to reduce the pressure on the brain; this can be decisive as to whether the patient will survive the repair phase or not.

Measures to be taken

- Any kidney collecting tubules SBS (syndrome), if active, should be resolved as quickly as possible (see p. 230ff).
- Cooling the head (cold showers, cold wraps, bags of ice).
- Take a walk in the cold air.
- Protect the head from sun and heat.
- Take organic dextrose ("quick energy"), possibly maltodextrine 19, a water soluble carbohydrate mixture (longer lasting) at short intervals, especially at night (strongest vagoto-

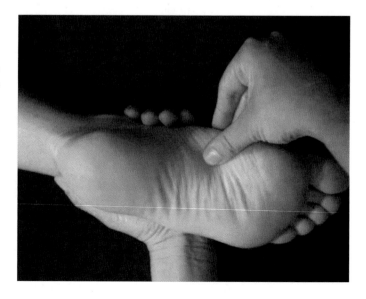

nia) - allow the dextrose to dissolve in your mouth.
- With sympathicolytic substances such as vitamin C, coffee or black tea, the vagotonia can also be reduced (see below).
- Ingest natural borax, dark beer (malt beer).
- Full or partial baths with sea salt, 0.9% or more concentrated (the sea is our home). Fluids are removed from the body through the pressure of osmosis as well.
- Head and facial lymph drainages.
- Foot and head are opposite poles of the body that influence one another. This can be used therapeutically: Warming or stimulating the feet relieves the head energetically > walk barefoot, take hot foot baths, foot massages.
- No salt infusions because salt binds water in the body.
- No glucose infusions if intake is possible orally (sugar in the blood binds additional fluids).
- Visualization: Starting from the head, energy flows over the spine into the legs and feet. My head becomes empty. My feet feel as though they are full of energy. Surround the head with blue light.
- Colloidal silver or MMS as necessary. In extreme cases, corti-

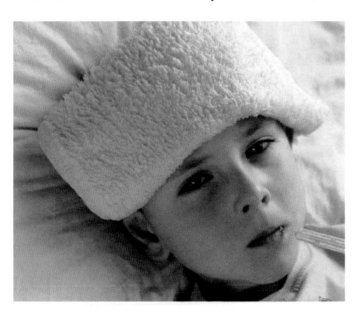

sone (Prednisolone) to reduce the vagotonia.

Therapy - repair phase at the body level

Inflammation should only be hemmed if suffering makes it unavoidable. Intense inflammation = intense repair > fast recovery. Taking anti-inflammatory measures could prolong the repair phase. If the pain is too great or the fever climbs too high, one should take measures to stimulate sympathicotonia.

Before reaching out for chemical substances I would use natural means. Natural healing has a treasure trove of remedies and methods for easing the repair phase symptoms (more details in the lexicon).

Painkillers work by exciting the sympathetic nervous system - the pain of repair is reduced because the vagotonia is correspondingly reduced. Chemical stress stimulus pulls the organ-

isms up from the vagotonic wave into sympathicotonia.
In severe cases, we must seek the assistance of intensive care physicians and surgeons.

Natural, general pain remedies

- A reasonable amount of movement and activity.
- Black tea, coffee. • Schüssler Salt No. 3
- Cold-hot treatments with emphasis on cold: cold-warm showers, "Kneipp" treatments, cool bags, cold showers.
- Hot spices, e.g.: pepper, chili, ginger, mustard, saffron.
- Willow bark tea: Willow is an ancient pain remedy. The bark of young shoots contains salicin (natural aspirin) and tannins.
- Teas made from peppermint, sage, thyme, arnica, wild daisies, celandine, pansies, or creeping thyme.
- Use refreshing, stimulating essential oils topically - i.e., peppermint, eucalyptus, sage, thyme.
- Cannabis.

Lymph drainage

works amazingly well and also eases pain. Rhythmically pumping hand motions improve lymph drainage and soothe the patient. From an energy perspective, lymph drainage has the effect of being relaxing (sedative), in other words, energy is reduced and inflammation is also reduced.

It is a good pain-relieving method, during repair phases in the musculoskeletal system (inflammations of the joints and after injuries, bruises, contusions, etc.).

During repair phases in the head and facial areas (e.g., toothache, neuralgia of the trigeminal nerve) and in the repair phase of internal organs, a good lymph drainage treatment is followed by increased urination.

Acupuncture, acupuncture massage, shiatsu, acupressure

By using these methods, therapists work with the patient's meridian system. The main principle is: If there is too much energy at one point, it is taken away. If there is too little energy, it is added. For the Chinese people, we are healthy when all of our meridians are totally filled with energy.

The healing-phases in the organs distinguish themselves by an abundance of energy (inflammation).Thus, somewhere else in the patient's meridian system there is an energy deficiency. The therapist tries with needle, stick, or finger pressure, to lead the energy from the inflamed area to the area with a deficit.

Cod Liver Oil

Without this home remedy (which has unfortunately fallen into oblivion), many people would not have survived the times of the great wars. Very helpful, particularly for emaciated (conflict-active, stressed) people. An ideal, cheap supply of the fat-soluble vitamins A, D, E can be found in a 1-2 tablespoons of cod liver oil daily.

Oil pulling

Put a tablespoon of cold-pressed sunflower seed oil into the mouth and swish it around the mouth and throat for about 10 minutes. Repeat this every morning on an empty stomach. Afterwards spit out the oil, which by this time will have taken on a milky-whitish color, as it is now loaded with toxins.

You can do this for four weeks as a "cure" or make it a once-a-week routine.

Natural antibiotic recipe

700 ml (23 oz) vinegar, two tbsp ea. of chopped garlic, chopped onions, grated ginger, grated horseradish, tumeric powder and two freshly chopped chili peppers. Fill a glass jar with the ingredients, close and shake. Continue shaking occasionally for two weeks and then afterwards, press the contents through a sieve and strain. Dosage: up to a max. of 6 tablespoons daily.

MMS (sodium chlorite NaClO2) by Jim Humble

A controversial substance, which I appreciate regardless. A strong oxidizing agent (the opposite of antioxidants), which we can use as a sympatheticotonic. I consider it to be a good substitute for CM antibiotics. From the perspective of the New Medicine, it can be used as a "mild antibiotic" for the attenuation of an intense repair phase. **Please note:** Before use, you must thoroughly inform yourself about the ingestion procedure (only recommended for adults). Due to its oxidative properties, I do not advocate long-term use.

Petroleum

Crude oil or petroleum (mixture of various hydrocarbons) is used in traditional medicine in Eastern Europe with success in treating various ailments. The mechanism of action is unclear, but you can risk a try. Because it is cheap and effective, it is discredited as outdated and toxic. (http://petroleum_de.lorincz-veger.hu)

Medication from the perspective of the 5 Biological Laws of Nature

Basically, it must be clear that everything in the body is there for a reason. Thus, we should think twice before making any chemical interventions.

Medications can be roughly divided into two groups:
- Stress-promoting medication (= sympathicolytic substances) like antibiotics, antirheumatics, cortisone, MMS and coffee. In this group, you'll find most of the CM medications.
- Sedative medications (= vagotonics) like anticonvulsants, sleeping aids.

Pain Medications

Active ingredient: paracetamol/acetaminophen
Trade names: Tylenol, Excedrin, store brands and can also be found in various cough and sinus medications, etc.
Effect: analgesic, antipyretic.
Good pain relief and not too many side effects.
Recommended for the attenuation of healing-phases.
The most recommended chemical painkiller - well-tolerated, central effect on the brain, no blood-thinning effect. However, for rheumatic complaints (bones, joints), it doesn't work as well as antirheumatic drugs.

Active ingredient: acetylsalicylic acid (aspirin)
Trade names: Bayer, Bufferin, Excedrin and store brands, etc.
Aspirin works well as an analgesic with few side effects (only harmful to the kidneys). From our point of view, the blood-thin-

ning property of aspirin is not desirable in most cases.
> Only conditionally recommended.
Active ingredient: diclofenac - antirheumatic agent
Trade names: Voltaren, Cataflam, Cambia, Zorvolex, etc.
Effect: analgesic, anti-inflammatory
> Recommended for attenuation of bone and joint pain during intense repair phases.
Active ingredient: ibuprofen - antirheumatic agent
Trade names: Advil, Motrin, Medipren, Nuprin, etc.
Effect: analgesic, anti-inflammatory, antipyretic.
> Recommended for attenuation of bone and joint pain during intense healing-phases.
Active ingredient: indomethacin - antirheumatic agent

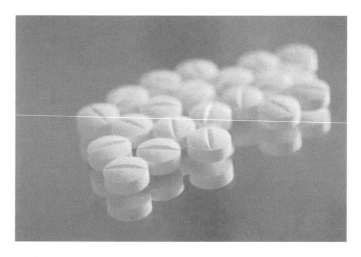

Trade names: Indocin, etc.
Effect: analgesic, anti-inflammatory
> Recommended for attenuation of bone and joint pain during intense healing-phases.
Active ingredient: morphine - strong painkiller
Trade names: Avinza, Astramorph, Duramorph, Kadian, etc.
Strongest sympathicotonic. Morphine is addictive. It paralyzes the intestines by causing continuous tension; it will break the morale of the patient.
Morphine is usually a one-way, dead-end street.
It shocks the vegetative nervous system and instantly shrinks the Hamer Focus in the brain. If the next dose does not come on time, the Hamer Focus will swell up again even faster. This leads to a breaking off of the connections between brain and nerves (synapses). In CM, morphine has been used very generously, because cancer patients "should at least be spared the suffering." Thus, it has become the "euthanasia drug." Morphine, as an intravenous therapy, is often given without any sort of agreement from the patient or family members. > Always ask, "What exactly is in there?" Even better: draw up a patient's decree (living will).
> Morphine is not recommended in general.
Morphine patch - active ingredient: fentanyl, buprenorphine
If anyone still needs morphine, they should be given morphine patches with semi-synthetic opiates. These have fewer side effects than real morphine and so there still is a "way back" (not a one-way street).

Cortisone

Cortisone effect: strong sympathicotonic - adrenocortical hormone.

Menacing, strong repair phases can be attenuated rapidly with cortisone. Dr. Hamer recommends cortisone during very strong repair crises to better survive the critical period just after the repair phase crisis.

During a syndrome, i.e., active kidney collecting tubules, cortisone is not to be recommended due to additional water retention (contraindicated). Cortisone can only be recommended in very severe cases, but use only for as short a period as possible.

Antibiotics

It only makes sense to take antibiotics when a healing-phase is too intense, a fever is too high or the pain is unbearable. They should only be taken as long as symptoms require. For example, if an infection of the middle ear has improved after taking antibiotics for two days, the patient should stop taking them at once. This approach is "strictly forbidden" by CM due to the danger of "building up resistance." Their argument that the patient must *"take the entire package in order to kill off all the bacteria,"* however, does not hold water: It is simply not possible to destroy a single strain or even all of them. If that were possible, we would be *"clinically clean"* and *"clinically dead."* Antibiotics damage the genes and should only be used in exceptional cases. A gentle alternative: take colloidal silver or MMS (see p. 62).

Anti-fungal drugs (Antimycotics)

> Using these drugs internally is very damaging and corresponds to a small dose of chemotherapy.

Anti-fungal medicines are not to be recommended!

Anti-viral drugs

> Not recommended because they are senseless and damaging.

Antihypertensive Medications (Blood Pressure Drugs)

Beta-blockers, ACE inhibitors, AT1 antagonists, calcium channel blockers, etc.

According to CM, hypertension is a risk factor for cardiovascular disease. Up until 2008, a blood pressure of 100 + age was considered normal. This prompted the WHO to suddenly fix the limit at 140. Since then, anything above that is now *"treated."* High blood pressure is no risk for the heart, blood vessels, or the brain. Blood pressure medicines have significant side effects and are not recommended for prolonged use. Only in exceptional circumstances is this sensible and only for a short time (see also p. 65).

Water pills (diuretics)

Only recommended if you have previously done everything to resolve the kidney collecting tubules conflict (see p. 230ff).

Cholesterol reducing medications

Not to be recommended due to their basic uselessness and strong side effects (see p. 38f).

Anticoagulants

Active ingredient: *apaxiban* - trade name: Eliquis
Active ingredient: *warfarin* - trade name: Coumadin
> The effects are similar to slight, continuous poisoning.

Coumarins (Coumadin, etc.) are also used as rat poison. It is only useful a few weeks after pulmonary embolism or thrombosis. It is not recommended as a long term medication.

Psycho-pharmaceuticals

Certainly there are exceptional cases, in which sleeping pills, antidepressants and tranquilizers, make therapeutic sense, i.e., to avert something worse.

> They are not to be recommended in general, because of their ineffectiveness, the danger of addiction, their personality-altering effects and severe side effects.

Chemotherapy (cytotoxics)

Dr. Ulrich Abel of the German Cancer Research Institute in Heidelberg: *"In the future, the dominance of chemotherapy research could turn out to be one of the most far-reaching aberrations in the clinical battle against cancer."*[32]

Radiation therapy

Because of its harmfulness, it is generally not recommended. It is recommended only in very rare cases, when a surgery is impossible because of inaccessible tumor location or if you can't calm down an extremely intense repair phase. For example, in an extreme bone repair phase in the spinal canal.

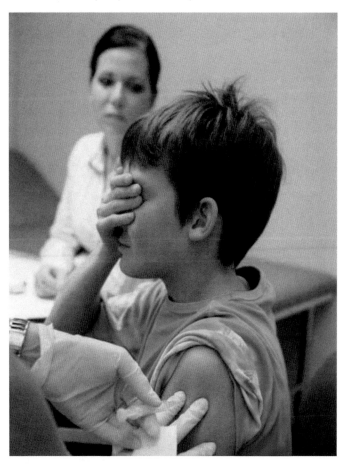

Hormonal contraception ("the pill")

32 Ulrich Abel: Chemotherapy of advanced carcinomas. A critical survey. 2nd updated edition, Stuttgart: Hippokrates Verlag, 1995. ISBN: 3-7773-1167-7

The pill makes the woman hormonally masculine. Due to this, she switches over to the right, "masculine" side of the brain (except in the cases of left-handed women or those who are already configured in this way). Shift of the active side of the brain (lateralization) produces "masculinization" as a result of the contraceptive effect.

From the viewpoint of the 5 Biological Laws of Nature, the pill is to be rejected, because it turns the normal brain relationship upside down. Conflicts can be activated or resolved by taking or stopping the pill (= "Russian roulette"). The pill increases the risk of cardiac infarction (heart attack), pulmonary embolism, and much more. All other methods of contraception are better.

Vaccinations and Inoculations

Even without the knowledge of the 5 Biological Laws of Nature, there is much to be said against vaccinations:

- There is no proof that they are effective.
- They go against the basic principle of medicine: "Above all, do no harm."
- Poisoning with aluminium hydroxide, the mercury alloy (thimerosal), formaldehyde, phenol, and recently also nanoparticles and many more.

The result: increasing rates of physical deformities, sterility, children with "Attention Deficit Syndrome" (ADS), allergies, mental deficiencies, and much more. The case for vaccinations is made by fear. Fear can only arise in combination with ignorance.

Our knowledge of the 4th Biological Law of Nature, which says that fungi, bacteria, and viruses (globulins), are our symbionts and "friends," liberates us from fear.

Recognizing this is simple: If there are no invaders from whom we must protect ourselves, then we no longer need inoculations. We can also safely abstain from many "hygienic precautions" of modern, everyday life.

What remains of the term "immune system," when the enemies out there are not even there at all? Just a term from the old school of medicine.

The biological reality of the situation is that there is a kind of "garbage collection system" for the disposal of toxins, waste products, and dead cells. Responsible for this task are the lymph nodes and vessels, the kidneys, liver, and spleen.

Summary:

Vaccinations - regardless against what - are not only useless, due

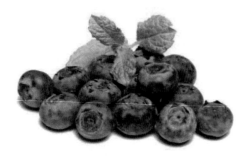

to their ineffectiveness, but also harmful due to poisonous side effects and the traumatic vaccination process itself (patient's fear, e.g., holding on > motor conflict).

LEXICON OF "DISORDERS"

Important instructions for use:

The lexicon is indexed according to the organs of the body, beginning with the nervous system and is ordered in the sequence normally used in professional medical literature.

It is advisable to begin study starting on page 230 with the Significant Biological Special Program (SBS) of the kidney collecting-tubules (fluid collection in the body). This forms the "background music" for many other "diseases" and is often referred to elsewhere (key word: *syndrome*).

For understanding diseases where muscles are involved (e.g., twitching eyelids), it is advisable to read the chapter beginning on page 307 first.

For almost all diseases, I have given examples of typical conflicts. Those beginning with ➜ are typical conflict situations. Those beginning with • have been taken from real events. In a few cases, I have changed the patient's gender or other details for the sake of privacy.

When printed in **bold**, the expressions "conflict-active," "repair phase" or "repair phase crisis" refer to the disease mentioned in the title. Please note that with recurring conflict, this classification is often inaccurate. > Always try to deduce for yourself, which phase the patient is experiencing.

There are therapy suggestions for every conflict. For diseases in the repair phase, "therapy" means attending to the patient's recovery.

The natural healing of tumors only works when they are small. > The description - conflict-active > repair phase > everything's better - only works with small tumors. Larger tumors have to be surgically removed/treated. (Nature will remove the individuals who can't find and implement solutions).

When it comes to the remedies recommended and their applications, I concentrate on simplicity, nativeness (overwhelmingly domestic herbs) and cost effectiveness (hardly any ready-made preparations). I have personal experience with most, but not all of these applications.

It is my wish to connect the New Medicine with natural medicine and the good aspects of conventional medicine. The patient seeking help does not care **what** helps; the main thing they want is that **it** helps.

For this, I will build bridges between disciplines. These bridges will be necessary until the separation of the medical disciplines is finally overcome.

The growing consciousness within the community can already be felt everywhere. In my opinion, this is an evolutionary step toward the New Age and the New Medicine.

GENERAL SYMPTOMS

High blood pressure (hypertonia, hypertension)

What is high blood pressure? Up until a few years ago, what is now considered "at risk" was still considered perfectly healthy: Until 2008, a blood pressure of 100 + age was okay. Then, the World Health Organization arbitrarily set the borderline value at 140/90. Since then, countless people have been continuously sedated with medications. The consequences: fatigue and the loss of strength, vitality and libido.

According to CM, high blood pressure is a risk factor for diseases of the heart and circulatory systems. This claim is both right and wrong.

It is right, in so far as conflict-active persons with stress-related high blood pressure suffer more often from heart attacks, strokes, and similar illnesses. It is wrong because the guilt lies with the stress and not the high blood pressure. For instance, through territorial-loss conflicts or conflicts stemming from being overwhelmed or outsmarted with regard to the heart.

Comparison: risk factor and oil pressure warning light. Assumption: cars with oil warning lights will have more engine damage than cars without an oil indicator light. - This is also both true and false.

> High blood pressure is not a danger to the heart, blood vessels, or brain; however, stress certainly is (= conflicts or triggers).

Possible causes

- **Medication, alcohol, and drugs:** The rise in blood pressure is based on the sympathicotonic effect. Especially: cortisone, adrenaline, antibiotics, immune suppressants, chemotherapy, etc.

- **General sympathicotonia - active conflict:** People, who are always "wired," and get upset about every little thing. Some are calm on the outside, but still tense on the inside. A lack of serenity = the most common cause of high blood pressure. The body is constantly in a state of alarm > narrowing of the blood vessels, tension in the skeletal muscles > high blood pressure. This is either linked to the situation (momentary stress) or longer lasting conflict activity due to one or more running, active conflicts.

- **Smooth vascular musculature:** The most common type of high blood pressure in the active phase: constant tension of the vascular musculature. Stress conflict: one believes that they can only get through life with conflict and stress (see p. 142).

- **Right heart muscle (myocardium) -** Conflict of being overwhelmed or outsmarted during the repair phase crisis: The left part of the heart must pump harder to compensate for the uncoordinated contractions of the right part of the heart > compensatory rise in blood pressure. Comes in sudden attacks (paroxysmal), usually occurring during a resting state (e.g., evenings on the couch). Possibly breathing difficulties due to involvement of the diaphragm (see p. 126ff).

- **Kidney parenchyma** in the active-phase or during persistent conflict activity: cell degradation (necrosis) in the kidney parenchyma > the organism raises the blood pressure so that the filter function can remain intact = "compensatory hypertonia" (CM: "renal hypertonia"). The blood pressure sinks to a normal level again when kidney cysts return to normal after about nine months. Up to that point, the cysts help the rest of the kidneys with filtering. In persistent conflict activity, the blood pressure remains high, because the filter tissue that was degraded has not been replaced by new tissue. This is because the repair phase is lacking (see p. 229).

  Example: A man suffers a liquid conflict when his mother drowns in a river. Since then, this river has always been a trigger. Unfortunately, he has to drive across the river every day to go to work = persistent conflict activity - chronic high blood pressure. (Archive B. Eybl)

- **Narrowing of the kidney arteries:** Persistent conflict according to Dr. Sabbah. One is boiling with anger on the inside and can't let off steam. The blood pressure receptors in the kidneys incorrectly register low blood pressure > impulse to raise blood pressure > increased blood pressure (possibly paroxysmal), dizziness, morning headaches (see p. 234).

- **Thyroid:** Raised thyroid hormone-level, during persistent conflict activity. Thyroid hormones make a person sympathicotonic > increased blood pressure, accelerated pulse rate, accelerated metabolism, weight loss (see p. 119f).

- **Adrenal cortex** with regard to cortisol in the repair phase: excess production of cortisol = CM's "Cushing's syndrome" (see p. 117).

- **Adrenal cortex** with regard to aldosterone in the repair phase or in persistent healing: raised aldosterone production = CM's "Conn's Syndrome" - falling potassium levels (hypokalemia), high blood pressure, muscle weakness (see p. 117).

- **Adrenal medulla** in the conflict-active phase: increase in dopamine, noradrenaline, and/or adrenaline production - hyperfunction of the adrenal medulla: sudden attack-like bouts of high blood pressure during stress with accelerated pulse, raised blood sugar levels, sweating, and trembling (see p. 118).

Therapy

According to the causes. Determine the conflict and family conditioning and resolve. Calm down and relax. Disengage from life as much as possible. Reduce activities. "Take your foot off the gas." Endurance sports, stretching gymnastics, no weight lifting, yoga, vegetable diet, vegetables rich in potassium like spinach, fennel, broccoli, cauliflower, beans, garlic, and many more. It only makes sense to take blood pressure medications in exceptional situations (on a case-by-case basis and only short-term) due to their fundamental pointlessness and the severe side effects (e.g. follow-up conflicts: impotence, lack of drive).

Low blood pressure (hypotonia)

Low blood pressure is, by and large, seen as positive from the perspective of the New Medicine and thus, doesn't require treatment. Although, values under 105/65 are often disconcerting: dizziness, black spots in front of the eyes when standing, lack of drive. The following causes come into consideration:

• **Side effects from blood pressure lowering medications:** Common situation among older people who do everything their doctor tells them.

• **Relaxed lifestyle:** People who enjoy a generally relaxed lifestyle, free of stress for the most part > low blood pressure - a good sign.

• **Withstood stress:** A person who has just gotten through a stressful (conflict-active) time. They relax, sleep well = repair phase > temporary low blood pressure.

• **Left heart muscle (myocardium)** - Conflict of being overwhelmed in persistent repair phase (recurrent conflict): The left half of the heart is weakened and doesn't pump sufficiently for the greater circulation, while the pulmonary (lung) circulation experiences (unnoticed) higher blood pressure. Main symptom: At rest, usually after stress, one feels their heart "beating in their throat" = repair phase crisis of the heart muscle (see p. 126f).

• **Adrenal cortex** in the active phase: reduced cortisol or aldosterone production = CM "Addison's disease": fatigue, nausea, brown coloration of the skin (see p. 116f).

Therapy

According to the cause. Determine the conflict and family conditioning and resolve. Often no need for treatment.

Due to a general state of vagotonia, people with low blood pressure, as opposed to those with high blood pressure, should show more commitment to life, get more involved, take a stand more often. *"Get living!"* Tightening up the family arrangement leads to a tightening of the vascular musculature. > Increased blood pressure.

Contrary to those with high blood pressure, people with low blood pressure should practice strength and speed training (muscle and blood vessel tension). (Less endurance training).

Make sure the diet has enough protein. (A purely vegetarian diet lowers blood pressure).

Sleep disorders (insomnia)

Possible causes

• **Severe conflict activity** (= stress): one or more conflicts can keep someone from being able to relax, even at night. Even though this endless thought usually doesn't result in anything constructive, one can't just turn it off. > Restless, light sleep, difficulties falling asleep and sleeping through the night, <u>waking up early in the morning</u>.

Biological function: The individual is kept awake in order to resolve the conflict. > Therapy: resolve the conflict!

• **Skeletons in the closet:** People who have trouble sleeping often fear coming in contact with their subconscious (repressed feelings, things left unsaid, taboo topics) - in principle, a form of conflict activity. Daytime corresponds with consciousness, night, the subconscious. Also, the fear of death can play a role: *"Sleep is death's little brother."*

> Address the taboo topic with courage, even when it seems very difficult. Come to terms with the reality of death and dying by reading, speaking and laughing about it etc.

• **Strong repair phase:** sleeping problems can arise even during vagotonia - not only due to the pain (repair) in the night. During the day, one is tired and looks forward to going to bed. However, <u>sleep only seems possible during the second half of the night</u>. During the day, you are tired again. There are two explanations for this phenomenon:

1. Nature wants to protect the vagotonia-weakened individual from being "easy prey" for predators (animals active at night). Sleeping during the day is safer > People who are in the repair phase should surrender to their fatigue during the day and allow themselves to take frequent *"naps."*

2. Nature makes sure that the nightly vagotonia does not cause an individual, who is already in a state of vagotonia, to fall into "super-vagotonia." This could possibly become critical. (Strong vagotonia = strong healing symptoms). Through this natural minimization of sleep, the person is kept in a tolerable vagotonia that is not too deep. By drinking coffee (or other sympathicotonics) in the evening, we can "outfox" nature. The body believes it is daytime and gives up the sleep inhibition. > In the repair phase, coffee helps a person to sleep better during the night (= paradox)!

• **Breathing disruptions (sleep apnea) at night due to mini right-heart myocardial infarction:** A coupling of the muscle of the right heart chamber with the diaphragm causes breathing to "stumble" > sleep disturbances. (See chapters on heart p. 126ff and diaphragm p. 209ff).

• **Breathing disruptions (snoring) at night due to a slackening of the soft palate** and disrupted air flow, usually occur among the obese. Loud snoring alternates with abnormally long breathing lapses > sleep disorder.

• **Hyperfunction of the thyroid, adrenal cortex, or adrenal medulla** > increase in sympathetic function > sleep disorders (see corresponding chapter).

Therapy for sleep disorders

• Do enough exercise to make the body tired in the evening. Spend the evening quietly (without TV or computer). Do not eat too late in the evening.

• Always go to bed at the same time and not too late.

• Perform a switch-off ritual: For example, take several deep breaths in bed, review the day, say farewell to the day, and then "switch off."

• Bach flowers: hornbeam, impatiens, olive; in the active-phase,

Star of Bethlehem.
- Place lavender sachets near the head.
- Make sure the feet are warm (foot bath, socks).
- Teas of valerian, melissa, hops, lavender, fennel, etc.

- Hildegard of Bingen: Eat two tablespoons of poppy seeds a day.
- Natural borax internally.
- CBD oil (cannabis oil).

Fatigue (Chronic Fatigue Syndrome - CFS)

When fatigue isn't caused by sleep disorders (see above), the following causes can be considered:
- **Medication side effects:** blood pressure medication, psychotropic drugs and many more. Often among older people who do everything their doctor tells them.
- **Withstood stress:** A person who has just gotten through a stressful (conflict-active) time. They relax, sleep well and are nevertheless tired during the day = repair phase. This type of fatigue should last a maximum of 6 months.
- **Adrenal cortex:** in the active phase: conflict - having deviated from the right path. Reduced cortisol or aldosterone production. Does not necessarily have to be diagnosed as "Addison's disease"

- there are also mild forms. Main symptom: stressed fatigue, poor appetite (see p. 116f). > Observe to see which situations cause the fatigue: e.g., the work week.
- **Heart muscle (myocardium):** chronic conflict of being overwhelmed: fatigue in the sense of having reduced performance (at work, sports) see p. 126ff.
- **Pericardium (heart sac):** chronic attack-to-the-heart conflict. > Heart weakness (see p. 129f).

Therapy
According to the cause. Determine the conflict, family conditioning and beliefs, resolve.

Overweight, obesity (adiposity)

Possible causes (combinations)
- **Obesity through conditioning**
- When a child or their ancestors (e.g., parents) have the experience that they will only be loved when they are fat, they will become fat unconsciously. Conditioning through statements like, *"You are as skinny as an starving man. Look at your sister, look at how beautiful and full her face is!"*
- When a child or their ancestors have the experience that losing weight is dangerous, the person will unconsciously refuse to lose weight even if they would like to: e.g., ancestor had esophagus cancer and died of malnutrition or an ancestor died of starvation, e.g., in a concentration/POW camp.
- The ongoing struggle with obesity and dissatisfaction with one's own body is usually carried on over generations and always has the same result: e.g., for her whole life, a mother repeats the phrase, *"Oh man, I've really got a big butt!"* Her daughter adapts to this pattern and the corresponding reality materializes - namely, a big butt. When her curves get rounder during puberty or pregnancy, she will think to herself, *"My God! Now I'm almost as fat as my mother!"* (= multi-generational vicious circle). Through this kind of programming, the Special Program will begin for the corresponding fat cells (see p. 282f). > *"I love my body the way it is - just like my fat mother/father. I may become just like her/him, but I can also become someone different, the person I want to become."*
- **Chronic conflict of the active kidney collecting tubules:** the most common cause by far. Refugee conflict: Fluid deposits, everything with caloric content is retained in order to get through the "lean times" > weight gain while eating very little. Few calories are needed. Dark urine, usually raised creatinine and uric acid values; fluid is also removed from the stool > hard stool, constipation. By filling up their body, a person creates reserves. Left alone, they effectively protect

themselves in this way from cold or further emotional disappointments, injuries, attacks (protective armor) (see p. 230ff).
- **Fatty tissue:** Conflict of feeling unattractive at the particular bodily locations > persistent repair > excess fatty tissue in the "problem zones" > formation of fatty tissue, cellulite (p. 283). The obese/unattractive condition can also be a part of a (usually unconscious) protective strategy: When someone is fat, they will be "left alone" by the opposite sex. This means that they are less likely to experience sexual violence. E.g., when ancestors or the person themselves were the victim(s) of sexual assault or abuse.
- **Alpha-islet cells (pancreas):** Fear-disgust or resistance conflict, chronic conflict-active phase > reduced function > constant low blood sugar (CM: "hypoglycemia, hyperinsulinemia") > constant hunger due to low blood sugar levels, craving for sweets, "hunger attacks" > weight gain (see p. 224).
- **Liver:** Early childhood starvation conflicts lead to a loss of "feeling full" or satiated. Later the person doesn't know when they have had enough. (See p. 216f)
- **Thyroid Gland:** Chunk conflict (see explanations p. 15, 16) of being too slow, persistent repair of the resulting condition > low production of thyroxine = thyroid insufficiency. (In CM, hyperthyroidism, myxedema, possibly Hashimoto's thyroiditis") > slowed metabolism - less energy is used up > weight gain (see p. 119f).
- **Adrenal cortex:** Conflict of having gotten on the wrong track, persistent repair > increased cortisol production = adrenal hyperfunction (CM: "Cushing's disease") "moon-face;" the symptoms are similar to long-term cortisone intake. (See p. 116f)
- **Lack of mobility:** If the balance between energy intake (eating) and energy consumption (movement) get out of kilter, the excess is stored in the form of fat. The body's need for mobility and a variety of motion is not met > regular exercise, sports, etc.

- **Malnutrition:** Low-fiber, "dead," cheap, mass-produced food (white flour, sugar, margarine, soft drinks, etc.) makes you fat and sick with the same amount of calories. > Nutritional switch to "living food," prepared with love.
- **Aspartame:** People want to become or stay slender with these zero calorie artificial sweeteners. However, if they knew that aspartame is given to livestock to fatten the animals up (it makes them hungry) and that it causes brain and nerve damage, they wouldn't touch it. Alternative: Stevia.
- **Low fat foods:** People wanting to lose weight are making a mistake if they believe that these will help. Valuable fats (e.g., butter, cold-pressed oils) don't make us fat.
- **Side effects of medication:** Cortisone, anti-depressants, tranquilizers (neuroleptics), "the pill" (chemical birth control), blood pressure medicines (beta blockers), insulin and more.

> Go through your medications and weigh the risks and benefits. Perhaps you can reduce the dosage or cut them out altogether ("medication vacation").

Therapy

According to the causes described above:

Recognize the entanglements and the thought patterns and throw them overboard. Be sure to "nurse" your new way of thinking on a daily basis, so it becomes anchored in your subconscious.

Anton Styger's morning ritual: You stand naked in front of the mirror, observe your body and say:

"Thank you (body) for being such a beautiful enclosure for my soul. Thank you letting me live inside you. You are strong, beautiful and I like you just the way you are. You and I will stay healthy until the end!" Afterward, clothe your body in divine, white light.

Underweight, lack of appetite, eating disorders (anorexia)

Put simply: The desire to eat is equivalent to the desire for life. Those who don't want to eat anymore will waste away. Possible causes:

- **Conflict activity:** Lack of appetite and the weight loss resulting from this problem are classic signs of an active conflict. Proper nutrition isn't a concern, because the person has other things to worry about. Further symptoms: restless thoughts, poor sleep, cold hands (see p. 9ff). Constant conflict activity saps a person's will (cachexia). One is thin and tense, but this is rarely fatal. The most common examples of cachexia that can end in death: people suffering from diagnosis shock (completely giving up) or the last days of a long life (one stops eating because they want to go). > Resolving the conflict.
- **Underweight through conditioning**
- *I will only be loved if I am thin* - can lead to eating disorders (e.g., anorexia): *"Don't eat so much or you will soon be as fat and ugly as Aunt Tracy!"*
- People with anorexia feel drawn by death. The cause can often

be found in the family system. The unconscious pattern is often, *"Better me than you."* (Someone becomes severely ill and the person wants to sacrifice their own life in the place of the other's). Also, *"I will follow you."* (E.g., someone has died and the person feels guilty because they are allowed to go on living).

- **Perfectionism** *"My body has to be perfect."*
- **Purity:** One wants to be pure and spotless like a virgin. One doesn't want to defile themselves with food/bad nutrition.
> Recognize the situation and break out of these patterns/habits.
- **Stomach mucosa:** Active territorial-anger conflict. One is especially nauseous in the morning, one has little appetite in general and loses weight. Usually accompanied by stomach pains, acid indigestion (see p. 190f). > Resolve the conflict.
- **Intestinal mucosa:** Chronic chunk conflict (see explanations p. 15, 16) > chronic bowel inflammation (enteritis) with tendency of diarrhea (Crohn's disease, ulcerative colitis). One has an appetite, but can't "digest" much of it. Bad nutrition conversion > weight loss > resolve the chronic conflict.

Colds, flu infections (influenza, viral bird and swine flu)

According to the 4. Law of Nature, no diseases are communicated from outside of the body. With this conviction, you can relax and don't have to worry about the various strains of the flu. CM makes an unnecessary distinction between "a dangerous, real flu" (= influenza or viral flus) and a "harmless flu-like infection." Seen from our perspective, we only pay attention to the symptoms (see below).

Why flu outbreaks usually sweep through the population during or at the end of winter: Most people are discomforted by cold or the cold times of the year. For our ancestors, the winter was often a threat and at least, a time of privation - this conditioning is embedded in our subconscious. > Cold (name "the common cold") = conflict or conflict triggers. The end of the winter = repair phase with the common symptoms as follows:

- **Pain in the limbs =** self-esteem conflict - repair phase.

- **Sniffles =** stinking conflict or scent conflict - repair phase.
- **Inflammation of the throat =** conflict of not wanting to swallow something, wanting to spit it out - repair phase.
- **Inflammation of the larynx =** shock-fright or speechlessness conflict - repair phase.
- Bird, swine, and other new influenzas are campaigns staged by the World Health Organization. The above symptoms can become dangerous illnesses or epidemics through conventional therapeutics such as Tamiflu, Relenza (chemotherapies that blocks a cell's ability to metabolize), vaccinations, and above all, through mass fear hypnosis.

I can't judge if you can rule out every infection. It is possible that infectious germs or parasites that cause sickness could actually arise in a completely polluted environment.

Hospital germs (MRSA)

We designate a group of staphylococcus bacteria that doesn't respond to antibiotics anymore as hospital germs because these germs have developed a resistance. From our view, this is unfortunate, because the (sometimes necessary) antibiotic option for attenuating an intense repair phase often no longer works.

The decisive factor is still: infections arise from within. This means: without germs introduced from the outside.

The standard situation: Someone receives a routine operation, e.g., on their knee. Despite being thoroughly disinfected, their knee becomes purulent within a day or several days following the OP. This is easily explained from the perspective of the New Medicine: this affects people who have a conflict with the opera-

tion itself, who fear that something will go wrong, fear a lengthy recuperation phase or fear the pain afterward. Simply put: they are OP conflict-active.

If the patient sees that everything went well after the OP (which is usually the case), their optimism returns = beginning of the repair phase. Their body now builds or breaks down tissue in a meaningful way, depending on which SBS has started. > Fever, infection (e.g. of the knee), blood sedimentation, elevated white blood cell counts, etc. The diagnosis is "MRSA."

> "After I decide to go through with a procedure/an operation I trust in the fact that, with God's help, everything will turn out all right and everything will soon be back to normal."

Loss of consciousness, prolonged unconsciousness (absence seizures)

According to the 5 Biological Laws of Nature, sudden losses of consciousness, often lasting only a few seconds, are the repair phase crises for separation, territorial or motor conflicts (epilepsy). If they occur regularly, the conflict is persistent. If the absence represents the main symptom - which isn't the rule - the following (additional) conflict aspect is present:

Conflict   The situation is unbearable, one wishes to blank it out/to "teleport" themselves/would like to disappear.

Example   • A 10-year-old girl has short, recurring absences at school. Cause: Her father is self-employed and is constantly taking on new projects. It's all too much for him. He would like to "make himself scarce." His daughter is carrying it for him and is making the family aware of the issue. (Archive B. Eybl)

Bio. function   Protection from an overwhelming reality. Escape to another "little world" where everything is quiet and peaceful.

Therapy   Determine and resolve the conflict, triggers and causal conditioning.

Lyme disease (lyme borreliosis)

In our view, the ring-shaped reddening of the skin attributed to Lyme disease is a separation conflict in the repair phase. With or without the tick bite - both are possible. The joint and nervous symptoms are mistakenly attributed to a tick bite. The reddening is a reaction to the introduction of foreign protein by the insect. In any case, a repair phase infection.

The screw-formed bacteria (spirochetes) don't have anything to do with the illness. This is also exactly what the medical medium Anthony William asserts and he wonders why the therapists and their patients jump on the spirochetes train without any critical deliberation.

I observed a patient with the typical ring-shaped reddening of the skin on their shoulder following a very small tick bite. Three weeks later, just as described in CM, massive bone pains set in, emerging from the very spot where she had been bitten and they spread over her whole body. The patient was not afraid of ticks or infections (in other words, no fear conflicts).

The interesting thing is, just before that, she had made a huge step forward regarding her self-esteem. This involved her elderly father, who for the first time, had opened up to her. The patient healed her borreliosis with natural remedies (teasel, oregano, anise, agrimony), but for the first two weeks she required painkillers (antirheumatics).

Another patient also had borreliosis without any demonstrable insect bite; two important people in his life had died three weeks prior (= separation conflict). When he overcame it, he contracted borreliosis on his right (partner) hip (= repair phase). Something else that argues against it being an infection: Why has there NEVER been any direct proof of Borrelia found in those affected? Many homeopaths believe that borreliosis is a result of vaccinations (vaccine damage). > For this reason, always determine the cause: Was there a vaccination before the onset of the symptoms? Were any antibiotics or other serious drugs administered?

Down syndrome (trisomy 21) affected children

Down syndrome is a chromosomal disorder in which three instead of two copies of chromosome 21 are present. It appears more often in children born to older women.

New Medicine's view: Unfortunately, reliable statements about the cause of the conflict still cannot be made. Nevertheless, the old adage, "Nothing comes from nothing," still applies.

Dr. Hamer reported on a Down syndrome child in his Golden Book, vol. 2, p. 445. Here, a hearing conflict and a motor conflict were identified as the cause:

During the pregnancy, the mother suffered from massive jackhammer noise in her office. After the birth, it was noticed that the child was extremely sensitive to noise and this is why Dr.

Hamer recommended that absolute quiet be the most important measure taken. The child developed excellently up to the present and in the meantime had finished high school. If trisomy was still present is unknown.

What commonly plays a role among women who have late pregnancies is the mother's doubt with regard to the child's health. These fears increase with the age of the mother - especially among those who are "well informed" by conventional medicine as opposed to younger, "happy-go-lucky" women.

→ *A pregnant woman sees another woman with a disabled child on the street and thinks to herself: "My God, what a tragic fate. Hopefully my child won't be like that."*

It is possible that these fearful ideas materialize and create exactly that which was feared most.

> *I remain confident and I look forward to my child. I will make myself comfortable and avoid noise (including ultrasound).*

Ancestor view: Disabilities can sometimes be explained by the family chronology (see p. 24f, family waltzes p. 27).

Spiritual view: My observations lead me to believe that parents/families that move forward positively with their child's disability receive a special radiant power, comparable to a lighthouse. It appears that these families win something: Through their child, they get an understanding of what life is really all about.

Depression, burnout syndrome

Depression + burnout are sometimes identical, sometimes not.

From the view of family energies:

• When a child (we are all the children of our parents) can't stand their parents anymore, they become sad/depressed. Someone who only takes what they want from their parents doesn't take them as a whole. Those who despise them cut themselves off from their power completely.

> *"You are my only father and the best one for me. Thank you."*

> *"You are my only mother and the best one for me. Thank you."*

• Some are depressed because their mothers or fathers were also. Depression is a part of our "basic psychological equipment" (see chapter on conditioning p. 24f). Here, you can also speak of solidarity.

> *„ "I don't have to carry this burden. I'll leave it with my dear mother/father."*

• A secret death-wish may lie behind depression.

Motto 1: *"Better me than you."* A child is helpless with regard to a beloved family member and thinks that they can take over their fate for them.

> *Be humble and recognize that no one has the right to intervene in the fate of another in this way.*

Motto 2: *"I will follow you."* A child believes that it's unjust that they are allowed to go on living while another family member must die.

> *"I'll stay a while and then I'll come too."*

• Depression as an unconscious strategy: 1) Get recognition (sympathy). 2) Take revenge - e.g., take revenge on mother.

Social view, many people in social occupations (e.g., companies, schools or hospitals) suffer from this because the system strictly limits their personal creativity. They feel they are running around like proverbial hamsters in a wheel, having no time for themselves and losing their energy, motivation and enjoyment of life.

Spiritual view: When we leave our prescribed path of development, don't follow our inner calling and only "function," living life from the outside, our life will have no meaning. Cut off from the divine flow of energy, we will be tired, unsatisfied and empty.

> *What is the meaning of (my) life? What sustains my happiness? This is the path I will follow!*

View from the 5 Biological Laws of Nature: Depression is usually the result of a territorial conflict or a territorial constellation

(see p. 313ff).

Sometimes a cerebellum constellation can cause depression: One feels listless and empty (see p. 314).

> Determine the conflicts and conditioning and resolve it.

Usually, someone goes through months and years of conflict activity until their reserves are used up. Then, the body pulls the emergency brake. Seen in this way, burnout is the (last) protective reaction. What happens after that depends on whether the person makes any significant change in their life. If they stay on the same path, they will remain sympathicotonic and permanently stressed, possibly with regenerating phases in between. In this case, no change can be expected.

It would be wiser for them to sit down and make an honest analysis of their life before making genuine, but often painful changes; just putting an end to stagnation can be a relief in itself. Every SBS has two phases and, after the conflict activity, there comes a long phase of regeneration (repair phase). On one hand, this brings us a hopeful perspective on the future. On the other hand, vagotonia takes its toll: chronic fatigue, tiredness, exhaustion, various illnesses and pain. That said, I also know of cases where only the repair phase - the time following a long period of overdoing it - is seen as burnout.

For this reason, we as therapists must be careful: The patient can be in chronic conflict activity, in a longer repair phase or in a condition in between.

> Locate the situation and change it as necessary.

Further causes

• Side effects of medication: High blood pressure medications dampen spirits and lower energy levels. When psychological drugs are taken over long periods, they can have the same effect as the symptoms for which they were proscribed.

> Reduce/stop taking ("medication vacation").

• Sleep disorders can increase depression (see above).

Therapy for burnout, depression

• An understanding of the 5 Biological Laws of Nature is good, but a little more is needed to overcome depression: above all, the readiness to make internal and external changes, the will to continue making personal development and the making or strengthening one's connection "above." Two tips for this direc-

tion: "Be thankful for everything that life has given you up to this point!" "Do good things for others!" Depressed people often concentrate too much on themselves and feel like a victim. Through giving, someone can break out of this role. Giving makes you happy. Whoever gives the gift of happiness will also be happy themselves.
- CBD oil (cannabis oil)
- Lavender tea
- Linseed oil (omega-3)
- Maca powder (5 g = 1 tablespoon/day), yam powder
- St. John's wort

- Nutmeg powder
- Vitamin B, Linseed oil.
- Colloidal Gold.
- For people over 45: natural (= nature identical) as hormones, e.g., as according to Dr. Lee, Dr. Platt and Dr. Lenard
- Communion with God and contact with nature (sun, wind, water, forests, mountains).
- Regular exercise in the fresh air.
- Be grateful for everything. Morning ritual by Styger (p. 68).
- Natural, alkaline nutrition, clean water.
- Minimize electro-smog (smartphone, cordless phone, etc.).

THE NERVOUS SYSTEM

Headaches, Migraines

The line between headaches and migraines is blurry. Typically, migraines are asymmetrical, involve high intensity pain and are accompanied by nausea or blind spots (scotomas). From the perspective of the New Medicine, head pain represents the repair phase and migraines a repair phase crisis. The good news is that through these, some of the conflict mass is depleted each time. After the conflict is resolved, no further symptoms should be expected.

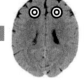

SBS of the Cervical/Cranial Bones

Headaches, migraines I

The most common type of head pain, usually symmetrical, comes from behind, combined with chronic tension.

Conflict	Moral-intellectual, self-esteem conflict. Perceived injustice, pressure to succeed, dishonesty. Belief that one has to do everything immediately or perfectly. Feeling stupid or unintelligent.
Vernacular	"Racking your brains." "Taking it on the chin." "Hanging your head."
Example	• *An office worker has been under stress the whole week because of too much work. She is really looking forward to the weekend. On Friday, as the tension subsides, the headache begins = repair phase of the self-esteem conflict.* Note: typical weekend migraine. (Archive B. Eybl).
Conflict-active	Functional impairment, cell breakdown in cervical vertebrae/cranial bones/ligaments/muscles.
Repair phase	Regeneration of the tissue, swelling, pressure on the bone skin > head and neck pain. So, the headaches appear in the context of a repair phase. Recurring conflicts cause an alternation between pain-free intervals and times of headaches.
Questions	With what and why do I put myself under pressure? Who do I want to impress? Why does only my performance count? What conditioning lies behind it (father, mother, teacher)? For further questions: see p. 288f.
Therapy	Determine the conflict, conditioning and belief systems and resolve them. Look for the love - there you will find the solution. Guiding principle: *"I trust in my abilities." "I can't do everything at once. - I will calmly accomplish everything I can and that's it." "What I can't change isn't going to upset me."* See also: therapy for headaches/migraines p. 73.

SBS of the Trigeminal Nerve

HFs trigeminus, base of cerebral cortex

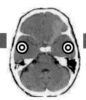

Headaches, migraines II, trigeminal neuralgia

Normally, migraines appear suddenly, are asymmetrical (usually only one side of the face) and are accompanied by intense pain. The fact that the most common form of migraines are caused by the trigeminal nerve was recognized by Angela Frauen-kron-Hoffmann. The following is derived from her excellent book, *1-2-3 Migränefrei* (see source list).

The trigeminus has three branches (see illustration p. 73): The upper, first branch, supplies the eye area, the second, essentially the nose and the third, the mouth and tongue. Usually the first branch reacts (migraines in the temple/eye area). As always, the content of the conflict reveals the function:

Conflict	Most common: 1st branch: Separation conflict with relation to face - one is not seen or recognized. The first and most important recognition (or just the opposite) takes place at birth - the mother receives/ sees the child. Adult conflict: losing face or prestige.
	2nd branch: Separation conflict with relation to smell - one is not "sniffed" (considered).
	3rd branch: Separation conflict with relation to mouth and tongue - one is not kissed ("licked").
Examples	➔ *A child is not beheld by the mother at birth. E.g., under anesthetic for a Cesarian section, the mother is too preoccupied with herself. The hospital staff take the baby away at first. In doing so, the "first recognition" is missing.*
	➔ *Real skin contact loss (e.g., through the separation from a partner).*
	➔ *Someone is made to look ridiculous or isn't taken seriously.*
	➔ *Someone is overlooked or skipped.*
	• *A 46-year-old is six when his mother dies. He can still remember exactly that his sister-in-law couldn't look at her. After becoming aware of this decisive situation, he is able to heal his migraine aura after over 30 years. (Archive B. Eybl)*
	• *The 48-year-old, right-handed, slim, childless patient works in an office. A year ago, the patient feels terrible as she sits alone in her apartment on the Friday before the Easter holidays: On this evening, she feels "extremely separated from everything - especially from her partner," who she really wants to be with after their relationship ended. She feels lonely, abandoned and desperate. = Separation conflict. One branch of pain runs to the jaw joint, another to the corner of the eye. (Archive B. Eybl)*
Conflict-active	Unnoticed reduction in sensitivity of the trigeminal nerve. Possibly dry skin in the nerve coverage area.
Bio. function	The separation should be "forgotten" through the reduction in sensitivity.
Repair crisis	Migraines or trigeminus neuralgia pain in the repair phase crisis during the repair phase. Restoration of the sensitivity. Migraine also occurs in a relaxed state after stress.
Note	Mother/child or partner side consideration. If the complaints are worse during stress and better at rest, a brutal separation conflict (affecting the periosteum) may be present. In this case, the region feels rather cold and one has cold feet. = Same conflict content.
Questions	When did the first migraine occur? What stress was there before it with regard to not being considered, being disgraced? How was the birth? How was I received? Did I receive enough recognition/love as a child? Do I often feel unnoticed? Do/Did I feel suddenly humiliated?
Therapy	Determine the conflict, triggers and conditioning and resolve if the migraines are recurring.
	Guiding principles: *"I am lovable." "I don't care what the others think about me." "What do I care about the opinions of other people?" "The way I am is okay; everybody makes mistakes."*
	For syndrome, resolve the refugee conflict. Quark compresses, cold water applications. Cold compresses with a decoction of chamomile and elder blossom tea. Gently apply dimethyl sulfoxide (DMSO), diluted lavender/St. John's wort oil at the site of the pain. Blue or violet light irradiation. Lymph drainage, possibly chiropractic treatment, osteopathy on the cervical spine (neck), hot foot baths. Internally: lavender and peppermint tea. Vitamin B preparations, cod liver oil, natural borax internally, possibly externally. Linseed oil. See also: repair phase on the brain level (p. 60). Pain medication. CM epilepsy medications (e.g., Carbamazepine, Oxcarbazepine) have many side effects, are hardly effective and therefore, their use doesn't make sense from the standpoint of the New Medicine.

E
C
T
O

– +

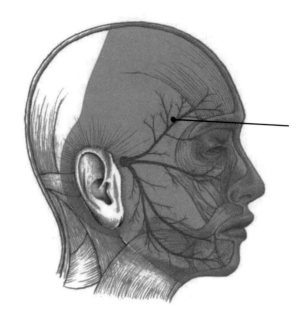

Trigeminal nerve - epidermis
Separation Conflict with Regard to the Face

Headaches

Further, possible causes for headaches

General healing symptom: The cause is the brain's need for more room (brain/cerebral edema). The pressure on the meninges causes headaches. The brain itself has no pain receptors. Light to medium headache = repair phase. Severe to extreme headache = repair phase crisis.

Following the consumption of certain foods or drinks: For some people, foods are conflict triggers (= allergy). Conflict activity is triggered through consumption. The affected organ must not necessarily be a digestive organ > repair phase = headache.

The result of being poisoned: Most medications, alcohol, nicotine, and other drugs, set the body under artificial stress, making them sympatholytic substances. If the sympathetic nervous system is stimulated, we feel "high." The effect of most medications is based on this autonomic shift. Repair phases and the pain associated with them are interrupted. When the poisonous effects diminish, the individual starts healing > repair after the poisoning > headache (for instance, analgesic-headache).

Hypoglycemia of the brain through any repair phase: During the repair phase, especially the repair phase crisis, the brain has a much stronger need for sugar. A low glucose level causes or increases the brain edema > headache. Thus, a regular application of organic glucose in the case of brain pressure symptoms is important for therapy.

Hypoglycemia of the brain, as a result of a fear-revulsion conflict or a refusal conflict, regardless of whether alpha cells or beta cells are affected, can cause a temporary hypoglycemia with headache, according to the phase. (See p. 224f)

Therapy headache/migraine

- The conflict is resolved! For recurring headaches, find out what the conflict and triggers are and resolve them.
- With syndrome: resolve the refugee conflict (p. 230f).
- Cold-water applications for the head and face, cold compresses.
- Walks in the fresh air (good for the oxygen supply).
- Dab diluted oils of lavender, frankincense, peppermint, or lemon balm on the temples.
- Irradiation with blue/violet light.
- Natural borax internally.
- Black cumin oil.

- Moderate amounts of alcohol, which acts as a diuretic substance by suppressing the antidiuretic effects of vasopressin (ADH). (Everyone knows the urge to urinate after drinking a beer).
- Colloidal gold.
- Lymph drainage, foot reflex-zone massage, acupoint massage, normal massage, chiropractic or osteopathy.
- Tea made from lavender, peppermint, rose leaves, violet blossoms and many more. Possibly, the painkiller paracetamol.
- Hydrogen peroxide (H_2O_2) 3% internally.

SBS of the Brain's Connective Tissue

Brain tumor (astrocytoma, glioblastoma, oligodendroglioma, ganglioglioma)

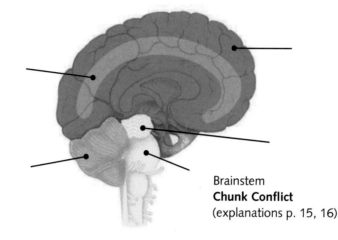

Cerebral White Matter
Self-Esteem Conflict

Cerebral Cortex
Social Conflict

Cerebellum
**Conflicts Related to:
Integrity Injuries,
Attitudes, Attacks and
Worry - among others**

Midbrain
**Chunk Conflict, Motor/
Peristaltic**
(explanations p. 15, 16)

Brainstem
Chunk Conflict
(explanations p. 15, 16)

About 50% of the brain's volume consists of brain connective tissue (= glia). The macroglia cells (astrocyte, oligodendrocyte, ependymal and plexus epithelial cells) are a part of the ectoderm and account for 80%. The other 20% are microglia cells (Hortega cells, mesoglia), come from scavenger cells and are mesodermal. The nerve cells (neurons) are completely dependent on the interaction with the glia. Without them, nothing would happen in the brain at all. The historical term, brain connective tissue, hardly does justice to the important function of the glia.

Functions of the macroglia: 1. Networking, stimulus conduction, nourishment, protection, isolation (blood-brain barrier) of the nerve cells. 2. Supplying the web-like mechanical structure.

Incidentally, the functions of the microglia are similar to the scavenger cells in the body: police, fire department and waste management for the brain.

Microglia tumors practically never occur. Our attention is therefore focused on the macroglia: From the functions, you can derive the following conflict content of brain tumors:

Conflict	1. Social conflict - one wasn't connected well enough, one doesn't feel sufficiently informed or protected by others, one didn't get enough help from others and therefore got into difficulties or, vice versa, one didn't provide sufficient help. 2. One can't deal with structures (e.g., social, economic systems) or fails in constructing sustainable structures (workplace, residence, family). The location of the tumor shows the tone of the conflict. E.g., in the white matter > self-esteem components, in the cerebellum > integrity-injury components.
Example	• A 21-year-old, left-handed patient is diagnosed with a "brain tumor" when she is examined in the hospital after having fainted briefly. A tumor is found in the right ovary relay. Thus, it is a loss conflict in the process of healing. The following occurred 6 years ago: Hexi, the patient's beloved poodle mix, is hit by a car. The poor animal lies there, whimpering with a crushed skull. In her shock, the girl, 15 at the time, does not go with her to the vet to have her put to sleep. = Conflict with loss components, that she should have provided support for her dog. In all the years since, whenever she sees a dog, she thinks of Hexi and how she abandoned her in his darkest hour (recurrence). The patient entered into the repair phase five months ago when she got a new dog named Akira. Since then, she no longer thinks about Hexi, but is often tired (vagotonia). The "brain tumor" shows the healing process. (Archive B. Eybl)
• A man comes to the realization that the system in which we live is dishonest. When he tries to get out of it by starting an alternative career (health products), he fails. After he changes things in his life several times, a tumor develops in his cerebral white matter. Due to pressure by his family, he submits to an operation. Nevertheless, he survives. (Archive B. Eybl)
Conflict-active	Unnoticed diminishing function of the brain's connective tissue or degeneration of glia.
Bio. function	1. Limitation/degeneration of the old network to make room for the new. 2. Limitation/degradation

E
C
T
O

– +

of the old structure so an alternative can be built (similar to an alternative system).

Repair phase   Repair phase: Increase in function and growth of the brain's connective tissue. Headaches, possible double vision, dizziness due to the swelling. Duration and intensity of growth dependent on the conflict size. Often, a **persistent conflict.** Estimating the length of the repair phase is difficult due to recurrences going unnoticed and the diagnosis shock.

Note   Brain tumors are being diagnosed more frequently, because patients are being scanned more precisely and more frequently (CT, MRI). Earlier, the patient just had headaches for three months. One didn't know why, but the patient was left to recover in peace. Today's policy is "action." Preventative examinations are also responsible for finding more and more tumors that may not result in any complications for the patient and would have been ignored in the past. Less than 2% survive the diagnosis "brain tumor." Most die of fear, chemotherapy and radiation.

This SBS is not the cause of all structures diagnosed as brain tumors: According to Dr. Hamer, a so-"brain tumor" is not an SBS itself, but represents a Hamer focus during or after an intensive repair phase. Thus, he explains brain tumors as not being their own SBSs.

In my experience, the SBS described here is running when the connective tissue doesn't stop growing for months and when the swelling cannot be explained by edema anymore = brain tumors with increasing swelling that would be diagnosed as "malignant" by CM.

Questions   When did the symptoms begin? (= Beginning of the repair phase, set off by something positive). What happened that was good? (E.g., good news, reconciliation, praise, vacation, retirement. > Based on the positive event, you can deduce the preceding conflict). Did I feel that I wasn't supported enough? Was there a lack of important information? Was there stress related to a structure/system? Why was that so important to me? What sensitized me to it (childhood, parents' emotions, pregnancy, birth)? What further conditioning in the family underlies it? What positive aspects can the diagnosis have?

Therapy   The conflict is resolved; support the healing. In the event that the symptoms do not improve, i.e., last longer than 6 months, you're dealing with a persistent conflict. > Determine the conflict, conditioning and beliefs and resolve them. Find out where the love is - there lies the solution. Knowledge of the 5 Biological Laws of Nature is decisive for someone finding their way out of the fear. For actionable measures, see repair phase - brain level, p. 60f. In the case of syndrome: resolve the refugee conflict. Cortisone to reduce the swelling as necessary. The surgical removal of brain tumors is only rarely advisable. Chemo and radiation therapy is not recommended based on the low survival rate. As a rule, the ideal therapy for every individual is the one that they trust the most. With this in mind, the decision for chemotherapy, although not to be recommended, should be accepted.

SBS of the Choroid Plexus

Brain tumor of the brain chambers - ependymoma, choroid plexus papilloma[1]

Conflict   1. Right side of the brain: cannot get something, Left side of the brain: cannot get rid of something.
2. Conflict that the brain dries up: One believes that they cannot think well enough.

Examples   • *For 1: A woman works reluctantly as a secretary at the social welfare court. = Conflict - she wants to leave. When she finds a new job, the ependymoma brain tumor, located in the left lateral ventricle, will break down by tuberculosis (ependymoma- tuberculosis).[1]* (Archive B. Eybl)
➔ *Someone cannot remember while learning or does not understand the math problems.*

Conflict-active   Function increase, growth of an arterial network adeno-ca = ependymoma or choroid plexus papilloma.
Bio. function   Enlarging the artery network so that more brain fluid can be produced/delivered.
Repair phase   Degradation of the tumor by fungi bacteria. = Ependymoma tuberculosis. Afterward, calcium deposits remain. A calcified choroid plexus can often be seen in the CT.
Therapy   Determine conflict or triggers and resolve them in real life if still active.

---

1   See Dr. Hamer, My Student Girl, pp. 469ff, Amici di Dirk Publishers, 2nd edition 6/2014, ISBN 978-84-96127-63-0

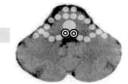

SBS oft the Pineal Gland (Pinealozytes)

Pineal tumor (pineocytoma, pineoblastoma)[1]

The pineal gland is a light-receiving organ which produces hormones. It's interaction with the retina converts the serotonin formed in the brain during the day into melatonin at night. It controls the circadian (day and night) rhythm and is considered the seat of the 3rd eye. - The gift of clairvoyance and intuition are attributed to this mysterious organ. According to Dr. Rick Strassman, it is a window into other areas of our existence.

The following is what little we know so far about the pineal gland from the perspective of the New Medicine:

Conflict	Chunk conflict (p. 15, 16): Too little light - it's too dark. Real or in the figurative sense. (The Light of God).
Examples	→ *One suffers from the absence of natural light (mine or night-shift workers, dark office).* → *One feels separated from God and forsaken by all the angels.*
Conflict-active	Increased light absorption and melatonin production. With prolonged conflict activity, enlargement of the gland by cell division. = Pineal tumor. Frequent complications: obstruction of the outflow of cerebrospinal fluid > liquid overpressure > intracranial pressure symptoms, possibly hydrocephalus.
Bio. function	Improvement of light reception - to cope with less light. More production of melatonin.
Repair phase	Tumor degradation by fungi bacteria. = Pineal tuberculosis > "brain sand" or calcification.
Note	Open questions: Why is the pineal gland calcified in almost all people? Does almost everyone experience this conflict? Is a life removed from God responsible or is the truth that calcification is a (positive) crystallization?
Therapy	Determine and solve conflict in real life if still active. Pay attention to a good sleep/night rhythm and get adequate sleep. As often as possible, "refuel" sunlight and nature. At sunset, look straight at the sun. Colloidal gold. Meditate, visualize, and be creative. Avoid fluorine, caffeine, sugar and all poisons. Guiding principle: *"I am always conscious about my divine descent. Its light shines in me. "*

---

1   See Dr. Hamer, my student girl, pp. 469ff, Amici di Dirk Publishers, 2nd edition 6/2014, ISBN 978-84-96127-63-0

SBS of the Muscle and Nerve Network

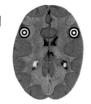

Paralysis of the facial nerve

Conflict	Motor conflict, made the fool. Fear of losing face or being humiliated.
Examples	→ *Somebody disgraces themselves in front of the family, in their circle of friends, or in front of their colleagues at work.* → *"Just look at yourself!" "Ugh! Look at them over there. "*
Conflict-active	Partial or general paralysis of the facial muscles. The most common symptom: on the affected side, the corner of the mouth hangs down. Light cases are common.
Bio. function	A paralysis of the facial expressions results in a "poker face" showing no emotions. In this way, the "game" can be won in the end.
Repair phase	Return of the feeling in the nerves. Note: Sometimes the paralysis does not show itself until the beginning of the repair phase or after the repair phase crisis = hot stroke (see below).
Repair crisis	Twitching, cramps In CM, facial paralyses are often seen as "strokes." Watch for "handedness."
Questions	When did the symptoms begin? Stress from losing face? Did I feel humiliated or disgraced? What conditioning in the family underlie this?
Therapy	See trigeminal neuralgia I.

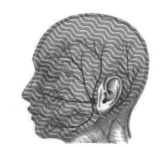

SBS of the Muscle and Nerve Network

 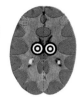

HFs sensory function (legs) in cerebral cortex

Stroke without documented brain hemorrhaging

In the following, we will deal with strokes in which there was no hemorrhaging found in CT/MRI scans. Upon closer inspection however, one will find Hamer foci or edemas in the motor area of the cerebral cortex.

As for the CM claim of an "insufficient oxygen supply to an area of the brain" (ischemic stroke): The blood vessels of all organs, including the brain, are arranged in a network. A potential vessel occlusion (blockage) is immediately detoured by so-called vascular redundancy (collateral circulation) and via new branches forming between adjacent blood vessels (neovascularization). Doctors often search for hemorrhaging to no avail and finally assign responsibility to some blood vessel arbitrarily because they can't find anything. Conclusion: "ischemic strokes" are questionable.

In the New Medicine, we know of two types of strokes. Both are caused, when paralyses occur, by motor conflicts. The first, less common form, is the so-called cold stroke = paralysis in conflict activity.

The second, much more common form is the so-called hot stroke. This happens during a fulminating repair phase after a very long period (several months, but usually years) of conflict activity.

Cold stroke[1]

E
C
T
O

(−+)

Conflict	Motor conflict. Fear of restriction. Conflict of not being able, allowed or willing to move.	
	Facial muscles: to be made a fool of.	
	Shoulder/back musculature: to be unable to avoid someone or something.	
	Leg and arm bending and pulling musculature (adductors):	
	To be unable to hold onto something or somebody, to draw him close, to hug him.	
	Leg and arm stretching and splaying musculature (abductors):	
	To be unable to escape from, push away, or fend off somebody or something.	
	Legs in general: To be completely at a loss. To be unable to get away, escape, or catch up. To be unable to run fast enough, climb, go up or down, dance, jump, keep one's balance, etc.	
Tissue	Voluntary (striated) musculature - cerebral cortex - ectoderm (innervation) and cerebral white matter - mesoderm (nutrition).	
Conflict-active	Paralysis is often just a weakness of the affected muscle group = cold stroke. Signs of sympathectomy such as cold hands, compulsive thinking, light sleep, weight loss, etc. CM normally does not call these paralyses strokes, instead, they go under names like MS (multiple sclerosis) or ALS (amyotrophic lateral sclerosis).	
Bio. function	The "play dead" reflex: Many animals pretend to be dead when being chased or when the situation is hopeless (e.g., fawn, mouse, snake). The pursuer then gives up or does not even see his prey. Carnivores - cats, for example - are only interested in "moving objects." When the danger has passed, the paralysis ends.	

Striated Musculature
Motor conflict

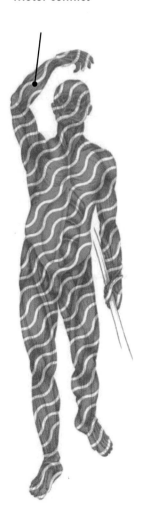

Repair phase	Recovery of nerve network. The paralyses only improve gradually because the nerve connections (synapses) in the brain have become overstretched (dissociated) by the healing edema.
Repair crisis	Convulsions, cramps, epileptic seizure or multiple seizures.
Note	Consider "handedness" (right or left) and side (mother/child or partner). The muscle groups most affected point to the conflict. For example, if the right adductors are affected in a right-handed patient, it is about the conflict of not being able to hold the partner (people other than the mother and child).
	Other organs and/or a brain relay can also play a role: If the person's speech is impaired, for instance, it is a shock-fright or speechlessness conflict in the repair phase. Memory gaps (absence seizures) can also lead to a diagnosis of stroke = separation conflict in the repair phase crisis.
Questions	When did the paralyses begin? (Conflict must have occurred before this). Accident, fall? Events in the family, relationships? What happened spiritually? What was going on in my head at the time? Did I want to run away? Was there someone I couldn't hold? Conditioning from the family (bad accidents, falls)?
Therapy	See remedies for paralysis, p. 309.

Hot stroke[1]

Same SBS as above or another SBS, for example, brain edema (repair phase) in the cerebral white matter > compression of the motor function in the adjacent cerebral cortex > motor skills cease to function > CM - "stroke."

Examples	• *From the beginning, the right-handed patient was brought up strictly by his dominant mother. At his first opportunity, he fled from home. He is an only child and felt responsible for his mother. If he did not visit her often enough, he felt guilty = motor conflict, not being able to shake off his mother. Two years after his mother's death, the 59-year-old patient had a stroke, which he barely survived = healing of the motor conflict. Especially affected were the abductors of the arm and leg on the left mother/child-side.* (Archive B. Eybl)
	• *For twenty years, the 45-year-old, right-handed patient worked for a company against his will = motor conflict, not being able to go in the direction that he wants to go, not being able to get away from the company. Finally, he resigned so he could open his own business (lifelong dream), but it never came to that. On the very day the business opened, he had a stroke = healing of the motor conflict. Mainly affected is the right partner-side.* (Archive B. Eybl)
Phase	**Repair phase:** Hot hands and feet, increased appetite, possibly fever, dizziness, and headache - signs of vagotonia. The most frequent symptom is a one-sided paralysis of the arm or leg.
	The Hamer focus in the brain swells up edematous and compresses its surroundings. After years or decades of conflict activity, the repair phase comes to the drama of a stroke. The price to be paid for the long-lasting conflict activity is usually incomplete recovery, sometimes even the death of the patient due to the brain edema. If a CT scan is made, this edema is often wrongly diagnosed as "intracranial bleeding."
Therapy	<u>In the acute phase:</u> The conflict has been resolved. Support the healing! See: repair phase at the brain level, p. 60f.
	<u>After the acute phase:</u> On the physical level, CM does the right thing: rehabilitation measures - physiotherapy, massage, swimming, etc. Practice, practice, practice, but with the right attitude!
	From a psychological point of view, the patient has indeed resolved one or more major conflicts; otherwise he wouldn't have had a stroke. However, the paralyses or other losses usually mean a new conflict for the patient, especially if rehabilitation progress begins slowly.
	For example, a motor conflict: *"My left leg is worthless now!"* Genital conflict: *"I can't even do anything in bed anymore." "My wife will start looking for somebody else!"* > Accept the situation as it is, but nevertheless, believe in healing and improvement.
	Resignation is just as bad as expectations that are too high.

---

[1] See Dr. Hamer, Charts pp. 138, 139, 143, 144

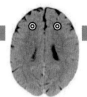

SBS of the Brain's Blood Vessels

Stroke through brain hemorrhage, cerebral hemorrhage (intercerebral hemorrhage, subarachnoid hemorrhage)

Bleeding between cranial bones and dura mater (= epidural hemorrhage) and bleeding between the dura mater and the arachnoid mater (= subdural hemorrhage) usually happens by accident (trauma) = no conflict.
A hemorrhage under the arachnoid mater (= subarachnoid hemorrhage) or in the brain itself (= intercerebral hemorrhage) usually occurs without external influences and is considered by conventional medicine to be the main cause of strokes (= hemorrhagic stroke). If a CT and MRI show that bleeding <u>actually</u> is present, the following conflicts may be present:

Conflict	Self-esteem conflict. According to Frauenkron-Hoffmann: Can't count on the intellectual support of the family when something's on the line or pressure from the family. Otherwise, one can't understand why a member of the family has gone away (represents the exiting blood).
Phase	Cell degradation (necrosis) during conflict activity in the arterial or venous wall, unnoticed as a rule. Through **recurring conflicts**, the weak points (weak blood vessels) can rupture quite easily. E.g., during physical exertion (high blood pressure is associated with this) or during a brain repair phase in the affected region > bleeding into the brain.
Bio. function	Like always, it is only to be recognized in the normally short, two-phase course. However, the cerebral hemorrhaging comes from a chronic process. Here, it reflects the body, what is going wrong internally (psyche).
Therapy	Intensive care medical treatment (hospital) at the signs of a stroke, rehab afterwards. Find the conflict and resolve it to prevent further episodes.

Inflammation of the brain (encephalitis)

According to CM, this is an infection by viruses or bacteria (e.g., borelia). The fact is, however, that the brain is the only germ-free region of the body. According to Dr. Hamer, a lumbar puncture (spinal tap) often leads to encephalitis.

Conflict	Depends on the part of the brain.
Tissue	Brain and/or meninges.
Phase	**Repair phase**: Every Hamer focus in the repair phase causes some sort of encephalitis, especially when several conflicts go into healing at the same time, which happens often (spring-cleaning of the brain). This has nothing to do with "infection."
Therapy	The conflict is resolved. Support the repair phase. See: repair phase at the brain level, p. 60f.

Meningitis (encephalomeningitis)

According to CM, meningitis is a viral or bacterial infection of the brain linings (meninges) and encephalomeningitis is an inflammation of the brain and spinal cord and their meninges. The primary symptoms are a strong headache and stiff neck; the stiffness of the neck points to a healing cervical spine. Skull bones and cervical spine have the same conflict content.

Conflict	Moral intellectual self-esteem conflict. (For examples and phases, see p. 295f).
Phase	**Repair phase:** The healing cranial bone or meninges builds tissue fluid, which lifts the linings of the brain (meninges) and presses them inwards toward the brain > strong headache.
Note	Further possible causes: Heat stroke causes similar symptoms (= real "heat-attack"). Intensified by syndrome. Difficult to differentiate from the normal repair phase of the brain.
Therapy	The conflict is resolved. Support the repair phase. See repair phase at the brain level, p. 60f.

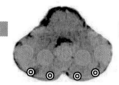

SBS of the Nerve Sheath
HFs in the cerebellum - topography still unknown

"Nerve tumor" (neurofibroma)[1]

In the peripheral nervous system, the nerve projections (axons and dendrites) are bundles of nerve fibers. They are surrounded by protective myelin sheaths, formed of so-called Schwann cells. A neurofibroma is a "tumor" of this connective tissue - like nerve sheath.

Conflict	Touch or pain conflict. Conflict of perceiving touch as painful, unpleasant, or undesirable.
	Explanation: The most intense contact is a pain attack (impact, strike, fall, etc.). Also, bone pain can start this SBS. To protect the organ, the organism can "turn off" the peripheral sensitivity (= pain).
Examples	→ *A woman is beaten by her husband.*
	→ *Someone hits their head in a very painful manner.*
	• *Neurofibroma on the spinal column: A 66-year-old, married retiree is on a ski vacation when one night, he suddenly feels violent pain in the area of the thoracic vertebrae. With an MRI, a hazelnut-sized neurofibroma is diagnosed between the 7th and 8th thoracic vertebrae. Due to the dramatic pain, it is removed in a risky surgery. Conflict history: 2½ years ago, he climbs an apple tree to clean a birdhouse that he had once attached at a height of 3 meters. Unfortunately, he slips and falls onto a big branch, on his thoracic spine "one storey down," and from there, to the ground. In doing so, he suffers the "worst pain of his life" = pain conflict. For two months, life is only bearable with the aid of pills = active-phase - growth of a neurofibroma. A little bump appears on his spine. Two and a half years later, the patient comes into healing, because he slowly forgets the accident. During his vacation, he distances himself from the place of the accident = beginning of the repair phase with degradation of the neurofibroma > inflammation, pain > surgery.* (Archive B. Eybl)
Conflict-active	Thickening of the myelin sheath at the affected spot via cell division of Schwann cells = neurofibroma. Thickening of the isolation layer leads to pain numbness (anesthesia). It is difficult to distinguish between this kind of numbness to pain and deafness in the active-phase of a separation conflict (see p. 271ff).
Bio. function	The thickening of the nerve isolation eases the intensity of the pain or unwanted touching and blocks off the pain.
Repair phase	Restoration of sensitivity with possible over-sensitivity at the beginning. The neurofibromas remain or are removed by bacteria. What remains is a bump.
<u>Neuropathy</u>	According to CM - a nerve disease. According to NM: convulsions, paralysis = SBS of the muscles, see. pp. 307ff. Numbness, tingling, pins and needles = SBS of the epidermis, pp. 271ff.
Questions	Is the location actually inflamed (healing) or "quiet" (active phase)? What happened at the location before (strike, impact, accident, spiritual injury)? Which conditioning plays a role?
Therapy	Determine the conflict and conditioning and resolve if possible (if it isn't already resolved).
	Find out where the love is - there you'll find the solution. Guiding principle: *"A protective coat shelters me. I only let those who are good to me get close to me!"* Externally, St. John's wort oil, meadow flower decoction. If inflamed, compresses of sour clay, pot-cheese, white cabbage leaves, etc. Lymph drainage massages. Hildegard of Bingen: oil of violet. OP is risky.

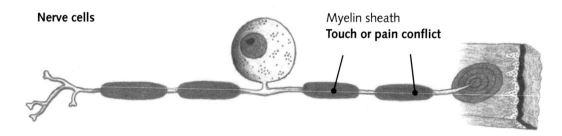

Nerve cells

Myelin sheath
Touch or pain conflict

---

1   See Dr. Hamer, Charts, pp. 45, 50

Hydrocephalus (water on the brain)

In the case of hydrocephalus, the ventricles for cerebrospinal fluid (CSF) (subarachnoid space) are widened because of a drainage disturbance caused by narrowing (stenosis), most often in the area of the 4th ventricle between the brainstem and the cerebellum.

Conflict	Active refugee or existential conflict and possibly more conflicts in the repair phase (= syndrome).
Phase	Repair phase: One or more Hamer focus(i) in the brainstem or cerebellum cause swelling due to a very intensive repair phase with syndrome.
Therapy	Resolve the refugee or existential conflict. Support the repair phase. See: repair phase at the brain level, p. 60f. In CM, during a shunt surgery, a small plastic tube is implanted into the brain so that fluids can drain. Surely, this is the last option that should be chosen when nothing else helps.

EYE

The eye is probably the most complex organ in the body. Tissue types from all three germ layers lie close together. All of the different structures of the eye serve a single purpose: sight. Dr. Hamer has discovered an unbelievable amount about the eye but much research remains to be done. According to the Ber-

lin ophthalmologist Dr. Kwesi Anan Odum, (contakt: k.odum@gomedus.de) the most intense emotional conflicts are reflected in the innermost regions of the eye, such as the optic nerve and the retina (increasing in intensity from the outer area inwards).

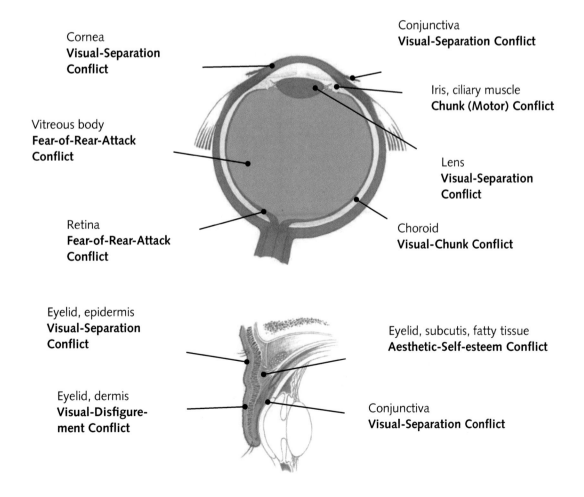

Cornea
Visual-Separation Conflict

Conjunctiva
Visual-Separation Conflict

Iris, ciliary muscle
Chunk (Motor) Conflict

Vitreous body
Fear-of-Rear-Attack Conflict

Lens
Visual-Separation Conflict

Retina
Fear-of-Rear-Attack Conflict

Choroid
Visual-Chunk Conflict

Eyelid, epidermis
Visual-Separation Conflict

Eyelid, subcutis, fatty tissue
Aesthetic-Self-esteem Conflict

Eyelid, dermis
Visual-Disfigurement Conflict

Conjunctiva
Visual-Separation Conflict

SBS of the Eyelid/Conjunctiva

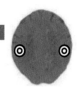

Inflammation of the eyelid (blepharitis), pink eye (conjunctivitis)[1]

E C T O

−+

Conflict	Visual-separation conflict, losing sight of someone.
Examples	• *While his parents were on vacation, a child was sent to his grandparents = visual-separation conflict. Two days after the parents came back, he contracts conjunctivitis = healing. (Archive B. Eybl)*
	• *The patient's partner suddenly developed a passion for a certain hobby, which did not please her at all = visual-separation conflict - the partner has distanced himself from her. She has lost sight of him. When the matter became unimportant to her, she contracted conjunctivitis = repair phase. (Archive B. Eybl)*
	• *For the last three weeks, the 49-year-old, right-handed patient has been suffering from severe conjunctivitis of both eyes. Conflict history: In the patient's family, everyone used to join together on All Souls' Day, which the patient found to be very pleasant. Unfortunately, for the last eight years, this meeting has no longer taken place = visual-separation conflict. Three weeks ago, for the first time, the All Souls' meeting took place again. The patient was very happy to see everybody again = beginning of the repair phase. His eye doctor had treated him in vain with antivirus medicine; in the hospital, he had been treated with cortisone. He is relieved as he begins to understand the psychic interconnections.*
	• *A 55-year-old man has just returned from vacation and has to go on another trip. He would rather stay at home with his wife, who is suffering from headache and dizziness = visual-separation conflict. On the last day of the trip, his eyelids become very swollen, so much so that he has to go to the eye emergency care as soon as he gets home = beginning of the repair phase. (Archive B. Eybl)*
Conflict-active	Cell disintegration (ulcer) in the conjunctiva or in the eyelid. Numbness to pain (hypoesthesia), dry eyes, scales.
Bio. function	The person, who has been lost from sight, should be forgotten temporarily through numbness and insensitivity.
Repair phase	Conjunctivitis, eyelid inflammation, restoration, pain, reddening, itching - actually a squamous cell cancer.
Note	The conjunctiva can also become inflamed through mechanical irritation, strong sun radiation or because of dry eyes - adaptation reaction. Consider parent/child, partner side or local conflict.
	Allergic conjunctivitis is again "started" by a trigger. E.g., someone lost sight of his love in spring, at the time of elevated flower pollen levels. > Seasonal pollen allergy.
Questions	Do other family members suffer from conjunctivitis? (Indication of family conditioning). Was this the first occurrence? If no: Determine the cause at the time. Which visual separation stress did I have before the inflammation? Who did I lose "out of sight?" Change of location, a move? Conflict with a family member/partner/friend? If recurring: What was stressful before the current episode? What was stressful before the last episode? (Work out similar situations). Why do I deal with these situations so poorly? (Determine conditioning, examine the childhood, infancy, birth and life of the ancestors after the separation situation).
Therapy	The conflict is resolved. Accompany the repair phase and avoid relapse. Find out where the love is, you will find the solution there. Cold compresses and possibly eye baths with decoction of eyebright or horsetail. Lymph drainage massage Schuessler Cell Salts: No. 3, 4, 11. MMS internally. Colloidal silver instilling internally and externally in the eye. Avoid sun and wind. Ingest Kanne Bread Drink (probiotic beverage). Hildegard of Bingen: Rebtropfen and Franconian Wine special recipe. Apply antibacterial eye drops, if the repair phase becomes too intense (painful).

MC (molluscum contagiosum)

Same SBS as above. MC causes wart-like growths on upper and inner lid of the eye with a central dipping.

Phase	Repair phase - **Persistent repair** of the upper lid caused by a visual-separation conflict.

---

1   See Dr. Hamer, Charts pp. 119, 132

Excessive repair > growth of warts.

Therapy | Questions: see above. Determine the conflict and resolve it in real life, if possible, so that no new growths appear. Guiding principle: *"I am bound to all of the people that I like. An invisible band binds us, even when we are not together."*
Surgical removal, if the warts are mechanically or aesthetically disturbing.

Pterygium

Same SBS as above. (See pp. 82) A pterygium is a growth on the conjunctiva that spreads from the edge toward the pupil and can restrict vision.

Phase | **Persistent repair** of the conjunctiva
Therapy | Questions: see above. Find conflicts and triggers, OP (outpatient) if the visual field is disturbed. Nevertheless, work on conflict resolution, otherwise it can grow back.

Pinguecula

Same SBS as above. (See pp. 82.) Yellowish colored thickening of the conjunctiva on the inner or outer corner of the eye (lid division).

Phase | **Persistent repair** of the conjunctiva
Therapy | Questions: see above. Also in CM, OP is seldom considered because patches only interfere mostly aesthetically.

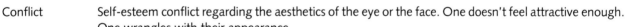

SBS of the Fatty Tissue

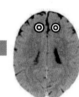

Wart-like fatty deposits on the eyelid (xanthelasma)

Conflict | Self-esteem conflict regarding the aesthetics of the eye or the face. One doesn't feel attractive enough. One wrangles with their appearance.
Example | ➜ *A woman examines her face in the mirror and notices that she has wrinkles around her eyes.*
Conflict-active | Unnoticed, local degradation (necrosis) of the fatty tissue.
Repair phase | **Persistent repair:** Reconstruction, i.e., building up fatty tissue. As with bones, the same happens with fatty tissue: Repair is generous and additional material is added (luxury group). Development of xanthelasma.
Bio. function | Increase in the fat covering. In the eyes of Mother Nature, *"being fat is good and attractive."* An animal that succeeds in adding fat is successful and desirable. An animal gets thin on its own when it becomes old and weak.
Note | Consider "handedness" (right or left) and side (mother/child or partner) or local conflict. Danger of a vicious circle, because the xanthelasma itself is regarded as disturbing and disfiguring.
Questions | When did the xanthelasma appear? What was stressing me at the time? Why don't I like myself? Why is my appearance so important? How do/did my ancestors think about their appearance? Were they also fixated on their external appearance? (Determine conditioning). What remains of life, the inner life or the body? What comes after death? What counts then?
Therapy | Determine the conflict or trigger and resolve it in real life, if possible, so that no new growths appear.
Guiding principle: *"I am satisfied with my looks and my eyes!"* *"The brightness of the soul is more important than my appearance!"* "Milky Way" therapy. Bach flowers: larch, crab apple. Surgical removal as necessary.

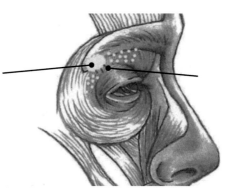

Lacrimal glands
Visual-Chunk Conflict

Lacrimal glands - excretory ducts
Visual-Recognition

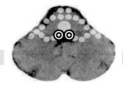

SBS of the Lacrimal Glands

Lacrimal gland tumor, lacrimal gland inflammation (dacryoadenitis)[1]

Each eye has one lacrimal gland, about the size of a hazelnut, and 20-30 small (accessory) lacrimal glands. The tear fluids they produce moisten, nourish, and cleanse, the conjunctiva.

Conflict	Visual-chunk conflict (see explanations p. 15, 16). To be unable to grasp (right eye) or to get rid of something (left eye). Simply: You cannot see something you would like to see or seeing something you don't want to see.
Examples	• A single, young woman suffers on the one hand, because she must regularly visit her aging parents, and on the other hand, an old friend at the same time - chunk conflict of wanting to get rid of the old friend (something uncomfortable) > cell division in the left lacrimal gland > weeping left eye. (See Claudio Trupiano, thanks to Dr. Hamer, p. 291)
Conflict-active	Growth of a cauliflower-like tumor (adeno-ca) of secretory quality on the lacrimal glands.
Bio. function	With more tear fluid, the sight impression can be better salivated and better ingested (or gotten rid of).
Repair phase	Inflammation of the lacrimal glands, tubercular-necrotic caseation of the tumor, purulent tears, pain, and possibly fever, night sweats.
Questions	What stressed me before the inflammation appeared? Which conditioning allows me to feel this way?
Therapy	By inflammation: the conflict is resolved. Support the repair phase and avoid relapse. Apply cold compresses and curd packs. Lymph drainage massages, MMS. Possibly antibiotics or surgical removal as necessary.

Drying up of the tear fluid ("cystic fibrosis" of the lacrimal glands, xerophthalmia, Sjögren syndrome, dry eye syndrome (DES))

Same SBS as above. For other causes of dry eyes, see p. 85.

Phase	Recurring-conflict - **persistent repair**. More and more glandular tissue breaks down and is replaced by inferior scar tissue > a drying up of the tear (lacrimal) fluids > dry eyes.
Therapy	Determine the conflict and conditioning and, if possible, resolve them in real life so that the remaining glandular function is preserved or the lacrimal glands can regenerate.
	Eye baths with eyebright, black cohosh (*Actaea racemosa*) and horsetail. Lymph drainage massage to stimulate fluid production.

---

1   See Dr. Hamer, Charts, pp. 18, 33

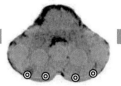

SBS of the Dermis | HFs in the cerebellum - topography still unknown

O L D   M E S O

+−

Styes (hordeolum) and chalazion

In the upper and lower eyelids, next to the eyelashes, lie the sebaceous glands: the so-called glands of Moll (which service the eyelids), the glands of Zeis (which are sweat glands), and the Meibomian glands (which prevent tears from drying up). An oily film prevents tear fluids from passing the edge of the lid. (The oil repels the watery tear fluid.)

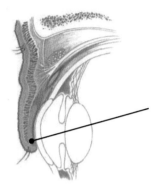

Sebaceous & sweat glands
**Visual-Disfigurement Conflict,
Conflict: Fear that the Eye Will Dry Out**

Conflict	Visual-disfigurement conflict. Damaged integrity of the eye or conflict that the eye is drying out.
Examples	➜ *A child sees the constant quarrelling of his parents - visual-disfigurement.* ➜ *A construction worker is hit in the eye by a metal splinter.* ➜ *Verbal attack with regard to appearance or the eye.* • *A city girl sees a mouse torn to pieces by a cat - visual-disfigurement. During the repair phase, the girl suffers from a stye.* (Archive B. Eybl)
Conflict-active	Thickening of the outer layer of the eyelid and enlargement of the Moll, Zeis or Meibomian glands (sebaceous gland cancer). Increased production of sebum.
Bio. function	Thickening of the corium/dermis of the eyelid leads to better protection of the eye. With more sebum, the eye can be better oiled.
Repair phase	Inflamed-tubercular-caseating degradation via fungi and bacteria, pain = stye. **Recurring-conflict:** Inflammation with inclusions of connective tissue (granulating inflammation) - chalazion.
Note	Consider "handedness" (right or left) and side (mother/child or partner).
Questions	Which sight was intolerable to me? (Determine the situation). Why can't I deal with it? Which event from my childhood does the situation remind me of? What brought me into the repair phase?
Therapy	The conflict is resolved. Accompany the repair phase and avoid relapse. If it is recurring, resolve the conflict and conditioning. Cold compresses. If acute: MMS, colloidal silver internally and instill in the eye externally. Bach flowers: if chronic, crab apple. Cayce: if chronic, hot castor oil packs. Compresses and possibly eye baths with eyebright, chamomile, and horsetail. Smear with honey. Lymph drainage massages, Schuessler Cell Salts: No. 3, 9, 11.

Dry eyes

Most often caused by a "modern" lifestyle, sometimes by conflicts:

• **Side effects of medication**: In particular, blood pressure medications, "the pill" (birth control), diuretics, anti-depressants, vasoconstrictive eye drops, etc.

• **Age-related estrogen deficiency**: One of the signs of aging is increased dehydration of the body due to a drop in hormone levels (especially estrogen). The mucous membranes are affected.

• **Working on the computer and watching television** cause a decreased rate of blinking > dry eyes for lack of moistening.

• **General sympathicotonia or deprivation of sleep** > dry eyes (moist eyes in vagotonia).

• **Not enough of the "charms of nature"**: light, water, wind, etc.

• **Lack of physical movement**: reducing the general metabolic rate, including the tear apparatus.

• **Conjunctiva** in the conflict-active phase: a feeling of dry eyes (p. 82).

• **Lacrimal glands** in persistent repair (p. 84).

• **Meibomian glands:** After too many conflicts, the sebum becomes limited > fat layer too thin (lipid layer) > dry eyes (p. 85).

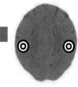

SBS of the Tear Gland Ducts | HFs sensory function - top of cerebral cortex

Inflammation of the lacrimal gland excretory ducts[1]

The main lacrimal gland's 10 -12 excretory ducts lead into the eyes from the upper sides.

Conflict	Wanting to be seen or to not be seen.
Conflict-active	Cell disintegration (ulcer), painful tension in the tear ducts > channel widening.
Bio. function	Better through flow of the tear fluid due to larger diameter > better sight.
Repair phase	Restoration of cell loss. Inflammation, possibly swelling of the ducts, with accompanying blockage of tear fluid > can give the impression of a lacrimal gland infection.
Note	Consider "handedness" (right or left) and side (mother/child or partner) or local conflict.
Therapy	The conflict is resolved. Accompany the repair phase and avoid relapse. Cold compresses, curd and flaxseed packs, lymph drainage massages.

E
C
T
O

(− +)

---

1   See Dr. Hamer, Charts, pp. 123, 136

SBS of the Eyelid Muscles

 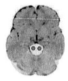

HFs in the midbrain - topography still unknown

Because of their vulnerability and importance, the eye is protected with two shielding systems: the inner shield is the iris musculature and the outer shield is composed of the upper and lower eyelids.

- According to CM, the voluntary (striated) eye-closing muscle (orbicularis oculi) is responsible for closing the eyes. Unconscious closing of the eyes (blinking) functions through a special nerve connection to the brainstem.
- Two muscles are responsible for opening the eyes. According to CM, the superior and inferior tarsal muscles are involuntary muscles, which unconsciously open the eye when we blink. The voluntary muscles, levator palpebrae superior and inferior, allow us to deliberately or consciously open our eyes or hold them open.

E
C
T
O

(− +)

E
N
D
O

(+ −)

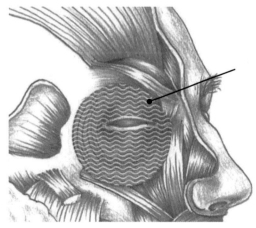

Eyelid-opening m.
Not being allowed to, not being able to, or not wanting to, hold the eyes open

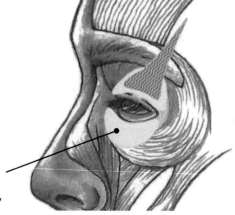

Eyelid-closing m.
Not being allowed to, not being able to, or not wanting to close the eyes

Inverted eyelid (entropion, trichiasis)

The task of the eye closing muscle (orbicularis oculi) is to close the eyelids. When this muscle is under increased tension, the eyelashes can turn inward and rub painfully against the connective tissue (entropion).

Conflict	Not being allowed to, not being able to or not wanting to close the eyes.
Examples	• A nearly 80-year-old, former entrepreneur, must earn extra money by working as a night watchman despite his age. His duty usually lasts the entire night - conflict of not being able to close one's eyes. When he comes home in the morning, his eyes drop closed from tiredness and he sleeps for a few hours. In the last 5 years of his career as a night watchman, an entropion has developed. The lower lids of both eyes have inverted, so that the eyelashes rub painfully on the connective tissue, which then becomes inflamed. When he reaches the age of 80, the patient really retires and can sleep every morning as long as he wants. The tension of the lids relaxes and the entropion retreats without a trace. (Archive B. Eybl) ➜ A long-distance driver must drive every night. ➜ A welder is distracted and looks into the glaring light.
Tissue/Phase	Eyelid-closing muscle (orbicularis oculi) - voluntary (striated) muscle - following completed repair or during **persistent repair** > increase of tension > eyelashes invert.
Questions	When did the symptoms arise? (Conflict must have happened before this). Worsening or getting better? (Getting better > conflict situation is getting better; getting worse > conflict situation is getting worse). Better or worse sleep in general? Sufficient sleep? Which situations cause stress? Is it better on vacation? (If yes, the conflict lies somewhere in daily life). Which conditioning pushes me to it?
Therapy	Determine the conflict and conditioning and, if possible, resolve them in real life. Find out where the love is - there you'll find the solution. Guiding principles: *"There's no harm in a little nap." "When I'm tired, I just lie down and close my eyes."* According to Richard Wilford: Dissolve saffron in milk and make an eye compress. Compress of tea made from horsetail, comfrey, chicory, or pot marigold (calendula). CM - OP if the conflict resolution fails and gentle measures do not help.

Outward-turned eyelid (ectropium)

Diminished tension in the eye-closing muscle leads to a limp, outward hanging lid (ectropium). This leads to weeping eyes because the tear fluids can no longer drain.

Conflict	Not being allowed to, not being able to, or not wanting to close the eyes. (For examples, see above).
Phase	**Conflict-active phase:** Muscle degeneration and paralysis > the eyelid falls limp toward the outside. Possibly incomplete closure (lagophthalmus) of the eye due to paralysis of the orbicularis muscle.
Therapy	Determine the conflict and conditioning and, if possible, resolve them in real life. Guiding principles: see above. Hildegard of Bingen: Lay fresh-from-the-morning-dew rose petals on the closed eye. Compresses or eye-baths of tea made from horsetail, eyebright, comfrey, or chicory. CM - OP, if the conflict resolution fails and gentle measures do not help.

Drooping eyelids (Ptosis)

Affected is the voluntary muscle, levator palpebrae.

Conflict	Self-esteem conflict of not being able to, not being allowed to, or not wanting to, keep the eye open. To have overlooked something. Not having been wide awake.
Example	➜ A mother tells her child, "Keep your eyes open! Next time, you're going to get hit by a car!" ➜ Somebody has to work at night and they are so tired that they cannot keep their eyes open.
Tissue	Eyelid lifting muscle, levator palpebrae - voluntary (striated) muscle - cerebral cortex - ectoderm (nerve supply = innervation) and cerebral white matter (nutrition).
Conflict-active	Drooping eyelid caused by paralysis or deterioration of the levator palpebrae muscle.
Repair phase	Restoration, eyelid tremor in the repair phase crisis. In persistent repair possibly incomplete eye closure.
Bio. function	Strengthening the muscles, so that the eye can be held open at decisive moments in the future (luxury group).

Note	Consider "handedness" (right or left) and side (mother/child or partner) or local conflict.
	The drooping of both eyelids can sometimes be caused by a general reduction in the sympathetic nervous system. In this case, it may not be an eyelid conflict, but, for example, a thyroid hyperfunction. (See p. 120)
Questions	When did the symptoms begin? (Conflict occurred shortly before this). What have I overlooked or carelessly ignored during this time? Was I reprimanded or can I not forgive myself for something. What has occupied my mind since then? Why do I react sensitively to this kind of stress? Conditioning from the family? Who acts in the same way?
Therapy	Determine the conflict and conditioning and, if possible, resolve them in real life.
	Guiding principles: *"I forgive myself for having overlooked something." "I only have two eyes." "I go to sleep and wake up when it suits me."* For further measures, see below.

Jittering eyelid (eyelid tremor)

Possible causes

1. Repair phase crisis of the orbicularis oculi muscle (see inward and outward-turned lids).
2. Repair phase crisis of the levator palpebrae muscle and/or the musculus tarsalis (see above).

| Example | • A 49-year-old, right-handed patient works for a gynecologist. Her working day starts at 7 a.m. and lasts until 10 p.m. Sometimes she has no lunch break because there is so much to do in the office. The patient is suffering from an extreme deficiency of rest and sleep - conflict of not being able to close one's eyes. During this period, the eyelid tremor starts up: during quiet moments, the lashes of the right upper lid (partner side) pull together trembling = repair phase crisis. It is the right eye, because her boss is responsible for the shortage of sleep and rest. Since then, this symptom appears again every time the patient gets too little sleep and rest. (Archive B. Eybl) |
| Therapy | If the symptoms return, determine the conflict and conditioning and, if possible, resolve them in real life so that the persistent repair comes to an end. Magnesium chloride ($MgCl_2$) foot bath. Rose leaves taken as tea or applied externally as decoction-compress. Internally: Magnesium, calcium, vitamin B complex, Schuessler Cell Salt no. 7. |

Weeping eyes (epiphora)

Possible causes

- **General vagotonia** > increased flow of tears.
- **Mechanical irritation,** wind, foreign bodies > the body tries to "rinse away" the foreign body.
- **Conjunctiva or cornea** in the repair phase (see pp. 82, 93).
- **Lacrimal glands** in the active-phase due to increased production of tear fluid = dacryorrhea (see p. 84).
- **Meibomian glands:** After too many conflicts, the sebum remain limited > too thin layer of fat> "overflowing" of the tear fluid (see p. 85).

- **Obicularis oculi** - Striated portions in an active-phase: the tears cannot be transported (see above).
- **Lacrimal gland excretory ducts** in the active-phase. (see p. 86).

Therapy

Depending on the cause: Compresses or eye-baths of tea made from eyebright and yarrow.

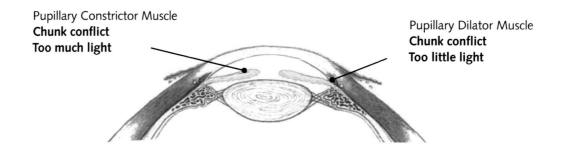

Pupillary Constrictor Muscle
Chunk conflict
Too much light

Pupillary Dilator Muscle
Chunk conflict
Too little light

SBS of the Iris Musculature

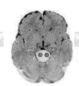

HFs in the midbrain - topography still unknown

The involuntary muscles of the iris (= "old intestinal muscles") form the eye's inner aperture system.
They regulate the amount of light that reaches the retina. There are two opposing players here: the pupil closing muscle (sphincter pupillae) and the pupil dilating muscle (dilatator pupillae).
The iris sphincter muscle is parasympathically innervated. It becomes tense during rest, thereby narrowing the sight opening. Tired and relaxed people have small pupils. The task of this muscle is to choke off the incoming light when it is too bright.
The iris dilating muscle is sympathetically innervated. It becomes tense when the individual is active. People, who are fully awake, under stress, and/or under the influence of drugs have large pupils. The task of this muscle is to widen the sight opening so that more light falls on the retina when it is dark.
From their tasks we can draw conclusions about their conflict content.

Night blindness, excessive pupil constriction (miosis)

Conflict	Chunk conflict (see explanations p. 15, 16). Right eye: Too much light. Not getting the chunk because it is too bright. 　　Left eye: Too much light. Not being able to get rid of something one does not want because it is too bright. Not being able to avoid something unpleasant or dangerous because it is too bright. In a figurative sense: You want to hide something from the eyes of others (under the cover of darkness). For some reason you dread the public eye. Not wanting to see the dark side. Fear of dark side in oneself or in other people.
Examples	➔ *Too much light due to an actual brightness-shock, such as being blinded by the sun or a welding machine.* ➔ *A simple laborer falls in love with a rich industrialist's daughter but she rejects him because he has too little to offer > not being able to have one's dream woman. The right eye is affected.* ➔ *A man hides that he has served jail time for theft from his employer. He is afraid that he wouldn't have a chance with the company otherwise. The matter comes to light nevertheless > too much light on the past. The left eye is affected.*
Conflict-active	Constriction of the pupil (myosis) due to constant tension in the iris sphincter muscle, possibly night blindness.
Bio. function	Narrowing of the pupil, so that less light comes in. Reducing the brightness so that the "chunk" can be taken better or what one rejects can be better eliminated.
Repair phase	Normalization of the pupil size.
Repair crisis	Convulsive pupil behavior.
Questions	When did the symptoms begin? What do I want to hide/keep secret in my life? Which "dark side(s)" am I not ready to face? Does this tendency lie in the family? Determine the exact conditioning.
Therapy	Determine the conflict and conditioning and, if possible, resolve them in real life.

Over-sensitivity to light, daytime blindness (hemeralopia), excessive widening of the pupils (mydriasis), unevenly shaped pupils

Conflict	Chunk conflict (see explanations p. 15, 16). Right eye: too little light. Not getting what one covets or wants because of the darkness. Left eye: too little light. Not being able to get rid of what one does not want because it is too dark, or not being able to prevent something unpleasant or dangerous because it is too dark. Frequently figuratively: Cannot put himself in the right light. One gets too little attention. Cannot see or find the spiritual, brightness and luminosity.
Example	➔ *At the job center, a hard-working, highly-skilled worker with years of experience must compete for a job with an unskilled worker - conflict that too little light will be shed on his good qualifications.*
Conflict-active	Constant tension of the pupil-widening muscle > pupil widening (mydriasis). Over-sensitivity to light > light shyness, daytime blindness, the pupils possibly become unevenly shaped.

Bio. function	Widening of the pupil, so that more light comes in. Therefore the "chunk" can be better received or what one rejects can be better eliminated.
Repair phase	Normalization of the pupil size.
Repair crisis	Convulsive pupil behavior.
Questions	When did the symptoms begin? Were did I not get enough attention? Where did I feel like I was standing on the sidelines? Was I given enough attention as a child? Further conditioning (similar parents, events, etc.)?
Therapy	Determine the conflict and conditioning and, if possible, resolve them in real life.

SBS of the Outer Eye Muscles

 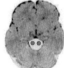

HFs in the midbrain - topography still unknown

Crossed eyes (strabismus)

Strabismus comes in varying forms: inwardly crossed eyes (esotropia), wall-eye
(exotropia) and vertical deviation (hypertropia). One or more of the six extraocular muscles are affected:
• The upper straight muscle (superior rectus) pulls the eye upwards.
• The lower straight muscle (inferior rectus) pulls the eye downwards.
• The inner straight muscle (medial rectus) pulls the eye inwards.
• The outer straight muscle (lateral rectus) pulls the eye outwards.
• The upper diagonal muscle (superior oblique) rolls the eye inwards and lowers it.
• The lower diagonal muscle (inferior oblique) rolls the eye outwards and lifts it.

Extraocular Muscles
Not wanting to see an unbearable situation anymore or not being able to escape someone/thing > Esotropia
Missing someone/thing and "searching" for them/it with the eyes > Exotropia

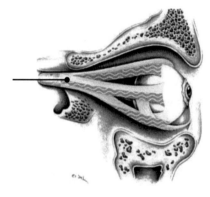

E
C
T
O

(–+)

E
N
D
O

(+–)

Examples
• *Parents take their 4-year-old son to the zoo and they come to the tiger cage. The path leads through a kind of cave in which the animals are behind bars. At the entrance, the little child suddenly becomes frightened. Thus, the mother takes him in her arms and carries him in - motor-eye muscle-conflict of not wanting to see the tiger. He clutches onto his mother and turns his eyes to the side, so he does not to have to look at the tiger.*
After the visit to the zoo, the boy is suddenly afraid of the dark. When he watches television, he avoids animal programs. A few days after the zoo visit, the parents notice that the boy often rolls his eyes uncontrollably and has developed a nervous tick (= repair phase - repair phase crisis): he throws his head back and to the left. At the same time, he turns his eyes away. The boy himself finds the tick disturbing, especially when watching television. The parents contact an eye clinic but the symptoms disappear on their own after three weeks. (Archive B. Eybl)
➜ *A child's parents get a divorce. The baby vainly searches for his mom or dad > outward strabismus or wall-eyes.*
➜ *A child is taken from his little spot right next to his mother and put to bed in the nursery too soon. He is afraid and searches with his eyes for his mother > strabismus.*
➜ *A baby has to watch, as he is crying and screaming, while the doctor gives him a shot.*
➜ *An infant lies in an incubator and must suffer from the glare of an incandescent light.*

Inwardly crossed-eye(s) (esotropia)

Conflict	Not wanting to see somebody or an unbearable situation. Not being able to escape a hopeless situation - the escape inwards! Those who are oriented inwards are usually affected here (receptive or introverted types).
Example	➜ *A child's parents separate. The mother/child eye is fixated for example on the mother - she is still there. The partner eye turns inward "to take the father into himself."*
Phase	**Persistent-active conflict** of the inner straight or outer straight muscle.

Outwardly crossed eye(s)/Wall-eye (exotropia)

Conflict	One misses someone or something and looks for him or it with the affected eye. "The outward search!" Not being able or wanting to see someone or something.
Example	➜ *A child's parents argue constantly - "First the parents diverge and then the eyes."* (Dr. Kwesi Odum). The wandering eye looks for the father in the distance, for example.
Note	The affected are usually outward-oriented (leader or extroverted) types.
Phase	**Persistent-active conflict** of the inner straight or outer straight muscles.
Note	The outer upright muscle is linked to the SBS of the kidney collecting tubules. (p. 226) > active kidney collecting tubules, for example, of the left kidney > pulling of the left eye outwards = diagnostic clue! The eye can be brought into the correct alignment consciously. (In this case, there is usually not a sight conflict but rather a refugee and existential conflict).

Vertical deviation (hypertropia), rolling of the eye(s) (zyklotropia)

Conflict	Not being able, allowed or wanting to see upwards or downwards. Not being able, allowed or wanting to see inwardly down or outwardly up or rolling the eye.
	In practice: Not being able or wanting to see someone or something located above or below. Fear that something dangerous will come from above or below (hypertropia).
Example	➜ *Hypertropia can mean that the child misses it's mother or father (looking up from below).* ➜ *While playing, a boy is hit on the head by a tree branch (danger from above) > hypertropia.* ➜ *A child sees some lying injured on the ground (fear from below) > hypertropia.*
Phase	**Persistent-active conflict** of the upper/lower straight muscle or upper/lower diagonal muscle.

Questions on crossed eyes

As always with children, we have to consider the family system. Children often carry symptoms for their parents. Were there symptoms at the same time that the eyes crossed? (Indication of the conflict's cause). In what direction does the eye cross? On the mother/child side or the partner side? (Indication of the person involved). When did the crossing happen for the first time? (The conflict must have happened before this). What happened at this time? (You may want to work with your calendar, diary). What affected the child? (E.g., parental quarrelling/divorce, stress with their teacher or in preschool). What was affecting the parents? (Relationship, quarrelling in the family, stress at work). Does the crossing get better during school breaks/vacation? (Then the problem lies in daily life, e.g., school). Is it worse during the day or in the evening? (During the day is an indication that preschool, school is stressful). Evenings is an indication that family, being at home is stressful). Recurring dreams? (Indication of conflict). Ask the child: What would you like the most? (Possible indication of the issue). Who would you like to have here/go away? (Indication of the issue).

Therapy for strabismus

Determine the conflict and conditioning and, if possible, resolve them in real life. Very important: eye training.[1] Spending time in nature instead of in front of the television or cell phone (in nature, the eye follows natural impulses > the eye muscles will be put to use in a healing way). Eye patches or bandages over the eyes only make sense for children and then, only where there is weakness in vision (amblyopia). Patches carry with them the danger of follow-up conflicts due to disfigurement and sight hindrance (it is better if they are only worn at home). An OP should be evaluated very critically, for instance, in order to prevent amblyopia.

---

[1] Books by Leo Angart, Mirsakarim Norbekov. See bibliography.

Nystagmus (dancing eyes)

With nystagmus, the eyeball twitches involuntarily outwardly or inwardly (most common), away from its correct position. Sometimes upward or downward twitching is possible as well. Sometimes the nystagmus happens in combination with eye crossing - not surprisingly, since both symptoms represent different phases of the extraocular muscles' SBS.

Conflict	For a nystagmus on a horizontal plane: Unable to see a danger from the side. Something from the side causing fear - I have to at least control it out of the corner of my eye. See also the conflict descriptions for crossed eyes.
Phase	**Repair phase, persistent repair** of the/an outer eye muscle(s).
Bio. function	Whatever is scaring someone should always be kept in sight.
Note	When someone has crossed eyes, after the conflict is resolved, nystagmus may appear - a good sign. However, when nystagmus lasts longer than three months, this means that the conflict is persistent > find and resolve the conflict.
Therapy	Determine the conflict, conditioning and belief systems to bring the persistent repair to an end. (See above for questions and therapy advice).

SBS of the Lenses

HFs sensory function - top of cerebral cortex

Clouding of the lenses (cataracts)[1]

Conflict	Very strong visual-separation conflict. Losing sight of someone.
Examples	→ *A woman is forced to move to a retirement home. She misses everything: her home, her personal possessions, her cat, her neighbors.* • *A patient's wife dies after 42 years of marriage.* (Archive B. Eybl) • *The marriage of a right-handed mother of two children ends. During the divorce proceedings, her husband arrogantly tells her that he plans to take the children away from her and that she won't be able to prevent it because he has enough money to pay for the best lawyer - visual-separation conflict, fear of losing sight of the children > sclerosis of the left lens.* (See Claudio Trupiano, thanks to Dr. Hamer)
Conflict-active	Cell degradation, no pain. Due to the thinning of the crystalline cells of the lens, more light can enter the eye.
Bio. function	The one who is moving out of sight can be seen better and for a longer period.
Repair phase	Restoration (cell growth) of the lost substance, which has occurred within the lens. Temporary clouding due to this (CM, = "cataracts") = sign of healing and repair.
Note	In **persistent repair** and because of recurrences, the lens gets cloudier and cloudier because the missing substance is replaced by inferior (scar) tissue. Consider "handedness" (right or left) and side (mother-child or partner). Artificial light plays a possible role in the cloudiness of the lenses (see macular degeneration).
Therapy	Questions: see above. Determine the conflict and conditioning and if there is persistent repair; resolve it in real life. The lens will regenerate itself if the conflict is resolved and stays resolved. Guiding principles: *"I am bound to all the people I like." "An invisible band binds us." "In my heart I am together with all those I love whether they are present or not."* Saying goodbye ritual. Eye training, eye baths with eyebright, also internally as tea. Acupuncture, acupoint, classical and facial lymph drainage massages. Unfortunately, an OP us usually unavoidable, but fortunately, eye surgeons do great work here.

---

1   See Dr. Hamer, Charts pp. 119, 132

SBS of the Cornea

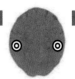

Thinning of the cornea (keratoconus), inflammation of the cornea (keratitis), corneal clouding[1]

Conflict	Strong visual-separation conflict. To lose sight of someone.
Example	→ *A single woman's son moves away from home.* → *A schoolgirl's favorite teacher is transferred.* • *A man has a major fight with his brother. He knows that their good relationship has now come to an end.* (Archive B. Eybl)
Conflict-active	Cell disintegration (ulcer) of the cornea. No pain. In persistent conflict activity, this can lead to a keratoconus = central curving forward and thinning of the cornea. Usually both eyes are affected, and it is almost always associated with myopia, because the light is refracted in excess.
Bio. function	The one who is out of sight should be forgotten temporarily.
Repair phase	Inflammation of the cornea, clouding of the cornea. Restoration of the tissue, pain, swelling, reddening. CM: "mycotic, bacterial or viral keratitis." In persistent repair: Arcus senilis/arcus lipoides, cornea band degeneration, iron deposits (hematocornea), copper deposits (Wilson's disease), clouding caused by the connective tissue (corneal pannus).
Note	Consider "handedness" (right or left) and side (mother/child or partner) or local conflict.
Questions	For keratoconus: Diagnosed when? (Conflict must have happened relatively long ago and still be active). Who did I lose out of sight? (Separation/going away/death of family member, partner, friend)? Why did that affect me so badly? (Conditioning: childhood, birth, pregnancy) Which family member is similar to me in this regard? (Examine for conditioning). For inflammation of the cornea: What happened that was good, shortly before the eye became inflamed? (E.g., reunion with someone I missed, good news, a good conversation) What separation was I suffering from before and since when? (To estimate the length of the repair phase, date precisely). Was this the first corneal inflammation of my life? (If no, also determine the conflict at that time - important for a permanent solution). Separation conditioning? (Infancy, birth)? With regard to the separations, which conditioning is there in the family?
Therapy	In cases of inflammation of the cornea and corneal clouding, the conflict is resolved. Support the healing process. In case of recurrences, determine the conflict and conditioning. Guiding principles: *"I am bound to all the people I like." "An invisible band binds us." "In my heart, I am together with all those who are dear to me, whether they are present or not."* Saying goodbye ritual, lymph drainage massage, MMS. Hildegard of Bingen: spring apple-tree leaves and onyx wine special recipes.
	Eye baths and tea: plantain and eyebright. Taking colloidal silver internally and externally instillation in the eye. Enzyme preparations. Eye bath tea: plantain and eyebright. In extreme repair phases: possibly antibiotic eye ointment.

Trachoma (Egyptian ophthalmia)

Same SBS as above. According to CM, the infection is caused by chlamydia. Chronic inflammation of the conjunctiva and cornea. It is a very common disease in developing countries.

Increased scarring that often leads to blindness (pannus trachomatosus or scar entropion).

Phase	Persistent repair or condition after many **recurrences**.
Therapy	Determine the conflict and conditioning and, if possible, resolve them in real life, so that the persistent repair comes to an end. See inflammation of the cornea. Improvement of living conditions (sanitation, clean water, etc.). See keratitis.

---

1 See Dr. Hamer, Charts pp. 119, 132

SBS of the Choroid

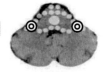

Choroid cancer (uveal melanoma adeno-ca), inflammation of the choroid (choroiditis), inflammation or tumor of the iris or the ciliary body (iritis, uveitis), nodules of the pupillary seam, coloboma, iris nevus, melanoma of the iris[1]

The choroid, iris, and ciliary body are made up of endodermal tissue = developmentally, the oldest part of the eye (the so-called eyecup originally). The choroid is basically intestinal mucosa tissue. The iris muscles (= old intestinal muscle) is coated with differently pigmented "intestinal mucosa" (different eye colors).

Conflict	Chunk conflict (see explanations p. 15, 16). Not being able to sufficiently identify what one wants (right eye), or not being able to get rid of seeing something unpleasant (left eye). Simply stated: one would like to see something but cannot (right eye); or one wants to avoid seeing something undesirable (left eye).
Example	• *A 17-year-old apprentice in the chemical industry goes to get sandwiches for his coworkers. While he is gone, his workplace is blown up by an explosion. When he comes back, he sees body parts lying all around. Two of his coworkers are dead and one is badly injured - conflict of not wanting to see the situation or wanting to see his coworker undamaged. Five months later, as he gets over the incident, both eyes become inflamed - beginning of the repair phase. In the hospital, he is diagnosed with a choroiditis in both eyes. Since the condition does not improve with cortisone, the doctors recommend chemotherapy. At this point, the family becomes familiar with the 5 Biological Laws of Nature. The young man gradually stops using the cortisone. After 8 months in the repair phase, everything returns to normal again. (Archive B. Eybl)*
	• *A 6-year-old boy is playing alone in his room as he gets the idea of pulling a plastic box over his head. Unfortunately, the box gets stuck and the child becomes afraid because it is dark in there - conflict of not being able to capture the coveted thing (right eye). He screams but his near-deaf grandmother in the next room cannot hear him because she is watching television. In the repair phase, a choroid inflammation of the right eye is diagnosed. Recurrences occur again and again. For instance, the child always becomes afraid when a sweater is pulled over his head. (See Claudio Trupiano, thanks to Doctor Hamer, p. 171)*
Conflict-active	Growth of a choroid tumor (adeno-ca), a tumor of the iris covering (CM: iris nevus, iris melanoma), a tumor of the ciliary body or the growth of so-called pupillary seam nodules (sarcoidosis: in principle, little intestinal polyps).
Bio. function	To produce more intestinal cells in order to be able to take up or eliminate the wanted or unwanted thing in a better way.
Repair phase	Tubercular caseating deterioration of the tumor. This process is called choroid tuberculosis or choroiditis. Tuberculosis lesion = white spots behind the retina which disappear over time. Caverns may remain. Inflammation of the iris, inflammation of the ciliary body, swelling, pain.
Questions	When did the symptoms begin? When was the tumor diagnosed? (Estimate the beginning of the growth - possibly a few months before - conflict must have happened at this point > count back the months). At the time, what couldn't I bear looking at anymore or didn't get to see anymore? What was going on in my life at the time/what changed? Why did this affect me so much? (Determine conditioning from ancestors).
Therapy	In the case of a choroid tumor: Determine the conflict and conditioning and, if possible, resolve them in real life. Guiding principles: *"There is a reason that it had to be like that." "One can only learn from it."* Attempts by CM to use radiation is risky and so is an operation. Better alternative: laser therapy (with smaller tumors). Tea/compresses: eyebright, dill, hibiscus, plantain, violet. Lymph drainage massages. Schuessler Cell Salt: No. 3, MMS. In extreme repair phases, possibly cortisone and/or antibiotics.

---

[1] See Dr. Hamer, GNM® Brain-Nerve Charts, HN II, columns 1 and 2

SBS of the Vitreous Body

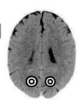

Vitreous opacity, increased pressure within the eye (glaucoma), posterior vitreous detachment (PVD) and bleeding, floaters[1]

In CM, the common German term "grüner Star" ("green stare") is used interchangeably with glaucoma and describe various conditions of the eye, especially the optic nerve - that sometimes, <u>but not necessarily</u>, are accompanied by increased pressure within the eye ("primary open-angle, narrow-angle, angle-closure and normal tension glaucoma").

In Dr. Hamer's opinion, the raised inner pressure comes from an edema in the vitreous body. In accordance with the 5 Biological Laws of Nature, we differentiate between the clouding of the vitreous body (= "green stare") in the active conflict stage and increased inner pressure (= glaucoma) due to an edema of the vitreous body during the repair phase.

Conflict	Fear-of-rear-attacks from "bad guys" (robbers, rapists, tax authorities, teachers, classmates, boss).
Examples	• *A patient divorces his wife. The wife is given custody and he may see the child only one day at a time - fear-of-rear-attack conflict. He feels that his ex-wife is robbing him of his child.* (B. Eybl) • *A 5-year-old boy suffers a fear-of-rear-attack conflict affecting both eyeballs because suddenly the lights go out in the apartment. Over the years, his fear becomes so intense, that when the lights are off, he suspects robbers and murderers are everywhere. He is diagnosed with reduced ranges of vision in both eyes - conflict-active phase. The boy does not come into healing until eight years later, when he has to ride his bike alone to his mother's friend's one evening. He realizes that it is not bad to ride in the dark. A few days later, he has an acute attack of glaucoma (edema in the vitreous humor). Three days later, the worst is over. Therapy: belladonna C 30.* (Personal archive Antje Scherret) • *The supermarket cashier is attacked from behind by a robber - fear-of-rear-attack conflict. Shortly afterwards, she notices that her range of vision has been reduced = active-phase - "wearing blinders" phenomenon.* (Archive B. Eybl)
Ocular Pressure	According to Dr. Odum, the inner eye pressure should be measured several times (as much as twice a day before and after stress) before being treated, except in the case where it rises to an extreme value of over 40. The thickness of the cornea should also be measured as this can affect the eye pressure measurement).
Conflict-active	Necrosis of tissue in the vitreous body and very rapid clouding (green stare). Limitation or elimination of the range of view (scotoma).
Bio. function	The opacity causes a "wearing-blinders phenomenon." The vision to the side, to the back and upwards is clouded. The pursued individual can fully concentrate on the flight forward (like a rabbit, which just runs instinctively without looking back).
Repair phase	Restoration of the vitreous body, rise of the inner eye pressure (glaucoma) due to edema. The pressure rises through constant production of fluid in the vitreous body and is naturally desirable, so that the eyeball stays full during the healing and does not "shrink up." The collagen in the vitreous body can condense > so-called floaters, possible lifting or bleeding of the vitreous body. Clouding of the vitreous body through persistent conflict.
Note	If the left halves of the vitreous body of a right-handed person are affected, it is about the partner. After many recurrences, one sometimes finds streaks of cholesterol or calcium phosphate in the vitreous body > seeing sparks (spintheropy). An SBS of the kidney collecting tubules (= syndrome) usually plays "background music" to a diagnosis of glaucoma **Retinal tear:** In the active-phase of this SBS, traction in the vitreous body can cause a tear in the retina (retinal detachment). Conflict aspect: something is pulling at a person.
Questions	With chronic, increased pressure within the eye: When did the symptoms begin? (Conflict previous). What am I chronically afraid of? Is it better when on vacation? (If yes > conflict from daily life). What stresses me in daily life? What worries/frightens me? What would I like to change? (Indication of the conflict) Which conditioning has sensitized me? (Pregnancy, childhood, ancestors)? In what condition is my trust?

---

1 Dr. Hamer, Charts, pp. 142,146 and Dr. Hamer®- Brain-Nerve ChartsHN II columns 3, 4

Therapy	In case of opacity of the vitreous body: determine the conflict and conditioning and resolve. Glaucoma: the fear-of-rear-attack conflict is resolved; support the repair phase: wear sunglasses, keep the head cool, darken the room, etc. See also: repair phase at the brain level, p. 60f. Resolve refugee conflict if necessary. Guiding principle: *"I am safe and taken care of."*
	Neck and face lymph drainages, acupuncture, acupoint massage. Hydrogen peroxide (H_2O_2). Eye baths and tea: eyebright. Take colloidal silver internally and instill in eye externally. Combination remedy Lymphomyosot to improve lymph circulation. Enzyme preparation. If all else fails, CM medications (Prostaglandin analogues, carbohydrase inhibitor).

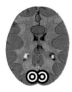

SBS of the Optical Nerve

Normal pressure glaucoma, damage to or "stroke" of the optical nerve

It is not certain if increased pressure within the eye poses a problem for the optical nerve. The fact of the matter is that the optical nerve is damaged just as often under normal pressure. According to CM, because of thromboses in the optical nerve's blood vessels, which in my opinion which is incorrect, the blood vessels are arranged as a network. If this were the case, blockages could always detoured collaterally (see p. 138).

Conflict	One does not want to integrate the information seen. One is annoyed. Self-esteem and self-respect component. = Intense eye(s) conflict. According to my experience, the person affected is usually hit by more than one thing at a time, pushing them over the limit they can handle.
Examples	➜ *"This is really getting on my nerves!"*
	• *A male nurse is unable to work anymore and goes to the job center. He is annoyed by all the paperwork and correspondence with the social security agency and the job center. He is diagnosed with a normal pressure glaucoma with damage to the optical nerve. (Dr. Odum)*
	• *The wife of the 68-year-old patient contracts Parkinson's disease. At the same time, his mother-in-law, who lives in the same house, becomes unable to care for herself due to dementia. Half a year later, the patient loses half of the sight of his right (partner) eye. Diagnosis: damage to the optical nerve due to stroke of the optical nerve. (Archive B. Eybl)*
Conflict-active	Cell reduction, decrease in function of the optical nerve, possibly also due to limited blood supply > disturbances in the field of view or loss of sight.
Bio. function	Blocking out the unbearable for the protection of the individual. *„Better to be half blind than to have to see that."*
Repair phase	Recovery depends on the conflict mass. Regeneration is usually incomplete.
Questions	When did the symptoms begin? (Conflict must have taken place some weeks before and have continued more or less until the present). What annoys/burdens me so much? Are there multiple, simultaneous unresolved problems? Which conditioning has led me into the dilemma? (E.g., perfectionism, wanting to do everything immediately, sloppiness)? Are there similar patterns among ancestors? (Indication of conditioning) Why am I doing it the same? Which new attitude was helpful? Which new internal and external changes?
Therapy	Determine the conflict and conditioning and resolve them in real life. Find out where the love is - there you'll find the solution. See also therapy for macular degeneration p. 97.
	Guiding principle: *"I couple myself with God's power and serenity. From now on, life will be easy."*

E
C
T
O

− +

Closed-angle glaucoma, open-angle glaucoma

The most difficult chapter of eye medicine - also for us:

- **Closed-angle glaucoma** = narrowing of the space between the iris and the cornea > disrupted drainage > increased pressure in the inner eye. The cause is an SBS of the iris in the active-phase (see p. 94) > swelling > narrowing of the angle.
- **Open-angle glaucoma:** First possibility: SBS of the vitreous body in the repair phase > increased intraocular pressure (p. 85). Second possibility: resistance to drainage in the scleral venous sinus canal due to cell growth or muscle contraction: visual-chunk conflict (see explanations p. 15, 16) that one cannot let go of/release something that has happened (e.g., a fight between grown children, daughter's unhappy marriage).

- **Another cause of increased inner pressure: SBS of the ciliary body:** Visual-chunk conflict > cell division in the active-phase > increased fluid production. Bio. function: Better vision through increased vitreous fluid. *Example: A man desires a woman, but she does not reciprocate. He produces more vitreous fluid for the "magnifying effect": In this way, he is subjectively closer to the one he adores. Diagnosis: glaucoma.* (Archive Dr. Odum)

Macular degeneration

In the center part of the retina - "yellow spots" in Latin: stains (macula lutea) - the vision cells lie extremely close together. This is where vision is the sharpest.

Most vision takes place in the macula.

In the case of macular degeneration, the cells in this area begin to die off. The patient can no longer see the object, the eye is fixed on sharply, although he can see the peripheral area well. Other symptoms: reduced strength of vision, sensitivity to being blinded by light, disturbances in seeing colors and contrast. CM differentiates between "wet" and "dry" forms of the disease. According to CM, the cause of macular degeneration is unknown.

Dry macular degeneration

During an ophthalmological examination, one sees so-called extracellular drusen = dead sensory cells. According to Dr. Odum, this is due to a persistent fear-of-rear-attack (neck) conflict with a special distinction: It has to do with negative expectations for the future and lack of self-esteem, guilt, shame and disgrace. The biological function of this conflict is to block out the threatening reality. Determine its cause. Questions: Symptoms since when? (Conflict some time before). What fear lies in the background? (Own future, career, retirement, future of the children, grandchildren)? Which life issues are haunting me? What can't I stand to see anymore? What is my greatest personal wish in life? (Indication of conflict and solution). Which hidden significance could the illness indicate to me? What am I being forced to do? What new realizations have I gained because of the illness?

Wet macular degeneration

An SBS of the choroid. (For this reason, see conflict p. 94 and dry macular degeneration). The choroid's blood vessels move into the degenerated retina. According to Dr. Odum, wet macular degeneration is a sight survival program. The choroid provides support for the dying retina by means of cell proliferation. Possibly other factors, such as "radiation" from LED lamps, television sets and computers, play a role. The unnatural and disharmonious glimmering light, with its high proportion of blue, may damage the eyes permanently. The lenses and the macula suffer most from this.[1]

Alternatives: incandescent light bulbs, as much natural light as possible, sunglasses only when necessary (e.g., in the high mountains).

Therapy for macular degeneration

- Determine the conflict and conditioning and resolve them in real life.
- Vital, alkaline foods, especially green vegetables, etc.
- Garlic and lemon drink cure, blueberries.
- Vitamins, minerals, trace elements (orthomolecular therapy)
- Hydrogen peroxide (H_2O_2) 3 % internally.
- Eye exercises (see bibliography), gymnastics.
- Acupuncture, acupoint massage, lymph drainages.
- Natural borax internally (www.institut-ernaehrungge sundheit.com).
- Breathing exercises.
- Amino acids, lutein, zeaxanthin, lycopene.

---

1   http://www.engon.de/c4/theorie/elampen.htm

SBS of the Retina

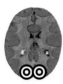

Reduced functioning of the retina, retinal edema, retinal detachment[1]

Conflict	Fear-of rear-attack conflict. Fear of a thing or a danger from behind that cannot be shaken off. *"Makes the hair on the back of your neck stand up."* According to Dr. Odum, also a guilt-shame theme.
Example	• *A patient lends an acquaintance a large sum of money. Suddenly, he is seized with the fear that he has fallen into the hands of a swindler - fear-of rear-attack conflict.* (Archive B. Eybl)
	• *An owner of a small construction company lets the firm deliberately go bankrupt in order to get a tax advantage. However, the tax authorities are onto his scheme. He is afraid of a financial audit nearly every day.* (Archive B. Eybl)
	• *A retired, 67-year-old woman suffers a fear-of rear-attack conflict when her doctor tells her the following: "You were a smoker in the past. Your breathing difficulties are dragging out so long that we need to find out whether something malignant has formed." The woman sees this as a cancer diagnosis. Later, when her fears are allayed, she comes into healing. Now a retinal detachment is diagnosed.* (See Johannes F. Mandt…Was Gesund Macht, p. 67).
	• *Someone finds out that his job at the company is "shaky."* (Archive B. Eybl)
	• *A patient has a car accident. He is afraid that he will lose his driver's license = fear-of rear-attack conflict.* (Archive B. Eybl)
Conflict-active	Clouding of the retina, partial occlusion of the range of vision (scotoma), reduced sight.
Bio. function	What one is afraid of should be made "invisible" by means of a temporary interruption in the functioning of the retina.
Repair phase	Edema between the sensory cell layer and the pigmented epithelium. It only rarely comes to a detachment of the pigmented epithelium from the choroid. Even rarer is a splitting of the retina (retinoschisis). There is usually a loss of sight in part of the field of vision ("blind spot," scotoma, flashes of light). The worsening of vision is dramatic if the retinal detachment is near the macula where vision is sharpest. Relapses cause callosity, that is, scar tissue is formed. Usually, a **recurrent conflict.**
Note	By all means, flashes of light should be looked into by an ophthalmologist. Syndrome aggravates the situation as it causes even more fluid to be stored! With the left half of the retina, the right-handed person looks to the right to the partner and with the right half of the retina, to the left to mother/child. If the left side of the retina of a right-handed person is affected, it is about the partner. If the right side of the retina is affected, it is about the mother/child. In contrast to the opinion of Dr. Hamer, I believe that diabetes really does aggravate diseases of the retina (diabetic retinopathy) as is maintained by CM. **Retinitis pigmentosa:** A loss of photo-receptors that begins at the periphery of the retina and moves inward so that the field of vision gradually narrows. Conflict: Putting something terrible out of sight by means of over-pigmentation. Persistent conflict! Retinal detachment (without edema) can also occur in the active-phase of a vitreous body SBS, if the vitreous body collapses and tears the retina.
Questions	Which stress was released before the retinal edema appeared? Fear lingers behind you? (E.g., mother-in-law, credit, tax authorities)? Which conditioning lies behind it? (E.g., insecurity, perfectionism)?
Therapy	The conflict is resolved. Support the healing. If it recurs, determine the conflict and conditioning. An edema of the retina does not need to be lasered immediately; one can wait until the excess fluid recedes. The two levels of the retina will then lay themselves together again if the conflict is definitely resolved and remains that way. Retinal detachments, however, should be taken care of in the conventional manner, for instance with laser treatment.
	If recurring, guiding principles: *"I am safe and taken care of."* Alkaline diet rich in vital elements, enzyme preparation. Garlic and lemon drink cure. Hydrogen peroxide (H_2O_2) 3% internally.
	Bach flowers: aspen, mimulus, star of Bethlehem. Neck/face lymph drainages, acupuncture, acupoint massage, enzyme preparations.

ECTO

−+

---

1   See Dr. Hamer, Charts, pp. 141,146

SBS of the Retina

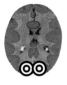

Red-green color blindness (color vision deficiency)

This is an "hereditary disease" and this is why we must place our focus on the ancestors. Those affected (10% of men, but only 0.5% of women) have difficulties distinguishing the colors red and green from one another.

Conflict	According to Frauenkron-Hoffmann: Not wanting to see something green or red. Ancestral conflict in connection with these colors. Stress during an ancestor's experience with these colors.
Example	• *An 8-year-old boy can't distinguish between red, green and violet. Mrs. Frauenkron-Hoffmann identified the following conflict for the color red: His parents decide to have the child when the mother is already 30. Unfortunately, they aren't successful for two years. Every time when the mother saw that she had her period (blood - red), she experienced stress - her time was running out. The other colors that he can't see also have something to do with his ancestors. As soon as the boy recognized the connection and understood that the stress is now over and didn't actually have anything to do with him, he could see all colors.* (www.biologisches-dekodieren.de)
Conflict-active	Impairment of the ability to see specific colors, usually from birth onward.
	Wether the problem lies with the retina (perception) or with the visual cortex (processing), doesn't play a main role for us.
Bio. function	Blocking out the color to protect the individual from the stress associated with it.
Repair phase	Restoration of color vision.
Note	Mrs. Frauenkon-Hoffmann explains why 20 times more men are effected by red-green color blindness in this way: Many of our male ancestors died on the battlefield (blood - red, field - green).
Questions	Which color(s) does it involve exactly? Is this vision deficiency also present in ancestors? (Indication that the conflict is to be sought there). Which stress ancestor(s) have with that color? Was there stress with blood at the time? Did someone die tragically on a battlefield (green). What do I think about with this color? Which role does this color/this associated something play with an ancestor(s)?
Therapy	Determine the conflict, triggers and causal conditioning and resolve them. See also Therapy p. 98.

Total color blindness (achromatopsia), day blindness (hemeralopia)

We categorize those people as color blind who can only see white-gray and no colors. Because color blindness is hereditary, we have to look for the conflict among ancestors.

Conflict	Light or daylight is dangerous, because one can be discovered. In the figurative sense: The light of recognition hurts. One doesn't want to see the skeletons in the closet - a test of honesty shouldn't be ruled out. Also: One's sight/judgement is limited to black or white. One has forgotten how diverse, colorful and many-facetted life is. One shuts out the light.
Examples	➔ *The soldier can only advance at night. He would be shot at the break of day.* ➔ *On the run: The hiding place is only safe at night. They'll be discovered during the day.*
Bio. function	Blocking out of all colors so that the individual believes they are safe. In white-gray, one feels better.
Conflict-active	Limitation of the ability to see colors, usually from birth onward.
Repair phase	A complete restoration is probably not so easy here. It depends on whether color receptors in the retina are present and functional.
Questions	Did ancestors also have this vision deficiency? Which stress did an ancestor(s) have once in the daylight? Did someone need the protection of the night? Dramatic war, criminal or refugee experiences? Have I or did my ancestor(s) suppress something monstrous? (E.g. murder, incest)? Has someone completely shut out the Light (of God) and sought their salvation in darkness?
Therapy	Determine the conflict, triggers and original conditioning and resolve them. See also treatment p. 97.

NEARSIGHTEDNESS (SHORTSIGHTEDNESS, MYOPIA)

In CM, one differentiates between two types of nearsightedness:

- By so-called axial nearsightedness, the eyeball, instead of being perfectly spherical, is slightly elongated. This results in the focus lying in front of the retina instead of on it > seeing in the distance is out of focus and blurred > nearsightedness. (An elongation of the eyeball by 1 millimeter results in a nearsightedness of about 3 diopters.)

- The second, rarer kind of nearsightedness is refractive nearsightedness. Cornea and lens refract the light too strongly. Here too, the focal point lies in front of the retina > nearsightedness. In the following, I describe three possible biological changes that occur with nearsightedness. After that, I present some conflict causes and case studies.

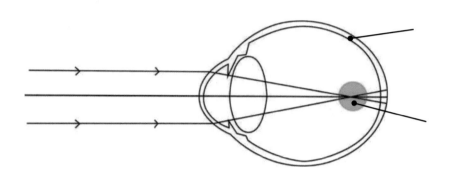

Eyeball too long

Focal point in front of the retina

SBS of the Ciliary Muscle

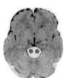

Nearsightedness caused by the ciliary muscle

According to CM, the ciliary muscle is an involuntary muscle. According to Dr. Hamer, it has involuntary and voluntary (striated) parts, which seems perfectly logical to me. In the following, I take both possibilities into consideration.

The ciliary muscle plays the main role in refractive nearsightedness. The interplay between this parasympathetic innervated ring muscle, the zonula fibers (suspension apparatus), and the lens is not easy to understand. In a tension-free state, the lens is a roundish, thick disk, which is connected with the ciliary muscle over the zonula fibers.

- When the ciliary muscle tightens, the inner diameter of the ciliary body diminishes > the zonula fibers, on which the lens hangs, relax > the lens takes on its original form of a roundish thick disk = nearsighted adjustment.

- When the ciliary muscle relaxes, the inner diameter of the ciliary body increases > the zonula fibers tighten > they pull on the lens > it becomes a flat disk = farsighted adjustment. Thus, the tension of the ciliary muscle behaves inversely to the tension on the lens. Tightened ciliary muscle > relaxed, thick lens. Relaxed ciliary muscle > tightened, flat lens. The "antagonist" to the ciliary muscle is the inherent tension of the lens.

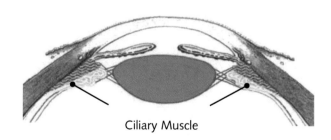

Ciliary Muscle

Progression	Involuntary part of the muscle: Increased muscle tension in the **active-phase** > better seeing up close (= bio. function) > nearsightedness, if the conflict is active for a longer period. Voluntary (striated) part of the muscle: Necrosis or paralysis in the active-phase. Refilling in the repair phase. **End of the repair phase** or in persistent repair: the ciliary muscle is stronger than before (luxury group) > nearsightedness.
Non-conflictive	It is very probable that nearsightedness can also happen with out a conflict with regard to the ciliary muscle and diagonal eye muscles: adjustment to constant near-vision use (school, computer, etc.).

E
C
T
O

– +

E
N
D
O

+ –

SBS of the Outer Eye Muscles

HFs in the midbrain - topography still unknown

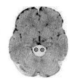

E
C
T
O

−+

E
N
D
O

+−

The role of the outer eye muscles is underestimated in CM: e.g., focusing on an image.

The New York ophthalmologist and founder of eye training, Dr. Bates (1860-1931), researched the cause of nearsightedness for more than 40 years. He observed that the vision among his students varied greatly. He noticed that patients, whose lenses had been removed could see fairly well nevertheless (accommodation). This is something that simply should not occur according to the textbooks.

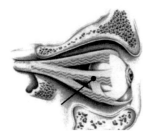

Inferior Oblique Muscle

His credo: *"The lens is not the main factor in the accommodation process."* He discovered that the lens, when focusing, was aided by the upper and lower, oblique eye muscles. These two muscles build a ring around the eyeball. When they tighten simultaneously, the eyeball is squeezed lengthwise > improvement of near sight. Permanent tension of these muscles results in nearsightedness!

Dr. Bates and representatives of modern ophthalmology schools start from the standpoint that near vision under stress leads to lasting tension of these muscles. The body does nothing other than accommodate the (somewhat unnatural) demand for permanent near vision **(nearsightedness - an adaptation process)**.

Eye training is an attempt to release the tension in these muscles.

This adaptation theory of Dr. Bates is confirmed by the fact that the numbers of nearsighted people increase with the level of civilization. In Japan, over 90% of the youth are nearsighted, among indigenous peoples, hardly any.

SBS of the Cornea

HFs sensory function - top of cerebral cortex

E
C
T
O

−+

Nearsightedness due to cone-shaped thinning of the cornea (keratoconus)

A persistent, active conflict of the cornea causes it to become thinner and thinner. This results in the loss of its regular curvature and it becomes cone-shaped, pointing to the front = keratoconus > usually linked to a distortion of the cornea. This type of myopia can be clearly diagnosed. It cannot be completely compensated with glasses. Due to the increased corneal curvature, the light is increasingly refracted > myopia.

Conflict	Strong visual-separation conflict. To lose sight of somebody.
Phase	**Persistent, active conflict**

Nearsightedness: conflict, examples, therapy

Conflict	<u>First possibility:</u> A person has the feeling that he does not belong. Someone or something is too far away. He misses somebody. *"I would like to have a certain something or someone within sight of me."*
Bio. function	A visual clinging to someone or something. The nearsightedness gives the illusion of being in a small, safe, and intact world.
Conflict	<u>Second possibility:</u> A person does not want to see something in the distance, because it frightens them.
Bio. function	Visually blocking something out. Subconsciously, one only wants to see in the near vicinity to feel safe or secure. *"What I cannot see in the distance cannot scare me."*
Type of person	Most often, people who tend to be introverted, fearful or hesitant are affected.
Examples	• *While a boy is attending a summer camp, the other boys gang up on him and beat him. After these three weeks, he is nearsighted. A test of his vision shows a diopter of minus 1.5. (Archive Dr. Odum)* • *A child has to go to kindergarten. He does not like it there and would much prefer to be at home with his mother. (Archive B. Eybl)*

Questions	When did the nearsightedness begin? (Conflict must be previous). What is frightening "out there?" Why? Why do I want to retreat? Did ancestors have similar tendencies? (Look for conditioning).
Therapy	Determine the conflict and conditioning and resolve them in real life.
	Avoid looking at things close up at an early age and avoid early learning pressure.
	Spend more time in nature rather than with television and books.
	Eye training (see bibliography.). Bach flowers: aspen and mimulus among others.
	Until 1850, one rightly assumed that eyeglasses made bad eyesight worse and thus, they were not prescribed.
	In any case, it seems sensible not to fully correct the eyes, so that room for improvement remains.

Farsightedness (hyperopia)

In the case of farsightedness, the eyeball is too short in relation to the refractive power of the seeing apparatus > blurriness when looking at objects up close.

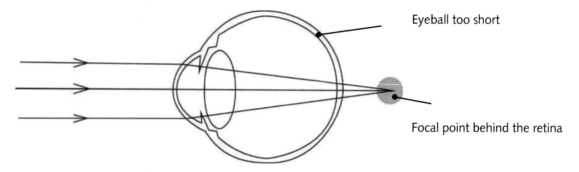

Eyeball too short

Focal point behind the retina

Possible causes

- **Farsightedness as an aging process?** Yes, this might be true for those over 45; however, this surely does not apply to young people, because they sometimes become farsighted too. The fact is that the rigid core of the lens becomes enlarged with age, which is a burden on the elastic outer layer. This causes the lenses to lose their overall elasticity > without elasticity, sharp eyesight (accommodation) is not possible!
- **SBS of the outer eye muscles:** Tension in the smooth eye muscles causes the eyeball to shorten = distance vision adjustment

(see p. 90f). In the case of a conflict, the tension can become permanent = farsightedness.
- **SBS of the ciliary muscle:** Weakness or paralysis of the ciliary muscle due to a conflict > tension in the zonular fibers > a tug on the lens > it causes it to become a flat disk = farsightedness.
- **Callosity:** Dr. Hamer explains farsightedness, as a shortening of the eyeball due to callosities in the rear (dorsal) part of the eyeball (see p 86).

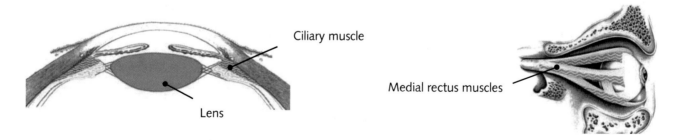

Ciliary muscle

Medial rectus muscles

Lens

Conflict	Not being able to see someone or something that is far away. Visual wandering and searching. *"I want to see whatever is out there carefully since it might be dangerous!"*
Example	• *A little boy always wants to carry his favorite toy around with him. Suddenly, his parents take it away from him. Within a short time, he develops farsightedness with a diopter of plus 7. The boy keeps looking and looking.* (Archive Dr. Odum)
SBS	Medial rectus muscles and/or ciliary muscle.
Bio. function	Good, long-distance eyesight in order to recognize someone or something more easily.

Phase	**Persistent active conflict.**
Type of person	Outward-oriented (extroverted) and energetic persons ("go getters") tend to be affected more often.
Questions	Farsightedness substantially before the age of 45? (> Look for the conflict's cause). What is frightening out there? What am I looking for in the distance? Which conditioning is this based on? (Parents, ancestors)?
Therapy	Determine the conflict or conditioning and, if possible, resolve them in real life.
	Eye training can decidedly improve or stabilize farsightedness. However, this requires commitment, diligence, and perseverance. (For books, see bibliography). *"As long as I live, I will remain curious and flexible." "I forgive myself and I forgive you."*

Age related farsightedness (presbyopia)

In CM, age related farsightedness is regarded as a normal part of the aging process. For most people, the ability to see up close begins to deteriorate after about the age of 45. There are excep-tions, however. Some people do not need glasses, even when they are old.

Possible causes
- **SBS of the lens:** Loss of elasticity in the lens due to conflict or age > without elasticity it is not possible for the eye to focus (accommodate) > (old age) farsightedness (See also: p. 92).

- **SBS of the ciliary muscle:** Weakness or paralysis of the ciliary muscle due to conflict or old age > the lens can no longer resume its original form of a roundish, thick disk > (old age) farsightedness.

Conflict	Fear of the future. One cannot see how things will turn out > "mid-life crisis."
Examples	➜ *Will my health hold up? Will I be able to support myself when I'm old? Is my job secure?* ➜ *What is going to happen to my mother/father? What will become of the children?*
SBS/Phase	Lens and/or ciliary muscle. **Persistent conflict.**
Questions	Do I suffer from separation conflicts? Am I often worried about the future? My personal pension? Job? Children, grandchildren? What do I see as my task in life? Can I actually change the things that I am worrying about? Then why am I worrying myself sick about it? What do I believe in? Am I confident?
Therapy	Determine the conflict or conditioning and, if possible, resolve them in real life. With eye training, the farsightedness can be decidedly improved.

Astigmatism

With astigmatism in CM, there is not a single focal point in front of the retina (nearsightedness) or behind the retina (farsighted-ness), but rather two or more focal points. This phenomenon is aptly called "lack of focal point."

Deformation of the cornea is the most common cause of astig-matism, but there are others: astigmatism of the lens (rare) and astigmatism of the eye background (retina).

Possible causes
- **SBS of the cornea** (thinning of the cornea p. 93).
- **SBS of the outer eye muscles:** Varying amounts of tension in the outer eye muscles that brace the whole eyeball, so that symmetry is lost (see strabismus). The asymmetry can affect the cornea or the retina.
- **SBS of the vitreous body:** A pulling of the vitreous body on the retina in the active-phase > distorted vision (see p. 95f).

Conflict	A person's internal vision - their expectations (of oneself or of others) - do not match reality. The two views cannot be brought into alignment.
Examples	• *A child has a natural inner vision of a strong father. The father, however, is a dialysis patient. Unfortu-nately, one day his mother takes him to the hospital where he sees his ailing father, who is dependent on dialysis.* (Archive Dr. Odum) • *The father of a patient - 5-years-old at the time - has become an alcoholic. He is drinking with his bud-dies and starts showing off his son's gymnastic stunts: "Hey look, he can do a headstand on a shot glass." For the boy, this is terribly embarrassing. He has to perform the stunt dressed only in his nightshirt. The real picture of his father does not match his inner vision.* (B. Eybl)

SBS/Phase	Cornea and/or external eye muscles. **Persistent conflict.**
Bio. function	The distortion of reality protects the individual from the "hard reality."
Questions	When did the symptoms begin? (First conflict must have been before this. The diagnosis usually takes place after the first symptoms > estimate when the SBS began). Which expectations didn't match up with reality at the time in question? Is the conflict still ongoing? What could be recurring? Why do I have such high expectations? Which conditioning has made me into who I am today? (Pregnancy, birth, parents)?
Therapy	Determine the conflict and conditioning and, if possible, resolve them in real life. Astigmatism can be improved considerably through eye training.

EAR

The external ear (auris externa) is made up of the auricle (pinna), the earlobe (lobulus auricula), and the outer auditory canal (meatus acusticus externus). The ear- drum or tympanic membrane (membrana tempani) marks the division between the outer ear and the middle ear (auris media). The air-filled, tympanic cavity of the middle ear, with its hammer (malleus), anvil (incus) and stirrup (stapes), is connected via the eustachian tube with the pharyngeal cavity. In the oval window (fenstra ovalis), the stirrup transmits hearing impulses to the snail-shaped cochlea of the inner ear, which is the actual auditory organ. The semicircular canal is where the sense of balance is located.

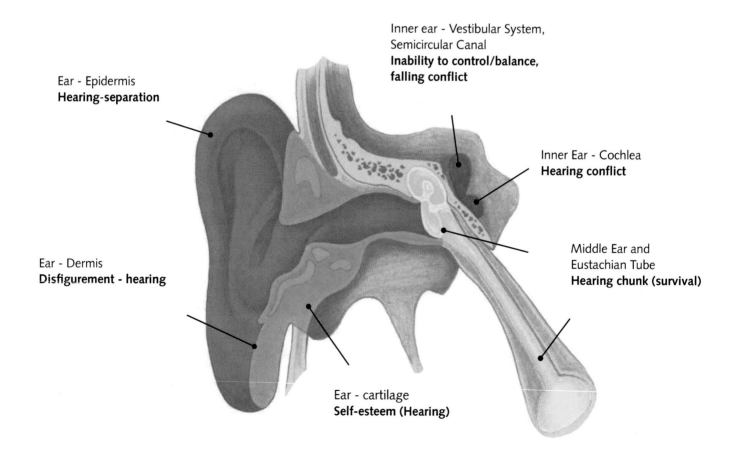

Ear - Epidermis
Hearing-separation

Inner ear - Vestibular System, Semicircular Canal
Inability to control/balance, falling conflict

Inner Ear - Cochlea
Hearing conflict

Ear - Dermis
Disfigurement - hearing

Middle Ear and Eustachian Tube
Hearing chunk (survival)

Ear - cartilage
Self-esteem (Hearing)

SBS of the Middle Ear

Middle ear infection (otitis media), inflamed ear polyp[1]

Conflict	Chunk conflict (see explanations p. 15, 16). Right ear: not getting hoped-for auditory information. Left ear: cannot get rid of an unpleasant, disturbing message or not having noticed (heard) something dangerous.
	I.e., not to hear something desired or not wanting to listen something undesired. Not getting or getting rid of information. One missed hearing something or doesn't hear something and suffered damage as a consequence.
Example	➜ *A child does not get the toy he wished for.*
	➜ *A baby wants to hear his mother's voice, but that is not possible in the nursery.*
	• *The 9-year-old daughter of a 36-year-old, right-handed married woman is doing relatively badly in school. One day, the daughter's teacher contacts the patient and says she thinks that the child's schoolwork leaves much to be desired = chunk conflict. She would rather hear something else, namely that the daughter's work had improved > right receptive ear is affected.*
	Resolution of the conflict: By chance, she runs into a friend, who has three children. She tells her that she has very similar problems with her children at school. A pleasant, and healing conversation, develops during which the patient pours her heart out to her friend. Shortly after the conversation, the middle-ear infection begins. (Archive B. Eybl)
	➜ *A woman learns from her girlfriend that her boyfriend was flirting with another woman = conflict, not wanting to hear this bad news (chunk conflict). In the repair phase, a middle-ear infection follows > here, the left ear is affected.*
Conflict-active	An increase in the functioning of the "primal-hearing cells." Growth of a flat-growing tumor (adenoca) of absorptive quality or a cauliflower-like growing tumor (ear polyp) of secretory quality - increased filling of the middle ear with "primal-hearing cells."
Bio. function	With more cells, there is better reception or rejection of what one hears.
Repair phase	A normalization of function: The tumor is broken down by fungi and bacteria; tubercular caseating = middle-ear infection (otitis media). Swelling, pain, possibly with perforation of the eardrum or the ear polyp bulging forward in the outer auditory canal with purulent discharge, fever, night sweats.
Repair crisis	Chills, severe pain.
Note	Repeated middle-ear infections can harm the auditory ossicles behind the eardrum and lead to permanent hearing loss.
Questions	Was this the first middle ear infection? (If no > determine the first episode, then identify the current one. If yes > a hearing conflict must have gone into the repair phase immediately before this). Which event led to the healing? (E.g., a good conversation, good news, the resolution of a quarrel - This healing event provides an indication of the conflict). What was stressing me beforehand? What couldn't I bear to hear anymore/What couldn't I hear anymore? Which conditioning is the cause? (Parents, pregnancy, childhood)?
Therapy	The conflict is resolved. In case of recurrences, determine the conflict and conditioning.
	Guiding principle: *"Life's not always a bowl full of cherries." "I can't have everything and I do not have to hear everything."* Lymphatic drainage, enzyme preparation, MMS, colloidal silver internally and externally. Drop vermouth-chamomile decoction or olive oil in the ear and cover with a wad of cotton. Steep mullein blossoms in olive oil for four weeks - drop into the ear. Onion compresses: lay finely chopped onion on the ear. Cover with curd cheese. Beat white cabbage leaves until soft and lay them on the ear. Enzyme compounds. Hildegard of Bingen: Oily "Rebtropfen" special recipe. CM antibiotics make sense for short-term treatment when symptoms are acute and severe, such as at night. Possibly only a single dose. Less recommended for chronic cases (see p. 63).

---

1   See Dr. Hamer, Charts, pp. 18, 23

Inflammation of the Eustachian tubes[2]

Similar to the SBS above

Conflict-active	Increasing closure of the Eustachian tube due to flat-growing adeno-ca of absorptive quality. Retracted eardrum due to insufficient ventilation > poor hearing.
Bio. function	With more cells, there is better reception or rejection of what is heard.
Repair phase	Tubercular, caseating reduction of the tumor through fungi or bacteria (mycobacteria). The discharge can flow off into the throat or middle ear and possibly take on the appearance of a middle ear infection. Swelling, fever, night sweats.
Therapy	The conflict is resolved. Support the healing. For therapeutic measures, see above.

2   See Dr. Hamer, Charts, pp. 18, 23

SBS of the Nerve Sheath | HFs in the cerebellum - topography still unknown

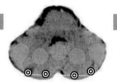

Tumor of the balance (vestibular) nerve - vestibular schwannoma - mistakenly "acoustic neuroma"

Dr. Hamer groups the acoustic neuroma with the brain stem (see p. 105f, middle ear infection), which seems correct, because the "tumor" lies in the brainstem (although it is on the border to the cerebellum). The reason I order this SBS, with the cerebellum - mesoderm, is because the tumor, when seen histologically, is made up of Schwann cells - thus a "nerve sheath tumor." It grows around the vestibulocochlear nerve (balance nerve) between the cerebellopontine angle, inner ear canal and the inner ear. Due to swelling, it can compact the vestibular (balance) nerve as well as the cochlear (hearing) nerve and trigeminal (facial) nerve.

Conflict	Likely a "balance-pain conflict." Painful/burdensome/negative information knocks one off balance.
Example	→ *One must work with a jackhammer every day.* • *Every time her grown daughter comes to visit, the right-handed mother hears a sermon about everything she has done wrong and what she should have done differently = balance-pain conflict. She can no longer listen to her daughter's harping and wishes she could have some understanding of her problems. Over the years, an acoustic neuroma develops on the left mother/child ear = active-phase. The patient's symptoms: deafness and dizziness. The neuroma is removed through surgery.* (Archive B. Eybl)
Conflict-active	Growth of a vestibular Schwannoma in the cerebellopontine angle. The longer the conflict lasts, the greater it becomes. Symptoms: deafness on one or both sides, disturbances in the sense of balance, dizziness.
Bio. function	Through the thickening of the nerve insulation, the unbearable information is blocked.
Repair phase	Inflammation > worsening of the symptoms. Break down of the tumor by bacteria. Restoration is possible, but only in the preliminary phase when the tumor is very small. After a certain size, its degeneration is unrealistic. The best possible scenario is a stoppage in growth.
Questions	Diagnosed when? (The conflict-active phase can already have been going on for months/years). What has been putting me off balance for a long time? What do I want to block unconsciously? What am I unable to "tune out?" If these questions remain unanswered: What bothers me the most in my life and has for a long time now? Which conditioning and character traits are the cause? (E.g. oversensitivity, absence of stability)? Which ancestors are similar? What made them become like that?
Therapy	Find out what the conflict and conditioning are and, if possible, resolve them. Find out where the love is - there you'll find the solution. Guiding principle: *"I have the power to change the things that are unhealthy for me."* If the tumor continues to grow or is already too big, an OP is unavoidable.

SBS of the Epidermis

HFs sensory function - top of cerebral cortex

Inflammation of the outer ear or auditory canal (otitis externa)

**E
C
T
O**

−+

Conflict	Wanting to hear something desirable or not wanting to hear something undesirable. Wanting or not wanting to have skin contact at the ear (local conflict).
Example	• *In a long telephone call with a friend, the patient gets an "earful" of verbal abuse. During his friend's diatribe, he was eating nuts. Since then, he is allergic to nuts (= trigger). One day after eating nuts, he suffers from itchy eczema in his ear during the repair phase. (Archive B. Eybl)* ➜ *Someone likes it when their cat lovingly rubs their ear. The cat dies = separation conflict of losing skin contact at the ear.*
Conflict-active	Cell reduction in the squamous epithelium of the outer ear or the auditory canal. Scaly, dry, numb skin, lessening of sensitivity, no pain.
Bio. function	Through lessening of sensitivity, the separation is more easily forgotten or the unwanted contact is "blocked out."
Repair phase	Inflammation of the outer ear or auditory canal. Replenishing and filling up of the squamous epithelium, over-sensitivity. Rash on the ear, itching ear canal eczema, scaling off of the outer skin (detritus) because new cells are pushing out from below.
Note	Consider "handedness" (right or left) and side (mother/child or partner) or local conflict.
Questions	When did it begin? (Previously, a hearing conflict must have been resolved). What didn't I want to hear? (Accusations, viscous words, criticism)? What stressed me? Did it have anything to do with a specific person?
Therapy	The conflict is resolved. Support the healing. If recurrent, determine the conflict and/or conditioning. Guiding principles: *"I do not expect anything." "I am happy with the way it is." "I say YES to life!"* Compresses and herbs: see middle-ear infection. Drops of the juice of the houseleek (sempervivum tectorum) in the ear. Sloughed off skin can lead to inflammation. Therefore, if necessary, clean the ear canal regularly with an ear bath or let the doctor clean it.

SBS of the Cartilage of the Outer Ear (Auricle)

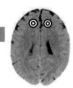

Inflammation of the outer ear cartilage (auricular perichondritis), gout

**N
E
W
M
E
S
O**

−+

Conflict	Self-esteem conflict with regard to the ear or the taking in of sound + active kidney collecting tubules.
Example	➜ *Somebody has a hearing impairment and can no longer follow the conversation at the table.*
Conflict-active	Cell degradation in cartilage, no pain.
Repair phase	Restoration of the cartilage. Inflammation of the auricular cartilage. Swelling, reddening, pain. In the case of syndrome, "gout tophus" on the auricular cartilage.
Bio. function	Strengthening of the cartilage so that sound can be better absorbed.
Note	With this SBS we are dealing with "gout in the ear." Consider "handedness" (right or left) and side (mother/child or partner) or local conflict. E.g., partner always sits on one side and gives you an ear full.
Therapy	The conflict is resolved. Support the healing. In the case of recurrences, determine the conflict and conditioning. Resolve any refugee conflict. Lay curd cheese or white cabbage leaves on the affected area. Cold compresses, cold showers. Spray the ear with tincture of frankincense or myrrh.

SBS of the Tympanic and the Stapedius Muscles

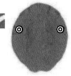

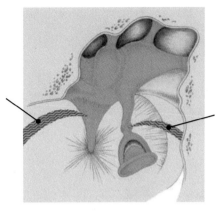

Tensor Tympani
Inability to dampen the noise

HFs motor function - top of
cerebral cortex

Stapedius Muscle
Inability to dampen noise

Deafness caused by the tympanic muscle and the stapedius muscle

These two muscles of the middle ear tense up in order to reduce the vibration of the eardrum, thereby protecting it from high sound levels. Sometimes, explosions and the like cannot be "intercepted," because the reaction time is too short. Thus, these and similar sounds can hurt the inner ear and cause deafness.

According to CM, voluntary (striated) muscles are involved here (one really can tense up the ear drum when a loud noise is expected). Normally, however, the two muscles behave involuntarily, as if they were smooth muscles. It is interesting to note that they also react in the same way (as if they were involuntary muscles) in the case of a conflict.

Conflict	Not being able to dampen the noise. (E.g., A wife complains constantly, someone with dementia constantly repeats the same thing, a coworker sings annoyingly the whole day long).
Examples	• *Thirty years ago on New Year's Eve, a firecracker exploded next to the now 67-year-old patient = conflict of not being able to silence the sound. For four months, he had trouble hearing with the right ear = active-phase with increased tension of the tympanic membrane and the stapedius muscle. After that, his hearing normalized again = repair phase. Since then, however, any loud noise - such as a truck driving by or the noise of a concert - causes several minutes of deafness = recurrence with muscle tension. Hearing tests show that the patient has excellent hearing.* (Archive B. Eybl) → *Someone works in a nightclub and suffers from constant noise.* → *Someone constantly "gets an earful" from their partner.*
Conflict-active	Increase in the muscle tension (hypertonia) of the tympanic muscle and/or stapedius muscle > deafness. Permanent deafness due to persistent conflict activity > constant tension. (Behaves like involuntary muscle?)
Bio. function	Damping of the sound.
Repair phase	Restoration of normal hearing.
Repair crisis	"Cracking" in the ear due to uncoordinated contractions of the aforementioned muscles.
Note	Behavior of involuntary muscles: Could it be that those striated muscles that also operate involuntarily (for instance the diaphragm, the outer eye muscles) might react like involuntary muscles in the case of conflict?
Questions	Was there a specific, extreme noise event or is something chronically annoying? (Office, particular people)? In which situations is it better/worse? (Indication of the conflict).
Therapy	Determine the conflict and conditioning and, if possible, resolve them in real life. Guiding principles: *"Now the noise does not bother me anymore. It could be worse. I am ready to hear everything again."* Bach flowers: beech, crab apple, lymph drainage massages, acupuncture, acupoint massage.

E
C
T
O

− +

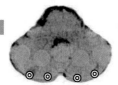

SBS of the Dermis

Ear canal furuncle (otitis externa circumscripta)

Inflammation of a hair follicle in the auditory canal

Conflict	Disfigurement conflict. Conflict of feeling deformed or disfigured. Also, feeling disfigured by what one has heard.
Example	→ *Somebody gets verbally abused.* → *The patient suffers from an overproduction of earwax. The partner complains about the bad smell coming from the ear = disfigurement conflict.* (Archive B. Eybl)
Conflict-active	A thickening of the dermis (corium) that usually goes unnoticed.
Bio. function	Better protection from disfigurement through thickened dermis.
Repair phase	Inflammation. Tubercular, caseating, stinking deterioration of the tumor (pus).
Note	Danger of vicious circle due to stinking ear. Sometimes histamines (see p. 152) or certain foods may be a trigger.
Questions	When did the symptoms begin? Which stress did I have before this? By what did I feel attacked? Is is based on my nutrition? (Trigger). Which stress did I have before the last episode of itchiness? (Self-observation).
Therapy	The conflict is resolved. Support the healing. In case of recurrence, determine the conflict and conditioning. Bathe the auditory canal or clean with an ear spoon to eliminate recurrences. DMSO (dimethylsulfoxide), H_2O_2 externally. If recurring, guiding principles: *"A crystal wall surrounds me." "That goes in one ear and out the other." "I will remain in my center."* Bach Flowers: crab apple, compresses and herbs (see middle ear infection).

O L D
M E S O

+−

SBS of the Inner Ear

Impairment due to the inner ear, sounds in the ear (tinnitus)[1]

Conflict	Not wanting the hear something. The most common hearing impairment SBS.
Examples	→ *"What I am hearing cannot be true!" I cannot believe what I'm hearing! This guy is pestering me!"* • *A youthful, 50-year-old, right-handed woman has been suffering from tinnitus of the right ear and dizziness for the last 5 days. Conflict history: The patient has a 53-year-old sister with psychological problems. Following a 4-month stay in a psychiatric clinic, her condition seems stable. Six days ago, the patient was invited by her sister to have breakfast together. She notices at once that her sister is in very bad shape again, as she constantly pokes around in her miserable past > hearing conflict: "I just can't listen to this anymore!" and falling conflict: "She will never stabilize!" To the patient, it is clear that her sister will never get out of this mess. Therapy: she tries to lay her sister's fate in the hands of God.* (Archive B. Eybl) • *A 41-year-old, right-handed man has a good position as the manager of a hotel. One day, his supervisor informs him that the hotel is about to be closed. It is clear to the patient that this means the end of his job > hearing conflict: "What I have just heard cannot be true!" Since this point he has suffered from tinnitus in both ears.* (Archive B. Eybl)
Conflict-active	Reduced functioning of the inner ear = deafness and/or humming, rustling, hissing, whistling, ringing in the ear = tinnitus. This causes further hearing reduction.
Bio. function	Blocking out of what is being heard through a reduced functioning of the inner ear. Tinnitus: one is warned when the same or a similar situation recurs. The tinnitus noise also helps to disrupt the unbearable quiet when someone is all alone. (The sound of the seashore in a shell pro-

E C T O

−+

---

1   See Dr. Hamer, Charts, pp. 141,145

	vides comfort and a sense of connection).
Repair phase	Often, one notices the tinnitus only after acute hearing loss: Here, there may be a chronic hearing conflict present, which just went into the repair phase (hearing loss) recently.
	Sudden deafness (see ISSHL below) followed by slow recovery of hearing, hearing impairment due to recurrences or persistent repair.
Note	Words, sentences or songs that repeatedly go through our heads also function according to this scheme (word - tinnitus, music - tinnitus = "stuck in the head").
Questions	For hearing impairment: since when? (Previous conflict, usually continuing up to the present). What could I no longer tolerate hearing, which situations got on my nerves? Am I resisting listening because it might hurt? (Criticism, objections)? Am I constantly transmitting and not receiving? Do/did my ancestors also have impaired hearing? Is there someone who I am similar to? (Indication of a family issue).
	For tinnitus: Since when? Which sounds/which situations does my tinnitus noise remind me of? In which situations does it get worse? (Indication of the conflict). When does it get better? (Weekends, vacation or mornings, when I am together with certain people? > Indication of the conflict).
Therapy	Determine the conflict and conditioning and, if possible, resolve them in real life. Guiding principle: *"It's a good thing that I heard that, but now, it's already forgotten."* Disconnect-ritual: "Say goodbye" to the hearing conflict with your heart and mind. Lymph drainage massages. Acupuncture, acupoint massage. Willfort: smoke ear with hyssop fumes. Tea: club moss, mistletoe, hyssop violets. Hydrogen peroxide (H_2O_2) 3% internally.
	In CM, in cases of acute tinnitus, high doses of cortisone are prescribed over several days. It makes more sense to practice the so-called tinnitus retraining therapy (TRT).

Acute hearing loss (sudden deafness)[2]

Same SBS as above. Sudden deafness ranging from slight hearing loss to total deafness, usually in just one ear and without pain. It can affect all or only certain frequencies.

Repair phase	Edema in the inner ear and in the hearing center of the meninges > short-term, severe reduction of hearing ability. In my experience, the order of tinnitus preceding acute hearing loss first isn't substantiated very often. Usually, it is the reverse (still unclear). What is clear is that the hearing conflict needs to be determined and resolved.
Therapy	The conflict has been resolved. Support the healing process. Guiding principles: *"Relax, the symptoms are temporary."* Alkaline food, lymph drainage massages, hydrogen peroxide (H_2O_2) 3% internally. In CM, circulation stimulating, blood-thinning medication and cortisone is administered. From the view of the New Medicine, this is only sensible as a short-term treatment. Personally, I would only apply the measures described above.

---

2 See Dr. Hamer, Charts, pp. 141,145

SBS of the Bony Labyrinth

Otosclerosis (otospongiosis)

Ossification can affect the oval window, the round window, the cochlea or the semicircular canals. The disease pattern is usually as follows: The normally moveable stirrup bone (stapes) becomes increasingly fixed in place > less transmission of sound waves > deafness.

Conflict	Self-esteem conflict that one has forwarded information incorrectly or carelessly (e.g., forgotten, misunderstood, erroneously divulged) and, in doing so, has exposed themselves or other(s) to danger. Conflict that one cannot handle coarse information - cannot integrate it.
Example	→ *Deafness following a hearing-conflict. The patient constantly hears a whistling in the ear.*
	→ *The doctor tell the patient, "Something is wrong with your ear!"*

N E W M E S O	Conflict-active	Degeneration of the bone (osteolysis) in the bony, osseous labyrinth.
	Repair phase	Restoration (recalcification), pain, otosclerosis, deafness through recurrent conflict or **persistent repair.**
	Bio. function	Strengthening, to be able to better forward the sound (= the information) later.
	Note	The ossification could also come from recurrent middle-ear infections (see above). Consider "handedness" (right or left) and side (mother/child or partner) or local conflict.
	Questions	When did the symptoms begin? (Conflict probably already took place months before). Which important information did I fail to forward or forward carelessly? Do I have problems with coarse/strong language? Who else in the family is similar? Similar incidents in the family?
−+	Therapy	Find out what the conflict and conditioning are and, if possible, resolve them in real life so that the persistent repair comes to an end.
		Guiding principles: *"I forgive myself - it must have a reason nevertheless." "Coarseness also is a part of earthly life - I want to adapt to it and integrate it."*
		Lymphatic drainage, acupuncture, acupoint massage.
		Natural borax internally. Garlic and lemon juice.
		With chronic condition, only a slight improvement in symptoms is expected (due to calcification of stapes).
		If necessary, CM surgery (implant - stapedotomy).

Hearing impairment (hypacusis)

Possible causes

- **Poisoning due to drugs or medication:** Antibiotics, diuretics, painkillers, acetylsalicylic acid (ASA) in high doses, psychotropic, chemotherapeutic substances, anti-malaria medication, iodine (as an additive to salt, toothpaste, etc.) can cause hearing impairment.

- **Cochlea hearing conflict:** Not wanting to hear something. In persistent conflict activity > hearing impairment due to reduced function of the inner ear and/or tinnitus. In the repair phase > impaired hearing due to edema of the inner ear (acute hearing impairment) see p. 109f.

- **Middle ear mucosa** or mucosa of the eustachian tube = hearing chunk conflict (see explanations p. 15, 16). Hearing impairment due to recurring infection. Scarring with calcium deposits in the middle ear > impaired functioning of the hearing bones.

- **Middle ear muscles:** Self-esteem conflict, not being able to silence a noise. Possible hearing impairment in the conflict-active phase.

- **Bony labyrinth:** Self-esteem conflict. Not being able to hear well. Impaired hearing in persistent repair or after many instances of conflict (recurrence).

- **Mechanical closure** of the outer auditory canal due to ear wax (cerumen). Noticeable worsening after coming in contact with water. Upwelling of ear wax.

Determining which of these various causes is the actual one isn't always clear.

The easiest is the explanation of the middle ear SBS: Here, several middle ear infections must already have taken place. Tinnitus is a clear indication of the second possible cause.

Therapy

- Determine the conflict and conditioning and, if possible, resolve them in real life.
- Mix dry mustard with water and paint it behind the ear (stimulates circulation)
- Garlic and lemon drink cure.
- Acupuncture or acupoint massage, lymph drainage massages.
- Natural borax internally.
- Hydrogen peroxide (H_2O_2) 3% internally.

Ménière's disease (MD)

CM's triad of symptoms for Ménière's disease is made up of the following symptoms: vertigo, one-sided hearing loss and tinnitus. Here, CM forms a single "disease" out of at least two separate SBSs in different phases.

SBS of the Semicircular Canals | HFs auditory function, lateral in cerebral cortex

Dizziness (vertigo) caused by a falling conflict[1]

Conflict	Falling or balance conflict. A person sees someone fall or falls himself. Also in the figurative sense: to lose one's grip or balance. To lose the ground beneath one's feet. Hang in the air. Fall in a hole. *"It made me fall off my seat!" "He fell down off his high horse!"* Further aspect: swindle comes from the German *schwindeln* (make) dizzy. Thus, this also includes the concepts (experienced passively or actively): lying, manipulation, twisting (truth), embellish/sugar coat, being unfaithful/disloyal.
Example	• *Due to her low and irregular income, the 40-year-old patient can barely afford an apartment. After hearing a lecture about the upcoming dramatic economic crisis, she has the feeling that she is losing the ground beneath her feet (= falling conflict). For two weeks, she was so dizzy that she can hardly walk or drive (= conflict-active phase). She resolves the conflict by deciding to move in again with her estranged partner. Immediately after she makes this decision, the dizziness ceases.* (Archive B. Eybl)
Conflict-active	Impaired function of the equilibrium organ (vestibular apparatus) > dizziness, possibly a tendency to fall. In my experience, the dizziness doesn't always occur immediately after the conflict, but rather after the first relaxation phase thereafter.
Bio. function	Dizziness causes someone to return to safe territory and avoid dangers = protection from further falls.
Repair phase	Disappearance of the dizziness.
Questions	1. Side effects of medication? (Check if the beginning of the symptoms corresponds with ingestion. > Discontinue use as necessary). 2. Dizziness since when? (Conflict previous). 3. Determine if the dizziness occurred in sympathicotonia (active falling conflict) or in vagotonia (pressure on the brain - general repair symptom). Headaches? (= Indication of vagotonia). Cold/warm hands? Poor/good sleep? Appetite? Thinking in circles? If in sympathicotonia: Falls, accidents in the period in question? Lost footing/rug pulled out from underneath - by what? If in vagotonia: How did I come into the repair phase? Which stress did I have before this? Do ancestors also suffer from dizziness? If yes, what similarities in character are there? Do I want to relive this pattern or will I take the liberty to go my own way?
Therapy	Determine the conflict and conditioning and, if possible, resolve them in real life. Consider "handedness" (right or left) and side (mother-child or partner). Avoid risk & stay on safe terrain. Guiding principle: *concentrate on safety in one's life.* "Grounding" activities such as gardening, handwork, walking (barefoot), strength training, grounding ritual, lemon-garlic drink cure. Bach flowers: clematis, aspen, cerato, scleranthus, honeysuckle. Tea: St. John's wort, mistletoe.

---

1   See Dr. Hamer, Charts, pp. 141,145

Dizziness - other causes

• **Poisoning with drugs or medication:** Antihypertensives (beta blockers, ACE inhibitors), pain killers (analgesics), epilepsy medication (antiepileptics), tranquilizers, antidepressants, cramp releasing medication (spasmolytics), antibiotics, antimycotics (anti-fungus medication), diuretics, anti-allergy medication (antihistamines), X-ray contrast media, etc. > Due to poisoning, the human body experiences artificial stress (sympathicotonia) > "success of the medication" > If the body neutralizes or expels the toxins later on, it actually enters a repair phase (vagotonia) > dizziness, headache.

• **Brain pressure = general healing symptom:** The interaction of the eyes, balance organs (inner ear), and muscle and joint receptors, is disturbed by the swelling in the brain (brain pressure) > dizziness.

• **Cervical spine or skull bone** in the repair phase (possibly in persistent repair), space requirement reaching into the inner-ear area > dizziness, see p. 295f.

• **Tumor on the hearing or balancing nerve** > dizziness.

• **High blood pressure,** see p. 65.

• **Hypoglycemia** see p. 222f.

PITUITARY GLAND (HYPOPHYSIS)

The bean-shaped pituitary gland (hypophysis) lies at the base of the diencephalon or interbrain.

The endodermal, anterior lobe of the pituitary gland - in principle, a hormone gland located in the brain - is distinct from the ectodermal posterior pituitary, which is part of the interbrain. Some of the hormones of the anterior lobe only have an indirect function: they stimulate the activities of other hormone glands. This includes the follicle stimulating hormone FSH and the luteinizing hormone LSH which causes maturation of the ova or sperm in the gonads, the adrenocorticotropic hormone ACTH which stimulates the adrenal cortex, and the thyroid stimulating hormone (TSH), which stimulates the thyroid gland. For each of these hormone functions, it must have had its own conflict and the conflict content must have something to do with the target organ. Unfortunately, I don't have much experience with the pituitary gland. For this reason, this chapter should be subject to reservations, because it is not substantiated in practice.

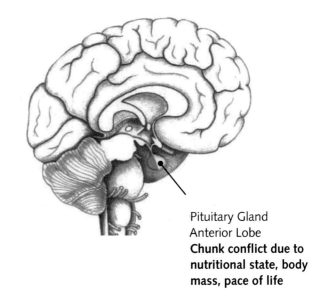

Pituitary Gland
Anterior Lobe
Chunk conflict due to nutritional state, body mass, pace of life

SBS of the Anterior Lobe of the Hypophysis

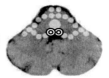

Tumor of the milk duct stimulating cells of the adenohypophysis (prolactinoma)[1]

Conflict	Probable chunk conflict (see explanations p. 15, 16): One is given cause to worry by superiors (family elders, parents, authorities) that one won't be able to support/feed their child or family.
Examples	➜ *The head of the family earns just enough to support his family, but he loses his job.*
	➜ *A single mother no longer knows how she can support her children.*
Conflict-active	Growth of additional, milk-duct stimulating cells = cauliflower-shaped adeno-ca of the hypophysis of secretory quality. Release of more lactotropic hormones (LTH or prolactin) > Because of the proximity to the optic nerve, a tumor, which is too large, can cause visual field defects.
	Effect in women: Increasing the milk secretion if she is breast-feeding. If she not breast feeding, possible milky discharge from the breast (galactorrhea), libido decrease, absence of ovulation and menstruation (amenorrhea).
	Effect in men: decreased libido, possibly impotence or infertility.
Bio. function	Production of more prolactin so the children and partner can be better nourished with more milk. A higher prolactin level promotes nurturing behavior and reduces sexuality and fertility. (Pregnancy and additional offspring is the last thing that this organism needs)!
Repair phase	If fungi or bacteria are present: a tubercular, necrotic degradation of the tumor > normalization of prolactin production > reduction of milk secretion. Inflammation, swelling, headaches, possible double vision.
Therapy	Determine the conflict and conditioning and, if possible, resolve them in real life if still active. Guiding principles: Realize that one is not alone in taking care of the family. There are relatives, friends, and social institutions that can help care for the family. *"There is enough to eat. Everybody will be taken care of. "* Bach flowers: elm, red chestnut, optionally pine. Consider surgery if the tumor creates a problem due to its size (e.g., compression of the optic nerve.)

E N D O

+−

---

1 See Dr. Hamer, Charts, pp. 17, 34

Tumor of the adenohypophysis (adeno-ca), gigantism (hypersomnia), enlargement of the extremities (acromegaly)[2]

Conflict	Chunk conflict (see explanations p. 15, 16) of being too small. Possibly also: One is "cut down to size" by superiors (parents, authorities) - feels like a "shrimp."
Examples	→ *A young animal is too small and does not get his share of his mother's milk.* → *A schoolboy is teased because he is the smallest in the class.*
Conflict-active	Increase in function, growth of a cauliflower-shaped adeno-ca of secretory quality > increased production of the growth hormone somatotropin. Conflict in the growing years > faster growth or gigantism. Conflict in adult years > enlargement of the hands, feet, lower jaw, chin, mouth, nose, sexual organs = acromegaly. Cardiovascular problems often occur.
Bio. function	Production of more growth hormones so that the individual grows.
Repair phase	Normalization of the somatotropin production. Due to inflammation, the tumor will grow even larger for a short time: swelling > headaches, impaired vision.
Therapy	Determine the conflict and conditioning and, if possible, resolve them in real life. Consider surgery, if the size of the tumor causes problems.

Short stature due to somatotropin deficiency

Phase	**Persistent repair:** Reduction of hormone producing tissue > deficiency of somatotropin > delayed development or short stature, insufficient buildup of muscular tissue, too much fatty tissue.
Therapy	Omission of the evening meal, athletic activities and sufficient sleep raise the somatotropin level. Basketball, volleyball: In these sports tall people have an advantage > small people come into conflict, which stimulates the somatotropin production > growth. Ingestion of high-quality protein, such as eggs. Linseed oil. Sunbaths.

Tumor of the adrenal gland stimulating cells (corticotropes)

Conflict	Chunk conflict (see explanations p. 15, 16) - one has to take a new direction in life because of being pressured/forced by an authority. Undesired influence on one's own path.
Conflict-active	Relatively rare tumor. Growth of additional adrenal gland stimulating cells > increased production of the adrenocorticotrophic hormone (ACTH) > Cushing's disease (p. 117).
Bio. function	With an increased cortisol or aldosterone level, one has a lot of energy. This enables one to find the right way for themselves or to continue on the right path.
Repair phase	Normalization of the hormone production, possible breakdown of the tumor by bacteria if present.
Therapy	Determine the conflict, conditioning and beliefs and resolve. OP if the tumor becomes too large.

Tumor of the thyroid stimulating cells (thyreotropes)

Conflict	Chunk conflict (see p. 15, 16) - one feels compelled to increase the pace of their life by external forces.
Conflict-active	Rare tumor. Growth of additional TSH cells > Hyperthyroidism or hypothyroidism.
Bio. function	Through increased thyroxine production by the thyroid, the individual is faster.
Repair phase	Normalization of the hormone production, possible breakdown of the tumor if bacteria are present.
Therapy	Determine the conflict, conditioning and beliefs and resolve. OP if the tumor becomes too large.

Hormone neutral tumor in the pituitary gland's anterior lobe

30% of pituitary adenomas produce no hormones (anymore). One of the SBSs described above has run its course and come to an end. The conflict has been resolved, the hormone production has returned to normal.

---

2   See Dr. Hamer, Charts pp. 17, 34

Abnormally short stature - dwarfism

If you can rule out these causes: Under or insufficient nourishment, vitamin deficiency (vitamin D), disturbances in absorbing nourishment (see colon), chemo-poisoning, radiation damage, etc., then the following causes may come into consideration:

- **Territorial conflict constellation(s)** (cerebral cortex) during the growth phase: simultaneously active Hamer foci on the right and left in the territorial areas bring about - in addition to physical changes - a cessation or delay in physical and psychic maturation (= retardation). Indicators: thin appearance, narrow shoulders, little muscle, late ovulation and/or late sexual maturation, so-called "baby face," (see p. 314f and literature from Dr. Hamer).

- **SBS of the bones** during the growth phase: long lasting, active, generalized self-esteem conflict - limitation of the bone metabolism and bone growth during the persistent conflict activity (see p. 286ff). Signs: anemia, bone and joint pain.
- **Testicles** - conflict activity during the growth phase: demise (necrosis) of testicular tissue, decrease in testosterone production due to persistent conflict activity > lack of drive, slowing of muscle and body growth (see p. 255f).
- **Pituitary gland -** persistent repair during the growth phase (see p. 114).

THALAMUS

The grape-sized, symmetrical halves of the thalamus are part of the diencephalon and it is considered the "Gateway to Consciousness." The core of the thalamus forwards all of the information that we should be aware of from the sensory organs on to the cerebral cortex. The thalamus filters this information with regard to its significance/insignificance. Without this filtering, we would be overwhelmed by sensory impressions. The conflict content is a result of the function: One cannot differentiate between what is important and what is unimportant and, thus, exposes themselves and/or others to danger. The thalamus also processes motor signals. The conflict content for this function is not entirely clear to me.

HYPOTHALAMUS

The hypothalamus lies under the thalamus in the area of the optic chiasm and the third ventricle. It is connected to the pituitary gland by the pituitary stalk. This small, unpaired organ is the most important link between the nervous system and the hormone system.

It produces various hormones (e.g., vasopressin and oxytocin) and is significantly involved in the control of the autonomic nervous system (circulation, respiration, body temperature, metabolism, sexual behavior).

■ SBS of the Hypothalamus

Hormonal and autonomic imbalance, hypothalamus tumor

Conflict	Giving up on everything. Throwing it all away. Along with the fear of death, the classic diagnosis-shock conflict.
Examples	• *A woman goes to the hospital to have a large lump in her breast examined. The doctor tells her flat out that she has only 4 months left to live. The woman has a nervous breakdown.* (Archive B. Eybl)
Conflict-active	Wide-ranging hormonal and vegetative imbalance: restlessness, sleeplessness, lack of appetite, sexual anomalies/disorders and much more.
	Hypothalamus tumors are extremely rare (adiposogenital dystrophy).
Bio. function	Only a completely new start can save a situation that is already in progress (similar to rebooting a computer). Through the shutting down of all values, the individual can achieve radically new insights.
Repair phase	Slow normalization of the hormone levels/the vegetative system, brain swelling.
Therapy	Determine the conflict, conditioning and beliefs and resolve them. Guiding principles: *"I will put everything that I previously did and thought to the test. What is live rally all about?" "Perhaps I may remain if I reestablish myself."*

ECTO

−+

ADRENAL GLANDS

The adrenal glands (glandula suprarenalis) are paired hormone glands located at the poles of the kidneys. According to Dr. Hamer, the stress hormones dopamine, noradrenaline, and adrenaline, are produced in the endodermal adrenal medulla. From the base substance cholesterol, the mesodermal adrenal cortex produces cortisol and aldosterone (also stress hormones) and male sex hormones.

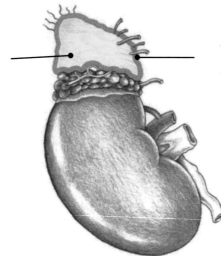

Adrenal Medulla
Too much stress

Adrenal Cortex
Conflict, being off track, wrong path in life

SBS of the Adrenal Cortex

Chronic Fatigue Syndrome (CFS), hypofunction of the adrenal cortex (adrenal gland insufficiency, Addison's disease)[1]

Conflict	Being thrown off course, taking the wrong path or having "bet on the wrong horse." Having made a wrong decision. Being on the wrong track/having fallen into the wrong hands.
Examples	→ *Distracted, an antelope loses contact with the herd (= mortal danger, start of the AC-SBS). Running further in the wrong direction, this program becomes active - it becomes tired. However, if by chance it runs in the direction of the herd, the brake is released - the cortisol turbo kicks in - and it gallops ever faster in the right direction. > In this way, it has the best chance of finding the herd again.*
	• *The young woman grows up in a sheltered environment. Due to marriage and quickly having three children, she finds herself in a difficult situation: The children keep her busy constantly and, in her opinion, her husband does not pay enough attention to her. It gets to the point where the partnership is in doubt = conflict of having chosen the wrong partner. In the hospital, she is diagnosed with adrenal gland insufficiency = active conflict. (Archive B. Eybl)*
	• *A man marries a woman of a different cultural background. At the wedding, he is confronted with these foreign customs, which he finds difficult to accept. He has the feeling he is making a mistake with this marriage. (See Rainer Körner, Biologisches Heilwissen, p. 257)*
Conflict-active	Tissue degradation (necrosis), reduced cortisol production > "stressed fatigue." Important SBS with chronic fatigue syndrome (CFS). The individual is forced to slow down when they are on the wrong path. In CM, acute adrenal hypofunction is called the Waterhouse-Friedrichsen syndrome. Chronic adrenal hypofunction = persistent conflict activity = Addison's disease > increased weakness and fatigue, lack of appetite (anorexia), nausea, weight loss, low blood pressure (hypotonia), low sugar levels (hypoglycemia), brown discoloration of the skin. In the repair phase of the relevant SBS, the cortisol values sink temporarily.

N E W   M E S O

−+

---

1 Dr. Hamer Charts pp. 67, 78

Repair phase	Filling out and restoration of tissue, increased production of cortisol or aldosterone.
Bio. function	An increased level of cortisol or aldosterone means an extra jolt of energy > despite vagotonia, the individual is extremely capable of performing. This way, they quickly get onto the right path and can compensate for the delay.
Questions	For fatigue: Since when? (Conflict previous). What did I change at that point in my life? (Changed partners, place of residence, job)? Did I make a decision that led me in the wrong direction at the time? What have I been wrangling with since then? Would I decide differently today? Fatigue only during the daily routine or also on vacation? (Indication of the conflict). Does the fatigue have anything to do with certain people? Did I make the decision myself? Do I support the decision? If no, why did I say yes at the time? Is there a similar pattern in the family? Am I carrying something inherited from my ancestors? If yes, will I allow myself to leave this pattern behind me?
Therapy	Determine the conflict and conditioning and, if possible, resolve them in real life. Guiding principles: *"I pause within and reorient myself." "I am allowed to decide anew." "I am free to determine my own way." "Now the journey can continue."* Grapefruit juice. If there is no improvement in the hormone levels and if the symptoms require it (persistent, unresolvable active conflict), CM hormone replacement therapy with cortisol or fludrocortisone (aldosterone).

Hyperfunction of the adrenal cortex with respect to cortisol (hypercortisolism, Cushing's syndrome) or with respect to aldosterone (hyperaldosteronism, Conn's syndrome)

Same SBS as above.
Chronic hypercortisolism resembles long-term cortisone therapy - high blood pressure, round and swollen face, bull neck, central obesity (abdomen), muscle atrophy = Cushing's syndrome.
Chronic high aldosterone level: high blood pressure, lowering of the potassium level (hypokalemia), causing weak muscles, possibly cardiac arrhythmia, constant thirst (polydipsia) and frequent urinary urgency (polyuria), especially at night = Conn's syndrome.

Repair phase	Restoration and refilling of tissue. Increased production of cortisol or aldosterone. **Persistent repair** = Cushing's disease (excess cortisol), Conn's Syndrome (excess aldosterone).
Note	In the active-phase of the corresponding SBS, the cortisol level rises briefly. Active kidney collecting tubules SBS probably also play a role in Cushing's Syndrome.
Therapy	Questions: see above. Determine the conflict and conditioning and, if possible, resolve them in real life so that the persistent repair comes to an end. Guiding principles: *"I am back on course and I can increase the tempo!" "God is guiding my ways." "Everything is okay again."* Bach flowers: hornbeam, oak. Surgery as necessary when symptoms require.

Tumor of the adrenal cortex

Same SBS as above! (See pp. 116-117)

Phase	Repair phase or **persistent repair** - restoration and refilling of tissue. A tumor that is as large as a fist develops; at the beginning there are fluid-filled cysts on the adrenal cortex > increasing growth of functional tissue = CM's "adenoma or cancer of the adrenal cortex," up to several kilograms in weight > increased production of cortisol or aldosterone = hyperfunction of the adrenal cortex.
Therapy	Questions: see above. Determine the conflict and conditioning and, if possible, resolve them in real life. Surgery if the size of the tumor causes problems in the surrounding areas.

SBS of the Adrenal Medulla

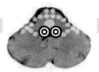

Tumor of the adrenal medulla (pheochromocytoma, neuroblastoma)[1]

Conflict	Extreme tension due to too much stress. Something seems impossible to get done, e.g., at work or school due to time constraints or personal reasons. "The going's getting tough."
Example	→ *Everything is getting to be too much. You do not know what to do first.* → *An employee is overworked; he has too many duties at the same time and is under pressure to do everything as quickly as possible.* → *Somebody caused a serious traffic accident.*
Conflict-active	Increased function, growth of an adeno-ca of secretory quality (= pheochromocytoma, neuroblastoma) > increased production of dopamine, noradrenalin or adrenalin - hyperfunction of the adrenal medulla. Symptoms: acute high blood pressure, racing heart, increased blood sugar, sweating, shivering.
Note	In the active-phase of the corresponding SBS, the adrenaline level also rises temporarily.
Bio. function	Extreme stress can be handled better. Extraordinary performance is made possible („natural-doping").
Repair phase	Function normalization, reduction of the tumor through fungi or bacteria (mycobacteria). Holes (caverns) in the tissue can remain. Persistent repair: hypofunction of the adrenal medulla. In the repair phase of the corresponding SBS, the adrenaline level also sinks temporarily.
Questions	When did the symptoms begin? (Look for the conflict in this time period). Questions to determine conflict activity: sleep, appetite, cold hands, dreams, high spirits and many more. What stressed me at the time (and probably up until today)? New job, demanding boss, partner stress)? What changed in my life? (Additional work, unhappy partner)? Why can't I handle it better? Have I spoken with the person it's regarding? What do I have to change inside myself so that it will get easier?
Therapy	Determine the conflict and conditioning and, if possible, resolve them in real life. Find out where the love is - there you'll find the solution. Guiding principles: *"There is nothing that can upset me." "Why should I get excited about that?" "Milky Way"* therapy. Bach flowers: olive, sweet chestnut. Surgery if the size of the tumor causes problems in the surrounding areas.

---

1   See Dr. Hamer, Charts pp.17, 27

THYROID AND PARATHYROID

The thyroid is shaped like a butterfly and lies underneath the larynx in front of the trachea (windpipe).

The main tasks of the endodermal parenchyma of the thyroid is to produce thyroid hormones (T3, T4 = thyroxine) and store iodine. The thyroid also produces the hormone calcitonin, which lowers the calcium level. Calcitonin is the antagonist to the parathormones of the parathyroid, which raises the calcium level.

From a historical development point-of-view, the endodermal thyroid and parathyroid once directed their hormones into the intestines; today they go directly into the blood.

The ectodermal excretory ducts of the thyroid once led thyroxine into the intestines.

One can imagine these excretory ducts as being like the gallbladder bile ducts, which transport bile from the liver into the intestines.

As far as I know, they no longer have a function but they still exist. Dr. Hamer discovered that they react with the so-called powerlessness conflict.

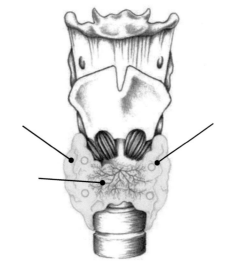

Thyroid Gland
**Chunk conflict,
to be too slow**

Parathyroid Gland
**Chunk conflict with regard
to muscle function**

Thyroid Excretory Ducts
Powerlessness conflict

SBS of the Thyroid Gland's Basic Tissue

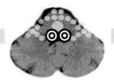

Enlargement of the thyroid, thyroid tumor (adeno-ca, autonomous adenoma, toxic lumps)[1]

Conflict	Chunk conflict (see explanations p. 15, 16). Not being able to grasp something (right thyroid) or not being able to get rid of something (left thyroid) because of being too slow. Simply stated: Conflict that one is too slow. Putting oneself under pressure to be faster or being put under pressure. Too little time for too many things.
Examples	• A retiree has worked for a family for years as a housekeeper. It is as if she were part of the family. One day, she is stunned when she is fired for being too slow! > She cannot hold onto her source of income because she is too slow. She develops a thyroid tumor in the active-phase. The tumor is surgically removed. (Archive B. Eybl)
	• An older employee feels that he can no longer keep up with the young people in the company. In his old-fashioned, thorough manner, he cannot keep up with the strict time limits. The firm's management would rather have a younger, more dynamic man in his position. They want him to retire. Soon afterwards, he is diagnosed with thyroid cancer > not being able to hold onto his job because he is too slow (chunk conflict). The tumor is removed. (Archive B. Eybl)
	→ Somebody has inspected a house that is for sale. A loan must be worked out with the bank. In the meantime, a cash buyer snatches up the house > not getting the house because of being too slow (chunk conflict).
	→ Somebody waits too long to sell his stocks and loses half his wealth as a result > not getting rid of the stocks because he did not sell quickly enough (chunk conflict).
Conflict-active	Increased function, growth of a compact, cauliflower-like adenoma tumor of secretory quality = "hard goiter (struma)" > increased thyroid hormone production > increased T3 and T4 levels in the blood > accelerated metabolism, and possibly breathing difficulties without coughing or hoarseness due to swelling. Possibly a recurring conflict.
Bio. function	With more thyroid hormones in the blood, the individual becomes quicker.
Repair phase	Function normalization, tubercular, caseating degradation of the tumor if fungi or bacteria are present > normalization of the thyroid hormone level. If no fungi and bacteria are present > the tumor is encapsulated. In this case, the thyroid hormone level remains high.

---

1   See Dr. Hamer, Charts pp. 20, 30

Questions	When did the tumor begin growing? (Conflict some weeks/months before). Did/do I feel I am too slow? Am I putting myself under pressure? Does everything always have to happen all at once? Goiter in the family? (Indication of family issue). What has conditioned me with relation to my conflict? (Parents, ancestors, childhood)? Which new, inner direction will I decide to take? What can I change externally?
Therapy	Find out what the conflict and conditioning are and, if possible, resolve them in real life if they are still active. Guiding principles: *"I am fast enough and satisfied with my speed. I set the tempo - no one else." "Haste makes waste!"* Bach flowers: impatiens, vervain. Hildegard of Bingen: lovage-mixture special recipe. Surgery, if the tumor causes a problem because of its size.

Hyperfunction of the thyroid (hyperthyrosis, Grave's disease)

Same SBS as above.

Phase	Conflict-active phase, usual **persistent-active conflict**. Increased thyroid hormone production caused by an increase in thyroid cells (adeno-ca). Symptoms: usually goiter, accelerated metabolism, ravenous appetite, warm and moist reddened skin, increased pulse, bulging eyes (exophthalmia), and wide open eyes, often weight loss due to high energy requirement, sensitivity to warmth, sleep disturbances, and lack of concentration.
Note	In the active-phase of the corresponding SBS, the thyroid hormone value goes up temporarily. By an SBS of the thyroid excretory ducts, there is also a slight increase in the amount of the thyroid hormone in the active-phase.
Therapy	Find out what the conflict and conditioning are and, if possible, resolve them in real life (see above). Avoid stimulants, such as coffee, black or green tea, iodized salt, iron preparations, and long sunbaths.

Acute inflammation of the thyroid (thyroiditis)

Same SBS as above.

Phase	**Repair phase** - degradation of thyroid tissue. Pain, reddening, swelling, possibly fever and night sweat. Even higher thyroxin levels temporarily due to the disintegration of the thyroid growth.
Therapy	The conflict is resolved. Support the healing process. Lymph drainage massages, curd cheese compress, apply cold compresses (e.g., cloth with salt water).

Hypofunction of the thyroid (hypothyroidism, myxedema)

Same SBS as above, if a thyroid inflammation took place. If not, an SBS of the thyroid excretory ducts is probably in progress (see next page). Symptoms: delayed development (in childhood), weakness, apathy, fatigue, sensitivity to cold, lack of appetite, constipation, dry, doughy, puffed-up skin (myxedema), sunken eyes (endophthalmus), reduced sweat production, slowed pulse and reflexes, low blood pressure, shallow breathing, weight gain, and high blood cholesterol levels.

Phase	**Persistent repair** or the condition thereafter. Excessive degradation of the thyroid tumor > falling of the thyroid values to levels under the norm > under-functioning of the thyroid.
Note	In the repair phase of the corresponding SBS, the thyroid hormone value sinks temporarily.
Therapy	Find out what the conflict and conditioning are and, if possible, resolve them in real life so that the persistent repair comes to an end. Medication with a thyroid substitute, if thyroid hormone production does not restart after the conflict resolution. However, if one begins medication early, the thyroid reduces production even more so that there is no way back > life-long medication is necessary. This is also true if one has opted for a total OP.

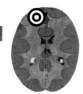

SBS of the Thyroid Excretory Ducts

Goiter without thyroxin level change (only TSH level + or -) (euthyroid goiter, euthyroid cyst, medial neck cysts)[1]

Conflict	Powerlessness or frontal-fear conflict (dependent on sex, "handedness," hormone levels and age). According to my experience, when it comes to powerlessness conflicts, the issue of being "too slow" always has something to do with it. Explanation: Powerlessness is a feminine-passive reaction to an approaching danger. One has to do something quickly, but feels powerless/helpless. One cannot stop something bad from happening. Time is running out. One doesn't do anything (but must) and is tense for this very reason.
Examples	Powerlessness conflict: (For examples of frontal-fear conflict; see p. 147f.) *"Something needs to be done urgently, but no one is doing anything!" "My hands are tied. I cannot do anything."*
	• *Over the course of a year, an intelligent, 9-year-old schoolgirl develops a moveable nodule just under the larynx. In the hospital, she is diagnosed via ultrasound with a 2 x 3 centimeter cyst (CM: "medial neck cyst" or "lymph angioma"). Conflict history: about three years before that, the little patient learns that her father is having an affair with her mother's best friend. After much "back and forth," her parents separate = powerlessness conflict on the part of the daughter. The little one longs to bring her father home to her mother. However, in this situation, she is helpless. Following two years of conflict activity, she slowly comes into healing, as it finally becomes clear to her that her father and mother no longer live together. She is fond of them nonetheless. Due to recurrences ("Why aren't Mom and Dad together anymore?"), the medial neck cyst described above develops. As the mother comes to understand that one thing is linked to the other, she wants to make a "family-campfire ritual" where the father is also present. (Archive B. Eybl)*
	• *A father receives a letter from the school informing him that his daughter is being expelled. The girl had been having repeated problems, but he hadn't expected an expulsion. (Archive B. Eybl)*
Conflict-active	Squamous epithelium tissue degradation (ulcer) in the thyroid excretory ducts, which are blocked in the meantime. Simultaneous slacking of the smooth muscle located underneath (ring-shaped portions) > increase in width. Painful pulling, slightly raised thyroid hormone production due to a functional linkage with the glandular tissue.
Bio. function	Widening of the ducts for better release of the thyroid hormones. > The individual becomes faster.
Repair phase	Restoration of the squamous epithelium, swelling but no pain, cyst development. This swelling is (also) diagnosed as a goiter or as a so-called medial neck cyst. In the case of syndrome, very large cysts develop. As these are not thyroid hormone producing cells (thyreocytes), but rather squamous epithelium cells, the level of thyroid hormones in the blood usually remains normal. (In CM: "euthyroid cysts of the thyroid" or "retrosternal or mediastinal thyroid cysts.") Possibly breathing difficulties due to swelling. Most often a **recurrent conflict**.
Questions	Symptoms/diagnosed when? (Conflict previous). Which situations am I powerless to face? Where do I think I have to do something? Which family pattern does my behavior prolongate?
Therapy	The conflict is resolved. Support the healing. In case of recurrences, find out what the conflict and conditioning is. Resolve the refugee conflict, if one is active. Guiding principles: *"I do not have to feel that I am responsible for everything." "I entrust it to God's hands." "Everything will be alright again!"* Bach flowers: rock rose, aspen, mimulus lymph drainage massages. Curd cheese packs, cold packs (e.g., cloth soaked with saltwater). Hildegard of Bingen: lovage-mixture special recipe. Spray the neck with colloidal silver, frankincense, and tincture of myrrh. OP, if the tumor causes problems due to size.

---

1 See Dr. Hamer, Charts, p. 124

Chronic inflammation of the thyroid (Hashimoto's thyroiditis)

According to CM, Hashimoto's is an autoimmune condition. Such a condition is not possible according to the 5 Biological Laws of Nature (see immune system, p. 18f). However, the disease pattern is real: It is characterized by a period of short, usually unnoticed hyperfunction, followed by lasting subfunction.

Phase	Thyroid subfunction due to **recurring conflict**. Symptoms: Tendency for constipation, listlessness (possibly diagnosed as depression), hair loss, dry skin, slow pulse. The TSH level is usually elevated, but sometimes also lowered.
Note	Determining which SBS (yellow or red group) is running is not always clear. It is advisable to take both possibilities into consideration in order to work out the individual conflict.
Q's/Therapy	See previous.

Hot lumps, cold lumps

Hot lumps, which can be determined through scintigraphy, are metabolically overactive areas of the thyroid tissue, usually associated with increased thyroid hormone levels. Cold lumps are metabolically underactive areas. They usually produce little thyroid hormones or none at all and thus, usually go hand in hand with underactivity.

Both SBSs come into question:
- **SBS of the thyroid gland** - recurrent conflict.
- **SBS of the thyroid excretory ducts** - recurrent conflict or persistent repair.

SBS of the Parathyroid Gland

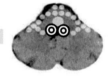

Tumor of the parathyroid gland (adeno-ca), increased parathyroid hormone (PTH) levels (hyperparathyroidism) and increased calcium levels (hypercalcemia)[1]

Conflict	Chunk conflict (see explanations p. 15, 16). Due to lack of sufficient muscle activity, not being able to get something (chunk) (right side) or expel something (chunk) not wanted (left side). Simply stated: One does not get something because of being too powerless, passive, inactive or lax.
Conflict-active	Hyperfunction - growth of a compact cauliflower-like (adeno-ca), of secretory quality. Increase in PTH producing cells = "hard goiter" (struma) > increased production of PTH (hyperparathyroidism) > increase in the calcium level due to depletion of bone calcium. By longer conflict activity, this can lead to decalcification of the bones (fibro-osteoclasis). Possibly recurrent conflict.
Bio. function	Increase in muscle activity through raised calcium levels.
Repair phase	Function normalization, tubercular-caseating degradation of the tumor, normalization of the PTH level or encapsulation if bacteria are not present. Parathormone level too low (hypoparathyroidism) due to persistent repair (excessive tumor breakdown).
Note	Not only calcium levels in the blood that are too low, but also levels that are too high can point to hypocalcemia.
Therapy	Find out what the conflict and conditioning are and, if possible, resolve them in real life if still active.
	Calcium supplements should always be combined with vitamin D (organically bound).

---

1   See Dr. Hamer, Charts pp. 20, 30

HEART

The approximately fist-sized heart lies behind the breastbone in the pericardial cavity or pericardium. The heart is made up of two halves: the strong-muscled left side and the thin-walled right side. Those are divided by a wall called the cardiac septum. Each of the two halves of the heart is divided into a fore-chamber (or atrium) and a main chamber (or ventricle). The chambers are connected via the mesodermal atrioventricular (AV) valves. The semilunar valves, which are also mesodermal, are found between the heart chambers and the large pulmonary and aortic arteries.

According to Dr. Hamer, the atria are mainly made of involuntary muscles and are controlled by the midbrain. The ventricles are made up of striated muscles and are controlled by the cerebral white matter (metabolism) and the cerebral cortex (motor) respectively. The pericardium (cerebellum-mesoderm) serves as protective wrapper and friction bearings. Its inner layer (epicardium) grows together with the surface of the heart. Its outer layer is the actual pericardium.

CM recognizes just one type of heart attack: Clogged coronary vessels restrict the supply of oxygen to the heart muscle tissue, which leads to their demise. If large areas are affected, the patient dies.

But why do post-mortem examinations of heart attack victims reveal "*pristine coronary arteries,*" while complaint-free, living persons have severely clogged coronary vessels (arteriosclerosis)? Why do stent-operated patients have no complaints at all, although their stents are already completely clogged after just a few years?

Once again, it was Dr. Hamer who cleared up this contradiction: He discovered that there are two types of heart attacks with differing conflict contents and differing control centers in the brain. One can die of both and one can survive both, depending on the severity and duration of the conflict.

The cerebral white matter-controlled conflict of being overwhelmed or outsmarted affects the heart muscle and causes the death of tissue in the active-phase.

The cerebral cortex-controlled territorial-loss conflict affects the coronary vessels and causes arteriosclerosis in the repair phase.

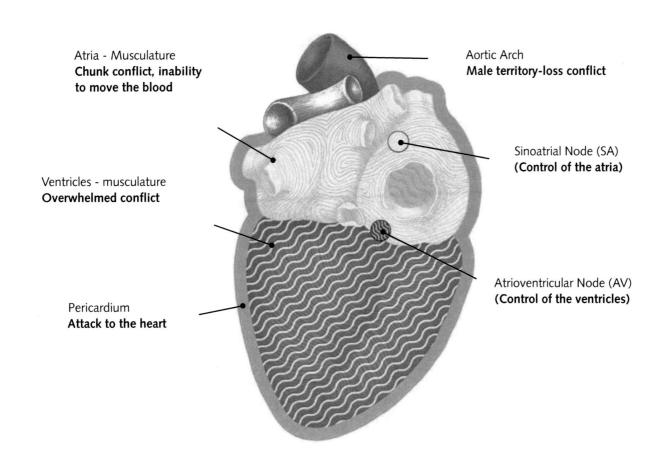

Atria - Musculature
Chunk conflict, inability to move the blood

Ventricles - musculature
Overwhelmed conflict

Pericardium
Attack to the heart

Aortic Arch
Male territory-loss conflict

Sinoatrial Node (SA)
(Control of the atria)

Atrioventricular Node (AV)
(Control of the ventricles)

Side note: The heart is not a pump

The technical data of the heart and blood circulation casts doubt on CM's pump theory: A pump, weighting 300 g (11 oz) and operating at 70 W, is supposed to push blood, which has five times the viscosity (thickness) of water, through thousands of kilometers - CM's estimate: 1000-100,000 km!) of vessels? 99 % of these are capillaries, which for the most part are so narrow that the red-blood cells are pressed into single-file in order to pass through.

As early as 1860, Chauveau and Lortet observed that during the systolic phase, the pressure in the left ventricle is lower than the aortic pressure, which, according to the pump theory, is impossible.

Bremer observed the blood circulation of very young chick embryos before the formation of the heart valves. He determined that the blood, without any apparent driving mechanism, moved forward around the chick's own vertical axis in spiral form. The spiral-forming stream of blood is only strengthened by the pulsating heart.

A medium alone, however, cannot generate a vortex: There must be two unevenly viscous materials. Blood contains oxygen, carbon dioxide, nitrogen, etc. It is likely that these gases play a role in the generation of the vortex.

The Austrian water researcher, Viktor Schauberger, came to similar conclusions about fluid dynamics by examining whirlpools in rivers like Chaveau, Lortet and Rudolf Steiner did when they were observing the circulation of the blood.[1]

Conclusion: The pumping capacity of the heart is only sufficient for a few meters. The rest - let's say 10,000 kilometers - is pushed forward by the blood by means of peristaltic vessel impulses, vortices, and largely unknown suction forces. The heart's role may be better understood as the organ responsible for giving the impulses and keeping the beat.

---

1   See Raum und Zeit 1998, article series "Das Herz ist keine Pumpe" No. 91, 92, 93.

SBS of the Coronary Arteries

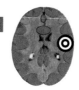

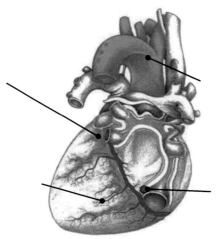

Coronary Arteries (red)
Male loss-of-territory conflict

Coronary veins (blue)
Female-sexual loss-of-territory conflict

Aortic Arch, Carotid Artery, Ascending Aorta
Male loss-of-territory conflict

Atrioventricular (AV) Nodes
(control of the ventricles)

Angina (pectoris) - chest pain/pressure/squeezing[1]

Conflict	Male loss-of-territory conflict or female loss-of-territory conflict (dependent on sex, "handedness," previous conflicts, hormone levels and age). Male loss-of-territory conflict means: loss of the entire territory or the contents of the territory. For example, someone loses his partner, his job or his rank. Someone loses his house, his business or his money. In the case of male loss-of-territory conflict, it is about the "external territory," in contrast to the female loss-of-territory conflict.
Example	For male loss-of-territory conflict (examples of female loss-of-territory conflict, see p. 165f):

• *A 50-year-old, right-handed man has a bad argument with his boss = loss-of-territory conflict. He feels that his territory has been taken away from him.* (Archive B. Eybl)

• *The father of a 9-year-old schoolboy is unfaithful. Afterwards, the marriage of the parents no longer functions - there is constant arguing = loss-of-territory affecting the coronary arteries of the boy. The intact family territory is gone.* (Archive B. Eybl)

ECTO

−+

---

1   See Dr. Hamer, Charts, p. 113

- *Whenever the early-retired teacher (left-handed, 56-years-old), thinks about her former boss, an authoritarian school principal, she gets angina. She has suffered from this affliction ever since one morning three years ago when she came to school too late and was confronted by the principal. On the outside, she was able to remain calm but inside she was extremely tense. On the way to school, she had a head-on collision, which she only survived by a miracle. Besides that, she was abandoned by her boyfriend, the "great love of her life," just a few days before. Because of this powerful combination, she suffered a male loss-of-territory conflict affecting the coronary arteries. (Archive B. Eybl)*
- *A 55-year-old, right-handed, professional printing worker has been suffering for the last 2½ years from cardiac arrhythmias (brief lapses). Conflict history: Five years ago, the old printing machine was replaced by a new one. The machine was the patient's sole responsibility and he grew attached to it. Now, the new machine is used by several coworkers at the same time. In addition, his salary has been reduced = territorial-loss-conflict affecting the coronary arteries. This has made the patient mildly depressed. Then, 2½ years ago, the patient was given a new job in the company and he came into persistent repair > cardiac arrhythmias. Therapy: decouple one's identity from company, strophanthin. (Archive B. Eybl)*

Conflict-active	Cell degradation (ulcer) of the sensitively supplied squamous epithelium on the inner surfaces of the coronary arteries (intima). > Increase in cross-section. The "hollowing out" of these vessels is practically never diagnosed because CM looks for narrowing (instead of enlargement). Squeezing pain in the heart (angina pectoris). Possibly recurrent conflict. An active territorial conflict has the tendency to make someone authoritarian, domineering; one underscores their power.
Bio. function	The luminal diameter of the coronary arteries is increased > better blood supply to the heart > increased heart performance in order to be able to win back the lost territory or territorial content. For instance, to be able to win back a job or partner (= second change through "BioTuning").
Repair phase	Repair and restoration of the squamous epithelium of the coronary arteries. Narrowing (stenosis) of the coronary arteries due to healing swelling = CM's "coronary heart disease" and/or "arteriosclerosis."
Repair crisis	Small heart attack (little conflict mass): Slowed, irregular heartbeat at rest or larger heart attack 2 - 6 weeks after the beginning of the repair phase, if not in constellation.
Questions	Chest pain since when? (Conflict occurred shortly before this). What territory is this about? (Partner, family, employment)? Does it feel better on vacation? (Indication of conflict in daily life). When is it the worst? (Focus of the conflict). Which stress is the hardest for me to deal with? Which feelings do I have during this stress? Similar feelings in childhood? (Determine the conditioning, e.g., mother wasn't there when I needed her the most or I was ignored during my childhood). Do ancestors also have heart problems? (Indication of family issue). Which similarities do I have with this/these ancestors? (Identify a common pattern).
Therapy	Determine the conflict and consider if one should resolve it, because when it has been singularly (without constellation) active for longer than 6 - 9 months, it may be followed by a heart attack. Consider: Should I focus on my development and take the chance of suffering a heart attack? My personal opinion is that it's worth the risk. When the conflict hasn't lasted too long, is low intensity or is a part of a constellation, the repair phase crisis is usually uneventful (e.g., short, stabbing sensations in the heart area while at rest). For your reassurance: The vast majority of us are in a safe constellation mode. In my experience, you can hardly control keeping conflicts unresolved anyway. (Goethe wrote: All theory, dear friend, is gray, but the golden tree of life is green.) Mental preparation: stay calm. Physical preparation: ouabain, in homeopathic form as g-strophanthin. All health inducing and strengthening measures, such as sufficient sleep, alkaline nutrition, etc. Heart strengthening foods: asparagus, honey, onions, red wine, red grape juice. Tea: rosemary, hawthorn, mistletoe, arnica, rose-blossom petals, etc. Hildegard: galangal powder and galangal-honey special recipe.

Heart attack coming from the coronary arteries (coronary heart attack), arteriosclerosis of the coronary arteries[2]

Same SBS as above.

---

2   See Dr. Hamer, Charts, p. 113

Phase	**Repair phase crisis:** 2 - 6 weeks after the beginning of the repair phase, the patient suffers a coronary infarction (CM: "heart infarction" or "heart attack"). Feelings of fear and the fear of death, intense chest pain, possibly extending into the back and the left arm, chills. Small heart attacks are much more common than a massive heart attack and are much less drastic in their effects. The pain does not come from the narrowing or closure of the coronary vessels, but from the strong sympathicotonic cramps of the vessel walls controlled by the cerebrum (according to Dr. Hamer: voluntary musculature) = local "vessel-muscle-epilepsy," which can also be generalized.
	With this type of heart attack, one finds "arteriosclerotic" coronary vessels, but no damaged or atrophied muscle tissue. Possible conscious absences (blackouts) or unconsciousness (syncope/fainting).
	The rhythm center for the slow heartbeat also lies in the male-territorial part of the cerebral cortex. This is why the pulse is irregularly slow during a heart attack. The pulse can drop to 3 - 4 beats per minute and is accompanied by very shallow breathing (earlier: "apparent death").
Therapy	If a heart attack is to be expected, see therapy on the previous page. Stay calm, procure ouabain. During/before a heart attack: ingest ouabain. If necessary, admission to a hospital for acute care. However, it is a judgement call, because CM's emergency care often does/administers much too much.
	Afterward: After intensive care for this SBS, CM will often try to perform bypasses or implant stents, which, from the perspective of the 5 Biological Laws of Nature, probably only make sense in the exceptional cases where one of the three major vessels is blocked. One must know that in the case of a blocked blood vessel, the body immediately forms parallel or bypass vessels (anastomosis) when a vessel is no longer passable due to injury or blockage = "natural bypass." A well-kept secret of cardiology is that stents or bypasses close up after a few months - nevertheless the patient continues to do well. See also p. 132f. > Consider these types of interventions very carefully.
	Even though the heart attack is a repair phase symptom, after surviving one, the patient should nevertheless work out the causal conflict in detail (see questions, p. 125). One should be sure that no recurrences are going to take place (because this would also mean further episodes). We can only be sure of this when we know the causes of the conflict. > *"I'm going to use my second chance."*

AV block (atrioventricular block)

Same SBS as above. (See pp. 124-125) AV block is an unnecessary CM term based on the false assumption that the drop in heart rate is due to a conduction disturbance between the atria and the ventricles.

From the view of the 5 Laws of Nature, the AV node, which controls the pulse rate of the ventricles, is directed by the right and left cerebral cortex and reacts to territorial conflicts. The AV node is the "sparkplug of the main chambers."

Symptom	Dramatic drop in the pulse rate (bradycardia) or cardiac arrest.
Phase	Repair phase - **repair phase crisis:** The pulse can sink very low, together with very shallow breathing (earlier "apparent death"). With longer conflict activity, it results in cardiac arrest.
Therapy	In CM, a pacemaker is implanted after emergency care. Pacemakers are probably useful in some cases: in chronic, recurrent, intractable conflicts. Their use must be considered carefully in each case.
	In my opinion - the symptoms should be the decisive factor rather than the patient's readings. (For additional therapeutic measures, see p. 132f.)

SBS of the Muscle-Nerve Supply

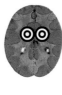

Myocardial infarction (infarction of the heart muscle)[1]

In the second type of heart attack, the heart muscle is affected, not the blood vessels.

Conflict	Conflict of being overwhelmed or outsmarted (cheated). Explanation: Being overwhelmed or outsmarted must also be seen in a social context, i.e., it has to do with other living beings (humans, animals). Being purely physically overwhelmed (e.g., sports, shovelling snow) is not enough. The fact that one has "too much to do" does not lead to a conflict of being overwhelmed or outsmarted. There needs

---

1   See Dr. Hamer, Charts, pp. 61, 72

to be a boss, for instance, that puts a person under too much pressure.

A common situation according to Ranier Körner: Someone wants to help another but cannot. > Helper syndrome: One can't stand to see others suffering and can't say "No."> Danger of burnout.

Examples

➔ *One "gets robbed blind by someone"* = conflict of being outsmarted.

• *The son of a right-handed patient is a "permanent student" = conflict of being overwhelmed, affecting the right heart muscle > cell degradation in the muscle tissue, myocardial infarction in the repair phase crisis during the repair phase. (Archive B. Eybl)*

• *A man has been together with a woman for 7 years when he realizes that she is just using him to support her = conflict of being outsmarted and three other conflicts. (Archive B. Eybl)*

• *A father learns that his son is probably going to lose his job, because he is unreliable = conflict of being overwhelmed - he cannot prevent the failure of his son. (Archive B. Eybl)*

• *A 64-year-old, right-handed, already divorced patient meets a man and falls in love with him. The beginning the relationship is very good, but as years go by her boyfriend gradually pulls away from her. He is often unfaithful and there are frequent arguments. The patient feels used and suffers from the rejection by her partner. Her weight drops to 49 kg (108 lbs). Conflict of being outsmarted or overwhelmed affecting the left partner-heart muscle. (Archive B. Eybl)*

• *A 54-year-old, right-handed man has a particularly good relationship with his grandson. He regards him as "his own child." They are like one in mind and spirit. When the boy is five years old, his daughter meets a man and decides to move far away to be with him = conflict of being overwhelmed by his grandson moving away affecting the RIGHT heart muscle (mother/child side - see note below). Three months later the man begins suffering severe heart attacks, which last for half a year = repair phase crisis = heart attacks. Then, everything is all right again. (Archive B. Eybl)*

Conflict-active

Demise (necrosis) of the heart muscle cells in one or several parts of the heart muscle = muscle atrophy. Athletic and physical performance drops more or less markedly. One should not burden oneself, for this could lead to a break (rupture) of the thinned-out heart wall - however, only during a massive conflict of being overwhelmed.

Repair phase

Restoration of heart muscle tissue in the affected area - beyond the original state = increase in muscle (CM: "myocarditis," "myocardial sarcoma").

Repair crisis

Smaller or more severe myocardial infarction (CM: "heart attack") according to the size of the conflict mass = local epileptic seizure of the heart muscle: increased, irregular heart beat (= CM: tachycardia dysrhythmia), heart trembling, ventricular flutter, ventricular fibrillation, possibly chills.

Light progression: increased pulse (tachycardia), "Heart throbbing, quaking in one's chest."

Infarction of the left ventricle: acute drop in blood pressure, so-called "circulatory collapse."

Infarction of the right ventricle: acute rise in blood pressure, due to the coupling of the muscle of the right ventricle with the left diaphragm (breathing assistance muscle) and the bronchial musculature, breathing is impaired: breathing pauses in the night (sleep apnea), respiratory distress, possibly respiratory arrest.

Bio. function

Thickening and strengthening of the heart muscle in order to better deal with future demands (= luxury group). The heart then has higher performance than before. (This only applies to a clean, two-phase process, not in the case of a recurring conflict).

Note

The cardiac system goes through a turnover during the course of embryonic development. For this reason, in the heart muscle and the other mesodermal parts of the heart (valves) the mother/child and partner sides are reversed. This means for the right-handed, a crisis of being overwhelmed or outsmarted with regard to the mother/child will affect the right heart muscle. With regard to the partner, it is the left heart muscle. For the left-handed, the mother/child relationship that affects the left heart muscle and in the partner relationship, the right heart muscle is affected.

With this kind of heart infarction, the coronary arteries are not "arteriosclerotic" - i.e., "pristine, unclogged blood vessels." In this, CM performs no stents or bypasses, yet they find perished or damaged heart muscle tissue (and don't know why).

We can also see this link between heart muscles and diaphragm in the so-called Roemheld syndrome. The heart muscle infarction can generalize, meaning the heart muscle convulsions can spread to the musculature of the musculoskeletal system > pattern of a "normal" epilepsy

Questions

To distinguish between coronary arteries and heart muscle: Was a coronary angiography carried out?

(If arteries are OK > heart muscle). Pain during the infarction? (If yes > coronary arteries) Decreased pulse during the infarction? (If yes > coronary arteries). When was the cardiac arrhythmia/infarction? (An overwhelmed conflict must have been resolved shortly before). First occurrence of the symptoms? (If no: Go back to the first episode and determine the conflict that happened/was happening at the time). What overwhelmed/stressed me? Did it have anything to do with helping? Why couldn't I deal with it? (Determine conditioning, e.g., during pregnancy, birth, childhood). Who "ticks" the same way in the family? (Find the conditioning). What formed this family member? Will I allow myself to leave this conditioning behind me? Is the conflict permanently resolved? (Estimation of recurrences). What do I definitely want to change in my inner/in my outer life?

Therapy	See p. 132f

Inflammation of the heart muscle (myocarditis)

Same SBS as above.

Phase	**Repair phase** - restoration of heart muscle tissue. Symptoms: weakness, fatigue, shortness of breath, possibly racing heart (= infarction).
Therapy	The conflict is resolved. Support the healing. Bed rest. Hydrogen peroxide (H_2O_2) 3% internally. Ouabain, possibly in homeopathic form as g-strophanthin (see www.strophantus.de)

Sudden cardiac death (SCD)

According to CM, during the autopsy, clogged coronary arteries are found in 80% of those who die from sudden cardiac death. This is a clear sign of a male territorial conflict affecting the coronary arteries.

The remainder - probably more than 20% - are thus attributed to crises of being overwhelmed in relation to the heart muscle. The characteristics of sudden heart death show that it occurs during the vagotonic phase, namely during sleep, in one's free time, while resting and in the recovery phase following sport activities.

Both kinds of heart infarction can occur here:

- Heart infarction coming from the coronary arteries (80%), loss-of-territory conflict - **repair phase crisis:** the center for the slow heartbeat (cerebrum right side) lowers the pulse rate toward zero > apparent or real death.
- Infarction of the heart muscle (about 20%), conflict of being overwhelmed - repair phase crisis.
- Sudden cardiac death during activity *(for example, an athlete collapses on the field):* usually a break (rupture) of the heart wall in the **active-phase** of a conflict of being overwhelmed > thinning of the heart wall > rupture through heavy strain.

SBS of the Heart Valves

Inflammation of the heart valves (endocarditis valvularis)

The four heart valves prevent the backflow of blood during and after a heartbeat. The tissue belongs to the mesodermal inner wall lining of the heart (endocardium).

Conflict	Self-esteem conflict related to the heart.
Example	→ *Somebody suffers from angina pectoris and other heart problems.* → *Somebody hears the diagnosis that something is wrong with his heart.* → *"My heart's no good anymore!"*
Conflict-active	Degradation of tissue (necrosis) in the heart valve tissue.
Repair phase	Restoration through increased metabolism and cell division = inflammation of the heart valve = filling up of "holes." Most often a **recurrent conflict.**
Bio. function	Strengthening of the valve.
Therapy	Questions: see below. See also p. 132f. CM: antibiotic therapy in the case of serious symptoms if necessary.

Ring calcification, narrowing (stenosis) of the mitral valve, calcifying aortic valve stenosis)

Same SBS as above. These diseases are regarded as being heart valve defects (mitral valve defect).

Phase	**Persistent repair.** Due to recurrences, scarred calcifications occur, usually at the edges of the valves. The scar tissue can diminish the tightness of the seal, reduce the closing function of the valves (valve insufficiency) or narrow the lumen (stenosis).
Note	A narrowing (stenosis) of the aortic valve hinders the thrust of blood from the left ventricle into the main circulatory system > this can cause the ventricle to widen (= pressure hypertrophy). The mitral valve lies between the left atrium and the left ventricle. If the mitral valve is narrowed (stenosis) or if the seal is not tight (insufficiency), the left ventricle is no longer completely filled up > the body increases the volume of the left atrium or ventricle (dilatation). Chronic mitral or aortic valve insufficiency becomes noticeable when a patient has difficulty breathing when strained (dyspnea).
Questions	When did the symptoms begin? (Conflict usually began long before the first symptoms). What was I thinking about my heart at the time? Was I sympathizing a lot with someone who had heart disease? Did I or did a loved one receive a serious diagnosis with regard to their blood or circulation? Were there those kind of worries during the pregnancy or in childhood? Have family members suffered from heart problems? If yes, am I similar to this family member? Do I carry these symptoms out of solidarity? (Work out the cause).
Therapy	Find out what the conflict and conditioning are and, if possible, resolve them in real life so that the persistent repair comes to an end. Guiding principles: *"I trust my heart." "I won't let anybody tell me anything else."* Read "The heart is not a pump" on p. 124. Hydrogen peroxide (H_2O_2) 3% internally. Ouabain, possibly in homeopathic form as g-strophanthin (see www.strophantus.de).Heart valve surgery, if the symptoms make it necessary.

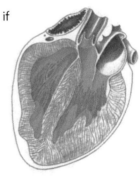

Heart Valves
**Self-esteem
conflict related
to the heart**

SBS of the Pericardium

Inflammation of the pericardial sac (pericarditis)[1]

Conflict	Attack-to-the-heart or anxiety about the heart (usually from a diagnosis).
Examples	➔ A real blow to or stab to the heart (blow, stab, electrical shock). Fear before a heart OP.

➔ *Mental attack: "You have a sick heart!" Or, "I have a bad heart." "I felt it deep in my heart!" Notification of a heart OP. May also be experienced vicariously.*

➔ *Pain in the heart region due to angina pectoris or heart attack (very frequent).*

• *A little boy loves his father, who has a heart condition, above all else. From the age of two years, he experiences, up close and personally, his father's attacks of angina pectoris. He is present when his father is taken to the hospital in an ambulance because of a "suspected heart attack" = attack-to-the-heart conflict, experienced as a proxy for his father. When he begins school, the conflict is resolved. The healing Hamer focus is diagnosed as a "brain tumor." The boy dies from the effects of CM treatment. (See Dr. Hamer, Goldenes Buch, vol. 1, p. 246).*

• *A 52-year-old farmer raises geese. Suddenly, in the middle of the night, the dog begins to bark. The patient runs outside to see what is going on. It is his neighbor, who is trying to steal his geese.*

---

1   See Dr. Hamer, Charts pp. 47, 52

At this moment, he is hit on the chest next to the left nipple with an axe = a real attack to the heart. 23 years later, after leaving his farm due to old age, he comes into conflict resolution with a major effusion of the pericardial sac. Over the intervening years, "his finger was on the trigger," i.e., conflict-active. (See Dr. Hamer, Goldenes Buch, Bd. 2, p. 488)

• *A 43-year-old woman wakes up at 3 AM because of a heart attack (repair phase crisis - right heart attack). She thinks she is dying. This happens several nights in a row. She is suffering from an attack-to-the-heart conflict.* (Archive B. Eybl)

Conflict-active	Cell division, growth of a pericardial tumor (= pericardial mesothelioma), usually unnoticed.
Bio. function	Thickening and strengthening of the pericardium in order to better fend off an attack.
Repair phase	Tubercular degradation of the tumor (pericardial tuberculosis) = pericarditis. Pain behind the breastbone, fever, night sweats. If the patient has no syndrome, the pericarditis is dry in the first part of the repair phase (pericarditis sicca). Afterwards, it is always moist (pericarditis exudativa). The border to the pericarditis effusion is seamless.
Repair crisis	Chills, severe pain.
Note	After the healing is complete, calcium deposits may remain. Following relapses, spotty or extensive adhesions of the pericardial layers (obliteratio percardii) can be found. A severe callosity of the pericardium (pericarditis constrictiva) leads to a lessening of cardiac performance due to reduced movement of the heart. Vicious circle due to diagnosis.
Therapy	The conflict is resolved, support the healing process. Guiding principle: *"My heart is only temporarily weak. The heart itself is all right. It is only momentarily inflamed, which is a good sign. Everything will be fine again."* Ouabain or in homeopathic form as g-strophanthin (info, sources of supply: www.strophantus.de). Lymph drainages, enzyme preparations, MMS. As necessary, CM pain medication. Hydrogen peroxide (H_2O_2).

Pericardial effusion (exsudative or transudative pericardial effusion)

Same SBS as above, but with **syndrome** (active refugee conflict - kidney collecting-tubules) in addition.

Phase	**Repair phase**: Buildup of tissue fluid between the two layers of the pericardial sac during the degradation of a tumor = pericardial effusion. In CM, this is often an indication of heart weakness (heart insufficiency). The heart is not weak, but rather, its motion is restricted in the full pericardial sac or, in the case of a pericardial tamponade, it can barely move > continually high pulse rate compensating for the reduced amount of thrust, labored breathing by strain. Usually a **recurring conflict**.
	In some people, the pericardial sac is separated into left and right parts; for others, it is open. Accordingly, there can be a right or a left pericardial effusion or an encompassing one (= circular pericardial effusion). The right pericardial effusion causes breathing difficulties, because the right side of the heart, which receives blood from the lungs, is impaired.
	Only in the case of syndrome (active kidney collecting tubules) can it come to a pericardial tamponade (massive effusion of the pericardium - one of the most frequent causes of heart-related deaths.
Note	The pericardial sac can also fill up with tissue fluid coming from the surroundings (usually the ribs or breastbone during healing). This kind of pericardial effusion is called transudative pericardial effusion. Here lies the danger of a vicious circle: A patient, who hears a diagnosis of pericardial effusion or "heart insufficiency" often sees this as a new attack to the heart.
Questions	Effusion since when? Which attack-to-the-heart conflict is being resolved? (E.g., diagnosis, heart ailments)? Are there indications of active kidney collecting tubules? (Water retention, weight problems, increased creatine levels)? Since when? (Possibly for a long time). What happened at the time? (Did I feel lonely as a child or shut out by my classmates)? Did my parents go through tight spots)?
Therapy	Resolve refugee conflict (kidney collecting tubules). Therapeutic possibilities, see p. 230ff. Guiding principles: *"I am safe and well provided for." "I am thinking about people who are completely alone and have no roof over their heads."* Visualization: The effusion drains away over the lymphatic system and becomes less and less. Do not take cortisone. If necessary, nonsteroidal, anti-inflammatory diuretic medications (diuretics). Puncture if necessary. See above also.

SBS of the Atrial Musculature

Atrial fibrillation (paroxysmal atrial fibrillation, arrhythmia absoluta)[1]

The atria of the heart are controlled by the midbrain via the sinoatrial nodes; the ventricles are controlled by the cerebral cortex through the AV nodes. The atria consist predominantly of smooth muscles related to the intestines. The intestine's principle of motion is rhythmically undulating (peristaltic) forward transportation. The rhythmic tightening and loosening of the atria corresponds with this principle.

Conflict	Chunk conflict (see explanations p. 15, 16) of believing that the heart cannot take care of the blood supply or does not pump enough. Fear that something is wrong with the heart. Possible substitution on behalf of a relative/friend. "Retired athlete or sports addict" conflict. Also in the figurative sense: conflict that someone can't keep the operation/business running (work or money turnover seen as pumping blood).
Examples	→ *Someone hears the diagnosis: "Narrowing of the carotid."* → *"Your coronary vessels are 80% congested!"* → *"We have found a blood clot in your daughter's brain!" (Substitute conflict)* • *A 61-year-old man is an avid mountain climber. In the course of a hernia examination in the hospital, the doctor measures his pulse and notices irregularities. Suddenly, he is regarded as an acute heart patient. Hectically, they put him on a stretcher and transport him to the coronary care unit, although he had just ridden his bicycle to the hospital. Twice, he is hooked to a 24-hour electrocardiogram > conflict, that the heart does not pump enough. He tells himself: "What is wrong?" Since then, the patient suffers from atrial fibrillation. (Archive B. Eybl)* • *An ambitious, 69-year-old, amateur racing cyclist is the oldest in his cycling group. This summer he had trouble keeping up with the others (pulse up to 190 according to his heart rate monitor). = Conflict that his heart can't keep up with his circulation needs. Since then he has atrial fibrillations. (Archive B. Eybl)*
Conflict-active	Strengthening and thickening of the smooth musculature of the atrium. Increased muscle tension.
Bio. function	With strong atrial muscles, the blood can be thrust forward more easily - thus, circulation is improved.
Repair phase	Normalization of the muscle tension. The thickened atrial musculature remains.
Repair crisis	Attacks of strongly accelerated peristalsis ("heart colic"). Atrial flutter, atrial fibrillation: racing heart, feeling disquieted. Up to 600 beats per minute, clearly diagnosed with the electrocardiogram, the so-called peristaltic waves being absent. Possibly chills. Usually a **recurring conflict**.
Note	Atrial fibrillation is among the most common heart rhythm disturbances, but it is not life-threatening. Sometimes it is seen simply as "an irregular pulse" or it is not noticed at all. Vicious circle: *"Something is wrong with my heart!"* > Often, an inner urge to always have control over the heart. (Blood pressure measurements, heart rate monitor, visits to the cardiologist, etc.)
Questions	Atrial fibrillation since when? (Conflict previous). Which stress did I have in relation to my heart or my circulation? Will I always remain top fit? (Sports addict conflict). Am I worried about someone else? (Substitute conflict). Do I have similar ancestors? Did my mother or father have problems with their heart/circulation during the pregnancy or in my early childhood? (Conditioning).
Therapy	The conflict is resolved. In case of recurrence, find out what the conflict and the conditioning are and resolve them. Guiding principles: *"My blood circulation functions perfectly." "I won't let anybody tell me anything else." "I'm going to slow down a little and enjoy life."* Ouabain, possibly in homeopathic form as g-strophanthin. (For information and sources see www.strophantus.de). For steps in the repair phase crisis, see heart attack. CM's current electrical cardioversion is rarely successful and, therefore, not recommended. The pharmacological (chemical) cardioversion using antiarrhythmic drugs is only sensible for short term use.

---

1   See Dr. Hamer, Charts pp. 37, 38

Cardiac insufficiency (heart weakness)

Possible causes

- **Pericardial effusion:** Attack to the heart: Heart insufficiency caused by reduced fullness of the heart (= diastolic heart insufficiency). Since the pericardium is filled with fluid, the chambers cannot fill up properly in the relaxed (diastolic) phase > performance drops even though the heart muscle is strong enough to pump. Effusion of the left pericardium "left heart insufficiency" > poor bodily circulation > lowered blood pressure, if severe: lung edema. Effusion of the right pericardium "right heart insufficiency" > weakened circulation in the lungs.

- **Heart muscle weakness** (= systolic cardiac insufficiency). SBS of the heart muscle (myocardium) in conflict activity > demise of heart muscle cells = myatrophy > weak performance (see p. 126ff).
- **Heart valve defects:** the most serious of these is a non-functioning aortic valve (see p. 128f).

Heart valve defect, heart valve leakage (heart valve insufficiency)

Possible causes

- **Cicatricial growths on the heart valve:** Persistent self-esteem conflict with regard to the heart > chronic heart valve insufficiency (see above).
- **Pericardial effusion:** Deformation of the heart due to pressure from the outside. Changes in the pericardial layers can cause tensile stress on the heart > temporary leakage of the heart

valve > heart valve "insufficiency" (see below).
- **Cell degradation or cell growth in the heart muscle** (myocardium). Shrinking of the heart muscle tissue (active-phase) and thickening in the heart muscle (repair phase) can "tense" the heart so that the heart valves leak temporarily or chronically (see p. 126ff).

Heart rhythm disturbances (arrhythmia)

Possible causes

- **Repair phase crisis of the coronary arteries:** decelerated, irregular heartbeat (bradycardia). Control of the slow heartbeat in the right side of the cerebral cortex = male territorial area (p. 124f).
- **Repair phase crisis of the coronary veins:** accelerated, irregular heartbeat (tachycardia). Control of the fast heartbeat in the left side of the cerebral cortex = female territorial area (see p. 165f).

- **Repair phase crisis of the heart ventricles:** accelerated, irregular or regular pulse, *"Heart pounding in one's throat,"* tachycardia (see p. 126ff).
- **Repair phase crisis of the atria:** atrial fibrillation (see above).

Therapy for heart attacks (both kinds)

The CM approach
Medicines that promote blood flow in the coronary arteries (nitroglycerin), tranquilizers against fear (benzodiazepines), pain medication (morphine) and beta blockers for stabilizing the heart rhythm. These are followed by a stent or balloon catheter surgery and/or anticoagulants (heparin and enzyme-containing medication).

Dr. Hamer is against this massive intervention. It seems better to accept the rhythm of "Mother Nature" and wait until the repair phase crisis has passed. However, one must honestly say that for lack of a New Medicine Hospital, we know very little about the right procedure in the case of an acute heart infarction.

The fact remains, CM's false assumptions have led to nonsensical therapies, which have not increased the chances of survival. According to my experience, and those of thousands of patients, the botanical hormone ouabain, also known as g-strophanthin, not only helps with heart attacks, but it also helps with all kinds of heart conditions.

It appears that this extraordinarily effective medication was removed from the market by the pharmaceutical industry during the 1960s for the sake of more profit.

As it stands in 2017, g-strophanthin is difficult to obtain except in homeopathic strengths. For information and sources see www.strophantus.de.

Follow-up treatment
In CM, anticoagulants are given. They "work" because they put the body under artificial stress (constant poisoning). Coumarins are used as rat poison and are even more damaging

than ASA. From the point of view of the 5 Biological Laws of Nature: **bed rest** is what is most important. Blood thinners for a few weeks maximum.

The current state of my knowledge according to the 5 Biological Laws of Nature

- Calm the patient and have them lie down with their trunk raised slightly.
- Give biological dextrose and maltodextrine 19 at short intervals.
- Cool the head: cold affusions, cold compresses, ice pack.
- Give ouabain/g-strophanthin.
- Possibly inject cortisone.
- Enzyme preparations (Wobenzym, for example), emergency drops (Bach Flowers).
- If breathing stops (right heart), injections of respiratory analeptics and cold affusions.

- Mental level > Guiding principles: *"It is good that I have resolved my conflict. Now I will get through the repair phase crisis as well. I will try to stay calm and relaxed, in spite of the pain." "I put myself in God's hands."*
- Bed rest, if necessary for six weeks. If one gets out of bed during strong vagotony, the blood can sink into the legs and lead to heart failure.

General heart-strengthening remedies

- Ouabain or in homeopathic form as g-strophanthin ingested best in combination with magnesium chloride ($MgCl_2$) - foot bath and hydrogen peroxide (H_2O_2) 3 % internally.
- Cod liver oil, linseed oil, colloidal gold.
- Teas: rosemary, hawthorn, mistletoe, arnica, rose petals and motherwort among others.
- Natural borax internally.

- Food: asparagus, honey, onion, red wine, red grape juice, among others.
- Garlic-lemon drink cure.
- Kanne Bread Drink.
- Hildegard von Bingen: galangal powder (Thai ginger), parsley-honey wine and galangal-honey special recipe.
- Breathing exercises.

BLOOD

Blood consists of over 40% solids (blood cells or corpuscles) and less than 60% of a watery fluid called blood serum. All blood corpuscles are made up of mesodermal tissue. This is no surprise, since the bones in which they are manufactured are also meso-dermal. Basically, we differentiate between red (erythrocytes) and white (leukocytes) corpuscles, as well as blood platelets (thrombocytes). See also: blood laboratory values on p. 37f.

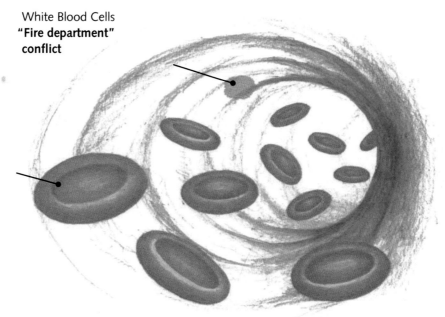

White Blood Cells
"Fire department" conflict

Blood Cells in General
Self-esteem conflict

Blood cells in a blood vessel

SBS of the Bone

Anemia (red blood cell deficiency)[1]

CM sees anemia as a shortage of red-blood cells (erythrocytes) or red blood pigment (hemoglobin).
Through this deficiency, the blood is thinner and those affected experience a loss of strength. Red stands for energy and combat - two important aspects of life (Mars energy).

Conflict	Generalized self-esteem conflict: little self-confidence and self-esteem, reduced will to live, little combat readiness, withdrawal/retreat. The cause can usually be found in childhood: One feels like they are not loved or valued enough by their mother. Women are disproportionately affected - at birth: *"Oh, it's just a girl."*
Examples	• *A child is delivered with the help of a suction bell. His condition is critical, so following delivery, he must remain in the hospital for two months. The mother is with him for part of the time and he is alone for the other part. When the boy is one year old, the parents begin to build a house as a "do-it-yourself" project. Now at the age of 9, he is often away from his mother again, staying at his grandmother's = generalized self-esteem conflict.*
	Unfortunately, the conflict recurs constantly because the boy has to go to school. On weekdays, he usually has cold hands; on weekends, his hands are warm. He always wants to sleep in bed with his mother. The red-blood corpuscles and the hemoglobin are lowered (restricted blood building = anemia). Moreover, he is too small for his age (restricted bone growth). The best therapy for the boy's self-esteem would be to allow him to be with his mother whenever he wants. (Archive B. Eybl)
	• *Following years of quarrelling with his wife, a married family father files for divorce. In court, the biased judge gives in to all of his wife's demands = generalized self-esteem conflict (bones) and ugly-genital conflict (prostate). At a physical check-up, his PSA is elevated (6.5). Now, the patient is at the mercy of CM's typical modus operandi: prostate surgery > impotence and incontinence > another self-esteem conflict > reduced blood cell formation > diagnosis of anemia > need for numerous blood transfusions. When the patient regains his self-esteem and enters the repair phase, he suffers from severe bone pain.* (Archive B. Eybl)
Conflict-active	Degradation of bone substance and, at the same time, reduced blood production (hemotopesis) in the bone marrow > reduction in the number of circulating blood cells **conflict-active phase** or during **recurring conflict** = anemia. Symptoms: fatigue, pale skin, feeling cold, problems concentrating. For laboratory values, see p. 37f.
Repair phase	In the first part of the repair phase, the anemia worsens, but only apparently, because the blood is "thinned" due to vagotonic widening of the vessels with additional serum (low hemocritic levels). In addition, vagotony intensifies the listlessness. The erythrocyte production is already underway at this point and for this reason the actual amount is already rising.
Bio. function	In the active phase: Whoever can't contribute anymore will be taken out of the running.
	After the repair phase: Whoever knuckled down and took up the fight will be stronger than before.
Note	Anemia can also be caused by a lack of dietary iron (malnourishment) and chronic bleeding (e.g., increased menstrual bleeding or bleeding from the esophagus, stomach or intestines).
Questions	Eliminate other reasons (extreme menstrual bleeding, other bleeding, iron deficiency). Anemia since when? (Conflict previous). Why is the self-esteem low? (Girl instead of a boy, childhood, teacher)? What is the parents' self-esteem? (Look for conditioning). What conditioned the parents? Am I going to fight if necessary?
Therapy	Find the conflict and conditioning and, if possible, resolve them in real life. Guiding principles: *"I am full of self-confidence! I love, value, and accept myself just as I am! I'm going to face life head-on and I want to fight for once!"* Awaken the Mars energy. 3x/week eat soup cooked with beef bone, fish, poultry. 1 tbsp of cod liver oil daily. Tea: elecampane (inula helenium), nettle, dead-nettle (utica), centaurium erythraea, sweet flag (acorus calamus), thyme, horsetail, ginseng. Food: beetroot, garlic, tomatoes, red wine, apple, black currant, honey, linseed oil (omega 3 fatty acids). Hydrogen peroxide

NEW MESO −+

---

1   See Dr. Hamer. Charts. pp. 65. 77

(H_2O_2) 3 % strength internally. Vitamin D3 (cod liver oil), natural borax internally (www.institut-ernaeh-rung-gesundheit.com). Bach flowers: larch, oak possibly, centaury. Hildegard of Bingen: Bertram powder (seasoning). Sunbathing, solarium, red light. Breathing exercises. Schuessler Cell Salts: # 2, 8. Spirulina alga. Garlic and lemon drink cure. If necessary, CM infusions with erythrocyte concentrate.

White blood cell deficiency (leucopenia)

Like the red blood cells, the white blood cells are also formed primarily in the marrow of the flat bones. They are called to inflammations (scene of the fire) and help there with the breaking down of foreign bodies and/or tissue respectively.

Conflict	Self-esteem conflict that one feels responsible for everything. One believes that they personally have to take care of all the problems (like the fire department and the white blood cells do) and, in doing so, reach the limits of their abilities. One always feels responsible for and tries to take care of everything. E.g., people who need physical care, the relationship problems of others, disputes at work). The typical conflict of first-born children or the siblings of handicapped people (early responsibility).
Example	• *A therapist who knows the 5 Biological Laws of Nature suffers through her son's very severe asthma attack. This causes her to have a substitute, self-esteem conflict in regard to the breastbone, because she cannot help her child and is powerless in this situation. In the active-phase, blood formation is limited. According to CM, she is diagnosed with leucopenia. The responsibility is best explained with her "susceptibility to infectious illnesses." As she recovers from this, she begins having severe pain at the breastbone and fourth rib = repair phase with an overproduction of white-blood cells. (See www.germanische-heilkunde.at/index.php/erfahrungsberichte).*
Conflict-active	Restriction of the blood production (hematopoiesis) in the bone marrow > decrease in white blood cells = leukopenia. If the blood formation does not start back up: **recurrent conflict**.
Repair phase	Small, unnoticed or actually diagnosed leukemia (see below and laboratory values p. 38).
Bio. function	At the end of the repair phase, more white blood cells are available. As such, inflammations in the body can be dealt with better. (Figuratively: One can take care of everything better).
Questions	Leucopenia since when? (Conflict since then and lasting up to today). Why do I believe that I'm always the one responsible? (Review childhood conditioning). Do I enjoy being used? Why?
Therapy	Determine and resolve the conflict and conditioning. Find out where the love is - there you'll find the solution. Guiding principle: *"I am easy-going and I put it in God's hands."* See above for therapy recommendations.

Leukemia, acute or chronic myeloid leukemia, chronic neutrophilic leukemia, chronic eosinophilic leukemia, polycythemia vera, mast cell leukemia, lymphoblastic leukemia, chronic lymphocytic leukemia, hair-cell leukemia)[2]

Same SBS as above. Leukemia is understood to be characterized by a large increase in the formation of white-blood cells, especially in their non-functioning early stages (myeloblasts).

Conflict	Self-esteem conflict (see above), but the conflict persists: I.e., one wrangles with taking on responsibility/taking care of everything, possibly with feelings of guilt. The diagnosis itself is then a real dilemma.
Examples	➔ *A child: "I am responsible for mommy and daddy fighting all the time!"* • *Eighteen months ago, a 50-year-old married woman is diagnosed with chronic lymphatic leukemia (CLL). Conflict pre-history: four years ago, the patient's husband suffered a brain hemorrhage - he lies in bed unable to speak. The hospital doctors explain to her that improvements are only possible during the first year. After that, everything will remain as is. After hearing this, she begins working day and night for her husband's rehabilitation. She hardly sleeps and pushes everything - her own job, housework and the children, to the edge of her limits = generalized self-esteem conflict. It all becomes too much > reduced production of blood cells in the spinal marrow. In addition to the burnout, she is diagnosed with anemia. Two years later, when her husband has almost fully recovered and can even ride a bicycle again, the patient falls into a deep vagotony. Always active and full*

2   See Dr. Hamer, Charts pp. 65, 77

of life before this time, she is now limp, tired, and has absolutely no energy. A diagnosis of leuke-mia is made based on a leukocyte level of 10,800 to 13,500 (normal values are up to 9000). This is followed by frequent blood tests and a sensible wait-and-see attitude on the part of CM (instead of chemotherapy). In the meantime, the patient has learned about the 5 Biological Laws of Nature and now sees her "illness" quite differently. (Archive B. Eybl)

• *A 30-year-old completes a trial period as a street sweeper. The hypercritical evaluation by his super-visor after three months: "I'm sorry, but you are not even capable of sweeping streets! Look for a job somewhere else!" = generalized self-esteem conflict. For six months, he is dejected and discouraged. However, he soon finds a new job as a salesman that suits him rather well = conflict resolution. In the leukemic repair phase, bone pain occurs throughout the body. (See Claudio Trupiano, thanks to Dr. Hamer, p. 253)*

• *A young mother refuses to breast-feed her two-year-old son, because she has a one-year-old daugh-ter, who has a greater need for the milk. The two-year-old, who was being nursed parallel to his sister, interprets this as "mother does not love me anymore" = self-esteem conflict with regard to the jaw. ("I am not allowed to suck anymore!") As the boy begins to recover from this rejection, he comes down with a 40-degree fever and sleeps for almost 48 hours. For six weeks, he shows all the signs of leukemia: He is so weak that he can hardly stand up, he has pain in his bones and especial-ly in his jaw, and he sleeps a lot. After six weeks, the little one has completely recovered. (See www. gnm-forum.eu/board)*

Phase	**Persistent repair** through recurrent conflict. Constant overproduction of white blood cells. Ahead of the leukemia, a leucopenia enters the active phase. Through the overproduction, many immature blood cells make their way into the blood stream. At the same time, the patient often has pain in their bones and all the signs of vagotonia (tiredness, headache, etc.). Exacerbated by syndrome (active kidney collecting tubules).
Bio. function	With many white blood cells, the individual can take care of problem areas better.
Questions	With children, usually a substitution conflict (shedding light on the parents' problems). When did the symptoms begin? (At the time, something large must have been resolved that was a heavy burden beforehand). Why have I taken so much upon myself? What conditioned me in this respect? What advantages to I get from having the illness? (I don't have to prove it anymore because I'm sick now - receiving attention/love).
Therapy	Determine the conflict and conditioning and permanently resolve. Find out where the love is - there you'll find the solution. Support the healing. Guiding principles: *"I don't need to carry this burden any longer - now it is easier." "I will keep my morale up even if it takes a long time." "God help me to remain patient."* Give in to theh fatigue and get a lot of rest. Hydrogen peroxide (H_2O_2) 3% internally. Natural borax internally. For advice on supporting the brain symptoms, see p. 60f. Blood transfusions if necessary.

Malaria - sickle-cell disease (SCD, sickle-cell anemia)

Malaria is caused by an infection by one-celled parasites (Plasmodiidae). The carrier is a specific type of tropical mosqui-to. The sickle-cell disease also occurs in areas prone to malaria and represents an adaptation to this disease. In its clinical picture, one finds - visible in a microscope - sickle-shaped, deformed red blood cells. The "disadvantage" of this disease is that some of the afflicted die (of so-called hemolytic crises). The "advantage" is that the survivors are hardly suscepti-ble to malaria anymore, because the malarial agent - the Plasmodiidae themselves - cannot tolerate this deformation of the red blood cells.

Conflict	for the species; the malarial pathogen has to be opposed somehow.
Conflict-active	Single individuals die.
Repair phase	Deformation of the red blood cells, to take away the ability of the Plasmodiidae to survive.
Bio. function	Defence against a life-threatening parasite to protect the species.
Therapy	In my opinion, the symptom-oriented measures taken by CM against malaria and the sickle-cell dis-ease are sensible, as are preventative measures against insect bites. Chemoprophylaxis is questionable. We don't yet know the psychic causes that allow the infection to manifest itself in individuals.

Anemia due to vitamin B12 deficiency (pernicious anemia)

A sufficient amount of vitamin B12 (cobalamin) is essential for the formation of blood. Cobalamin is produced from food by intestinal bacteria with the help of a stomach protein (intrinsic factor) and is absorbed through the small intestine. Symptoms: the same as those of ordinary anemia: fatigue, weakness, pale skin.

Possible causes

- Active self-esteem conflict (bones) + active territorial-anger conflict (stomach ulcer). (see p. 134 and 190f).
- The stomach's gastric parietal cells, produce too little intrinsic factor > recurring-conflict or persistent repair of the stomach's mucosa - conflict of not being able to digest something (chunk conflict, see p. 15, 16, 192).

- A disturbance in the absorption of vitamin B12 in the small intestine (malabsorption syndrome): recurring-conflict of the small intestine mucosa. Chunk conflict of not being able to digest something, usually with a starvation aspect (see p. 15, 16, 196f).
- Missing stomach or small intestine following a surgery.
- Vitamin B12 deficiency due to malnutrition.

Therapy

According to the cause.

Tendency to bleed (bruising, nosebleeds), hemophilia

Blood clotting represents one of the most complex biochemical processes in the body and cannot be definitively assigned to just one SBS. The liver, spleen, kidneys, bone marrow and blood vessels act together in concert here and for this reason, we have to speak of an SBS-complex. The body's goal is to have blood that is thin enough to flow easily, yet in the case of bleeding, clots quickly at the location of the bleeding. Hereditary hemorrhagic telangiectasia also belongs to this clinical picture.

The transition from a tendency to bleed to a blood disorder is a fluid one. Inherited hemophilia almost always affects men.

Conflict	1. Conflict that one was too closely connected with the family or a group and was therefore exposed to danger. One wants less family instead of more (distancing). Conflict that one should have gone their own way (divergent from the family way). 2. Conflict that one - themselves or an ancestor - endured such unbearable suffering that they wished to bleed to death.
Examples	• *A female patient is happy that she doesn't have much contact with her family. > Constant bruising, nosebleeds.*
Conflict-active	Reduced blood clotting. The severity of the clotting disorder corresponds to the intensity of the conflict.
Repair phase	Improved blood clotting. The blood becomes thicker through more blood coagulation factors.
Biol. sense	1: The body tries to effect a looser arrangement between family members (blood cells). 2: To have a painless death in the case of being wounded.
Questions	How do I stand in relation to my group or family affiliation? Bad experiences? What are my thoughts on bonds and freedom? What conditions me in this regard? What were my ancestors like? Circumstances of my ancestors' deaths? Was someone wounded/tortured? How do I feel myself in relation to this topic? How do I feel when I see war movies/people suffering?
Therapy	Determine and resolve the conflict and conditioning. The CM therapies for the tendency to bleed and hemophilia are recommended without a doubt.

Bleeding diathesis (hemorrhagic diathesis) - further causes

- **Bones: self-esteem conflict** in the active-phase: the hematocrit value sinks due to insufficient production of blood cells > thinning of the blood. At the beginning of the repair phase, the blood thins even more because of the widening of the vessels and inclusion of serum in the bloodstream > low-grade bleeding tendency (see p. 287ff).
- **Blood vessels: self-esteem conflict:** Due to persistent conflict, the blood vessel walls become brittle and are prone to bleeding. Usually capillaries are affected > dark red spots (petechiae): see p. 140ff

- **Kidney collecting tubules: refugee conflict** in the active-phase > fluid retention not only in the tissue, but also in the blood. Thinning of the blood, sinking of hematocrit > low-grade bleeding tendency (see p. 230ff).
- **Spleen: blood self-esteem conflict** in the active phase: Blood platelets are "caught" and "stored" by the spleen > the number of blood platelets circulating in the blood sinks > bleeding tendency (see p. 150).
- **Blood-thinning medications:** Phenprocoumon and aspirin among others. Chemotherapies also effect blood clotting.

Thrombosis tendency (thrombophilia), clotting tendency (hypercoagulability)

A very important SBS - better said, an SBS-complex (because again here, several organs are working together). The blood clotting tendency is common and represents the opposite of the tendency to bleed. Here, the blood tends to form clots, which is unfavorable, because this increases the likelihood of venous thrombosis, strokes, myocardial infarctions, lung embolisms and infarctions - a decisive factor in life expectancy. The thrombosis conflict issue also occurs more often than that of the bleeding tendency.

Conflict	Not-sticking-together-enough conflict (solidarity conflict). The feeling that the family/group has to stick together better, so that one's self or someone from the family/group isn't exposed to danger. Typical for families that live in a foreign country: one is alone in a foreign land and has to stick together as a unit.
Examples	• *A 50-year-old woman has already experienced two venous thromboses (clear indication of this SBS-complex). Originally from France, she moved to Austria with her husband and raised four children. Due to her strong homesickness, she felt the need to keep her family very close together. On every birthday and holiday, the entire family is rounded up - only then is she happy. = Conflict that one has to keep the family close together.* (Archive B. Eybl)
Conflict-active	Increased production and release of blood coagulation factors (thrombin, among others) in the liver. Blood coagulation factors are protein molecules with a high binding capacity (like flour in the gravy). > Encourages plasmatic blood clotting and the formation of "red" thromboses when the blood flow is slowed (e.g., in the case of varicose veins or atrial fibrillation).
Bio. function	Improved connection between blood cells. - An attempt by the body to intensify the connection between family members (blood cells).
Repair phase	This SBS is more or less always running in the background. I assume that with the resolution of the conflict, a slow improvement of the flow properties can be expected. In any case, the chances of experiencing thrombosis should decrease.
Note	The break-up of families and nations is unfortunately being driven by the forces at play in the world (small children into nurseries, elders into nursing homes, individualization, the promotion of alternative lifestyles and multicultural identity). The almost universal use of blood thinners by older people (one of the most proscribed medications) is its counterpart at the medical level. > Destruction of the organic connections.
Questions	Why is the cohesion of my family in danger? Did we have to leave our homeland/region/move away from the family in the countryside into the city? Would I like to have a better sense of being connected? (More contact with family members, getting together more often, more correspondence)? What has conditioned me in this regard? (History of the ancestors; ask my parents)? What can I learn from this? What do I want to specifically change to resolve the conflict?
Therapy	Determine and resolve the conflict and conditioning. Find out where the love is - there you'll find the solution. Alkaline diet, regular endurance training outdoors, water treatments, sauna, proanthocyanidin (grape seed extract), garlic, hydrogen peroxide (H_2O_2) borax internally, CM blood thinners are prescribed too quickly. In my opinion, long-term medicating is rarely sensible. Phenprocoumon (brand name Marcumar) suppresses vitamin K in the liver and inhibits the production of coagulation factors. Coumarins (Marcumar) are also used as rat poison. Aspirin (acetylsalicylic acid) is less harmful.

AIDS

AIDS is not it's own "disease," but rather a composite complex arbitrarily compiled of about 30 different symptoms from lung infections to foot fungus by the AIDS propagandists at the WHO. AIDS is also not an "infectious disease." The HI virus has not yet been substantiated, nor have its disease causing properties ever been proven - by the way, this goes for all other so-called "infectious diseases."

AIDS or HIV was invented in 1983 by the physicians Montagnier and Gallo.

If we take a look back today at the events as they took place, we can literally watch this cash cow being led to slaughter.

"Shortly after the establishment of an HIV antibody test on the world market, Dr. Gallo and his colleagues at the National Cancer Institute published the discovery of an HIV-inhibiting substance. The whole world was amazed by the scientific achievements that followed: the discovery of the "fatal AIDS pathogen - HIV" came first, then the development of a selection test for the "HIV-infected" and finally, the presentation of a "cure." This cure is known as azidothymidine or AZT for short, zidovudine biochemically with the trade name of "Retrovir."[1] It goes without saying who the beneficiaries (profiteers) were and are (for the AIDS tests, see p. 41f).

According to Dr. Hamer, a positive HIV test can be the result of

---

1   See Dr. med. Heinrich Kremer, Die stille Revolution der Krebs- und AIDS-Medizin, 1. Aufl. 2001, Ehlers Verlag

a trigger caused by smegma (= foreskin secretions). This means that the affected person experienced a conflict while the odor of the male member "hung in the air" and was consequently stored in their subconscious mind.

Why do people die of AIDS?

- As a result of the diagnostic shock: fear-of-death conflict > lung cancer, territorial-fear conflict > bronchial cancer, indigestible-anger conflict > colon cancer, etc.
- As a result of social isolation (desocialization) and the conflicts it brings. *For example, "Watch out when you're with him - he has AIDS!"*
- As a result of an actual disease, which was present before the diagnosis and through which, now becomes more significant.
- From the multi-chemo cocktail.

Those who survive for a long time are consistently those people who refused therapy, who somehow were able to accept the diagnosis, who recognized it as nonsense or at least doubted it or repressed it in their minds.

Therapy

- For the patient, the most important thing is to recognize AIDS for nonsense that it is, to leave the fear behind, and to stop the toxic therapy administered by CM.
- With the knowledge of the 5 Biological Laws of Nature, look at the individual symptoms as one does with every other patient, try to find the corresponding conflict and to resolve it.
- After the long consumption of chemicals, it is necessary to purify the body: avoidance of the "pleasure poisons," exercise in fresh air, consumption of organic foods, water treatments, sauna, etc. Hydrogen peroxide (H_2O_2), 3 % strength internally, natural borax internally (www.instituternaehrung-gesundheit.com), garlic and lemon drink cure. Linseed oil, omega 3 fatty acids, etc..

Polycythemia

Polycythemia is characterized by an increased number of red-blood cells in the circulating blood due to an increased rate of new formation in the bone marrow.

Possible causes

- **Bone SBS:** at the end of the repair phase, the number of blood cells is increased for a short time.

- **SBS of the lung or heart:** insufficient lung or heart performance > adaptation to inner oxygen shortage.
- **Exposure to high altitudes** > adaptation to ambient oxygen shortage in the environment (high altitude training, mountain climbing).

BLOOD VESSELS

According to CM, arteriosclerosis is the cause of heart attacks, strokes, pulmonary embolisms and other serious "illnesses." These "deposits" are considered to be the response to micro-injuries on the inner walls of the blood vessels or as "metabolic disturbances" and "mistakes of nature."

From the viewpoint of the 5 Biological Laws of Nature, this is not a matter of mistake; rather, it is a matter of (sometimes overreaching) repair measures that the body takes in the framework of a Significant Biological Special Program or SBS.

We have to look carefully at where the calcification is situated, for there are two conflict possibilities: certain arteries (those that develop from the branchial arches) react to territorial conflicts; all the other arteries and veins react to self-esteem conflicts. According to Dr. Sabbah, blood and blood vessels react to conflicts concerning the family.

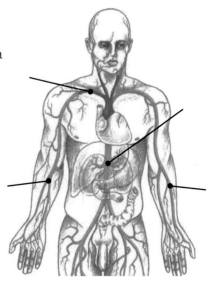

Aortic Arch, Carotid Artery, Ascending Aorta
Male loss-of-territory conflict

Abdominal Aorta
Self-esteem conflict, belief that the blood does not circulate well enough

All Other Arteries
Self-esteem conflict cut off from the flow of life or restricted by life's circumstances

Vascular Musculature (Blood Pressure)
Tension (stress) conflict

SBS of all Other Arteries

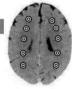

Hardening of the arteries (arteriosclerosis) of all other arteries[1]

Conflict	Self-esteem conflict with regard to the blood supply. Specifically: insufficient circulation conflict: 1. One feels cut off from the flow of life or the family. Life is passing one by. 2. One believes they have to make more effort (e.g., athletes) or more sales (businessman). 3. One feels constricted, like in a corset (by family, the conditions of their life, etc.).
Examples	• *A patient's husband forbids her to use their car to visit girlfriends or get on the internet. Due to this chronic recurring conflict a massive atherosclerosis forms in the right (partner) leg artery - and only there. (Archive B. Eybl)* • *An assembly worker works all day long with the attitude: "It should be going faster!" = Self-esteem conflict. After an extremely stressful period at the end of the year, he is diagnosed with an occlusion of the leg artery (= repair phase) > OP. (Archive B. Eybl)*
Conflict-active	Degradation of cells (necrosis) in the inner layer of the artery (intima), generally unnoticed.
Repair phase	Restoration and thickening of the inner walls by means of cell division. Pain, swelling = inflamed arteries (arteritis). Local thickenings as a remaining condition. Due to **recurring conflict**, plaque builds up, the vessel lumen get smaller = arteriosclerosis.
Bio. function	Strengthening of the arterial wall, so that the blood flow can circulate better.
Note	Nutrition plays an important role in the pathogenesis and treatment of vascular diseases. Consider "handedness" (right or left) and side (mother-child or partner) or if it is a local conflict.
Questions	Diagnosed when? (Conflict probably already long before). Left or right-hander? Which part of the body? What does one do with this part of the body? Am I affected by a cardiovascular disease (my own or in the family)? What are my biggest health worries? Do I feel cut off from life or my family? Was there a fight that isolated me? Am I carrying something from my ancestors? Why do I feel this way?
Therapy	See p. 144.

Intermittent claudication = peripheral artery disease

Same SBS as above.

Phase	**Recurring-conflict** or persistent repair: Excessive repair of the vessel wall > build-up of arteriosclerotic plaque in a large leg artery > decrease in the diameter of the vessel > obstruction of blood supply to the leg > leg pain and/or cold extremities due to oxygen shortages > walking must be interrupted with pauses because the muscles run out of oxygen = cramps in the calf of the leg.
Note	Probably combined with a brutal-separation conflict regarding the periosteum > bad circulation > shortage of supply to leg tissue (cold feet, pain in sympathicotonia). In the case of occlusion of large vessels, the shortage of oxygen can cause the outer appendages of the extremities to turn a dark color or to die off completely (gangrene).
Therapy	Questions: see above. Determine the conflict and conditioning and, if possible, resolve them in real life. Gymnastics, exercise, water treatments, classic/acupoint massages, lymph drainages. Hydrogen peroxide (H_2O_2) 3% internally and externally. Spirulina algae. Cod liver oil. For the rest, see: therapy for arteriosclerosis above.

Hemangioma (infantile hemangioma (IH))[1]

Usually on the face or the lips. 75% of cases are from birth onward and appear as a reddish-blue growth. As opposed to birthmarks like stork bite or a port-wine stain (firemark), larger and deeper-seated blood vessels are also enlarged and there is a tendency that the growth may grow further. > For this reason, attempt conflict resolution.

Conflict	Family self-esteem conflict with relation to speaking (lips), thinking (head), hearing (ear). In children, the cause always lies with the parents/ancestors.

---

1   See Dr. Hamer, Charts pp. 67, 79

Phase	**Persistent repair** or recurring conflict: rapid cell division in the wall of a blood vessel = hemangioma.
Questions	Were ancestors also afflicted by this symptom? How did the pregnancy proceed? What touches/moves me? Is there stress in the family regarding the topic in question? Do I have the same beliefs as my ancestors? Similar situation in life? What would serve to resolve the conflict?
Therapy	Find out what the conflict and conditioning are and, if possible, resolve them in real life so that the persistent repair comes to an end. Hydrogen peroxide (H_2O_2) 3% internally. Vitamin D3. CM beta blockers if necessary.

Aortic aneurysm (dilation) or narrowing (stenosis) of the abdominal aorta

Conflict	Self-esteem conflict of believing that the blood doesn't flow through fast enough or well enough. According to Dr. Sabbah: Conflict with a member of the family who wants one to do something in particular.
Example	➜ *During an examination, someone learns that the aortic blood vessels are badly clogged.* • *A patient has survived a heart attack. Afterwards, the doctor tells her that her heart performs only at 45%. She believes that not enough blood is circulating through her body. In the repair phase, it comes to an almost total occlusion of the abdominal aorta.* (Archive B. Eybl)
Phase	In a **persistent, active conflict**, tissue in the arterial wall is lost > weakness > aneurysm. In **persistent repair**, the aorta's inner skin thickens due to cell division > increasing narrowing (stenosis). Occlusion (blockage) of the aorta after countless recurrences.
Note	Normally, aneurysms are found in the abdominal aorta. Segments usually become arteriosclerotic = indication of a longer-lasting conflict. Bulges occur because of thinned, weakened arterial walls. Many aneurysms remain undiscovered because they are not noticed. If such an aneurysm breaks (ruptures), the patient's life is acutely threatened, because they bleed to death in the abdominal region (hemorrhage) > immediate surgery.
Therapy	Questions: see above. Find out conflict, conditioning and beliefs and resolve. Guiding principle: *"My blood circulates just as it should."* Hydrogen peroxide (H_2O_2) 3% strength internally and externally. Vitamin D3 (cod liver oil). Spirulina algae. By rupture: emergency surgery.

Vascular dilation in the face: telangiectatic rosacea, rosacea, rhinophyma

Rosacea and then a rhinophyma can develop out of telangiectatic rosacea. These three clinical pictures are superlative forms of the same SBS. The resolution of the conflict can bring about repair/improvement at every stage.

Conflict	Self-esteem conflict that one is not recognized/accepted by the family (blood relatives). According to my experience, when the nose is affected (rhinophyma), the patient feels like they are not, but should be, present enough at the center (of the family/the action). (Nose = center of the face).
Example	➜ *Someone feels excluded from the family.* • *A 60-year-old mother of three children is divorced from her husband. Unfortunately, she is not invited to some family events. She feels like an outsider - no longer at the center of the family, a place she had happily enjoyed. She developed rosacea on her nose.* (Archive B. Eybl)
Phase	**Recurring-conflict:** Weakening of the capillary vessels (new-mesoderm) during conflict activity (daytime), restoration in the repair (nights). Vascular dilation (telangiectatic rosacea) after months > over the course of several years (rosacea) > possible development of an enlarged, red nose (rhinophyma).
Bio. function	Through the reddening of the face/red nose, one attracts attention to themselves (like a red light). One shows the relatives that they have the same (related) blood flowing in their veins.
Questions	Where does the conditioning, that I don't feel accepted, come from? Who acts similarly in the family? Which internal reorientation(s) would be sensible and helpful? What can I change externally?
Therapy	Determine and resolve the conflict and conditioning. Find out where the love is - there you'll find the solution. Alkaline diet. Blood vessel remedy: proanthocyanidin (grape seed extract), ginkgo, horse chestnut, removal by laser as necessary AND conflict resolution.

SBS of the Smooth Vessel Musculature

HFs in the midbrain - topography still unknown

Raynaud syndrome (Raynaud's phenomenon)

In people with Raynaud syndrom, individual fingers or the fingertips suddenly turn white as if they were dying. This happens especially in cold weather.

Conflict	Not wanting to touch death or cold (animal) corpses.
Phase	**Recurring, active conflict/repair phase crisis.** Tension in the vascular musculature > insufficient supply to tissue > white discoloration, pain during sympathicotonia.
Note	The vascular musculature (new-mesoderm) also plays a role in this syndrome.
Example	• *The now 53-year-old woman worked reluctantly in her parents' butcher shop until she was 25. She was disgusted, always having to work with the meat. = Intense separation conflict in relation to having to touch the raw meat (animal corpses). In cold weather, she regularly suffered from Raynaud syndrome. At 43, she made the transition to her dream-job, massage therapist. Since then, the symptoms have not returned. (Archive B. Eybl)*
Questions	When did the symptoms begin? Experience(s) with dead people/animals? Corpse experience(s) with ancestors? Dead life forms?
Therapy	Determine the conflict, triggers and conditioning and resolve them if possible. Warmth treatments. Guiding principle: *"I recognize what was and make complete peace with what has happened."*

High blood pressure due to blood vessel tension

The most common type of high blood pressure. Lower or higher blood pressure is exceedingly family-specific. From this, we can conclude that we are dealing with a family issue, i.e., a conflict that usually goes back over generations.

Conflict	Tension (stress) conflict. One believes that you can only get through life by exerting force, by being a "mover and a shaker." One lets oneself be put under pressure or puts others under pressure. Dr. Sabbah: The family (blood represents the family) has to withstanding pressure/duress. In some families, there is the one who enforces order and the others who suffer under it. Through this friction, the blood pressure rises, at least on one side of the equation.
Conflict-active	Ongoing tension in the smooth musculature > increased blood pressure.
Bio. function	With the tension in the blood vessels, the flow of blood (family life) will be ordered more strictly. E.g., when someone stands up quickly, they don't experience a sudden drop in blood pressure. One is always ready to deal with any situation.
Repair phase	Blood vessel tension returns to normal as well as the blood pressure. Possibly fluctuating blood pressure during the repair phase crisis.
Note	Often, a performance mentality that spans multiple generations. People who are "wound-up" and get upset over every little thing. Many seem calm on the outside, but are still tense on the inside = lack of serenity.
Questions	Why do I think that I have to be involved in everything? How do I deal with the opinions of others? What are the unspoken rules in the family? Which member of the family is the judge? Does discipline make sense?
Therapy	Less judgement, order and discipline. More tolerance of others: "Let them be." Seen from conflict perspective, the positive effects of endurance training on high blood pressure are easy to see: One runs/hikes away from one's constraints and into the expanses where there are no pressures or requirements > relaxation of the vascular musculature > decrease in blood pressure. See also p. 65.

E
N
D
O

SBS of the Leg Veins

Inflammation of leg veins (phlebitis, thrombophlebitis)[1]

Conflict	Ball-and-chain self-esteem conflict. Restriction of personal freedom. One carries around the (old) burden. Conflict that one can't go back (just like the blood) or one feels that their family is a heavy burden.
Example	• *A young woman becomes pregnant and sees the child as a burden or "ball-and-chain." Her freedom is suddenly limited. Day and night, she feels chained down. In the active-phase, cells break down. The restoration = inflammation of the veins in the repair phase.* (Archive B. Eybl) • *The patient feels like he is "imprisoned" at the workplace. He is constantly thinking about everything that he is missing out on "outside." Varicose veins develop on his right (partner) leg.* (Archive B. Eybl)
Conflict-active	Cell degradation (necrosis) in the inner layer of the vein (tunica intima).
Repair phase	Restoration and thickening of the inner layer by means of cell division. Hot-reddened veins, pain, swelling = inflammation of the veins.
Repair crisis	Strong pain, chills.
Bio. function	Strengthening of the venous walls.
Note	Strong swelling is often wrongly diagnosed as thrombophlebitis (occlusion due to thrombus + inflammation), although it is usually just a normal inflammation of the veins coinciding with syndrome. Consider "handedness" (right or left) and side (mother/child or partner) or local conflict.
Therapy	The conflict is resolved. Support the repair phase. Wear support stockings, keep leg elevated, cold affusions, swimming in cold water, lymph drainage. Enzyme preparations, Schuessler Cell Salts: No. 1 and 3, alkaline diet, eat buckwheat often. Borax internally. Hydrogen peroxide (H_2O_2) internally. Hildegard of Bingen: Nettle juice and hemp compression special recipe. CM's heparin injections are useful.

Thrombosis of the leg veins (thrombosis, phlebo-thrombosis)

Same SBS as above.

Phase	**Recurring-conflict** - persistent repair. A leg vein thrombosis occurs when a vein, narrowed by arteriosclerosis, comes into the repair phase: swelling + arteriosclerosis plaque + **syndrome** = occlusion (leg thrombosis).
Therapy	Find out what the conflict and conditioning are and, if possible, resolve them in real life so that the persistent repair comes to an end. Resolve the refugee conflict if active. Guiding principles: *"I am free and independent." "I have the right to enjoy my freedom."* For measures to take, see inflammation of leg veins. CM's heparin injections are useful.

Varicose veins (varices)[1]

Same SBS as above.

The German word *"Krampfader"* (cramp artery or varicose vein) comes from the old high German "krimphan," from which the English words *crimp* and *cramp* are also derived. Crimped veins would perhaps describe the symptoms better.

Conflict	Ball-and-chain self-esteem conflict (see above).
Example	• *A 59-year-old patient is looking forward to the freedom she will have when she retires. She is already planning trips and other activities. Two years after the beginning of her retirement, her mother becomes disabled. Although her mother is in a home, nothing will come of the patient's plans,*

---

	because she has a bad conscience, when she doesn't visit her mother often. She perceives her mother as a "ball-and-chain." The conflict partly comes into healing when she is able to manage the situation better. Over the years, she gets varicose veins. (Archive B. Eybl)
Phase	**Recurring-conflict,** persistent repair - the veins gradually inflame > thickening of the veins. The vein valves are also affected by this SBS, which leads to scarred degeneration > leaky valves cannot hold up to the columns of blood (blood moving vertically against the flow of gravity) > widening, thickening, and twisting of the veins = varicose veins.
Note	Dr. Hamer says that where there is thickening of the veins, the involuntary (smooth) vessel muscles could also play a role: thickening in the conflict-active phase, through which nature balances out the thinning of the vessel walls. The involuntary (smooth) muscles remain thickened after the conclusion of the SBS > thickened "crimped vein." Consider "handedness" (right or left) and side (mother/child or partner) or local conflict (also injuries).
Questions	Did the varicose veins appear gradually or all of a sudden? (Suddenly would be an indication of a specific event as a cause). What makes me feel like I am tied down? (Child, invalid)? What do I miss? (Travelling, free days)? What would be the price of freedom? Which character traits can I develop through these limitations? Do my ancestors have varicose veins? Which common pattern is there? Which specific limitations did my ancestors experience specifically? Do I have to go on carrying this burden?
Therapy	Find out what the conflict and conditioning are and, if possible, resolve them in real life so that the persistent repair can come to an end. Guiding principles: *"I am as free and independent as a bird on the wing." "I let go of everything that is weighing me down." "I can do or not do whatever I want."* Physical exercise, sport, gymnastics, swimming, etc. Do not sit or stand for too long, elevate legs often. Keep body weight down. Kneipp applications, cold water treatments. Lymphatic drainage, massage. Support stocking. Hydrogen peroxide (H_2O_2) 3% strength internally and externally. Alkaline foods, especially buckwheat, linseed oil (omega 3). Colloidal silver internally and externally. Schüssler Cell Salts: No. 4, 9, 11, garlic and lemon drink cure. Cayce: Apply mullein leaves poultice and drink mullein tea. Liniments or poultice with cold, oak-bark decoction. OP, if complaints make it necessary. Do not have surgery at a stage that is either too early or too late. The measures above are also good for the recovery period after surgery.

Venous ulcer (open leg ulcer)

Conflict combination

- **Brutal-separation conflict,** afflicting the **periosteum** - active-phase or recurring-conflict > poor blood circulation - insufficient supply to the leg-tissue > cold feet, pain during sympathicotonia. (See p. 294f.)
- If the **veins** are affected (more frequent): **"ball-and-chain"** conflict - recurring-conflict > poor blood transportation due to degenerated veins and valves > vein inflammation, varicose veins, usually affecting the inner sides.
- **If arteries** are affected (rarer): **self-esteem conflict** regarding the blood supply and the localized area - recurring- conflict > poor blood supply - insufficient supply of oxygen - demise of tissue > usually the foot and/or leg outer sides are affected.
- **Disfigurement conflict** regarding the dermis (*"Just look at those varicose veins!"*) - persistent repair or recurring-conflict. Thinning of the dermis due to caseation.

Note
Worsening due to over-acidification, lack of exercise, constant standing, and being overweight.

Therapy
- Resolve the conflict, so that the repair phase can start.
- Alkaline diet, light, especially buckwheat , spirulina algae.
- Exercise, gymnastics and, if needed, bandaging to provide relief.
- White cabbage poultice (pounded until soft) on the affected area.
- Hildegard of Bingen: artemisia-honey special recipe or bryony special recipe.
- Colloidal sliver, natural borax internally and externally.
- If necessary, compression stocking.
- Hydrogen peroxide (H_2O_2).
- Vitamin D3, petroleum cure.
- For further measures, see varicose veins.

SBS of the Coronary Arteries

Arteriosclerosis in the coronary arteries, left and right carotid, ascending aorta, subclavian artery (A. subclavia dextra), and aortic arch

E
C
T
O

−+

Conflict	Male loss-of-territory conflict or female loss-of-territory conflict (depends on "handedness," hormone levels, and previous conflicts, see p. 165f and 247f for examples).
Tissue	Inner vessel walls - ectoderm. These vessel sections are descendants of the branchial arches and are lined with sensitive squamous epithelium.
Conflict-active	Functional limitation, simultaneous slackening of the underlying smooth musculature (ring-shaped portions). Later, cell degradation (ulcer) from the inner surface (intima) of the affected vessel (stumps): These vessel "caves" are practically never diagnosed because CM looks for vessel diameter narrowings (instead of enlargements). Pain in the conflict-active phase due to gullet-mucosa-pattern = angina pectoris.
Bio. function	The inner diameter (lumen) becomes greater > improvement of blood flow. Heightened performance in order to be able to retrieve the lost territory or territory contents. For example, to be able to win back one's job or partner (= second chance).
Repair phase	Repair and restoration of the squamous epithelium from within = CM's arteriosclerosis. This is often tied to persistent repair. Healing swelling > local vessel tightening (stenosis). Due to conflict recurrences or triggers, the layer (plaque) becomes thicker and more compact. With time, the plaque deposits harden the vessels = a complete picture of arteriosclerosis. Usually a **recurring conflict.**
Note	The most important principal substance for this repair is cholesterol. This fat-protein substance is the basis for almost all hormones and other important materials in the body (see p. 38). Arteriosclerotic narrowings (stenoses) of the carotid artery are diagnosed via ultrasound. Patients often become unnecessary fearful, since mild stenosis is normal with age. Deposits in the carotid are seen as a risk factor for stroke, which is not true from the viewpoint of the 5 Biological Laws of Nature. In CM, the health effects of a blood clot (embolism or thrombosis) are overestimated. Healing scabs (embolisms) can really clog the vessels, for instance, in the case of a lung embolism. However, in most cases the body sends the blood through parallel or neighboring vessels (anastomosis). After some time, the body dissolves the clot by itself (= "recanalization"). Problematic are embolisms in thick, main arteries, e.g., the legs.
Therapy	If chronic: Find out what the conflict and conditioning are and, if possible, resolve them in real life so that the persistent repair can come to an end. Alkaline diet, healing foods: apple, garlic, buckrams (Allium ursinum), spelt, buckwheat. Hydrogen peroxide (H_2O_2) internally. Borax internally. Ginkgo leaves, enzyme preparations, Schuessler Cell Salt no. 1. Blood-thinning medications are not recommended, unless they are used for a short period of time.

LYMPHATIC SYSTEM

Unlike the circulatory system, the lymphatic system is a "one-way street." In the venous angle (Pirogoff's angle)- which is located in the groove at the center of the collarbone - the clear fluid called "lymph" flows into the blood.

The lymph nodes are lined up on the lymphatic vessels like strings of pearls. The lymph nodes are the production site and "home" of the lymphocytes.

The lymph system can be described as the waste channeling system of the body. Its duty is to collect metabolic end products, cell waste and excess tissue fluids, which are then eliminated through the kidneys.

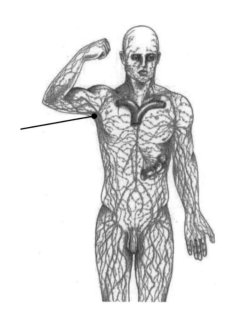

Lymph Nodes, Lymph Vessels
Self-esteem conflict regarding not being able to clean something, unable to remove a burden, unable to get rid of something unpleasant

SBS of the Lymph Nodes

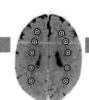

Lymph node inflammation or swelling (lymphadenopathy, lymphadenitis, mononucleosis), the lymphatics (lymphangitis), lymph node cancer (malignant lymphoma, Hodgkin's disease)

Conflict	Self-esteem conflict, not being able to remove or purify something in the affected drainage area. Not getting rid of a mess. Dr. Hamer: "Local self-esteem-collapse conflict." In actual sense: it's usually a tumor that's scary and one wants to get rid of. In a figurative sense: A burdensome thing one could not remove; unable to get rid of or purify something unpleasant or uncomfortable.
Example	• *A woman is terrified day and night because of a tumor in her right breast > Growth of the axillary lymph nodes, so that the tumor can be removed more effectively.* In CM, one now speaks of "metastases." (Archive B. Eybl) ➔ *Someone can't get rid of the poison that is splashed over him.* ➔ *Unpleasant work piling up - coming in faster than going out.*
Conflict-active	Degradation of cells (necrosis) in the lymph nodes - "holes" like in "Swiss cheese." Usually goes unnoticed as there is no pain if the conflict was felt locally; only local lymph nodes are affected. If the conflict was generalized, lymph nodes throughout the body or the spleen may feel affected.
Repair phase	Restoration and replenishing of cells through cell division (mitosis) in the lymph nodes > the diagnosis in CM: "malignant" = Hodgkin's disease. Inflammation of the lymph nodes, pain, swelling, and reddening. Increase in symptoms in the case of syndrome. After completion of the healing, the lymph nodes remain larger than before.
Bio. function	Strengthening and enlargement of the lymph nodes leading to higher capacity (luxury group).
Note	Consider "handedness" (right or left) and side (mother-child or partner) or local conflict. Lymph nodes and white blood cells (lymphocytes) work "hand in hand," for this reason see also p. 135.
Further causes	For swollen lymph nodes: repair phase "upstream." Any inflammation (= repair phase) is associated with increased metabolism and fluid formation in the intercellular space. The lymph nodes in the drainage area swell because plenty of fluids and waste products must be removed. No separate SBS of the lymph nodes (no division), but "high-tide" in the corresponding lymph section. For example, thick neck lymph nodes by the tonsils, throat or purulent tooth inflammation. Thickness of the inguinal lymph nodes with knee joint inflammation (see corresponding organ chapter).
Questions	Lymph node swelling since when? (The conflict must have been resolved shortly before this=). Where?

NEW MESO

−+

NEW MESO −+

What happened at this location? (OP, inflammation, pain, worry about a diseased organ)? Is it a substitution conflict? (Someone else is sick and one would like to remove it or there are accusations that one wants to be cleared up). In the case of children, always keep the parents/ancestors in mind. Which beliefs are at the root of it?

Therapy   The conflict is resolved. Support the repair phase, avoid recurrences. Elevated body positioning, rest. Lymphatic drainage, cabbage leaves poultice. Schuessler Cell Salts: No. 2, 4, and 10. Complex remedy Lymphomyosot. Teas: spiny restharrow (Ononis spinosa), elderberry, fenugreek. Spirulina algae. Garlic and lemon drink cure, colloidal silver internally and externally. Vitamin D3. Hildegard of Bingen: Columbine leaf special recipe. Lymphoma: Very large or aesthetically disturbing lymph nodes should be surgically removed - without chemo or radiation.

SBS of the Branchial Arches

Non-Hodgkin's lymphoma, cysts on the side of the neck (lateral neck cysts, branchiogenic cysts)[1]

In CM, non-Hodgkin's disease is called lymph gland cancer. However, Dr. Hamer has found out that it is not the lymph nodes that are affected by this "disease." Rather, it is the branchial arches. The branchial arches are an ancient building block of nature from the era of aquatic creatures. The branchial facilities of fish and amphibians, (which are also found in human embryos), develop into the gills.

In human beings, there are six branchial arches. These little, non-functioning pipes lie in the central compartment of the mediastinum and reach approximately from the neck to the diaphragm. They are lined with squamous epithelium and react with pain in the active-phase, following the gullet-mucosa pattern. Except in embryology or in the context of the cranial nerves (branchial arch nerves), CM virtually ignores these passages.

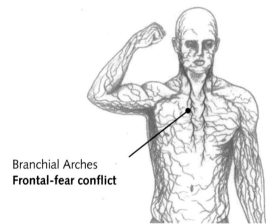

Branchial Arches
Frontal-fear conflict

ECTO −+

Conflict   Frontal-fear conflict. Fear of approaching, inescapable danger coming towards us and we cannot evade it; a conflict of powerlessness (dependent on "handedness," hormone levels and previous conflicts).

Examples   For frontal-fear conflict (for examples of powerlessness conflicts see p. 121):

➜ Fear of cancer.
• *A young woman does not like children. Every time she sleeps with her boyfriend, she fears she will become pregnant = frontal-fear conflict > cell degradation in the branchial arches in the active-phase, non-Hodgkin's lymphoma in the repair phase. (Archive B. Eybl)*
• *A 46-year-old, right-handed woman suffers from a frontal-fear conflict when her husband contracts kidney cancer. She becomes very interested in the subject and reads about the 5-year survival rates in the literature. She thinks to herself: "If he survives the five years, then he made it." Her husband survives the five years, and he is healthy; the patient comes into healing. Her neck swells up on both sides, she becomes weaker and weaker and has a dry cough. By means of a CT and an unsuccessful mediastinum endoscopy, a non-Hodgkin's lymphoma is diagnosed. Two years ago, her husband's cancer came back > frontal-fear conflict recurrence. They both know about the New Medicine, try everything, but his condition keeps getting worse. Existential conflict (syndrome), because of fear for the husband > the patient swells up with fluid. Two months before the death of her husband, the pressure on her neck is so strong that she goes to the hospital for an examination. Through a CT scan of the thorax, it is determined that the superior vena cava is completely closed off because*

---

[1]   See Dr. Hamer, Charts p. 111

of pressure from the branchial arches. At this point, her heart capacity is only 25%. (Archive B. Eybl)

Conflict-active	Functional limitation and later cell degradation (ulcer) in the branchial arches, simultaneous slackening of the underlying, smooth musculature (ring-shaped portions) > increased cross-section. Later, cell degradation (ulcers) in the branchial arches, slight pain in the neck.
Bio. function	Better flow-rate and better breathing through widening of the branchial arches (only to be understood through developmental history).
Repair phase	Restoration of the squamous epithelium accompanied by swelling, inflammation. Pain during the repair phase crisis. In CM, this is termed "non-Hodgkin's lymphoma," "lateral neck cysts" or "small-cell bronchial carcinoma." In the repair phase crisis, possible migraines or headaches (forehead). Through a **recurring-conflict**, cysts develop and become relatively large, especially during syndrome.
Questions	Tumor diagnosed when? (Look for conflict previously). Which danger did I experience? Was there an accident? What changed in my life at the time? (Ask about problems in career, relationship, family). Which beliefs led me into this situation? What is the earliest conditioning related to this issue? (Pregnancy, birth, childhood)? What were my parents feelings in this regard?
Therapy	With a tumor diagnosis, determine the conflict and conditioning and resolve if active. Lymph drainage massages, breathing exercises. Hydrogen peroxide (H_2O_2) 3% strength internally. Tumors in the mediastinum area are not operable, and are treated by CM relatively unsuccessfully with chemo - not recommended.

SBS of the Adipose Tissue

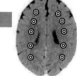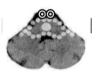

Lymphedema, cellulite on the legs, elephantiasis

Conflict	Self-esteem conflict of feeling unaesthetic on the legs and buttocks.[1] + **syndrome**
Examples	→ *A woman has heavy legs and feels unattractive because of them.* → *A child feels in the womb that the mother is dissatisfied with her legs and buttocks and that she feels abandoned > similar conflicts later in life.*
Conflict-active	Breakdown of adipose tissue (adipose tissue necrosis).
Repair phase	Restoration of the adipose tissue. In nature, there is no such thing as being too fat! A fat person is beautiful and desirable, because he or she is successful in getting food. Being thin happens through neglect. In persistent repair, a new buildup of adipose tissue varies. Usually a multi-generational conflict.
Bio. function	Increase in adipose tissue, thickening of the fat layer, because "fat is beautiful." Danger of a vicious circle.
Note	Getting out of this SBS is very difficult, because the daily frustration of glancing in the mirror or critical inspection of the "problem zones," puts one into a vicious circle. Possible accompanying causes: • **Desolate venal system**: SBS of the veins - "ball-and-chain" self-esteem conflict (see p. 143). When the return circulation from the legs is blocked, the lymphatic system has to step in as an "overflow system." The capacity limit is reached quickly. > Liquid remains in the inter-cellular space. • **Overeating and/or "junk" diet, lack of exercise**: In other words, constant standing or sitting, insufficient natural cold and warm stimulation, and effeminacy. **Always in combination with active kidney collecting tubules. Without syndrome, no fat legs.**
Questions	Why do I feel that I'm not beautiful? (Demeaned by father or mother)? Did my mother think she was beautiful? My grandmother? (No > family issue that wants to be healed, e.g., through open discussions, through meditation, family constellation) What is my attitude when I eat food? (Feelings of guilt, shame)? Is it possible that I gain advantages by being overweight? (E.g., being left alone by men, not being seen as a rival, a protective shield so that no one comes too close to me)? Which role does the

---

1   See Dr. Hamer, Charts pp. 60, 71

	body play at all in relation to the meaning of life?
Therapy	Find refugee conflict and self-esteem conflict and solve for real - e.g., get rid of the mirrors in the house. Accept body fully.
	Movement, exercise, swimming and do other sports instead of sitting.
	Support stockings by acute discomfort. Food restrictions or change in diet.
	Hydrogen peroxide (H_2O_2) 3% strength internally and externally.
	Vitamin D3.
	Kneipp treatment, lymph drainage, massage.
	Complex remedy: Lymphomyosot.

Swelling following acute injury or surgery

Following a sprained joint, strain, torn ligament, bruise, contusion or surgery, the affected area swells up = repair-metabolic increase. The injured structures are "put under water" in order to optimize the supply of nutrition, remove waste and to prevent tissues from sticking together.

The swelling limits movement (like a natural cast) > immobility = biological function. Strong swelling with syndrome!

Therapy
- Elevation, ice pack, lymph drainages.
- Cold compresses with curd cheese or clay soured with vinegar.
- Only gentle movement or light stretching.
- Enzyme preparation.

SPLEEN

The fist-sized spleen lies on the left side of the body underneath the diaphragm. For a long time, the spleen's function was not understood, as its removal seemed to have no physical effects worth mentioning. Today, we know its main purpose: the removal of old or damaged blood cells (via filtering and "devouring" = phagocytosis) as well as the storage of blood cells, especially thrombocytes for bleeding emergencies.

CM agrees with Dr. Hamer in that the spleen belongs to the lymphatic system and that it is, in principle, a large - although blood perfused - lymph node. The lymph system and the spleen are entirely made up of mesodermal tissue.

A healthy human being has a thrombocyte count of between 150,000 and 350,000 per liter.

Red Pulp:
Self-esteem conflict with regard to the blood.

White Pulp:
Self-esteem conflict, not being able to remove or clean something.

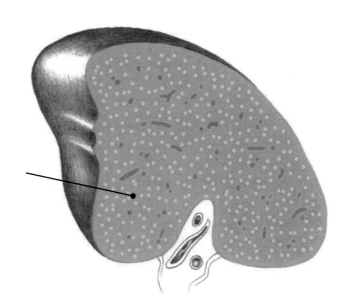

■ SBS of the Spleen ■

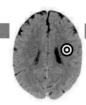

Spleen enlargement (splenomegalia), inflammation of the spleen (splenitis), splenic abscesses, splenic cysts

Conflict	1. Red Pulp: Self-esteem conflict in regards to the blood
	2. White Pulp: Self-esteem conflict, for not being able to remove or clean something
Examples	➜ *A human or animal is wounded or is bleeding = self-bleeding conflict.*
	➜ *Someone gets a "blood cancer" diagnosis or a blood transfusion. = Self-esteem conflict in relation to the blood.*
	• *A young woman has, because of an intestinal SBS lasting 5 weeks, large amounts of blood in the stool. = Self-bleeding conflict. Platelet count declines at this time to less than 5000 = active-phase. In the repair phase, the spleen swells. (Archive B. Eybl)*
	• *A very health-conscious woman has a complete blood count done. The blood lipids are increased. Fearful, she goes back to the doctor and wants to determine the values again and again. > "Something is wrong with the blood." = Self-esteem conflict in relation to the blood. (Archive B. Eybl)*
	• *The 28-year-old student is almost finished with his studies, only his thesis remains. Although the subject is fixed, he writes nothing for several months. "I should already be done with it, but I do not know where to begin." = Conflict, not being able to move something forward. Cannot "remove" the thesis from his to-do list. Healing comes when he finally overcomes the writer's block and completes the first pages > cell division in lymph nodes and spleen (white pulp). CM finding: "Numerous consistently pathological lymph nodes to 4 cm in diameter…the spleen with a longitudinal diameter of 14, 5 cm, is well above the norm…massive generalized lymphadenopathy." The patient knows the 5 Biological Laws of Nature, and can deal calmly with the diagnosis. By themselves, after the conflict resolution, the lymph nodes decrease by half their size. (Archive B. Eybl)*
Conflict-active	In the first place: Necrosis of the spleen tissue - empty spaces are created for storing blood cells. The number of blood platelets (thrombocytes) in the circulating blood sinks; they are "captured" and "stored" in these empty spaces. In the area of the injury, however, the thrombocytes assure fast blood coagulation. Secondly: cell degradation in the white pulp (spleen necrosis) - holes like "Swiss cheese." Only if the conflict was felt as generalized is the spleen affected - otherwise, only the lymph nodes react in the affected area (see p. 146f). The active-phase is mostly unnoticed - no pain.
Repair phase	Increased metabolism, cell division = inflammation of the spleen (splenitis). This causes the spleen to swell up (splenomegalia). Afterwards, the spleen remains enlarged
	A splenic abscess may occur during the repair phase through a recurring-conflict.
	Splenic cysts indicate a completed SBS or a recurring process.
Bio. function	At the end of the repair phase, the spleen is larger than before. > 1. This leads to better blood storage capacity and filter capacity. > From that point onwards, the body will be better able to deal with heavy bleeding and, in case of poisoning for instance, the body can remove more damaged blood cells from circulation. 2. Improved lymph node capacity.
Questions	1: Determine the phase: Blood count? (Thrombocytes increased/decreased)? Inflammation, pain? (> Repair phase). Which event brought on the repair phase? Splenic cysts: Have I ever experienced severe bleeding? Did I ever sympathise with someone who was bleeding/bled to death? Am I reading much too much into my blood count? Can I deal well with accidents? Were there dramatic bleeding incidents with my ancestors that have conditioned me? Dreams? 2: Enlarged lymph nodes in the body? Yes > What am I not able to remove? (Tumor, problem)?
Therapy	For inflammation of the spleen or an abscess, the conflict is resolved. > Support the repair phase. Lymph drainage massages, spleen compresses: wrap the abdomen in a warm, damp cloth with a dry cloth over it and go to bed (possibly soaked in salt water), garlic/lemon drink cure. Tea: fenugreek, fennel seed, kidneywort, toadflax, deadnettle, absinthe. H_2O_2 3% internally.

NOSE AND SINUSES

It is said, that of all the senses, the sense of smell has the strongest direct connection to the subconscious. Perhaps this is the reason why the nose reacts the fastest to an SBS in comparison to all other organs and why triggers (allergies) are so frequent here. The nasal cavity (cavum nasi) is connected to the four hollow sinuses between the nose and eyes (sinus paranasales) by narrow canals. The sinuses of the cheeks (sinus maxillaris), the sinuses of the forehead (sinus frontalis), the sinuses behind the eyes (sinus sphenoidalis), the ethmoidal cells (cellulae ethmoidales), also between the nose and eyes, and the nasal cavity are lined with endodermal intestinal mucosa and the ectodermal squamous epithelium that lies over it.

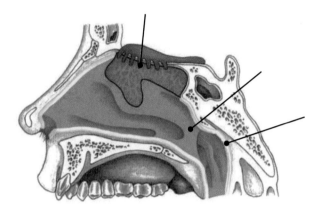

Olfactory Mucosa
Stinking conflict or territorial-scent conflict

Nasal Mucosa (ectodermal)
Stinking conflict or scent conflict

Nasal Mucosa (endodermal)
Chunk-stinking or scent conflict

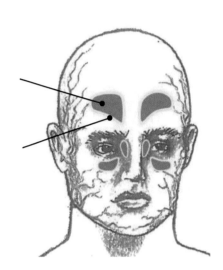

SBS of the Epithelial Layer of the Nasal Mucosa   HFs olfactory bulb in the cortex

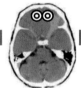

Cold (rhinitis), sinus infection (sinusitis)[1]

Conflict	Stinking conflict: Not wanting to smell something. *"This situation stinks!" "To get a nose-full." "Something stinks about it."* Also, scent conflict: The scent cannot be picked up. Not scenting (sensing) what or when something happens. (A dog lifts up his nose to pick up the scent. When he picks up the scent, he can assess the situation).
Examples	→ *Somebody is a non-smoker and is being subjected to heavy smoke by his friends.*
	• *Somebody feels that he is being bullied at work. He cannot put up with his colleagues anymore > "This situation stinks!" (Archive B. Eybl)*
	• *A 31-year-old patient is cutting firewood in immediate vicinity of a manure pit. Suddenly, the farmer comes with the tractor and begins to mix and pump away the liquid manure. An unbearable stench spreads over the patient's workplace, but he can't quit and escape the stench cloud because has to finish the work. = Stinking conflict. Two days later, he comes into healing = a cold. (Archive B. Eybl)*
	• *The pupils in a primary school class learn at the end of the school year that they will get a new teacher next year. = Scent conflict: "Not knowing what to expect." Three weeks into the new school year, some of the students come in healing as they realize that the new teacher is as nice as the old one. > Collective rhinitis. (Archive B. Eybl)*

ECTO
−+

---

1   See Dr. Hamer, Charts, pp. 122, 134

• The students at a high school are under pressure just before the Christmas holidays. Many of them flunk the math test. Stinking conflict: "These written tests stink!" During the holidays, half the class becomes ill = repair phase. (Archive B. Eybl)

Conflict-active	Limited functioning and later, cell degradation (ulcer) of the squamous epithelium mucosa in the nasal cavity or sinuses. The longer the conflict lasts the deeper the damage to the substance. Dry mucous membrane, no bleeding, possibly dry scabs. Usually, these symptoms remain unnoticed.
Bio. function	For stinking conflict: Blocking out the unbearable stench through functional limitation.
Repair phase	Restoration, swelling, and narrowing of the nasal cavity, breathing noises (Stridor nasalis). Itchiness, possibly nosebleed, and runny nose (cold). Aggravated by syndrome.
Repair crisis	Sneezing, nosebleeds, possibly a feeling of being cold or chills.
Questions	When was the last cold? (Something good must have happened, e.g., finally the weekend, a good conversation). Which stress did I have before this? (Couldn't stand something anymore or wasn't able to assess something properly)? Also determine the circumstances of the cold before latest one and, if possible, the very first one: Which common theme appears? Are they related to a certain person or to situations? Why do I have a problem dealing with this (the trigger)? Which conditioning or beliefs lie behind this? (E.g. "I'm just too stupid." "Nothing goes right when my mother-in-law is involved." "I have to plan everything or it won't work out right"). When did the belief system form? Does it come from the parents or ancestors? How can I separate myself from it? Can I change the external conflict situation? How? Which new attitudes do I want to develop/cultivate?
Therapy	The conflict is resolved. Support the healing. If recurrent, find out what the conflict and triggers are and resolve them. Guiding principles: *"It could be worse. It just stinks sometimes." "I will not take it so seriously and will enjoy life." "Even if I don't know what the future holds, I know that everything will turn out well, because I trust in God."* Tea: marshmallow, peppermint, sage, ivy, elderberry, marjoram, yarrow. Saltwater nasal rinsing, salt water or tea inhalations. Colloidal silver internally. Essential oil blend for Inhalation: cajeput, eucalyptus, lavender, thyme. Lymphatic drainage, hot foot baths, walks in cold air. Vitamin D3, Schuessler Cell Salts: No. 3, 8, 10. Hildegard of Bingen: pelargonium mixed powder- and fennel dill special recipe, tanacetum powder. If chronic: red light irradiation. Chemical nose sprays only if necessary (for example, before bedtime) and only for a few days. There is a threat of damage to the nasal mucosa and constant swelling when treatment is stopped.

Histamine intolerance

Histamine is primarily found in mast cells (type of white blood cell) and as a tissue hormone. One can also encounter high concentrations in certain foods: in fermented foods and drinks (cheese, olives, sauerkraut; wine, beer and vinegar). Histamine usually works as an allergy amplifier.

Conflict	Being-on-alert conflict: The world is unpredictable. One always has to pay attention, so that nothing happens. Often found in combination with choleric/aggressive people. "You always have to be on guard."
Example	*• A man's coworker is aggressive and unpredictable. The patient always tries to neutralize his fits of rage through "friendly persuasion." Over this period in time, he develops a histamine intolerance. When his coworker was fired, the symptoms disappeared. (Archive B. Eybl)*
Phase	Histamine **amplifies repair phase symptoms** and manifests itself primarily on the mucous membrane of the nose, eyes and intestines. Also, every neurodermatitis (epidermis) is amplified by histamine. Analogy: In the tissue, histamine lights a "fire" (inflammation) corresponding with the "fiery aggression" that is experienced in a conflict.
Questions	When did it begin? (Date as accurately as possible, work with a calendar if necessary). Which organ? (In the case that conjunctiva (eye) is affected: combination of visual-separation and being-on-alert conflict). Why/from what do I have to protect myself? Why am I on alert so often? What has conditioned

ECTO

me? Do my ancestors also have allergies? Is there a common pattern? Which belief system should I leave behind me? Which new attitude could be helpful? Meditating on something? Can I change the actual situation?

Therapy	Determine the conflict, triggers and conditioning and resolve. If that doesn't work: avoid situations of the type. Avoid foods that contain histamines. If necessary, short-term use of antihistamines.

Allergic "cold" (runny nose), hay fever, dust mite allergy (allergic rhinitis)

Same SBS as above. According to CM, allergies are caused by hypersensitivity of the immune system. The body's own defense cells (T and B-lymphocytes) are said to suddenly turn against harmless substances like pollen, excrement, and house dust mites. Actually, allergies are always based on triggers (see p. 24). The nose is often affected. In the case of anaphylactic shock, there was the danger of death during the conflict.

Examples	• *A 66-year-old retiree has suffered for the last 34 years from an extreme pollen allergy affecting the nose and throat membranes, as well as the conjunctiva of the eye. The allergy begins every year in May and can only be tolerated with the injection of cortisone and other strong medications. Conflict history: Forty years ago the young man, 24 at the time, and his wife wanted to have a child. Following a premature birth, the child died. Five years later, the head of obstetrics promises to do all that he can so that they are successful this time. When the woman gets pregnant again, she stays at the clinic starting from the third month so she can stay in bed until the child arrives. After 6½ months - on the 15th of May - she has another premature birth. Stinking conflict regarding the mucosa of the nose. Not being able to "swallow" the premature birth - related to the mucosa of the throat and visual-separation conflict - affecting the conjunctiva (eye). As a trigger, the May pollen becomes anchored firmly in the subconscious. The child weighs 1.5 kg (3.3 lbs) and is brought to another hospital where he is laid in an incubator. The doctor is not sure "whether he will survive the transport."The son is now 35 years old and suffers, probably due to the birth trauma, from the same pollen allergy as his father.* (Archive B. Eybl)

• *Allergic to wine: "The first time" - A schoolboy is in love with one of the girls in his class. One evening, during a vacation week, the young couple are allowed to go out and celebrate by themselves. Together, they buy two liters of white wine and drink it all. The girl takes the drunken schoolboy by the hand and leads him to a mattress on the floor. They want to sleep together but the boy is too drunk = stinking conflict. Whenever he drinks wine, allergic sniffles are triggered in the repair phase.* (Archive B. Eybl) |
Phase	The length of the conflict activity can vary between just a few seconds and several days. Usually, the conflict activity lasts briefly and then the repair phase lasts longer = **persistent repair** - allergic cold.
Note	An additional conjunctivitis points to a visual-separation conflict, a swollen throat to a conflict of not-wanting-to-swallow-something, tightened bronchi to a territorial-fear conflict or shock-fright conflict. (A conflict can start more than one SBS.)
Questions	See also above. When did it begin? Work out the accompanying circumstances: Pollen trigger? Which? In which month is it in the air? Which stress was experienced outside? (Find the correspondence with the time of the conflict). Triggered by cold/heat? (Time of year, gets better on vacation or while travelling)? Dust mite trigger: Stress in the house at the time in question? Moving house? Food trigger? (Stress while eating/drinking, argument at the table/in a restaurant/in the cafeteria)? Am I the only one in the family with allergies? (Determine the family issue)? What sensitized me? (Pregnancy, birth, childhood)? > Questions for the mother: what stresses her? Will I allow myself to leave this conditioning behind me? What could help? (Discussion, healing-regression meditation)?
Therapy	Find the conflict and conditioning and, if possible, resolve them in real life. If this fails, you can try a CM desensitization. Antihistamines are useful in acute or threatening conditions, but not for long-term intake. Before that, the gentle measures on p. 152 should be tried.

SBS of the Lamina Propria of the Nasal Mucosa

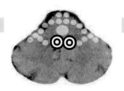

Purulent cold, nose polyps, suppuration of the sinuses (e.g., empyema of the frontal sinus)

Colds with yellow pus and suppuration of the sinuses indicate that either remaining pockets of endodermal intestinal mucosa or mesodermal connective tissue (the lamina propria underneath the epithelium) are being degraded. Nose polyps are bulges of this endodermal mucous membrane. They can develop in the nasal cavity or in the sinuses and hinder breathing.

Conflict	Chunk-stinking conflict. Not wanting to smell something: *"This situation stinks."* *"To get a nose-full."* *"Something stinks about it."* Also, scent conflict: not being able to sense something. Not being able to sense what will happen.
Examples	• *A young woman frequently has trouble with her parents. Most visits end disharmoniously. With her partner, she also suffers several bitter disappointments = stinking conflict - "Having it up to here (nose) with the constant arguing!" After three years of almost constantly purulent sinuses, the patient is suddenly symptom-free when the relationship with her parents suddenly takes a turn for the better = resolved conflict.* (Archive B. Eybl) • *An executive staff member of a technical office must look on as her boss makes one wrong decision after the other and steers the company in the direction of bankruptcy. More and more customers turn away. Once a month, she has a purulent nose and sinus infection. "I have had it up to here (nose) with this mismanagement!" = recurring stinking conflict. After the company goes bankrupt, the patient finds herself an interesting new job (= completely resolved conflict) and from that point on has no more sinus infections.* (Archive B. Eybl)
Conflict-active	Increased function, growth of a flat-growing tumor of absorptive quality or a cauliflower-shaped tumor of secretory quality (nasal polyps).
Bio. function	With more cells in the mucous membrane, one is better able to analyze and/or eliminate the smell.
Repair phase	Function normalization, inflammation of the sinuses, reduction of thickening of the mucosa or polyps by fungi or bacteria. Yellow-pus "cold" (runny nose), possibly fever and night sweats. During conflict activity, the nose may run due to increased production of clear nasal secretions (mostly **recurring-conflict**). Chronic discharge from the sinuses can cause sinus (forehead) headaches.
Repair crisis	Pain, feeling of being cold, possibly chills.
Therapy	Questions: see previous page. The conflict is resolved. Support the healing process. In the case of recurrence, find out what the conflict and conditioning are and resolve them. See also: measures on p. 152. When conflict resolution is not possible, nasal polyps above a certain size should be surgically removed (infundibulotomy) because of the possibility of respiratory obstruction.

SBS of the Olfactory Epithelium
HFs olfactory bulb in the cortex

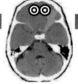

Loss or impairment of the sense of smell (anosmia or hyposmia)[1]

Colds cause insufficient air to reach the olfactory-mucosa (regio olfactoria) at the roof of the mouth.

There is also an impairment of the sense of smell with a cold, i.e., a conflict of the olfactory-mucosa (fila olfactoria). That is what this SBS is about:

Conflict	Stinking conflict - not wanting to smell something. *"This situation stinks."* *"I've had it up to here (nose)"* *"Something stinks."* Also, a scent conflict: not being able to sense/scent/sniff something. Not being able to sense/scent/sniff what or when something will happen to the person. (Dog stretches his nose up to sniff. He picks up the scent, he can assess the situation). This olfactory mucosa conflict probably has a territorial component, which is likely to differentiate it

---

1   See Dr. Hamer, Charts, pp. 141, 145

<table>
<tr><td rowspan="6" style="writing-mode: vertical">E C T O
−+</td></tr>
</table>

from the rest of nasal mucosa SBSs (territory-scent conflict).

Examples • *A mother gets a phone call from her son, her only child. He hurriedly tells her that he and his girl-friend are getting married. He says that the wedding will be kept to a minimum and so she will only be invited to the dinner after the civil ceremony = scent conflict affecting the olfactory muco-sa. During the conversation there is a foul, sour smell from the kitchen's garbage can in the air. For two weeks, the patient has this foul smell in her nose. She thinks that something about her clothing must have this smell and asks others whether they smell it too = smell paranoia in the active-phase. Note: here, we have a so-called smell-constellation, i.e., there is one Hamer focus to the right and one Hamer focus to the left of the olfactory bulb in the cerebral cortex. (Archive B. Eybl)*

Conflict-active Impaired functioning of the olfactory mucosa (hyposmia or anosmia) without cell degradation. Aromatic material cannot be discerned completely or only to a limited extent. One can smell pungent odors like ammonia or vinegar because they stimulate the other nose membranes.

Bio. function The blocking-off of unbearable stenches.

Repair phase Restoration of sense of smell - no cold.

Repair crisis Sudden loss of smell, analog to a sudden loss of hearing = sudden, brief impairment of the sense of smell.

Note In constellation, there is smell confusion (smell paranoia, e.g., cacosmia).

Therapy Questions: see above. Determine the conflict and conditioning and, if possible, resolve them in real life. Find out where the love is - there you'll find the solution. See cold (rhinitis), p. 153.

Nosebleeds

Possible causes

• Tendency toward nosebleeds in the repair phase, especially during the repair phase crisis of a stinking or scent conflict. The healing sores of the nasal mucosa bleed.
• Very strong nosebleeds due to thinner blood. See: tendency to bleed p. 137.

Therapy
• Depends on the cause.
• Bleeding: Bow the head slightly forward, close the nose with thumb and forefinger for 10 minutes, cool the back of the neck.
• Hildegard of Bingen: dill-achillea powder special recipe.

LARYNX

The larynx lies at the junction of the throat and the windpipe. It is made up of three cartilages, which are bound with muscles and ligaments. One protrudes as the so-called Adam's apple.

The two tasks of the larynx
1. Swallowing: when we swallow, the epiglottis closes the windpipe and leads the chewed food into the esophagus.
2. Making sound: with the help of the vocal chords, the larynx plays a role in the production of sound and language. The inner surfaces of the larynx and vocal chords are lined with squamous mucous membrane, under which lies voluntary (striated) and involuntary (smooth) muscles. The larynx is small. However, from the viewpoint of the 5 Biological Laws of Nature, it is an important organ, since conflicts of the larynx belong to the spectrum of territorial conflicts.

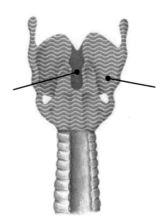

Larynx Mucosa
Shock-fright conflict or speechlessness conflict

Larynx Muscle
Shock-fright conflict or speechlessness conflict (motor)

SBS of the Larynx Mucosa

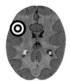

Inflammation of the larynx (laryngitis), cancer of the larynx (larynx carcinoma or papilloma)[1]

Conflict	Shock-fright or speechlessness conflict or territorial-fear conflict (dependent on "handedness," hormone levels, and previous conflicts). One is startled because of a sudden threat or noise. One cannot speak loud enough or scream (teacher and football coach conflict). *"So scared I couldn't scream." "To be scared to death." "Deer in the headlights, (rendered rigid and mute)." "The words are stuck in my throat."* Typically, the shock-fright conflict is the feminine-passive reaction to a threat. The territorial-fear conflict would be the male-active reaction. (Females tend to react with passive fright while males tend to react by attacking).
Examples	The following are examples of shock-fright conflicts: (examples of territorial-fear conflicts see pp. 161f)

→ *In a conference, somebody urgently wants to say something, but is unable to say a word.*

→ *Someone is put under pressure (be it for time or an appointment).*

• *A pregnant woman drives head-on into another car. She is thrown out of her car. She greatly fears losing her baby = shock-fright conflict. Degradation of mucosa cells in the active phase, restoration in the repair phase = laryngitis. (See Gisela Hompesch, Meine Heilung von Krebs, p. 57)*

• *A person is surprised with bad news over the telephone = shock-fright conflict. (Archive B. Eybl)*

• *The husband of a 60-year-old, married, left-handed retiree has been suffering with heart problems for the last several years. In the last months, they have been getting worse. Now, her husband is constantly asking the patient to do things and take care of things for him. She feels that her husband is robbing her of her personal freedom and time = shock-fright and territorial-fear conflict. The problem is that he is really starting to need more care and cannot manage by himself - her personal freedom is getting smaller and smaller. As her husband is sent off to a rehab-spa for a few weeks, the patient comes into healing (at least for the time being) > laryngitis and tightening of the larynx. (Archive B. Eybl)*

• *Four years ago, an entrepreneur turns over his company to his successor. He steps down just one step at a time, since the continuation of his life's work means a lot to him. One day, an old business friend with whom he has worked closely for the last thirty years contacts him and regretfully tells him that he wants to end their cooperation at the end of the year = shock-fright conflict (larynx), territorial-marking conflict (bladder) and chunk conflict (colon). Four days later, he comes into healing because he makes it clear to himself: "It is no longer your firm. It's none of your business. And it's not your fault, so don't drive yourself crazy!" (See www.germanische-heilkunde.at)*

Conflict-active	Functional limitation, cell degradation later in the squamous mucosa or the vocal cords. Simultaneous slackening of the underlying, according to Dr. Hamer, striated musculature. The voice may be weakened or altered. The conflict-active phase, however, usually proceeds without symptoms. No pain.
Bio. function	Through limited vocal ability and poor enunciation, one withdraws and has time to think (passive reaction).
Repair phase	Restoration of the larynx mucosa = laryngitis or cancer of the larynx: swelling, reddening, pain, alteration of the voice, rough voice, hoarseness or loss of voice. Strong swelling: the difficulty breathing in, along with syndrome. Cough due to "healing-itch." Often, **recurring-conflict.**
Repair crisis	Coughing attacks involving the larynx musculature, pain, feelings of being cold, possibly chills.
Note	Cancer of the larynx is diagnosed in the repair phase. Usually in combination with syndrome.
Questions	When did the inflammation of the larynx begin? (A territorial conflict must have been resolved shortly before this. E.g., through a vacation, reconciliation/discussion, a reunion). What was stressing me before this? What was I unable/not allowed to say? Was this the first episode? (If no, then work out the original conflict, because the later episodes are based on this one). What has conditioned me, making me unable to deal with the issue? (Early experiences in childhood, the mother's stress during pregnancy/birth or ancestral stress in similar situations > listen to the ancestors' story. Which new attitude is called for? Am I ready to leave the past/old issues behind me?
Therapy	The conflict is resolved. Support the healing. If recurring, find out what the conflict and conditioning are

---

1   See Dr. Hamer, Charts p. 124

and resolve them. Guiding principles: *"It can't cost me more than my head." "I am calm, for I trust in my divine guidance." "Next time I'll speak freely."* Walks in cold air. Compresses with curd cheese or salt water. Tea: mallow (Malva sylvestris), blueberry, lungwort, sage with honey. Schuessler Cell Salts: No. 3, 4 and 8. Colloidal silver internally. Vitamin D3 (daily dose of cod liver oil). Hildegard of Bingen: horehound and mullein-fennel special recipe

Vocal cord polyps

Same SBS as above. The main symptom of vocal chord polyps is persistent hoarseness. Sometimes cough.

Phase	**Recurring-conflict -** persistent repair: excessive restoration of the mucosa > growth of vocal chord polyps.
Therapy	Questions: see above. Find conflict and conditioning and resolve them so that the persistent repair comes to an end. Possibly removal via surgery, should the conflict resolution not change anything.

Stuttering (stammering)

Conflict	According to Frauenkron-Hoffmann: One is afraid (shock-fright), but doesn't scream - doesn't let it out.
Bio. function	Winning time - one has more time to give an answer.
Phase	**Conflict-active.** The impulse to stutter comes exclusively from the brain (no organ changes).
Therapy	Questions: see above. Determine and resolve the conflict and conditioning (e.g., ancestors didn't put things into words, repressed important words). In a regression, the screaming in the specific situations should be made up for. > Good prospects for recovery, because the brain's "switch" must only be flipped.

SBS of the Laryngeal Musculature

Constriction of the larynx - laryngeal asthma[1]

With asthma or constriction of the larynx, inhalation is impaired. This leads to prolonged and heavier breathing (gasping for air when inhaling). The SBS of the vocal cord musculature - what we're talking about here - is often coupled with an SBS of the laryngeal mucosa. In this case, there is both laryngitis and asthma at the same time.

Conflict	Motor shock-fright, speechlessness or territorial-fear conflict and additionally an active conflict on the opposite side of the cerebral cortex. (For examples see p. 156).
Conflict-active	Cerebral cortex-controlled restriction ·of innervation. Motor paralysis. Simultaneously, cerebral white matter controlled cell degradation from the laryngeal muscles (muscle necrosis). > Muscle weakening > end result "weak voice," (usually unnoticed).
Bio. function	Widening of the laryngeal lumen through relaxed laryngeal musculature in order to breathe better.
Repair phase	Restoration of the laryngeal musculature and return of innervation. Possibly laryngitis at the same time.
Repair crisis	Laryngeal asthma attack: coughing cramps or constant tension of the laryngeal musculature lasting from a few minutes to several days; feeling of being cold.
Note	The attack occurs only when the opposite right half of the cortex is conflict-active or also in the repair phase crisis (= constellation). It comes to a life-threatening "severe acute asthma" if the bronchial-muscular area (right cortex) is in an repair phase crisis at the same time as the larynx muscle area. With allergic laryngeal asthma, a conflict starts up briefly due to a trigger (CM: "allergen"). In the repair phase crisis, there is another asthma attack.
Therapy	Questions: see previous page. Determine the conflict and conditioning and, if possible, resolve them in real life. Guiding principle: *"I am quiet and calm and trust in my guidance."* Walks in cold air. Shred and eat radishes or hollow out radishes, fill with brown sugar or honey and swallow the juice that comes out. Vitamin D3. Tea: horehound, hibiscus, raspberry leaves, cowslip, English plantain, coltsfoot, Iceland moss, violet with honey. Bach flowers: rescue drops, aspen, cherry-plum. Cayce: mix horehound

---

1   See Dr. Hamer, Charts p. 124

syrup with whiskey and swallow in small doses. CM: inhalers (ingredients cortisone, anticonvulsants): Useful for acute attacks. Long term use is not recommended because of side effects.

Cough coming from the larynx, laryngitis with cough (croup = diphtherial laryngitis, pseudocroup = subglottic-stenosing laryngitis)[1]

Same SBS as above (conflict constellation). According to CM, croup and pseudocroup differ by the fact that for the "real croup" one can prove a diphtheria bacteria. Through the New Medicine, we know that one could prove bacteria even if it is called pseudocroup.

Therapy | Questions: see p. 256. As necessary, mucolytic and expectorant medications (secretolytics, expectorant). Dramatic coughing fits: remain calm. If nothing helps and if necessary, administer cortisone (inhaler). Note: Most synthetic cough syrups contain the morphine derivative codeine (addictive).

Diphtheria

According to CM, diphtheria is caused by the poison (toxin) of the Corynebacterium diphtheriae. The clinical picture is diverse: larynx, pharynx, nose and tonsil infection, swelling of the lymph nodes and fever.

The diagnosis "diphtheria" doesn't bring us very far. A more sensible course, like always, would be to examine the patient's symptoms and determine the conflicts.
Phase: one or more different SBSs in the **repair phase.**

LUNGS, BRONCHI AND TRACHEA

The lungs (Lat. pulmo), which are enclosed in the pleura, fill up nearly the whole chest cavity. The lungs are connected together by the windpipe (trachea) and the two main bronchi. The right lung is made up of three pulmonary lobes (lobi), and the left lung is made up of two. The smallest units of the lungs are the 300-400 million microscopic endodermal air sacs called alveoli, which together constitute a breathing surface of 80-100m². The alveoli are where the actual taking in of oxygen and giving off of carbon dioxide take place.

The wind pipes and bronchial tubes are made of cartilage and are lined with ectodermal epithelium. They belong to territorial areas controlled by the cerebral cortex.

The endodermal mucus producing goblet cells sit everywhere in the windpipe and bronchial tubes and provide the breathing apparatus with moisture.

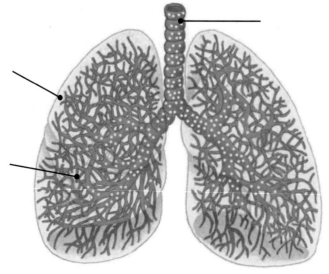

Alveoli
Fear-of-death conflict

Bronchial Mucosa
Territorial-fear conflict

Goblet Cells (yellow)
Fear-of-suffocation conflict

SBS of the Alveoli

Adeno-ca in situ of the lung, pulmonary tuberculosis (PTB), pneumonia (Pneumocystis pneumonia, pneumocystis carinii pneumonia, staphylococcal pneumonia, Klebsiella pneumonia, Legionnaire's disease), pulmonary abscess[1]

We can survive for relatively long periods of time without food or drink. Without air, we are dead within three minutes. In nature, not getting air means the same as the end of life. This is why the alveoli trigger a fear-of-death SBS.

Conflict	Fear-of-death, fear of dying or death. State of panic.
Examples	→ *Often due to a diagnosis or prognosis shock: "Your tumor is very malignant! Perhaps we can still stop its growth!"*
	• *An 11-year-old boy shares a bedroom with his siblings in the family farmhouse. As the youngest, he must sleep in the bed nearest the door. Unfortunately his older brother is an alcoholic. At 24, he still lives at home. The whole family is afraid when he comes home drunk at night, because he is extremely aggressive and unpredictable. One night, as he returns totally drunk, he attacks his younger brother with a kitchen knife = fear-of-death conflict. The boy can hardly be calmed down and after that he is allowed to sleep between his parents in their bed. Repeatedly, he is forced to face dangerous situations with his brother. Even the mother is helpless against him. As a security measure, they decided to turn on the light at night when the brother comes home. When the youngest boy is 15, his brother moves away for a job = conflict resolution. He is now diagnosed with an open tuberculosis of the lung = repair phase. Immediately, the boy is sent to a home far away for fear of contagion. He feels desperately abandoned there. His body weight goes up to 85 kg (190 lbs),(water retention due to an active conflict of feeling abandoned (refugee)). (Archive B. Eybl)*
	• *A sturdy young man is a non-smoker who enjoys diving in his free time. He is diving with his best friend when an accident occurs: Coming up from a dive, his friend develops a lung embolism and dies right there in the water in the arms of the patient = Fear-of-death conflict regarding his friend. An alveolar adenoma develops, because it is about someone else and not himself. After a month of difficult breathing, he is diagnosed with a cancer by CM. (See Claudio Trupiano, thanks to Dr. Hamer, p. 180).*
	• *The Olivia Case: A reporter from the popular news magazine, Spiegel-TV, is following Olivia, who is walking next to Dr. Hamer and calls out to them from behind: "Mr. Hamer, what will you do if Olivia dies the day after tomorrow?" At that moment, Olivia suffers a fear-of-death conflict. (See Pilhar, Olivia - Tagebuch eines Schicksals)*
Conflict-active	Increased functioning, cell proliferation in the alveoli, alveolar cancer of secretory or absorptive nature, mostly symptomless. In the case of fear of death for another person, a single (solitary) pulmonary nodule appears. For fear of death concerning oneself, several (multiple) pulmonary nodules appear.
Bio. function	With more alveolar tissue, air can be better utilized in emergencies > better exchange of gases > better chance of survival.
Repair phase	The normal biological process is the tubercular-caseating degradation of the tumor through tubercles = pulmonary tuberculosis (PTB) (CM-diagnosis: pneumonia, lung abscess) > bloody phlegm, bloody cough (hemoptysis), fever, and heavy sweating at night, bad breath (halitosis). Caverns remain. If no fungi or bacteria are present, the tumor becomes encapsulated with connective tissue and is closed off from the metabolism. However, the principle also applies here: A long period of conflict activity may allow the emergence of such large tumors that their size exceeds the body's ability to repair itself. > OP necessary. Tuberculosis has become rare in industrialized countries, because almost everything is found in the active-phase; thus, it rarely comes to tuberculosis in the lungs.
Repair crisis	Intense pain, chills, bloody phlegm, bloody cough.
Questions	First determine if you are dealing with adeno-ca (fear-of-death) or bronchial-ca (territorial-fear). (Examine the CM biopsy results). Bloody sputum? (Indication of an adeno-ca in repair). Night sweats? (Indi-

---

1   See Dr. Hamer, Charts p. 21

cation of repair, likely adeno-ca). Last lung x-ray when? (Indication of the time of the conflict). Coughing, night sweats when? (Indication of (partial) resolution). What panic did I have? Was I afraid for myself? For others? (Family member, friend)? Why did I react so sensitively? (Experiences in childhood, the mother's stress during pregnancy > find out all details). What new attitude would heal me?

Therapy
Determine the conflict and conditioning and, if possible, resolve them in real life. Find out where the love is - there you'll find the solution. Tuberculosis is not a trivial matter. The lung tissue temporarily loses stability. The areas of the pulmonary nodules "collapse." In the vernacular, "moth-eaten,"< no exertion, lots of rest, at least as long as the nighttime sweating lasts. Guiding principles: *"I understand how it all fits together." "I am patient and trust in nature." "Everything will be all right."* Clean, nutritious, protein-rich foods. Hydrogen peroxide (H_2O_2) 3% internally. Tea: horehound, club moss, comfrey, rosemary, thyme, English plantain. Hildegard of Bingen: elecampane root wine, bay leaf- or hedge rose-elixir special recipe. OP, if the tumor grows - better earlier than later.

Deterioration of the alveolar tissue (pulmonary emphysema)

Same SBS as above. With an emphysema, the exchange of gases is reduced. This causes chronic respiratory distress (dyspnea) and shortage of oxygen (hypoxia).

Phase
Recurring-conflict - The condition remains after many repair phases: if pulmonary nodules are degraded, holes in the tissue (caverns) normally remain (seen as circular shadows on an x-ray). Advancing emphysema causes more and more alveoli to lose their ability to function.

Therapy
Questions: see previous page. Find out what the conflict and conditioning are and, if possible, resolve them in real life so that the SBS comes to an end. Guiding principles: *"I am safe." "The danger has passed." "I am safe in God's hands."* Breathing exercises, stretching, gymnastics, yoga. Hydrogen peroxide (H_2O_2) 3% internally. Hildegard of Bingen: lungwort tea. Bring the herb to a boil and allow it to stand in the water. Drink it on an empty stomach for several days. Linseed oil. (See also: the lung remedies on p. 168).

Enlargement of the lungs, lymph nodes and connective tissue nodules (pulmonary sarcoidosis, Besnier-Boeck disease)

Same SBS as above. (See also: pp. 159-160). Conflict possibly has a self-esteem-component: "I can't breathe well enough." In CM, this is seen as a so-called systemic illness of the mesoderm, with the lungs being the primarily affected organ. From the viewpoint of the 5 Biological Laws of Nature, there are no such "systematic illnesses" and thus, we look at the symptoms: enlargement of the lymph nodes on the lung stem points to a repair phase (CM: sarcoidosis stage 1). The conversion of functional lung tissue into connective tissue points to relapses (CM: sarcoidosis stage 3).

Example
• *The bike-riding student starts crossing a traffic light too early and is nearly run over by a car. Although nothing happens, he "sees his life flash before his eyes" = fear-of-death conflict. The conflict recurs daily, since he crosses the same intersection everyday while riding to the university. After two years, he goes to the doctor because he has trouble breathing and coughs when he exerts himself. Diagnosis: sarcoidosis of the lungs. He is treated with 35 mg of cortisone per day but his lung volume remains at 70%. The conflict is resolved when he learns about the 5 Biological Laws of Nature and avoids the traffic light as his "therapy." The sarcoidosis retreats almost completely.* (See www.germanische-heilkunde.at/index.php/erfahrungsberichte)

Phase
Recurring-conflict affecting the alveoli > formation of scar tissue.

Note
It is possible that the diagnosis of sarcoidosis is based on multiple bronchial scarring (this would be a recurring territorial-fear conflict).

Therapy
Questions: see previous page. Find out what the conflict and conditioning are and, if possible, resolve them in real life so that the recurring conflict comes to an end. Guiding principles: see above. See also lung remedy below. Breathing exercises, gymnastics, outdoor exercise. Hildegard of Bingen: millet mixed powder special recipe. In CM, for asthma, emphysema and sarcoidosis, the same drugs are given (bronchodilators, cortisone). In acute cases (repair phase crisis) they are practical and they are undoubtedly useful. Long-term intake is not recommended due to the side effects.

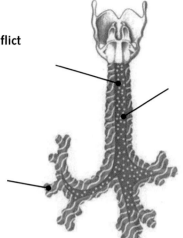

Bronchial Mucosa
Territorial-fear conflict

Bronchial Goblet Cells
Suffocation-fear

Bronchial Musculature
**Territorial-fear conflict
(motor)**

SBS of the Bronchial and Tracheal Mucosa

Bronchial tumor (bronchial epithelial cancer)[1]

Conflict
Territorial-fear or shock-fright conflicts (dependent on "handedness," hormone levels and previous conflicts). A person is afraid of losing his territory (e.g., partner, job) or his position in the territory (position, level). *"To have a terrible or mortal fear." "I was scared to death." "I am terrified!"*

The territorial-fear conflict is an active/male reaction to a threat to his territory. The shock-fright conflict is a passive/female reaction to the same thing (typically, the male reacts with attack, the female with passive fright).

Examples
• *A woman has a husband, who is always being unfaithful. She is never sure whether or not he is having another affair = territorial-fear conflict with degradation of cells from the bronchi in the active phase. She comes into healing when she separates from him and meets another man who loves her passionately and deeply. With this new partner, she is sure that he is true to her. Restoration of the bronchial mucosa = bronchitis or a bronchial ca. (Example from Ursula Homm)*
• *A family father has a job in a small plumbing company and is two years away from his retirement. He has a good, friendly relationship with his boss. One day, the boss decides to join up with a new business partner. The new partner cannot stand the patient. The relationship worsens and the patient is afraid of being fired. This would be very bad, as he still has two young daughters to raise and moreover, he wouldn't be able to get a new job at his age = territorial-fear conflict. Before he goes into retirement, in other words, two years later, his fear of losing his job dissolves. He begins to cough and thinks he has bronchitis. When his symptoms do not improve he gets a lung x-ray. The diagnosis: "cancer of the bronchi." This causes him to have a fear-of-death conflict. Finally, the patient dies after receiving all possible therapies. (See Claudio Trupiano, Danke Doktor Hamer, p. 327.)*
→ *Also, often a threat to one's "time territory." For example, someone is put under time or schedule pressure. Someone's time is "robbed" from them or someone else decides what will be done with their time.*
• *A 26-year-old, left-handed man starts up a small company with a friend. After a while, they begin to have major arguments about how their presence at the firm should be regulated. The patient wants to take advantage of his entrepreneurial freedom with flexible, need-oriented working hours. His partner insists on an exact work schedule = territorial-fear conflict regarding the larynx (left-hander). After an unpleasant separation from his business partner, the patient can choose his own hours, and the conflict seems resolved. Unfortunately, a trigger remains: whenever he is pressured with private or business appointments, he subconsciously remembers the old stress and reacts with territorial-fear. The day after the appointment, he has a congested larynx and a hoarse voice = repair phase of the larynx mucosa. (Archive B. Eybl).*

**E
C
T
O**

− +

---

1 See Dr. Hamer, Charts p. 111

E
C
T
O

− +

> • *For the last 30 years, a 47-year-old mother of two has met with her "best friend" twice a week. In the last half year, however, her friend has suddenly stopped seeing her. After several futile attempts to contact her, she gives up, disappointed = territorial-fear conflict - "My friend is leaving my territory." She comes into healing when her friend phones her to wish her a happy birthday and she confronts her on the matter. Now, she can close the books on the subject. A week later, she contracts pneumonia.* (Archive B. Eybl)

Conflict-active	Functional limitation; later, cell degradation (ulcers) of the bronchial mucous membrane, usually unnoticed. Simultaneous slackening of the, according to Dr. Hamer, striated musculature. The affected area can be anywhere from the beginning of the trachea into the smallest branches of the bronchi = CM's "ulcerating bronchial cancer."
Bio. function	Expanded bronchi due to lax ring musculature. This allows the person to improve their intake of air, so they can defend the territory more effectively. One can "scream" everyone else out of their territory - shout louder during a dispute.
Repair phase	Restoration of the bronchial and/or tracheal mucosa = inflammation of the bronchi (bronchitis), pneumonia, bronchial cancer: swelling, reddening, cough, possibly bloody sputum, and pain; strong swelling with exhaling difficulties during syndrome. Due to the swelling, an entire section of the lung can be cut off temporarily from the breathing process (= insufficient-ventilation atelectasis). As soon as the swelling is reduced, the air passage opens up again, that is, the atelectasis disappears again. Longer lasting bronchitis is due to a recurring-conflict.
Repair crisis	Cough and/or coughing cramps due to participation of the bronchial musculature, chills.
Note	Bronchial cancer is usually diagnosed in the repair phase, often together with syndrome.
Questions	When did the symptoms begin? Which territory is this about? (Partner, residence, workplace)? What stressed me at the time in question? What am I thinking about when I can't sleep? Dreams? (Indication of the conflict). What keeps me from dealing with the issue better? Was one of my ancestors confronted with a similar situation? What is continuing on, down through the generations? Which conditioning sensitizes me? What beliefs lead me to the dilemma? Am I ready to start over?
Therapy	If still conflict-active: Determine and resolve the conflict, conditioning and beliefs. Enzyme preparation, lymphatic drainage. Hildegard of Bingen: ground ivy elixir special recipe. Vitamin D3 (cod liver oil), hydrogen peroxide (H_2O_2) 3% strength internally. See also lung remedies p 168. If necessary: OP, if the tumor is too large and/or large bronchial branches are affected.

Inflammation of the bronchi (bronchitis)

Same SBS as above.

Phase	**Repair phase:** Restoration of the squamous mucous membrane. Pain, narrowing of the bronchi (stenosis) or closure (atelectasis) due the healing-swelling, breathing noises (stridor). Expectoration of phlegm (sputum). Cough = repair phase crisis of the bronchial musculature. The cough's biological purpose is to expectorate the mucus.
Note	By recurring-conflict or in persistent repair, CM speak of "chronic hypertrophic bronchitis." A "bronchial cancer" might just as well be diagnosed, should a lung x-ray be taken.
Therapy	The conflict is resolved. Support the healing and avoid relapses. Saltwater or tea inhalations. Tea: horehound, marshmallow, Iceland moss, mallow, primrose, mullein, elderberry. Colloidal silver internally. In the repair phase crisis, black tea or coffee. Possibly CM - cortisone, anticonvulsants. See also: lung remedies p. 168.

Bulging or widening of the bronchi (bronchiectasis)

Same SBS as above. (See pp. 161-162). According to CM, chronically recurring inflammations can degrade the structure of the bronchial wall. Symptom: expectoration of large amounts of phlegm upon arising in the morning.

Phase	Recurring, **persistent-active conflict** with local cell degradation from the bronchial mucosa > a thinning and subsequent bulging out of the membrane. During the periods between the repair phases, there is increased phlegm with coughing in the repair phase crisis.
Therapy	Questions: see above. Find conflict and conditioning and resolve them in real life, in order to prevent relapses. See also: lung remedies on p. 168.

Inflammation of the trachea (tracheitis), tracheal cancer (tracheal-epithelial cancer)

Same SBS as above. (See pp. 161-162). With regard to conflicts, the mucosa of the trachea belongs to the bronchi.

Phase	**Repair phase**: Restoration of the squamous mucous membrane. Pain under the breastbone. Possibly narrowing of the trachea (tracheal stenosis) due to repair-swelling especially with syndrome. If the cell degradation was long and intense, the healing can also take a long time. This is possibly the manifestation of a recurring conflict. In both cases, tracheal cancer may be diagnosed.
Therapy	The conflict is resolved. Support the healing. Avoid recurrences. In the repair phase crisis, possibly CM: cortisone, anticonvulsants. If necessary: surgery. See: lung remedies on p. 168.

SBS of the Bronchial Musculature

Narrowing of the bronchi (bronchial asthma), spastic bronchial inflammation (spastic bronchitis)[1]

Bronchial asthma causes difficulties in exhaling > slow and heavy exhalation. If the mucosa and muscles are affected, the condition is accompanied by bronchitis <u>and</u> bronchial stenosis.

Conflict	Territorial-fear conflict or shock-fright and speechlessness conflict in the repair phase crisis. Additionally, an active conflict or a repair phase crisis on the opposite, left, cerebral cortex side. (For conflict explanation, see p. 161).
Examples	• *When he was a child, a 33-year-old, right-handed, asthmatic patient had to listen to the intense arguing of his parents. The parents then separated = territorial-fear conflict affecting the bronchi, shock-fright conflict affecting the larynx, and stinking conflict affecting the mucous membranes of the nose. All three conflicts led to cell degradation in the active-phase and restoration in the repair phase. The patient has several triggers: dampness or warm-damp weather, arguments, separations, and disharmony of all sorts. Due to the triggers, he repeatedly comes into conflict activity and then into repair with the symptoms of asthma and sniffles.* (Archive B. Eybl)
	• *A 60-year-old, right-handed retiree with two grown children has had a cat allergy, since his 18th birthday. Whenever he is near a cat for longer than half an hour, the bronchi tighten up and he cannot breathe properly - although he loves cats! Moved to tears, he recalls the original conflict 40 years ago: His favorite cat often stole food from the table. Once, his mother caught the cat "in the act" and hit it so hard that the cat slunk into the cellar. After that, the cat had nothing to do with any family member other than him = territorial-fear conflict. Subsequently, he always went down into the cellar and pet his cat. It then licked his temples with gratitude. Later, the cat died.*
	Additional finding: The patient has a basal-cell carcinoma (skin cancer) on the temple, just on that spot = for the last 40 years, a hanging-separation conflict - the skin contact with the cat was broken off. Note: The patient's cat allergy is based, like all allergies, on a trigger. For this man's subconscious, cats are an alarm signal: Watch out! Something bad could happen again > start-up of a bronchial SBS > relaxation of the bronchial musculature in the active-phase > cramping up in the repair phase crisis = CM: "asthma." (Archive B. Eybl)
Conflict-active	Degradation of the bronchial musculature (muscle necrosis) > muscle weakness. Simultaneously, cerebral cortex-controlled reduction of innervation > motor paralysis. In the case of a coupled conflict, simultaneous degradation of bronchial mucosa - all largely symptomless.
Bio. function	Widening of the lumen in the bronchi due to "relaxed" bronchial musculature > get air better and faster.
Repair phase	Restoration of bronchial musculature and return of innervation, tickling irritation in the throat. With coupling, simultaneous bronchitis with expectoration.
Repair crisis	Bronchial asthma attack: coughing fits, longer exhalation and/or exhalation together with coughing, lasting from several minutes to a maximum of three days. Narrowing (tightening) of the bronchi and/

---

[1]   See Dr. Hamer, Charts pp. 111, 112

	Note	or trachea, possibly with wheezing sounds (stridor trachealis) when breathing.
		An attack occurs when a conflict is active on the opposite, left half of the cerebral cortex or also in the repair phase crisis. Only this constellation makes bronchial asthma possible.
		By allergic bronchial asthma, the conflict is started up briefly due to a trigger (= CM's allergen).
	Therapy	Questions: see p. 162. Determine the conflict and conditioning and, if possible, resolve them in real life. Guiding principles: *"I am safe." "I am in the hands of God."* Breathing exercises, dancing, singing. Hydrogen peroxide (H_2O_2) internally. Vitamin D3 (cod liver oil). In the repair phase crisis black tea or coffee, possibly: CM cortisone, antispasmodic and bronchodilators. Long-term use is not recommended because of side effects.

ECTO

−+

SBS of the Goblet Cells

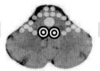

Goblet cell tumor (adeno-ca), excess phlegm (mucus) in the bronchi[1]

From a developmental standpoint, goblet cells are descendants of the intestinal mucosa glands. They are responsible for the lubrication and moistening of the air passages.

ENDO

+−

Conflict	Chunk conflict (see explanations p. 15, 16): not being able inhale, moisten the air. In practical terms: suffocation fear, blocked airways (foreign objects, artificial respiration). *"I'm not getting any air." "I'm struggling for air."*
Examples	• *For the last year, a 28-year-old mother is so congested that it causes her to vomit regularly. Her only son was born prematurely and suffers from respiratory problems among others. One night, he nearly suffocated in her arms - she called an ambulance much too late. Since then, she always listens in the night to hear if her little one is breathing normally. Substitute suffocation conflict for her son affecting the goblet cells. When the connection was explained to her, she was able to completely accept her son's difficulties and, for the first time, appreciate herself as the good mother that she is. Relieved, she subsequently spent several nights soaking the sheets with sweat and coughing up yellow sputum. Afterwards, her symptoms were gone.* (Archive B. Eybl)
	→ *The umbilical cord of an infant is cut too soon > insufficient oxygen supply to the baby.*
	→ *While having an asthma attack, a person thinks he is suffocating.*
	→ *A person is exposed to an extreme amount of dust or smoke (fire dept., mining, stone cutting, etc.).*
Conflict-active	Increased function, cell proliferation of the goblet cells (goblet cell tumor) = in CM: chronic cartarrhous bronchitis, intrabronchial goblet cell adeno-ca, goblet cell hyperplasia = excess phlegm due to increased production of mucus.
Bio. function	Better breathing and/or dust expulsion due to more bronchial mucus.
Repair phase	Normalization of function. If fungi or bacteria (mycobacteria) are present > tubercular-caseating degradation or small goblet cell "tumorlets." Expectoration of yellow (purulent) mucus, fever, night sweats, halitosis.
Note	This SBS is rare. It is difficult to draw the line between this disease and bronchitis (territorial-fear conflict), which is also accompanied by excess mucus. Decisive sign: proof of bacteria (laboratory), expectoration of yellow, purulent sputum, night sweats accompanying goblet cell carcinoma degradation. This SBS would explain why asthmatics, who are regularly afraid of suffocating, often suffer from extreme congestion.
Questions	Congestion since when? (Conflict previous). Suffocation fear from what? (Own asthma or that of a loved one, dusty workplace, artificial respiration, etc.)? What has sensitized me? What did my parents/ ancestors experience? (Miners, lung disease)? Did the pregnancy or birth play a role?
Therapy	Determine the conflict and conditioning and, if possible, resolve them in real life. Tea: horehound, anise, fenugreek, speedwell, linseed, ground ivy. Vitamin D3 (cod liver oil), black cumin. Colloidal silver internally. Hildegard of Bingen: special recipe: blackberry elixir.

---

1   See Dr. Hamer, Charts p. 21

Cystic fibrosis (CF = mucoviscidosis, drying up of the bronchial mucus)[1]

Same SBS as above.

Phase	**Persistent repair**, usually recurring in infancy > more and more goblet cell functional tissue is "melted away" - converted to connective tissue. This causes less mucus to be produced or its production stops altogether = mucoviscidosis.
Therapy	Find out what the conflict and conditioning are and, if possible, resolve them in real life so that the persistent repair can come to an end and the goblet cells can regenerate. Lymph drainages, acupuncture, acupoint and classic massage, colloidal silver internally. See also: lung remedies below.

Coronary Veins (blue)
Female-sexual loss-of-territory conflict

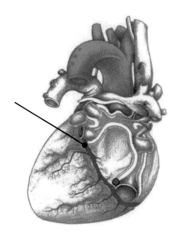
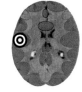

SBS of the Coronary Veins

Occlusion of the lung artery (pulmonary embolism, thromboembolism)[1]

This "disorder" should actually belong to the chapter on the heart, because the lung only receives the effects of a heart SBS. According to CM, the blood clot (thrombus) that leads to a lung embolism is transported from the leg veins. However, Dr. Hamer found out that in a pulmonary embolism, the thrombus originates in a venous shank of the coronary vessels (coronary veins). According to my experience, this explanation does not account for all lung embolisms. In all likelihood, some of the blood clots do break away from the deep leg veins (SBS of the Veins s. p. 143f). For individual cases, a diagnosis based on the symptoms shouldn't pose a problem. The following describes a clot departing from a coronary vein: The blood supply of the heart: Via the coronary arteries, the heart muscle is supplied with oxygen-rich blood. After the gas exchange in the heart's muscle tissue, the coronary veins take the oxygen-poor blood into the right atrium. From there, it goes into the right ventricle and then via the pulmonary artery (albeit with oxygen-poor blood) into the lungs for new oxygen enrichment. Now the decisive point: If any clot is released from the coronary veins, it will becomes lodged in a pulmonary artery = lung embolism.

Conflict	Female loss-of-territory conflict or sexual-frustration conflict of not being mated. *"It breaks my heart!"* Also, possible male loss-of-territory conflict (dependent on "handedness," hormone levels and previous conflicts). The female territorial conflict always has a partner-related or sexual aspect. It is about the "inner territory." The partner is the "territory" of the woman. That is why it is better if the man takes the woman into his territory. Then, the man has his territory and the woman has her partner. If the man moves in with the woman, the woman has her partner, but the man has no territory.
Examples	➔ *A woman is abandoned by her husband, mistreated, or forced into having sexual intercourse.* • *A 15-year-old, right-handed schoolgirl sleeps with a boy for the first time. Unfortunately, the condom breaks. She takes the "morning-after" pill, since she is afraid of getting pregnant. What really upsets her, however, is that the boy tells everybody about what happened. Even the girl's mother hears about it from "the grapevine." Female loss-of-territory conflict with regard to the coronary*

---

1   See Dr. Hamer, Charts p. 126

veins and the cervix, in the active-phase: cell degradation in the coronary veins. Four weeks later the girl comes into healing, with restoration of cells to the coronary veins. For months, she repeatedly has absence seizures with tachycardia (racing heart rate). (Archive B. Eybl)

• *A 32-year-old patient with a Christian upbringing has a partner who loves her, but does not want to get married "out of principle." = Female loss-of-territory conflict. After 10 years of "living in sin," he proposes to her. After the proposal (= beginning of the repair phase) the woman becomes weaker and weaker and suffers from increasing shortness of breath. Six weeks later she has an embolism and two month long episode of bleeding from the cervix = repair phase. (Archive B. Eybl)*

• *A now 35-year-old, right-handed woman is two and a half when her father "says goodbye" to his wife and daughter. His departure is preceded by violent arguments, her mother often having to protect her from his aggressive behavior. She meets her father once, later on, but she will never forget it. As a seven-year-old, she is playing in her mother's restaurant, when her father comes in and says, "Hello, I am your father." He then seats himself at the bar with his back toward her. When she is nine, she learns that her father has died = female loss-of-territory conflict in addition to a fear-disgust conflict. (Shortly afterwards she is diagnosed with diabetes.) The patient has regular angina pectoris (= active territorial conflict) when stressed. When she climbs stairs, she has the feeling her heart is being "constricted." Additionally, she suffers from severe menstrual complaints. (Archive B. Eybl)*

Conflict-active	Functional limitation, simultaneous slackening of the underlying smooth musculature (ring-shaped portions). Later, cell degradation (ulcer) on the inner surface of the coronary veins (intima). > Cross-sectional enlargement. Possibly mild, constrictive chest pains (angina pectoris). Usually, (but not always), accompanied by simultaneous cell degradation in the mucosa of the cervix. Often, **a recurring conflict.**
Bio. function	Due to the breakdown of the cells, the lumen of the coronary veins increases > better flow of blood from the heart > higher heart capacity for being able to win back the lost territory (e.g., the partner).
Repair phase	Repair and restoration of the epithelium of the coronary veins. Formation of scabs (plaque).
Repair crisis	Three to six weeks after the beginning of the repair phase, the pulmonary embolism occurs: gasping for air, fear, and a sense of impending doom, possibly chills. In the repair phase crisis, there is a cramp-like spasm (= local epilepsy) of the voluntary (striated) vessel musculature below the epithelium. This causes scabs to break loose and course with the blood via the right side of the heart into the pulmonary arteries = lung embolism. Larger pieces quickly get stuck the larger vessels, smaller ones can reach the smaller branches of the pulmonary arteries. The blockage of the flow of blood in the smaller and middle-sized vessels is not a problem, because bypassing vessels (anastomoses) insure the blood supply. The blood clots usually dissolve within weeks without therapeutic measures (recanalization). However, this is problematic on the brain level: repair-swelling of the Hamer focus and then acute shrinkage during the repair phase crisis.
Note	The rhythm center for the rapid heart beat lies in the relay for the coronary veins and the cervix. Due to this, we sometimes find high heart rates (tachycardia) during the repair phase crisis, possibly with lapses (tachyarrhythmia). Fatal ventricular fibrillation is also possible, if the conflict has been active for too long.
Questions	Which territorial conflict was resolved 3 - 6 weeks before the embolism? (Partner, friend, house, etc.)? What stressed me? (In the conflict-active period, one must have been manic; now, calm again). Was menstrual bleeding absent during this time? (Yes > indication of conflict activity). Which emotions accompanied the conflict? How did I even get into these difficulties? Which beliefs lie beneath this? What conditioned me? (E.g., childhood experiences)? Are there parallels to ancestors? (Try to learn the life stories of your ancestors). Which reorientation could help prevent recurrences? Which old patterns/habits and beliefs will I throw overboard?
Therapy	The conflict is resolved. Support the healing. Nevertheless, analyze the conflict to prevent recurrences. Assert a calming/reassuring influence. Possibly administer cortisone at the end of the repair phase crisis. Peace and rest. Avoid recurrences. Vitamin D3 (cod liver oil). Hildegard of Bingen: horseradish-galangal special recipe, Portuguese lavender elixir special recipe. Natural borax internally. Hydrogen peroxide (H_2O_2) 3% internally. Blood thinning medication as necessary in the acute phase. In the case of cervical bleeding, however, these have a negative side effect of increasing the blood flow. > Administer for a limited time if possible, and only if there is no cervical bleeding.

SBS of the Branchial Arches

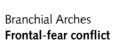

Small cell bronchial (lung) cancer

In CM, this kind of tumor is seen as a bronchial tumor. However, as Dr. Hamer found out, we are dealing with an SBS of the branchial arches or with callus (bone fluid) leaking from an injured bone in the area. Vertebrae, ribs or the sternum come into question. (See osteosarcoma p. 292).

Due to its inaccessible location in the middle of the chest cavity, this tumor is considered inoperable by CM and hardly curable.

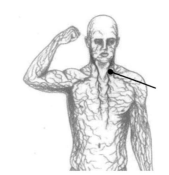

Branchial Arches
Frontal-fear conflict

Conflict	Frontal-fear conflict. Fear of an unavoidable danger coming towards you. (See also: non-Hodgkin's lymphoma, p. 147f.)
Examples	• *A 43-year-old, right-handed, happily married patient has a 12-year-old son. One day, the father has to have a meniscus surgery. When he wakes up from the anesthesia, his wife informs him that his son is hospitalized, having badly injured his head diving head first into water. The next day, he learns that his son will have to undergo surgery. His life is in danger > still in the hospital, the patient suffers a frontal-fear conflict because of the oncoming danger (the surgery) and a fear-of-death conflict - both conflicts in substitution for his son. He feels the urge to jump out of the window if the boy should die (high conflict-intensity). In the repair phase, he feels a downwards pull in the left ear toward the neck and breastbone with strong pressure and squeezing. Just above the collar bone, a cyst has developed (= branchial arches in healing). He also sweats heavily during the night and coughs blood (= alveoli in healing). The hospital's explanation of the symptoms is a diagnosis of an alveolar cancer and a small-cell bronchial cancer.* (Archive B. Eybl)
Repair phase	Cell division, restoration of the branchial arches = CM: small-cell bronchial cancer. This progression is described on p. 147f under non-Hodgkins lymphoma.
Questions	Did I feel an indication of this under my breastbone, possibly long before the diagnosis was made? (= Beginning of the conflict). Which danger is this about? Is the issue permanently resolved? (Exclude the possibility of recurrence).
Therapy	The conflict is resolved. Support the healing. Guiding principles: *"The danger is over. I am safe."* Lymph drainages. It is crucial to overcome the shock of the diagnosis and leave the fear behind.

Water in the lungs (interstitial or alveolar pulmonary edema)

It is typical for patients with water in the lungs to only sleep in a sitting position - at least in this position they have the upper part of the lungs to breathe. We can hear the typical rattling noise as the patient breathes. This serious symptom is a sign of poor general health. Principally, the kidney collecting tubules are always involved with this. The following causes come into consideration:

• **Pulmonary edema due to poisoning:** Irritant gases (chlorine, ammonia, hydrochloric acid, etc. = acute pulmonary edema), drugs (heroin, methadone), chemo-poisoning > destruction of the alveoli and capillaries > leakage of fluid into the lungs = pulmonary edema.

• **Weakness of the left ventricle (heart failure):** Overwhelmed conflict > backflow of blood into the pulmonary circulation> leakage of blood plasma in the pulmonary capillaries > water in the lungs = most common cause of lung edema (see p. 126ff).

• **Repair phase bronchial mucosa:** Territorial-fear in repair: Inflammation of bronchial mucosa = bronchitis > pulmonary edema during syndrome (see p. 161f).

• **Repair phase alveoli**: Fear-of-death conflict: Inflammation of the alveoli lung tuberculosis > exudation ofpus and water > pulmonary edema during syndrome (see p. 159f).

Therapy

In accordance with the cause. Both acute and chronic pulmonary edema need treatment. Definitely consider: therapeutic measures for kidney collecting tubules p. 231f.

Chronic obstructive pulmonary disease (COPD)

COPD is a collective term for various chronic diseases of the lungs. This mainly includes emphysema and chronic bronchitis. The diagnosis is, in our view, relatively meaningless, except for the term "chronic" > recurring SBS of the alveoli and/or recurrent SBS bronchi. For therapy, see the respective SBS. If applicable, cannabis oil.

Whooping cough (pertussis)

According to CM, whooping cough is caused by the bacterium Bordetella pertussis, and is one of the so-called pediatric diseases. Whooping cough comes from either the larynx or the bronchial muscles.

- **Cause larynx: repair phase crisis** of the laryngeal musculature or irritation (= tickle, urge to cough) of the laryngeal mucosa in the repair phase = shock-fright conflict.
- **Cause bronchi: repair phase crisis** of the bronchial musculature or irritation of the bronchial mucous membranes in the repair phase = territorial-fear conflict.

In both cases, the coughing has a biological function of expectorating the phlegm generated by the inflammation. Whooping cough attacks are especially serious in combination with syndrome.

Therapy

The conflict is resolved. Support the repair phase.

By attack (repair phase crisis): stand up, go where it is cool, drink cold beverages, tea, coffee, possibly CM: cortisone, antispasmodic, bronchodilators.

Tea: hibiscus, ivy, thyme, English plantain, peppermint.

By recurring-conflict: breathing exercises, sunbaths, solarium, sauna, infrared cabin, damp chest compress.

Black lung disease (pneumoconiosis; silicosis, asbestosis)

This is one of the most commonly occurring occupational illnesses. To a certain extent, dust is intercepted by the mucous membranes of the nose, throat, windpipe, and bronchi. With the help of the cilia (tiny hairs), these particles are transported outward or coughed up. The smallest or thin, fibrous particles, however, can make their way as far as the bronchioles and remain there. The very smallest particles can even enter the alveoli. There, the body builds connective tissue around them, which, in and of itself, is not harmful. If, however, over the years and decades, dust is continually inhaled, this scar tissue takes up more and more space so that the performance of the lung is eventually diminished. One speaks of a fine-particle-induced "pulmonary fibrosis" > not a conflict but damage caused by dust. The growths of connective tissue are often interpreted as "cancer."

Dust inhalation can also be perceived as an attack conflict as can the diagnosis "black lung." (See p. 170.)

Therapy

Stop breathing in dust. Guiding principle: *"My lungs are full of light and energy."* Breathing exercises, gymnastics, sport for cleaning the lungs. See also: lung remedies.

Smoking and the lungs

It is clear that smoking is not healthy. It pollutes the breathing passages with tar and soot. Nicotine and other ingredients are taken up by the body and they poison it gradually from within. Nicotine, like all drugs, makes us temporarily sympathicotonic = "high."

For the *"good feeling"* that comes from smoking, we pay a high price: the loss of freedom (due to addiction), loss of vital energy due to a bad conscience and local and general contamination. However, the commonly accepted maxim, "Smoking leads to lung cancer," is wrong. The signal for cell division in the bronchi and alveoli comes from the brain. There is no cell division without the brain ordering it to happen. Why is it that lung cancer is diagnosed more often in smokers?

- Smokers' lungs are examined more often because of contamination - symptomatic coughing or as a "precaution."
- Doctors intentionally examine smokers more often for lung cancer. Swollen, inflamed, sooty, scarred bronchial epithelium is designated as "cancer."
- Many smokers believe that they will get cancer because they smoke. Mandatory warnings reinforce this belief. Whoever continues smoking with this on their mind will eventually suffer a fear-of-death conflict and be responsible for their own undoing.

Therapy

Quit smoking. If possible, quit without being forced to do so. Brutal withdrawal harbors considerable conflict potential.

Guiding principle: *"I am free and independent! This is real quality of life."*

Lung remedies

Regular breathing exercises, aerobic exercise. Tea: horehound, lungwort, fir needle, agrimony, sage, plantain, knotgrass. Pelargonium root extract (Kaloba®).

Cayce: horehound syrup. Hildegard of Bingen: goat's milk. Hydrogen peroxide (H_2O_2) 3% internally. Sunbathing. Vitamin D3 (cod liver oil). Cannabis oil (CBD oil).

PLEURA

The pleura lines the chest cavity. It is controlled by the cerebellum and is made up entirely of mesodermal tissue. The pleura has two layers: the outer layer (pleura parietalis) is attached to the chest cavity, while the inner layer (pleura pulmonalis) forms the outer layer of the lungs. The very thin space (pleural cavity) between the two layers is filled with a fluid that allows the lungs to glide during breathing.

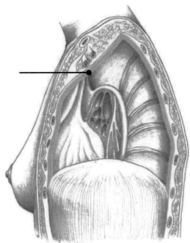

Pleura
**Attack-to-the-chest
or chest cavity**

SBS of the Pleura

Cancer of the pleura (pleura mesothelioma, pleura cancer)[1]

O L D   M E S O

+ −

Conflict	Attack-to-the-chest conflict. Real attack/threat or imagined threat. Fear concerning the lungs, heart, ribs and thoracic spine.
Examples	→ *Severe pain in the chest cavity (lungs, chest, heart, ribs, thoracic spine).* • *A person is diagnosed with a roundish shadow on the lung (lung cancer) = attack-to-the-chest conflict. During the conflict-active phase he develops a pleura mesothelioma. (Archive B. Eybl)* • *Fifteen years ago, a thin woman gets breast cancer (adeno-ca). Having become acquainted with the 5 Biological Laws of Nature she lets the tumor be and lives very well with it. Unfortunately, 6 years ago, she allows a biopsy to be taken. Afterwards the breast does not heal shut and for three years she lives with an open wound. At this point she becomes frightened and suffers an attack-to-the-chest conflict > growth of a pleura mesothelioma. After the breast is surgically closed (skin closure), the patient comes into healing with a pleural effusion. (Archive B. Eybl)*
Conflict-active	Cell proliferation in the pleura. Growth of a pleura mesothelioma. Either flat or patchy growth, depending on the kind of attack perceived. Possibly a recurring conflict.
Bio. function	Protection of the chest cavity by thickening of the pleura.
Repair phase	Tubercular, caseating degradation of tissue: inflammation of the pleura (pleuritis), pain, fever, night sweats, breathing difficulties, chest pain, pleural effusion due to syndrome.
Repair crisis	Chills, severe pain.
Note	Most cancers diagnosed in the pleura can be attributed to diagnosis shocks and are interpreted by CM as "metastases." - The prognosis is correspondingly poor.
	With knowledge of the 5 Biological Laws of Nature, there will be fewer cases of pleural tumors in the future and fewer people will die of them.
Questions	Symptoms since when? (Determine the phase, because complaints normally begin after the onset of the repair phase). Which type of attack did I experience? (OP, diagnosis, physical fight, accident, etc.). Can I handle diagnoses in general? Which conditioning is this based on? (Childhood, ancestors)?

---

1   See Dr. Hamer, Charts pp. 47, 52

Therapy	Determine the conflict and conditioning and, if possible, resolve them in real life. The most important therapy is the knowledge of the biological interrelations. Guiding principles: *"I am surrounded by a wall of crystal." "I am safe and protected." "Nobody and nothing can do any harm to me."* Lymph drainages, acupoint massage, breathing exercises. CM treats with surgery, chemotherapy and radiation and is content with extending their life expectancy prognosis by three months. Right after the surgery, mesothelioma usually grow back into the OP wound. Our view (and the view "from the view of the pleura") is that this is logical, because the surgery represents another attack. > Not recommended due to low chances of success.

Pleurisy, accumulation of pus in the pleura (pleural empyema), pleural adhesions (fibrinous or granulomatous pleurisy)[2]

Same SBS as above. (See p. 169)

Phase	**Repair phase**: degradation of the pleural tumors. Inflammation, severe pain while breathing, especially with dry pleuritis - fever, night sweats. Growths due to chronically recurring-conflicts (triggers).
Therapy	The conflict is resolved. Support the healing. The greatest problem is the pain. Cannabis works gently and relieves pain. Damp chest or whole-body wraps with brine, enzyme preparations, lymph drainages, colloidal silver internally. CM pain medication if necessary.

Pleurisy or adhesions caused by dust (e.g., asbestos pleurisy)

Same SBS as above. (See p. 169)

Phase	**Repair phase or persistent conflict**: degradation of a pleural tumor. Although the pleura has no direct contact with dust, it can co-react to the conflict: The inhalation of dust is unpleasant for everyone. Constant or intensive inhalation can lead to a dust-attack conflict to the lung. *"This dust is toxic and I have to breathe it in all the time!"* > growth of a pleura mesothelioma > inflammation of the pleura in the repair phase with pain, Fever, night sweats. Pleural callosities (plaque) due to this usually being a **recurring-conflict.**
Therapy	For recurrences: Determine the conflict and conditioning and, if possible, resolve them in real life. It is likely that it will be necessary to avoid any source of dust. Massages, lymph drainage massages, enzyme preparations, breathing exercises for cleaning and strengthening. CM pain medication.

Collection of fluid in the pleura that comes from the pleura itself (exsudative pleural effusion)[2]

Here the protein content is about 30 g/l. SBS same as above (see p. 169), but in addition - **syndrome**.

Example	• *A patient is found to have cysts of the branchial arches. CM's diagnosis: "non-Hodgkin's lymphoma." He is told that they must do major surgery on his chest cavity in order to get to both sides = attack-to-the-chest conflict. After the surgery, the patient dies of massive pleural effusions on both sides.* (See Dr. Hamer, Goldenes Buch Vol. 2, p. 135)
Phase	**Repair phase or persistent conflict**- fluid is collected between the inner and outer layers of the pleura, due to the degradation of the tumor = "sweating out" of the pleura. To a certain extent, this is normal because fluid forms during every inflammation. In combination with syndrome, however, the effusion can become threatening. Exudative pleural effusions are rich in protein. This is where the problem with punctures lies. Due to repeated draining of fluid, the body loses large volumes of protein > lowered albumin level. Low blood protein content leads to a drop in the colloid osmotic pressure in the blood system which promotes fluid collection = 1st vicious circle. At the psychic level, a puncture can set off another vicious circle that is even worse if the painful and risky puncture procedure (pneumothorax danger) is perceived as an attack-to-the-chest conflict = 2nd vicious cycle. Nevertheless, punctures are sometimes unavoidable. Usually a **recurring-conflict.**

---

2   See Dr. Hamer, Charts p. 47, 52

Therapy	The attack conflict is resolved. Support the healing. Address the kidney collecting tubules conflict, if present. Lymph drainages. Salt water baths or wraps. Cannabis (CBD) oil, enzyme preparation. Tea: stinging nettle, horsetail, goldenrod. Intake of biologically valuable protein (e.g., eggs, quark). Hydrogen peroxide (H_2O_2) 3% internally, vitamin D3 (cod liver oil). Puncture (tap) only as a last resort. Possible albumin infusions. No infusions with salt. Gradual lengthening of the intervals between punctures.

Collections of fluid in the pleura that comes from the surroundings (transudative pleural effusion)

Through transudative pleural effusion (protein content of less than 30 g/l), fluid seeps from inflamed surrounding tissues into the pleural cavity. This can be the case with a weak heart (cardiac insufficiency p. 126ff), low blood protein levels (hunger edema), or with healing ribs, breastbone, thoracic vertebrae, lungs or bronchi. There is significant accumulation of water only during syndrome.

Conflict	Not an SBS of the pleura, but another SBS (usually bone) combined with **syndrome.**
Example	• *A woman with breast cancer undergoes radiation and chemotherapy. This makes the breast small and unsightly, which results in a local self-esteem conflict with respect to the breastbone. As she enters the repair phase, the healing bone presses the resulting fluid into the pleura = transudative pleural effusion.* (See Dr. Hamer, Goldenes Buch Bd. 2, p. 364)
Therapy	See exudative pleural effusion and causative SBS above.

LIPS, MOUTH, AND THROAT

The mouth and pharynx (throat) are the first part of the digestive tract and at the same time they serve as sound and speech-forming organs. Over the deep-lying, endodermal "intestinal mucous membrane" lies the ectodermal epithelium, which migrated from the outer skin. Most SBS of lips, mouth, and throat, take place in this superficial mucosa.

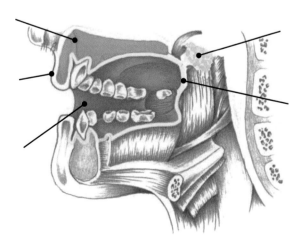

Hard Palate
Self-esteem conflict

Lip Epidermis
Separation conflict

Mouth & Pharynx Mucosa
Separation conflict

Tonsils
Chunk conflict

Oral Submucosa
Chunk conflict

SBS of the Superficial Lip and Oral Mucous Membrane

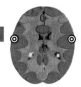

Aphthous stomatitis (canker sores)

Aphthous ulcers, also known as canker sores, are painful, dot-like ulcers of the mucosa in the mouth.

Conflict	Separation conflict regarding the lips, mouth, or tongue. To become separated from somebody or wanting to become separated. Wanting (or not wanting) to have contact (e.g., kissing, touching). Also applies to food or dietary restrictions. Not wanting, being allowed to or being able to say something. Also not wanting to have said something.
Examples	→ *"I can't spit it out." "Talk 'till one's blue in the face; burn one's tongue."* • *A woman has suffered from aphthous ulcers of the mouth for the past 50 years. As a child, she was severely beaten for having eating nuts from her neighbor's garden = mouth-separation conflict. Since then she has been allergic to nuts, reacting with aphthous ulcers in the repair phase. When she recognizes the connection, she says to herself: "The nuts cannot do anything to me!" = conflict resolution. The ulcers disappear for good. (See Dr. Hamer, Was ist die Neue Medizin?)*
	• *A 45-year-old, right-handed, married patient is an avid gardener. Her husband appears with a pair of heavy-duty scissors, intending to prune the grapevine. The patient sees this and says, "You know you have to use the hedge clippers for that!" The man hands her the scissors and says, "Here are the scissors - do it yourself!" = separation conflict of not being able to reach (touch) the partner with words (with the tongue). She steps back without saying a word, as if she was struck by lightning and says to herself, "I will never criticize anything again because he doesn't get it anyway." = Active-phase with cell reduction of the tongue mucosa and pain. Two days later, after she has forgotten the whole matter, she develops an aphthous ulcer on the right side of the tip of her tongue (partner side) = repair phase with restoration of the mucous membrane. (Archive B. Eybl)*
Conflict-active	Increase in the sensibility of the oral mucosa. Development of smaller or larger defects in the mucosa (aphthous ulcers). The longer the conflict lasts, the deeper they become. Pain is in the active-phase and repair phase crisis. Usually a **recurring-conflict.**
Bio. function	Increased sensibility so one doesn't say anything inconsiderate or senses more when kissing/eating.
Repair phase	Restoration of the oral mucosa, inflammation, swelling, reddening. Active phases and repair phases can quickly switch. Sometimes small inflammations of the deep-lying, endodermal oral mucosa will also be diagnosed as aphthous stomatitis. In this case, pain and halitosis during the repair phase (see SBS of the oral submucosa - trench mouth, p. 174).
Repair crisis	Severe pain, bleeding.
Note	Consider "handedness" (right or left) and side (mother/child or partner).
Questions	When did the symptoms begin? (Conflict shortly before). The three most important questions: Speaking/kissing/eating? (Usually it's about speaking)? In which situations is it better/worse? Does the conflict have to do with someone? Why do I react so sensitively to this issue? With regard to this, which burdensome experience of my ancestors do I carry on? (Ask about the family history). Will I allow myself to let this go?
Therapy	Determine the conflict and conditioning and, if possible, resolve them in real life. Guiding principles: *"My words are long since forgotten." "In the future, I will say what is on my mind right away."* Diluted hydrogen peroxide (H_2O_2) internally, gargle with of sage tea, tea tree oil, colloidal silver, EM, DMSO.

Squamous cell skin cancer (tumor) of the lip, mouth, gum or tongue[1]

Same SBS as above.

Vernacular	*"It's on the tip of my tongue!" "I could bite my tongue!" "Speak until one's blue in the face."*
Examples	• *A married, left-handed woman sees her 4-year-old grandson throw a stone through a relative's window. The patient thinks she should inform the parents about this incident. Her husband, however, is against it, because he doesn't want to start an argument = conflict of not being allowed to say something. Two weeks later, the patient finds the courage to write the mother an e-mail = conflict resolu-*

E
C
T
O

− +

---

1   See Dr. Hamer, Charts pp. 122, 135

tion. Two days after that, a 1.5 cm swelling appears on the right side of the patient's mouth (mother/ child side) = repair phase. After two weeks, the swelling subsides. (See www.germanische-heilkunde.at)
• Within a few weeks, a 67-year-old, right-handed, married mother of five, develops an approximately 8 mm wart (tongue papilloma) immediately behind the tip of the tongue = conflict of not being able to say something, in persistent repair. Conflict history: Her husband has a hot temper. For the patient, however, a peaceful and harmonious co-existence is important. She is always trying to "smooth things over." Often, she is about to say something, but it stops, so to speak, "on the tip of her tongue." After brief consideration, she holds her tongue to avoid irritating her husband. Later, through a fortunate coincidence, he discovers a new hobby in cooking. Now, the patient is starting to say what she thinks more often. (Archive B. Eybl)

Phase	Repair phase or **persistent repair**: Restoration of the epithelium (= squamous cell ca). White coating (leukoplakia), swelling, possibly bleeding without pain. Pain (e.g., burning tongue) in the active-phase and in the repair phase crisis. Larger, more problematic tumors can only arise through long-lasting conflict. Often a **recurring-conflict.**
Therapy	Determine and resolve the conflict, conditioning and beliefs. For questions, therapeutic advice: see previous page. OP if necessary, without chemo or radiation.

Scarlet fever (affecting the mouth)

Same SBS as above (see p. 172) and other SBS. The primary symptom for scarlet fever is inflamed, reddened mucosa of the mouth and tongue - the typical "raspberry tongue" - and inflamed tonsils:

Examples	➡ *A child insists on having a sweet but does not get it.* ➡ *A child is weaned from his pacifier.*
Phase	Inflamed mucosa of the mouth, "raspberry mouth": repair phase of a separation conflict - restoration of the squamous epithelium-mucous membrane. Inflamed tonsils: repair phase of a chunk conflict (see explanations p. 15, 16). Skin rash: repair phase of a separation conflict.
Therapy	The conflict is resolved. Support the healing. Avoid recurrences. See aphthous therapy on previous page.

Fever blisters (herpes simplex, herpes labialis)

Same SBS as above. (See p.172)

Examples	➡ *A child does not want to be kissed by his aunt. Nevertheless, he gets a big "smooch" from her every time. > The child wants to be separated.* ➡ *Someone stuffs himself and regrets having overeaten afterwards > wanting to undo the lips' contact with so much food.* • *A man sips a beverage with a straw. Afterwards, somebody tells him that a cat had just licked the straw. The man is disgusted = lip separation conflict. In the repair phase, he gets a fever blister. Note: It wasn't true at all, a cat hadn't licked the straw. Someone was playing a trick on him. (See www.germanische-heilkunde.at/index.php/erfahrungsberichte). Also: This is a good example of how conflicts can be entirely subjective and based on one's imagination.* • *A woman notices, with distress, that her thoughtless words have deeply hurt her partner = conflict of wishing that one hadn't said something. Whenever this happens, she gets a fever blister two days later = repair phase. (Archive B. Eybl)*
Phase	**Repair phase:** fever blisters, swelling, scabs, hardly any pain. In repair phase crisis pain, bleeding.
Note	Pain during cell degradation (ulcer), in other words before the fever blister appears. Consider mother/ child or partner side or local conflict.
Therapy	The conflict is resolved. Support the healing. If relapses occur, find out what the conflict and conditioning are and resolve them. Guiding principle: see above. Hydrogen peroxide (H_2O_2) internally. Apply salve, e.g., propolis salve (acts as a sealant), hyssop salve: add a few drops of hyssop oil to a basic natural salve, DMSO, colloidal silver.

Fissures (cracks) in the corner of the mouth (rhagades)

Conflict	Separation conflict that one doesn't open their mouth at the right moment. It was necessary to say something, but one remained silent. Teacher at school: *"Say something, why don't you?!"*

E
C
T
O

−+

E C T O		
	Example	• A 25-year-old saleswoman has been suffering from a crack in the corner of her mouth since she has been together with her new partner. He tends to blow every little thing out of proportion. To keep from angering him any more and out of plain fear, she remains completely silent during these situations. = Conflict of not being allowed to open her mouth. (Archive B. Eybl)
	Phase	Painful fissures in the **conflict-active phase**, crusting and scabbing in the repair phase.
–+	Bio. function	Increasing the sensibility of the mouth > the attention is directed to the lips so that one will finally open their mouth (wide).
	Therapy	Determine and resolve the conflict, conditioning and belief (system). Practice expressing opinions freely. Apply ointment to the corners of the mouth, e.g., with propolis salve.

SBS of the Oral Submucosa

Trench mouth, thrush (candidiasis), leukoplakia, geographic tongue[1]

Acute necrotizing ulcerative gingivitis (ANUG), commonly known as trench mouth, is a typical pediatric illness: The oral mucosa is coated with a yellowish-white, stinking film.

Conflict	Chunk conflict (see explanations p. 15, 16) of not being able to grasp something that one wants to have or not being able to spit out or expel something that one wants to get rid of. Simply stated: Conflict of not getting what one wants or not being able to get rid of something one doesn't want.
Examples	• A young woman has been wanting to switch to a vegetarian diet for years, but never succeeds. She always ends up eating hot dogs or other fast foods due to lack of time = chunk conflict of not getting the right nutrition. One day, her partner and her decide to become vegetarians = beginning of the repair phase with painful oral thrush of the gums. (Archive B. Eybl)
• In the beginning, a new mother has breast-feeding problems. For the first few days, the baby remains hungry = chunk conflict of not getting the food (milk). When the child finally gets full, it develops thrush (candidiasis) > a very common situation. (Archive B. Eybl)
Conflict-active	Growth of a lawn-shaped flat tumor (usually unnoticed) under the squamous epithelium of the oral mucosa = adeno-ca.
Bio. function	To produce more mucous with more (intestinal) glandular cells, so that the "chunk" can better slip in or out of the pharynx.
Repair phase	Tubercular caseating degradation of tissue - white patches, so-called plaques, appear. In CM, this can sometimes be diagnosed as leukoplakia. Halitosis = trench mouth.
Therapy	The conflict is resolved. Support the repair phase and avoid relapses. See also: p. 180.

Cancer of the palate (palatal adeno-ca)[1]

Conflict	The same conflict as with SBS of the oral submucosa. See above.
Example	• Someone thinks he has won the lottery, but the lottery license shop has incorrectly registered his ticket. Chunk conflict of not being able to get the jack-pot. (See Dr. Hamer, Charts, p. 19)
Conflict-active	Growth of a cauliflower-like tumor of secretory quality or a flat-growing tumor (adeno-ca) of absorptive quality under the epithelial mucosa of the mouth.
Bio. function	To produce more mucous with more (intestinal) glandular cells, so that the "chunk" can better slip in or out of the pharynx.
Repair phase	Stinking tubercular caseation of the tumor. Degradation via fungi, or bacteria (mycobacteria). Possible white patches (leukoplakia), pain, halitosis, rotten taste in the mouth.
Therapy	Questions: see tonsillitis. Find out what the conflict and conditioning are and, if possible, resolve them in real life if they are still active. OP if necessary. See also: p. 180.

---

1   See Dr. Hamer, Charts pp. 19, 31

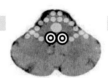

SBS of the Tonsils

Tonsil infections (angina, tonsillitis, angina tonsillaris), tonsil cancer (adeno-ca), pharyngeal polyps[1]

Together, the adenoids (pharyngeal tonsils) and the tubal, palatine and lingual tonsils form Waldeyer's tonsillar ring. The tonsils are lymphatic sensors that determine if something about to be swallowed is fit to swallow. With increasing age, the tonsils shrink, because they have fulfilled their task (childhood learning and conditioning phase).

Conflict	Chunk conflict (see explanations p. 15, 16), not being able to sufficiently verify an incoming chunk. Put simply: one can/may not verify (assess) if the thing that one is swallowing is good or bad. Conflict that one is confronted by accomplished facts (without being allowed to verify them). *("You'll eat everything!")* One cannot just "row their boat gently down the stream" of life, rather, one <u>wants</u> to do everything their own way. *("I want..., I want...")*
Example	→ *A child is forced to eat something he doesn't like. > Thus, their instincts are violated by force. Conflict that one cannot judge what is good for them for themselves.*
	• *A girl is weaned from the breast at the age of six months. She suffers a chunk conflict with respect to the tonsils and the sub-mucosa of the oral cavity. Three months later, when she is accustomed to not receiving breast milk, she gets oral thrush and shortly thereafter tonsillitis = repair phase of the two chunk conflicts.* (Archive B. Eybl)
Conflict-active	Increasing the sensibility of the brainstem through enlargement of the tonsil's surface area = enlarged tonsils, pharyngeal polyps. Possibly difficulty with swallowing or breathing.
Bio. function	The enlarged surface area and increased sensibility makes a better assessment of the food "chunk."
Repair phase	Normalization of function, stinking, tubercular caseation of the tumor via fungi or bacteria = tonsillitis. Tightening of the pharynx due to healing swelling. Aggravated by syndrome. Pain, swelling, halitosis, purulent tonsils, tonsil abscess, and night sweats.
Note	Increasingly, patients are being diagnosed with "tonsillar cancer" instead of tonsillitis or enlarged tonsils. A portion of the tonsil consists of lymphatic tissue > combination tonsil SBS + lymph SBS (for this reason, see p. 145f).
Questions	In the case that a child is affected: When did they have their first tonsillitis? (Find the original conflict, but keep in mind that it could also be a substitution conflict - a parent has a conflict and the child carries (materializes it in themselves) > ask about the child's and the parent's stress) E.g., didn't get a toy/favorite food, parents fight. What brought on the repair phase? (E.g., got the food/toy). What was the conflict situation for this episode? (Work out the similarity to the original conflict). Which event sensitized the child? (Conditioning, e.g., through the character of the parents, pregnancy, birth).
Therapy	In the case that it is recurring: Determine and resolve the conflict, conditioning and belief (system). Guiding principles: *"I am open for surprises - life is wonderful." "Sometimes you get something you weren't expecting - I want to accept and appreciate my gifts."*
	In children, tonsillitis tends to stop by a certain age, when they learn to accept the things they don't have the power to change. (E.g., that they have to listen to the parents, that they don't get an ice cream immediately). If the patient is a child with a substitution conflict, the parent(s) should resolve the conflict and then explain to the child that they do not have to carry it anymore (see p. 32ff).
	Gargling with colloidal silver.
	If necessary, use chinstrap while sleeping so that the mouth is closed. This offers a chance to improve recovery for enlarged tonsils.
	Surgery if the conflict recurs repeatedly and the tonsils are too abscessed.
	See also: p. 180.

---

1   See Dr. Hamer, Charts pp. 19, 32.

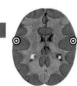

SBS of the Pharyngeal Mucosa

Inflammation of the pharynx (pharyngitis)

Common SBS with "infections," colds, the flu.

Conflict	Separation conflict, not wanting to swallow something, wishing to spit it out again (e.g., hostilities, accusations, insults). *"That is hard to swallow!"* Also, separation conflict of not being allowed to swallow a certain food - for example, when on a diet.
Examples	➜ *A woman must "swallow" a lot at the company where she works. On vacation she comes down with laryngitis during the repair phase.*
	➜ *A child is not allowed to eat sweets. Instead, he should eat his vegetables > not wanting to swallow the vegetables.*
	➜ *A person is constantly being reproached by his partner > wanting to spit out the accusations > cell reduction of the pharyngeal mucosa in the active-phase and restoration in the repair phase.*
	• *A schoolboy must study math every day; otherwise he will not pass > not wanting to "swallow" the learning material. As vacation approaches, he enters the repair phase > pharyngitis.*
Conflict-active	Increased sensitivity, later cell degradation (ulcer) in the pharyngeal squamous epithelium with pain.
Bio. function	Through the high sensibility, one has a better sense of what they want to swallow and what not.
Repair phase	Restoration of the mucosa defects = pharyngitis. Swelling, difficulty swallowing, aggravated by syndrome.
Repair crisis	Severe pain, possibly lasting several days, chills.
Questions	Inflammation since when? (Resolution of the conflict, e.g., through a discussion, relaxing on the weekend, through attending to others). What did I not want to swallow before? Was this the first episode? (If no, go back and locate the first time this conflict was experienced = original conflict). What has conditioned me? (E.g., childhood).
Therapy	The conflict is resolved. Support the healing. In case of a relapse, find out what the conflict and conditioning are and resolve them.
	Guiding principle: *"I only swallow what is good for me!" "I won't let anybody force something upon me that I don't want."* See also: p. 180.

E
C
T
O

– +

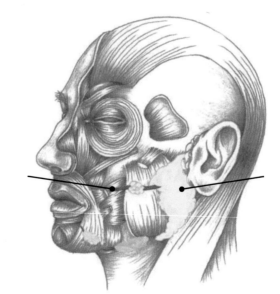

Salivary Gland Excretory
Ducts (Mumps)
**Not being allowed to
or not wanting to
eat something**

Salivary Glands
Chunk conflict

SBS of the Salivary Glands

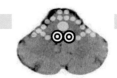

Tumor or inflammation (sialadenitis) of the parotid, sublingual and submandibular salivary glands[1]

Most people affected by sialadenitis are between the ages of 20 and 50. Up to 80% of the cases are parotitis, the other salivary glands are only involved in approximately 20% of the cases.

Conflict	The same conflict as with the SBS of the oral submucosa (see above).
Example	➜ *A child must eat all their food, even though they are already full.*
	➜ *A child wants a certain toy, but does not get it. This often happens in kindergarten, when an only child suddenly has to share with other children.*
	• *A father of a very underweight, young son says he thinks the boy is suffering from bulimia nervosa (binge eating followed by vomiting). He can't think of anything else > Can't ingest the chunk, felt in substitution for his son. In the active phase, a tumor of the salivary gland develops. (Archive B. Eybl)*
	• *A 44-year-old patient leases a small farm from a farmer, so that he can live there with his family. When the key is handed over and the family wants to move in, the farmer shows up drunk and is very unfriendly. He says that before they can move in, they must "wash the windows." Over the following months, the patient can take little pleasure in the house, because the landlord is constantly meddling = chunk conflict of not being able to savor (insalivate) the "house-chunk." In the end, they communicate only through their lawyer and the lease is canceled at the first opportunity. During this time, a tumor of the parotid salivary gland develops on the right side. The patient is familiar with the 5 Biological Laws of Nature and accepts the diagnosis serenely. Within 6 years, the tumor disappears completely - by itself - without inflammation. (Archive B. Eybl)*
Conflict-active	Increased function, growth of a cauliflower-life tumor (adeno-ca) of secretory quality. Enlargement and increase in capacity of the salivary gland. Possibly a recurring conflict.
Bio. function	Production of more saliva, so that the "chunk" can be ingested in or be expelled.
Repair phase	Function normalization, tubercular caseation, stinking saliva, halitosis, pain, inflammation, reduction (melting away) of the tumor via fungi (mycosis) or bacteria = inflammation of the salivary gland, Fever, night sweats.
Repair crisis	Severe pain, chills.
Therapy	Find out what the conflict and conditioning are and, if possible, resolve them in real life if they are still active. Guiding principle: *"I don't expect anything. I can't have everything. I fully accept everything the way it is."* Soften white cabbage leaves and apply. Oil pulling. Chew chewing gum to stimulate salivation and the purification of the gland. See also: p. 180.

Dry mouth (mucoviscidosis of the salivary glands)[1]

Same SBS as above.

Phase	**Persistent repair** or the condition thereafter. Scarred degeneration of the glandular tissue due to recurrences > insufficient production of saliva. More common are the other reasons listed below.
Note	The frequent dryness of the mouth following menopause usually goes hand in hand with a lowering of the estrogen level (dryness of the mucous membranes). Increased dry mouth with active kidney collecting tubules. Radiation or radiation therapy can damage the mucous membrane and lead to dry mouth. Also, medications like antihypertensives, anti-depressants, diuretics and alcohol abuse can cause these symptoms. Dry mouth can be an indication of diabetes.
Therapy	Find out what the conflict and conditioning are and, if possible, resolve them in real life so that the persistent repair can come to an end. Oil pulling and lymph drainage massage, so that the juices start flowing again. Gargling with natural salt solution, Symbioflor 1, or EM.

---

1   See Dr. Hamer, Charts, pp. 20, 31

Salivary gland cysts

These usually appear in the small salivary glands distributed throughout the mouth. For example, they can be caused by a bite on the upper lip > mucus collects and then solidifies (mucocele). If there is no injury: same SBS as above.

Phase	Completed healing or **state following relapse**. The completely removed tumor leaves an empty space (cyst). With syndrome, the cyst can be "pumped up" again.
Therapy	The conflict is resolved. Avoid relapse and resolve refugee conflict, if still active. OP if necessary.

SBS of the Hard Palate

Cleft lip, jaw or palate (harelip, orofacial cleft)

One of the most common birth defects: An incomplete joining of the left and right nose or upper jaw plates in the embryonic stage. As with all hereditary diseases, our focus is directed to the parents and family.

Conflict	According to Frauenkron-Hoffmann: Self-esteem conflict, one doesn't need a palate, because they are unable to get/swallow a chunk anyway. Substitute conflict (look among the parents/ancestors). Resignation with regard to survival/getting by.
Conflict-active	Limited connection of the tissue halves during embryonic development.
Repair phase	A closure of the cleft - making up for the development - is probably only possible during pregnancy. Restoration after birth without an OP cannot be ruled out, but is yet to be documented (own research).
Bio. function	A biological function for the individual is not recognizable. This defect should bring the issue to the family's attention and, like every handicap, has the potential of providing great learning and developmental opportunities for all.
Questions	Did any ancestors already experience this birth defect? Does this issue correspond with any of the ancestors? Was there conflict/resignation during the pregnancy in the sense of: *"I/we am/are not going to get through this anyway?"*
Therapy	Determine and resolve the cause of the conflict and original conditioning so that the issue is healed within the family. This procedure undoubtedly also requires the healing after the (probably necessary) OPs.

SBS of the Branchial Arches

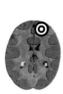

Side (lateral or branchiogenous) neck cyst or fistula

We normally think of the lymph nodes when the neck swells. In rare cases, however, this can be a lateral neck cyst. They are usually situated on the anterior surface of the sternocleidomastoid muscle, also known as the sternomastoid or SCM.

Conflict	Frontal-fear conflict. Fear of an inescapable danger coming head-on. (See also pp. 147, 167.)
Phase	**Repair phase**: Restoration of the squamous epithelium. During the repair swelling, the fluid can collect in cysts. If a cyst opens outwards, it is called a lateral (branchiogenous) neck fistula. Usually **recurring conflict**.
Therapy	The conflict is resolved. Support the healing. Avoid recurrences. Lymph drainage massages.

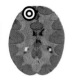

SBS of the Thyroidal Excretory Ducts

Medial neck cysts (thyroglossal duct cysts)

These cysts are found on the existing remains of the thyroglossal ducts, on the center line of the body between the base of the tongue, the larynx and the thyroid. Powerlessness conflict or frontal-fear conflict (see p. 121).

Phase	**Persistent repair:** healing swelling of the thyroid's excretory ducts. Therapy: See also p. 180.

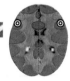

SBS of the Salivary Gland Ducts

Inflammation of the parotid salivary gland ducts (mumps)[1]

According to CM, mumps affects the parotid salivary glands. However, according to Dr. Hamer, mumps is an inflammation of the parotid salivary gland excretory ducts.

Conflict	Not being able to, not being allowed to, or not wanting to eat something (moisten it).
Example	➔ *A child is forced to eat everything. "You will eat everything on your plate!"*
Conflict-active	Functional limitation, later, cell degradation (ulcer) in the squamous epithelium of the duct, painful pulling sensation.
Bio. function	Larger diameter > better excretion of saliva, better insalivation of food.
Repair phase	Swelling and reddening of the ducts. Possible occlusion and build-up of secretions = mumps - they look like an inflammation of the glands. Aggravated by syndrome.
Note	It is hard to tell the difference between mumps and an inflammation of the parotid salivary glands. Consider "handedness" (right or left) and side (mother/child or partner) or local conflict.
Therapy	The conflict is resolved. Support the healing. Avoid recurrences! Chew gum to stimulate salivation and the purification of the gland. See also p. 180.

1   See Dr. Hamer, Charts, pp. 123, 136

SBS of the Tongue Musculature

Paralysis of the tongue

A complete paralysis practically only occurs in the case of a stroke (paralysis of the hypoglossal nerve), but in these cases, one is also dealing with the underlying conflict. A partial paralysis manifests itself with the outstretched tongue leaning toward the paralyzed side.

Conflict	Motor conflict of not wanting, being allowed or being able to say something. Wishing that one had not said something. *"I should have bitten my tongue." "If I just wouldn't have said anything."* Not being able to reach something with the tongue (e.g., lack of food).
Phase	Paralysis in the **conflict-active phase**. Slow restoration in the repair phase. With a hot stroke, the conflict is already in the repair phase. (Paralysis through the enlargement of the synapses in the motor cortical center).
Questions	Paralysis since when? Conflict-active indication (compulsive thought, poor sleep, cold hands) or repair phase indication (psychically resolved, headache, warm hands) in the context of a hot stroke? Which stress was there in regard to speaking/speech? Did I say something wrong/I shouldn't have said or was I afraid to speak? Why am I sensitized here? Similar characteristics in ancestors?
Therapy	Find out what the conflict and conditioning are and resolve them in real life. Guiding principle: see above.

Sialolithiasis (salivary (duct) stones)

This is most often found (in 80% of cases) in the excretory ducts leading from the parotid salivary glands.

Possible causes

- **Recurring inflammation of the salivary gland -** persistent repair or condition following persistent repair. At the end of every tubercular repair, calcium deposits remain. Scarring degeneration of the glandular tissue due to recurrence > thickening and clumping of the saliva and deposition of minerals > salivary stones.

- **Recurring inflammation of the excretory ducts -** persistent repair of the excretory ducts and condition following persistent repair. Repeated inflammation and congestion in the excretory ducts > clumping, thickening > mineral deposits > salivary stones.

Remedies for inflammations in the mouth and throat

- Tea: fenugreek, chamomile, agrimony, sage, burdock root, anise, common mallow, horsetail, etc.
- Oil pulling (see p. 61).
- Gargle with colloidal silver.
- Swedish bitters - "pull" or swish in the mouth, gargle and then swallow.
- Vitamin D3 (cod liver oil).
- MMS, DMSO.
- Gargling remedy: Natural salt solution, diluted or concentrated, swish in mouth for 10 min. then spit out.
- Gargling remedy: Boil nut shells and oak bark and then allow them to steep for several hours; then drain and store in a cool place. Swish in the mouth and gargle several times a day.
- Symbioflor 1, EM (see p. 59) or bread drink (Brottrunk) for symbionts
- Curd cheese compress for the neck. Lymph drainage massages.

Tooth Enamel
Not being allowed to bite

Tooth Dentin
Self-esteem conflict not being able to bite

Jawbone, Periodontium
Self-esteem conflict, not being able to bite

Oral Submucosa
Chunk conflict

TEETH AND JAW

Every tooth is made up of a dental crown (corona dentis), a neck (colum dentis) and a root (radix dentis). What we see externally in a healthy set of teeth is only ectodermal tooth enamel, which covers the mesodermal dentin lying below it like a glaze. In turn, the dentin covers the and nerve and vessel-filled tooth pulp (pulpa). The teeth are connected elastically to the jaws with the mesodermal cementum. There is a layer of old, endodermal intestinal mucosa between the mesodermal jawbone and the ectodermal oral mucosa.

According to Dr. Hamer, teeth "function" strictly according to the 5 Biological Laws of Nature.

Although this might be true in theory, experience in this field tells a different story.

According to my own experience and after numerous talks with New Medicine dentists, I had to rewrite this chapter: Firstly the diet is much more important than we thought, and secondly the restoration (re-calcification) has a literal "flaw."

In the best case, i.e., if one permanently resolves their bite conflict and keeps to a proper diet, cavities will not increase in size, the affected areas (and the remaining teeth) harden. The black, decayed areas harden from the inside out and even regain a hardened surface.

If you do nothing (without a dentist), cavities will not get better; they will get larger.

Conclusion: conflict resolution AND a change in diet! Good, professional dental care is advisable - also for aesthetic reasons.

Where was recovery observed?
- In the jawbone, periodontal apparatus and gums.
- In small cavities in the dentin and enamel. Larger cavities do not fill up again.

Diet and teeth
Proper nutrition is as important for healthy teeth as psychological balance. In his great, in-depth book, "Cure Tooth Decay," (see source list) Ramiel Nagel shows that tooth decay goes hand in hand with the introduction of modern industrial food.

In his view, neither bacteria nor their acid excretions cause caries, but malnutrition and stress. Nagel's nutrition recommendations for the regeneration of teeth and gums in short form:

Avoid sugar (e.g., cakes, chocolate, soft drinks, sweet fruit), isolated starch (white flour, bread, pasta). These short-chain carbohydrates cause blood sugar spikes that interfere with the calcium-phosphate balance.

Favor natural, vitamin rich foods. Especially important: Natural calcium and phosphate (e.g., in vegetables, unpasteurized dairy products, fish), naturally bound vitamins A, D and C (e.g., in liver, fish, eggs, unpasteurized butter, cream, cheese, avocado, herbs and fruit).

Oral hygiene, brushing the teeth
All New Medicine dentists I have interviewed say that hygiene, care and healthy food are all crucial to healthy teeth.

Also, well-cared for teeth and pleasant breath can improve a person's self-confidence and interpersonal relations.

- I personally brush my teeth with a salt solution (sea salt or Himalaya salt dissolved in water and stored in a bottle or glass jar). I take a tablespoon of salt solution into my mouth and brush my teeth as usual. If the gums are sensitive, one can dilute the solution at the beginning.
- Cayce: Brush the teeth with a solution of bicarbonate of soda and table salt.
- New Medicine dentists recommend using fluoride-free toothpastes.

Should one wait patiently when they have a cavity?
No, because larger cavities do not regenerate themselves. Any sensible dentist will try to drill out only what is necessary and preserve as much of each tooth as possible. By undetermined pain, one should first wait and see before unnecessarily "sacrificing" a tooth. Below are the biological relationships regarding the teeth:

The purpose of the teeth
- Incisors: biting, snapping and snarling.
- Canines: sicking, seizing, capturing and holding on.
- Bicuspids: chewing.
- Molars: grinding.

The conflict content based on the aforementioned:
- Both incisors: not being able to or allowed to bite, snap, or bare one's teeth.
- Canine teeth: not being able or allowed to sic, seize, capture or hold onto.
- Bicuspids: not being able or allowed to chew.
- Molars: not being able or allowed to grind.

"Not being able to" means: One doesn't dare, is too weak, too cowardly, too shy, or too cautious. One cannot bite, because it is outside of one's possibilities (e.g., worker/boss, pupil/teacher). Tissue affected: dentin - self-esteem conflict - cerebral white matter - mesoderm.

"Not being allowed to" means: Somebody or something prevents one from biting (e.g., "political correctness" or "rules of propriety"). Affected tissue: tooth enamel - separation conflict - cerebral cortex.

SBS of the Tooth Enamel

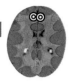

Surface cavities affecting the tooth enamel[1]

Conflict	Not being allowed to bite, small variations in conflict according to localization (see above).
Examples	→ *An employee is always being "bossed around" (bitten) by his superior; however, he may not bite back, or he will lose his job.*
	• *A woman is put under pressure by her partner to finally defend herself against her sister's attacks. However, the patient wants to avoid arguments.* (Archive B. Eybl)
Conflict-active	Cell degradation in the tooth enamel (ulcer). Development of cavities = enamel defect, pain.
Bio. function	The person or thing should be rendered "unbiteable" due to temporary hypersensitivity. - One doesn't want to bite anymore, because biting hurts.
Repair phase	Restoration only of minimal defects. False sensitivity to hot/cold or sweet/sour. For large cavities, a full restoration is unrealistic. In the best case, the cavity will stay the way it is - or it will even get larger, if it is not treated.
Therapy psyche	To avoid new cavities, think about a possible psychological reason. Determine the conflict and conditioning and, if possible, resolve them in real life. Questions: see next page.
	Guiding principle: *"I have the right to defend myself!" "I don't have to put up with anything and from now on, I'm going to sink my teeth into life!"* Alternate strategy: Absolute forgiveness.
	Always think positively about your teeth and imagine them being healthy and shiny.
Tooth therapy	Let a dentist fill the tooth - avoid amalgam fillings! If necessary, CM painkillers - short term.
	Nutrition according to Nagel (see also p. 183): Omit sugar and white flour. Consume more vitamin-rich foods. Cod liver oil 1 tbsp/day. Beef bone or fish soup with vegetables at least 3 x/week, soft boiled or raw eggs often.
	Mouthwash with sage, clove, blackberry, frankincense or tincture of myrrh or EM. Natural Borax, hold in mouth as long as possible before swallowing.

1   See Dr. Hamer, Teeth Charts, columns 1 - 6

E
C
T
O

− +

SBS of the Dentin

Deep cavities affecting the dentin[1]

Conflict	Self-esteem conflict of not being able to bite, to defend oneself or to assert oneself. Small variations in conflict according to localization.
Examples	→ *A weak boy is regularly beaten up at school by his stronger classmates.*
	→ *At work, a man must always acquiesce to the will of others. He is too weak to get his own way.*
	• *A 53-year-old, left-handed man has an older brother who is very aggressive. During his childhood and youth, the patient was always an easy victim when his brother came home drunk = bite conflict - "I would like to bite back, but I don't dare, or I will come out on the short end!" > Damage to the dentin on the molars (partner side) in the active-phase.* (Archive B. Eybl)
	• *The sister of a right-handed patient always knows better. During their few telephone conversations, her sister always holds monologues = conflict of not being able to bite her sister because it would disturb the family peace. The patient tries to accept her sister the way she is and thus comes into healing. The dentin of the right molar is affected.* (Archive B. Eybl)
	• *The parents of a 6-year-old boy are constantly quarreling. The father always loses his temper and*

N
E
W
M
E
S
O

− +

1   See Dr. Hamer, Teeth Charts, columns 3 and 4 (orange group)

begins screaming = bite conflict for the boy: "I would like to tell my father off, to bite him!" > Break-down of tooth dentin. Almost all of his teeth form cavities. He wishes for harmony between his mother and father. Unfortunately, the situation continues for years. Later in life, he lives with his own family in the same house, so the conflict continues to receive sustenance. (Archive B. Eybl)

• I am left-handed and when I was 24 years old, I decided to begin an apprenticeship as a masseur. It was not easy to get a position, but I finally found a very promising one with a renowned acupoint masseur in Salzburg. Quickly, I saw through the secret of my teacher's business success. He persuaded people that their pelvis was lopsided and that this was the cause of all their illnesses. My admiration of my boss quickly turned into aversion. I wished I could bite him and grind him to a powder. However, I couldn't, since I knew that no one else would take me on as their apprentice after that. The conflict activity lasted for six months - finally it came to a discussion and our parting ways. Two weeks after my dismissal, I was lucky enough to find a new position. The toothache came at night - the dentist diagnosed a deep cavity. "It is already affecting the nerve." > Root canal treatment. (Personal experience B. Eybl)

Conflict-active	Formation of holes (cell breakdown) in the interior of the tooth - the dentin - usually only visible with x-ray, no pain. Consider "handedness" (right or left) and side (mother/child or partner). Usually a **recurring conflict.**
Repair phase	Inflammation, toothache, especially at rest or in the night. Restoration (recalcification) only in very small defects. Aggravated by syndrome (kidney collecting tubules).
	If the inflammation goes into the dental pulp, the pain can be excruciating.
	According to New Medicine dentists: in the best case, recalcification only at the border to the healthy tissue > the cavity solidifies and does not get any bigger.
	Experience shows that a cavity will continue to increase in size if one doesn't truly resolve the conflict and decisively change their diet.
Bio. function	Strengthening of the dentin
Questions	Which tooth is affected? (Molars - grinding, incisors - open conflict). Handedness, side of the mouth? (Right for right-handers > partner side, left for right-handers > mother/child side). Pain since when? (A bite conflict must have been resolved when the pain began: E.g., prevailing against an antagonist, finally expressing oneself clearly, bringing a project to an end). Did it appear suddenly? (Yes: sudden conflict resolution shortly before. No: Drawn-out/gradual conflict resolution). Pain at rest/nights? (Yes: Clearly an acute repair phase). Now, one should be able to clearly determine the conflict. Questions: What stressed me before this? Who did I want to bite? Where was I unable to get my way/"bite-through?" How do I deal with conflict/disharmony? Do I always give in? Do I avoid it? At what age were my teeth still intact? (Indication of the beginning of the bite conflict - but consider the lead time)! What is my diet like? (Determine if the diet plays a role). Conditioning: How do the members of my family deal with conflict/differences of opinion? (Culture of conflict). Was I programmed to "bite my way through?" (Ambition, successful parent(s)). Did my ancestors have important experiences with regard to "giving in/backing down," violence/biting or "biting-through." (Look for conditioning).
Therapy: psyche	To avoid new cavities think about possible psychological reasons > Determine the conflict and conditioning and, if possible, resolve them in real life. Guiding principles: *"I am strong and brave!" "I'll bite if necessary!"* Imagine the situation or the adversary and bite with satisfaction.
	Different strategy: forgiveness. Think positively about your teeth and imagine them being healthy and shiny. Bach flowers: larch, centaury.
Therapy: tooth	Dietary changes according to Nagel: omit sugar, white flour. Eat more vitamin-rich foods. Cod liver oil 1 tbsp/day, beef-bone or fish soup with vegetables at least 3 x / week, soft boiled or raw eggs often.
	By all means, have large cavities filled by a dentist. In case of smaller cavities, one can possibly wait. CM painkillers if necessary. Preserve every natural tooth if possible. If a root canal or extraction is necessary, antibiotics are usually prescribed as a precaution measure. These are unnecessary from the perspective of the New Medicine.
	Lymph drainage massages, oil pulling. Tea/mouthwashes: comfrey, horsetail, possibly restharrow, chamomile. Xylitol, DMSO. Rinse mouth with salt water, EM, colloidal silver. Hydrogen peroxide. Natural borax - hold in mouth before swallowing.

Parodontitis (atrophy of the gums)

Same SBS as above.

Example	• A 46-year-old cheats on his wife and pays for it with prostate cancer. (See p. 259). That is not all: after he confesses to his wife, she becomes, understandably, distrustful. She wants to go everywhere with him and is always checking up on him. The patient feels guilty toward his wife and no longer dares to be demanding. He accepts all the limitations placed upon him = active self-esteem, bite conflict. > Subsequently, he develops extensive, advanced parodontitis, the upper jaw being affected more then the lower jaw. His once white teeth become discolored and are now yellowish-gray. In addition, the dentist finds a decrease in their vertical dimensions (the teeth have sunken). A root planing is carried out. Therapy: When the couple sees the connections, they decide that they should renew their marriage vows with a little ceremony - from now on, he will remain faithful and she puts an end to the whole matter in her mind. Two years later : the relationship is rosy again and the patient's teeth are solid again. (Archive B. Eybl)
Conflict-active	Degradation of cementum. The tooth neck appears longer, because the apparatus that holds the teeth in place (periodontium) is receding = parodontitis. The teeth may possibly take on a yellowish discoloration (= indication of a lack of tooth vitality). No pain. Chronic periodontitis is a result of recurrent conflicts.
Repair phase	Inflammation, bleeding (while brushing), pain, restoration.
Bio. function	Strengthening of the periodontal apparatus
Therapy	Questions: see previous page. Find the conflict and conditioning and if resolve them in real life. If this succeeds, repair pain (good sign) will follow. Stabilization of the tooth with adhesive or bracket until the tooth is stable and the healing is complete. Be patient - the healing process often takes longer than one would like. Natural, nutritious, alkaline diet, linseed oil.
	Dietary changes according to Nagel: omit sugar, white flour. Eat more vitamin-rich foods. Cod liver oil 1 tbsp/day, beef-bone or fish soup with vegetables at least 3 x/week, soft boiled or raw eggs often.
	Bach flowers: larch, centaury, tea/mouthwash: comfrey root, horsetail, blackberry leaves, sage. Rinse the mouth and/or brush the teeth with salt solution, hydrogen peroxide, DMSO. Oil pulling. Cayce: for susceptibility to parodontitis and cavities, clean and massage the teeth and gums with ipsab powder (= prickly-ash, North American "toothache tree"). Natural borax - hold in mouth for a long time before swallowing. Xylitol. Zeolite powder internally.

Dedentition (tooth loss)

Same SBS as above. (See pp. 182 - 184)

Phase	**Persistent-active conflict.** Atrophy of the periodontal apparatus > loss of teeth.
Therapy	Find the conflict and conditioning and resolve them in real life so that no more teeth fall out!

Jaw cysts

Same SBS as above. (See pp. 182 - 184)

Phase	**Recurring-conflict**, usually with syndrome. Restoration and degradation phases repeat themselves > formation of hollow spaces (cysts).
Therapy	Determine and resolve the conflict, conditioning and belief (system). Change diet (see p. 183).

Jaw Tumor (odontoma, myxoma, osteosarcoma)[2]

Same SBS as above. (See pp. 182 - 184)

Example	• A 50-year-old, married, right-handed woman fulfills her long-time dream: With a considerable sum (her entire savings), she opens a flower boutique together with a partner. Now, she is self-employed. Unfortunately, her project turns out to be a mistake, because shortly after opening, there is a dispute with the landlord. The business also doesn't take off as hoped. = Bite conflict - she would like nothing more than to tear the landlord to shreds and she isn't succeeding professionally. After two years, she finally pulls the emergency brake, leaves the partnership and writes off the money. = Beginning of the repair phase: She experiences tooth and jaw pain (right side) and chronic fatigue. When the

pain doesn't improve, she is taken to the hospital where a jaw tumor is diagnosed. An operation follows immediately. (Archive B. Eybl)

Phase **Repair phase** or persistent repair (recurrent conflict), possibly with syndrome. Restoration of the jawbone after previous cell degradation. Severe pain.

Therapy The bite conflict is resolved, support the repair phase. If recurring, determine and resolve the conflict, conditioning and beliefs. If necessary, resolve refugee crisis. Change diet (see p. 183). Attention: Do not puncture > danger of callus leakage > resulting in a "sarcoma." Lymph drainage. See also: repair phase at the brain level, p 60f.

Dental calculus (tartar)

Not only poor dental hygiene can be the cause of solid dental tartar:

1. Dental calculus forms increasingly in the area of bad, loose teeth. During repair phases of the periodontium, dentin or the jawbone, fibrocartilage callus finds its way into the oral cavity via the salivary glands or directly out of the gums. This "liquid bone" mixes with dental plaque and hardens on the outside of tooth necks > yellowish deposits = tarter.

2. One often finds tarter in the area were the salivary gland excretory ducts enter the oral cavity = indication of salivary fluid imbalance (tendency toward crystallization). According to Nagel, tartar forms due to too much free calcium or an imbalance between calcium and phosphate.

Phase Buildup during the repair phase or **recurrent conflict** (same SBS as above).

Therapy Determine the conflict and conditioning and resolve them in real life so that no new tartar forms. Improve oral hygiene, change diet (advice on p. 183) Mechanical removal as a part of regular prophylaxis.

SBS of the Jaw Muscles

Grinding of the teeth (bruxism)

Some of us have taken the words *"Clench your teeth!"* too literally. Teeth-grinding is usually noticed only by the partner because it occurs in the context of repair phase crises during deep sleep. The grinding wears the teeth down unnecessarily, therefore, something should be done about it.

Conflict Motor conflict: not being able or allowed to snap, grind or "bite one's way through." One believes that they must bite their way through. Issues: doggedness, uptightness, fanaticism.

Example ➜ *During the day, someone wishes to bite often, but does nothing, because they are too cowardly > at night they enter the repair phase and grinds their teeth during repair phase crises. At night, one does (biting) what they didn't do during the day.*

Phase Repair phase crisis in the context of the repair phase > cramping of the jaw muscles (masseter, temporal, medial pterygoid) during relaxation (at night) - teeth-grinding = "chewing muscle epilepsy." Usually a **recurring-conflict.**

Questions Grinding since when? (Ask partner, parents. A bite conflict has been ongoing at least since then). If it was especially heavy: What happened the day before? (Indication of the conflict). How is it on vacation? (If better > conflict in daily life). Ancestors/family members also affected? (If yes: work out the family issue).

Therapy Find out what the conflict and conditioning are and, if possible, resolve them in real life so that the persistent repair comes to an end. Guiding principle: *"No more 'grin and bear it.' If need be, I'll bite!"* Imagine the situation or the adversary and bite. Immediately address everything bothersome or what one disagrees with and then bury it. Thereafter, reconcile with the situation internally or personally with the person in question. Bach flowers: agrimony. Occlusal bite block/splint ("night-guard"), so the teeth don't get worn down grinding in the night.

SBS of the Oral Submucosa

Periodontal abscess (tooth fistula)

Conflict	Chunk-bite conflict: In right side of the mouth: not being able to bite/get a food chunk (something desired or good, for example, certain foods, a good job, a car, because you do not dare). In left side of the mouth: Not being able to get rid of something undesirable or uncomfortable because you cannot prevail. (For example, a man feels stuck in a situation where he cannot "bite his way through"). According to Frauenkron-Hoffmann: One doesn't have enough confidence to address/approach the problem directly and chooses a "diplomatic detour" instead.
Example	• *A single-mother is tormented by her teenage daughter. She would rather avoid confrontations. - She can't bite her way though.* (Archive B. Eybl)
Conflict-active	Increased function, growth of a tumor (adeno-ca) under the oral squamous epithelium (usually unnoticed).
Bio. function	With more glandular cells, more mucus is produced, so that the chunk glides in or out of the throat better.
Repair phase	Normalization of function, tubercular, caseating degradation. Foul taste in the mouth, possibly local excretion of pus, halitosis, night sweats (tuberculosis). Usually a **recurring-conflict.**
Repair crisis	Severe pain, possibly chills.
Therapy	Support the healing. In the case that the abscess recurs or doesn't go away, resolve the conflict and conditioning. (Questions: see p. 183.) Oil pulling therapy, lymph drainages, gargling with colloidal silver. Tea/mouthwash: anise, blueberries, mallow, honey. Gargling with (H_2O_2). Natural borax - hold in mouth for a long time.

Gingivitis and parodontitis - inflammation of the gums, parodontium

Possible causes

• **Inflammation of the superficial, ectodermal oral mucosa -** repair phase. Superficial, visible reddening, swelling, bleeding, but without pain (except during the repair phase crisis). No night sweats, no halitosis (see 172ff).

• **Inflammation of the deep-lying endodermal oral submucosa -** repair phase. Inflammation from underneath, halitosis, stinking pus, night sweats (see above).

• **Inflammation of the periodontium** - repair phase: deep inflammation, loose tooth or teeth, pain, non-stinking pus (= callus). No night sweats, mini-leukemia.

• **Calcium deficiency/improper diet** (see p. 183).

Therapy

Improve diet, especially by taking vitamins D and C (see p. 183). Gargle with colloidal silver, sage tea, tincture of frankincense or myrrh, MMS, EM, hydrogen peroxide (H_2O_2). Regular dental prophylaxis.

Gum proliferations (gingival hyperplasia, epulis)

Each of the following three causes is possible
• Oral submucosa : Persistent conflict activity
• Oral mucosa: persistent repair

• Periodontal apparatus: persistent repair

ESOPHAGUS

The approximately 25 cm (10 in) long, muscular food pipe - the esophagus - transports food pulp from the pharynx to the stomach using peristaltic (undulating) motions.

The esophagus is composed of endodermal intestinal mucosa with involuntary muscle underneath.

In the upper two-thirds of the esophagus, ectodermal epithelium, composed of voluntary (striated) muscle which migrated from the mouth, lies over the old intestinal mucosa (ectodermal squamous epithelium and voluntary striated muscle usually make a pair).

In the illustration below, you see two ectodermal areas located in the otherwise endodermal digestive tract: The lesser curvature of the stomach along with the pyloric sphincter and the last inch of the rectum and anus.

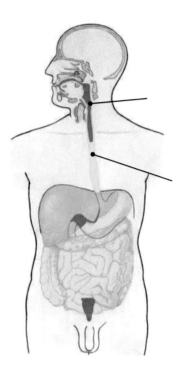

Superficial Esophageal
Mucosa (upper two-thirds)
**Not wanting to swallow
something**

Esophageal Submucosa
(lower third)
**Chunk conflict, not being
able to swallow something**

SBS of the Esophageal Submucosa

Endodermal esophageal cancer (adeno-ca)[1]

This cancer normally develops in the lower third of the esophagus. It can also occur in the upper two-thirds, as a "leftover" of the old intestinal mucosa or below the squamous mucosa (submucosal).

Conflict	Chunk conflict (see explanations p. 15, 16). Not being able to swallow something. One wants to swallow something but is prevented from doing so. One wants something but does not get it.
Example	→ *Someone is left empty-handed in terms of money, inheritance, pension, even though they counted on it.* • *A 70-year-old, married retiree likes most of all to spend time tending to his leased garden. As he returns from a summer vacation, he finds a backhoe digging up the garden = conflict, the garden (= chunk) can't be ingested - he can no longer "embody" it. In the active-phase, a "malignant" adeno-ca develops. The patient has trouble swallowing. Fortunately in the meantime, he has been promised a new garden = beginning of the repair phase with night-time coughing and spitting up of caseated pieces of the tumor. (See Claudio Trupiano, Danke Doktor Hamer, p. 161)*
Conflict-active	Increased function. Growth of a cauliflower-like tumor of secretory quality or a flat-growing tumor of absorptive quality. Narrowing of the esophagus, swallowing difficulties. Possibly only pureed or liquid food can be swallowed = esophageal stenosis.

1   See Dr. Hamer, Charts, p. 21

Bio. function	Secretory quality: To produce more digestive juices to break down the chunk that is stuck in the esophagus so that it can actually be swallowed.
	Absorptive quality: To be able to absorb the chunk through improved up-take of nutrients.
Repair phase	Normalized function and/or tubercular caseation of the tumor. Degradation via fungi or bacteria. Inflammation of the esophagus (esophagitis, esophageal thrush). Pain behind the breastbone. Danger of unnoticed bleeding (black stool, "occult blood"). Night sweats, fever. Aggravated by syndrome. Possibly scars, diverticula (bulges where the tube has been weakened) or so-called esophagus rings and membranes may remain.
Repair crisis	Severe pain, bleeding, chills.
Questions	Complaints since when? (Conflict previous). What am I not allowed to incorporate/take in/embody? (Sum of money, something important to me, a better life)? Why is it so important to me? (Work out conditioning, e.g., early childhood experiences of not getting something). Why is this thing more important than my life? What is my attitude toward ownership/possessions? What is the meaning of life?
Therapy	Determine the conflict and conditioning and, if possible, resolve them in real life. Guiding principles: "I am satisfied with what I have." "There is a reason why this has happened." "That's it, done!" If necessary, OP without chemo or radiation.

"Varicose veins in the esophagus" (esophageal varices)

Same SBS as above. In CM, this is seen as congestion in the portal vein system. This hypothesis is questionable - more than likely, this is an SBS of the esophagus.

Phase	**Recurring-conflict** or the condition thereafter. Extremely dilated submucosal veins in the lower third of the esophagus = blood vessel scar tissue.
Therapy	Identify the conflict and conditioning and, if possible, resolve them in real life so that the SBS comes to an end. In the case of acute, threatening hemorrhage: OP (rubber band ligation or sclerotherapy).

SBS of the Esophageal Ectodermal Mucosa

Ectodermal esophageal cancer (ulcer-ca)[1]

This type of cancer only grows in the upper two-thirds of the esophagus.

Conflict	Not wanting to swallow (accept) something, wanting to spit something out again. One would rather just vomit and rebel - but they don't do it.
Examples	→ "It's a hard pill to swallow." "That's going to be hard for me to swallow."
	→ "That's hard to swallow!" (E.g., accusation, loss of work, stroke of fate.)
	• A very honest postman is accused by his boss of having embezzled a package containing a large sum of money = conflict of not wanting to swallow the accusation. Growth of an esophageal cancer in the active-phase. It is diagnosed in the repair phase. (See Dr. Hamer, Krankheit der Seele, p. 296)
	• The patient is a glassblower and comes back to his workplace following a vacation. He is stunned to learn that an apprentice has taken his place. He has a big row with his supervisor = not wanting to accept the fact. (See Dr. Hamer, Krankheit der Seele, p. 218)
Conflict-active	Cell degradation in the epithelium (ulcer-ca), pain.
Bio. function	By increasing the diameter of the esophagus, the chunk can be better expectorated or vomited.
Repair phase	Restoration of the mucous membrane. Inflammation of the esophagus (esophagitis, herpes or cytomegalic esophagitis, glycogen acanthosis, no pain, but swelling and swallowing difficulties). Aggravated by syndrome. The patient can be left with scars, diverticula or so-called esophageal rings and membranes. Possibly a recurring conflict.

---

1 See Dr. Hamer, Charts pp. 122, 135

Repair crisis	Pain, possibly heavy bleeding > melena (tarry stool), chills.
Questions	Study the histological findings and determine if it is an adeno-ca (yellow group) or a squamous cell-ca (red group). Determine if one is in vagotonia or still in the active phase: sleep in the early morning, hand temperature, fever, appetite, dreams? Estimate the time period of the conflict. If in the active phase: What don't I want to swallow? (Determine the exact situation). Do I generally acquiesce a lot? What is stressing me? Are there taboo topics? (These are often a source of conflict). What conditioning makes me sensitive to this issue? (Childhood experiences, experiences of the parents/ancestors)? Which belief(s) has paved the way for the conflict? (E.g. Being everything for everyone. One is only loved when one is well-behaved. It's better not to be conspicuous). Are/were there similar conflict situations among my ancestors? (If yes, resolve the family issue through healing thoughts/meditation/prayers).
Therapy	Identify the conflict and conditioning and, if possible, resolve them if they are still active. Guiding principles: *"I will only swallow what's good for me." "I won't let anyone force anything down my throat anymore." "I am at peace with everything."* If necessary, surgery without chemo or radiation.

Inflammation of the esophagus (esophagitis)

This could be either of the two SBSs described above

- Inflammation of the upper two-thirds of the esophagus: repair phase. One found something revolting.

- Inflammation of the lower two-thirds of the esophagus: repair phase. One wasn't allowed to incorporate something.

STOMACH

The stomach takes the food pulp from the esophagus and sends it on through the pylorus to the duodenum. Glands in the mucous membranes of the stomach produce gastric juices (pepsin and hydrochloric acid), which break down proteins. Like most of the digestive canal, the stomach (ventriculus) is made up mainly of endodermal tissue, with the exception of the pylorus and the lesser curvature - those are covered with ectodermal squamous epithelium.

Stomach Mucosa - Squamous Epithelium
(Lesser Curvature and Pylorus)
**Territorial-anger/
identity conflict**

Stomach Mucosa -
Columnar Epithelium
**Inability to digest
something**

Duodenum
**Territorial-anger
conflict**

SBS of the Superficial Mucosa of the Stomach

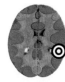

Heartburn I, hyperacidity of the stomach, inflammation of the gastric mucosa (gastritis), stomach-epithelial cancer (stomach ulcer-cancer), stomach ulcer[1]

Conflict	Territorial-anger conflict, less often - identity conflict (dependent on "handedness," hormone levels and previous conflicts). One is sour (like the gastric juices). One boils with rage or is angry on the inside.
Examples	→ *Usually dealing with aggression. Either it's one's own anger coming from someone else.*
	→ *Boundary disputes with neighbors, a mother-in-law's encroachments," problems with coworkers.*
	→ *One is forced to accept a subordinate role or "back down."*
	• *A man regards a new colleague at work as competition.* (Archive B. Eybl)
	• *A 34-year-old woman shares an office with a nice colleague. Suddenly, they are joined by three new coworkers of various nationalities who ignore the rules: The kitchen and toilet are dirty and the standard working hours are not observed = territorial-anger conflict. After a few weeks, the conflict is resolved when her friend tells her about another job opening in another company. Since then, she is more relaxed about the situation. In the repair phase and/or repair phase crisis, the patient becomes very sick to her stomach.* (See www.germanische-heilkunde.at/index.php/erfahrungsberichte)
	• *A now 41-year-old patient has a violent father, under whom he suffers to this day. His father beats his mother regularly and he himself has been berated and put down ever since he was a child. All the time he hears "...you loser!" = territorial-anger conflict > cell degradation in the stomach mucosa. Repeatedly, he has mild heartburn = active-phase. Seven months ago, a child runs into the patient's car. He is not at fault, but out of his subconscious, the conflict comes up again: "...you loser! " = recurrence > After the accident, he has had severe heartburn for half a year = active-phase. The patient is always slightly conflict-active, because he lives with his family at the parents' farm, practically next door to his father. The best therapy would be to move away from the farm, but that is out of the question for the patient.* (Archive B. Eybl)
Conflict-active	Increased sensitivity, later, cell degradation in the affected area of the squamous epithelial mucosa of the stomach. The longer the conflict lasts, the deeper the tissue defects (ulcers) become. Paralysis of the underlying voluntary (striated) muscles, leading to a greater stomach lumen. According to Frauenkron-Hoffmann, if someone is repeatedly angered or feels like they're being attacked, the gastric juices respond to the "thing" that can't be digested, producing acid reflux. (A prophylactic stomach acid attack).
Bio. function	With increased sensitivity, one has a better sense of what is digestible or indigestible (sickening).
Repair phase	Restoration of the stomach mucosa's squamous epithelium. Bleeding stomach ulcer, possibly some blood in the stool (occult blood).
Repair crisis	Severe colicky pain, heavy bleeding (tarry stool), loss of consciousness (absence seizures), stomach colic, and possibly chills.
Questions	When did the symptoms begin? (Conflict directly beforehand and also precisely during the symptoms). What stressed me during the heartburn? (Review all situations in the recent past). Symptoms for the first time ever? (If no, analyze the time period in question = initial territorial anger). What conditioned me, so that situations like these make me so angry? (Childhood experiences, pregnancy, parent's experiences - these are also subconsciously mine). Work out any similarities with ancestors > become aware > ask myself the question: Am I ready to leave this pattern of behavior? What do I want to change on the outside?
Therapy	Identify the conflict and conditioning and, if possible, resolve them in real life so that the stomach mucosa can regenerate. Find out where the love is - you will also find the solution there. Guiding principles: *"No anger in my heart." "There isn't anything that can upset me." "If necessary, I will fight!"* Alkaline powder, but better if organically bound - i.e., eat lots of fruits, vegetables and wild herbs (especially apples, carrots, potatoes, boiled cabbage). Kanne Bread Drink. Willfort: 3-week treatment with freshly-squeezed cabbage juice - drink 0.5 - 1 l (16 - 32 oz) over the whole day. Colloidal silver internally.

E
C
T
O

−+

---

1 See Dr. Hamer, Charts, p. 115

Segment and reflexology massage, acupuncture. Hildegard of Bingen: fennel seeds and leaf, mosquito plant (Mentha polegium), sage, muscatel-sage elixir.

Acid neutralizing remedies (antacids - mostly sodium bicarbonate) are harmless drugs, which may even benefit the organism if it is too acidic in general (with active kidney collecting tubules SBS). The situation with antacids (proton pump inhibitors, H2-antihistamines) is quite different. These are harmful in the long run. See also: stomach remedies on p. 193.

Perforation of the stomach wall - gastric ulcer > peptic ulcer disease

Same SBS as above.

Phase	**Persistent, active conflict**, causing the ulcer to become increasingly deeper. > Stomach perforation that can be life threatening (acute abdomen > peptic ulcer disease).
Therapy	Questions: see previous page. Identify the conflict and triggers and, if possible, resolve them in real life, so that the mucosa of the stomach can regenerate. Surgery if necessary. See above and stomach remedies p. 193.

Stomach displacement (gastroptosis), partial stomach paralysis stomach (gastroparesis), stomach prolapse into the duodenum (gastroduodenal prolapse)

Same SBS as above. (See p. 192)

Phase	**Conflict-active phase:** sinking of the stomach or prolapse into the duodenum due to a paralysis of the voluntary (striated) muscles of the stomach.
Therapy	Questions: see previous page. Identify the conflict and conditioning and, if possible, resolve in real life.

SBS of the Gastric Sphincter

HFs in the midbrain - topography still unknown

Heartburn II, regurgitation of gastric juices into the esophagus (reflux, esophageal reflux, Barrett's esophagus), cardia insufficiency

With heartburn, the esophagus becomes inflamed by gastric juices entering the esophagus (esophageal reflux).

First, we have to consider territorial-anger (p. 190f), then this SBS:

Conflict	Not being able to disgorge something bad that has been swallowed or not being able to take up or accept something good that has been swallowed.
Example	• *A 20-year-old, introverted man feels ill-at-ease in larger groups. In spite of this, he regularly attends soccer practices and goes out drinking with his colleagues in bars. There, the loud ones have the say. He often has to swallow things he doesn't like at all = conflict of not being able to disgorge or spit out what he has had to swallow. Since he was 16, he has experienced a trigger whenever he has been forced onto the defensive or whenever he drinks alcohol > heartburn. (Archive B.Eybl)*
Conflict-active	In sympathicotonia, the cardia opens > rise of the gastric juices into the esophagus > heartburn, persistent-conflict: a "burning" of the esophagus. Persistent-conflict: "burning" of the esophagus > reflux esophagitis.
Bio. function	Dilation of the cardia: so that what is bad can be better disgorged or what is good can be better swallowed.
Repair phase	Normalization of tense muscles. In the repair phase crisis, stomach or esophageal cramps occurring in fits.
Therapy	Questions: see p. 190. Determine the conflict and conditioning and, if possible, resolve them in real life. Guiding principles: *"From now on, I'll only swallow what's good for me. Otherwise I will refuse."* Eat alkaline foods. See also: stomach remedies. Acid blockers, possibly proton pump inhibitors short-term.

SBS of the Gastric Mucosa

Stomach cancer (adeno-ca), stomach polyps, parietal cell proliferation (hyperplasia), thickening of the stomach wall, diffuse hyperplasia of the stomach mucosa[1]

Conflict	Chunk conflict (see explanations p. 15, 16), not being able to digest something. Trouble with the mother-in-law, siblings, children, boss, etc. *"I don't have the stomach for/can't stomach it." "It turns my stomach."*
Examples	→ *Somebody isn't given the pay raise they were promised. Someone must sell his car for far less than its value, although they need the money badly. A man's mother-in-law, who lives in the same house with him, gets on his nerves every day.*
	• *A 45-year-old, married mother of two works as an exercise therapist at a social organization. She finds the work entirely unsatisfying and meaningless = indigestible-anger conflict. When she gets a new job, she comes into healing with night sweats and stomach pain. CM diagnoses a metaplasia of the gastric mucosa.* (Archive B. Eybl)
Conflict-active	Increased function. Growth of a cauliflower-like tumor of secretory quality up to the size of a grapefruit, or a flat-growing adeno-ca of absorptive quality (CM: a "thickening of the stomach wall" or a "hyperplasia of the mucosa"). In principle, polyps are cancer (cell growth) as well. In CM, the size alone often determines whether the diagnosis is a "malignant cancer" or "harmless polyp."
Bio. function	Production of more digestive juices in order to better break down (secretory quality) or absorb (absorptive quality) the firmly lodged chunk.
Repair phase	Function normalization, tubercular-caseating degradation of the tumor with light bleeding, pain and night sweats or encapsulation of the tumor if no tubercular bacteria are present. One can live symptom free for decades with an encapsulated tumor, assuming the food pulp has enough space and the passage is clear.
Repair crisis	Heavy bleeding and pain, chills.
Note	Diagnostic tip: acid blockers only help with an SBS of the superficial mucous membrane, not with an SBS of the deep-lying mucosa.
Questions	First, based on the symptoms, determine if the conflict is active or in the repair phase: If active or recurring: Diagnosed when? (Conflict probably began much earlier). What happened at the time period in question? Which stress situations where there? What changed in my life? (Career, relationship, friends, life situation, information that was hard to bear)? Which conditioning lies at the bottom of the conflict? (Childhood, pregnancy, parent's/ancestor's experience)? Which beliefs play a role?
Therapy	Identify the conflict and/or trigger and, if possible, resolve them in real life if they are still active. Guiding principles: *"I will make peace with myself and my family." "What has happened is all right - it had a purpose." "With my new knowledge, I'll make a new start in life."* If applicable, surgery without chemo or radiation. See also: p. 193.

Gastritis with fever and night sweats, stomach thrush[1]

Same SBS as above.

Phase	**Repair phase:** tubercular-caseating, necrotic degradation of the tumor with acid-resistant fungi and bacteria (mycobacteria) > "thrush" or "candidiasis."
Therapy	The conflict is resolved. Support the healing. If recurring, resolve the conflict and conditioning.
	Colloidal silver internally, Schuessler Cell Salts: No. 5, 8, and 9. See also: p. 193.

---

[1] See Dr. Hamer, Charts, p. 22

Stomach bleeding, tarry stool, stomach colic, vomiting blood

- **Inflammation of the squamous epithelium** (gastritis) - Repair phase: the healing stomach ulcers bleed. No pain, tarry stool. In addition to the loss of blood, a "stomach coma" (= repair phase crisis) can be dangerous. Heavy bleeding and colic in the repair phase crisis.
- **Adeno-ca** - Repair phase: tubercular, caseating, necrotic degradation of the tumor by acid-resistant fungi and bacteria (mycobacteria). Bleeding, fever, night sweats. Heavy bleeding in the repair phase crisis: hyperperistalsis, possibly vomiting. Blood in the vomit.

Therapy

The conflict is resolved. Support the healing. For heavy bleeding, monitoring via hemogram (blood count) > If necessary, administer transfusions temporarily.

Warning: Blood-thinning medications (anticoagulants) increase blood loss.

Stomach remedies

- Tea: centaury, absinthe, sweet flag (Acorus calamus), marjoram, fennel, bitter root (Gentiana lutea), hops, raspberry leaves
- Chew your food thoroughly, enjoy your meals, and "decelerate/slow down"
- Bach flowers: holly, willow
- Swedish bitters, nut-schnapps, Kanne Bread Drink
- The stomach is treatable with therapeutic massages (in the area of the left shoulder blade)

- Infrared therapy (red), warmth
- Reflex-zone massages and acupuncture
- Best time for therapy according to the organ clock: 7-9 a.m.
- Zeolite powder
- Willfort: three-week health cure of drinking 0.5-1 l (16-32 oz) of freshly-squeezed white cabbage juice

SMALL INTESTINE - DUODENUM

The approximately 25 cm (10-15 in) long duodenum receives the food pulp from the pylorus, the "stomach's gatekeeper." The beginning of the duodenum widens into the duodenal bulb. The middle of the duodenum narrows to the papilla. Here, the ducts of the gallbladder and pancreas join. The duodenal bulb is lined with ectodermal squamous epithelium. However, the parts that are further "downstream," such as the rest of the small intestine, are made up of endodermal tissue.

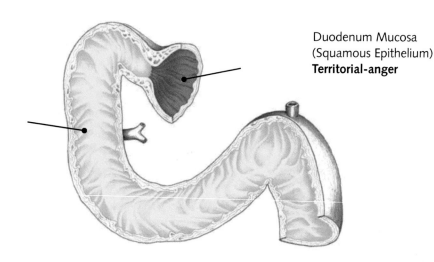

Duodenum Mucosa
(Squamous Epithelium)
Territorial-anger

Remaining Small Intestinal Mucosa
Inability to digest something

SBS of the Superficial Duodenal Mucosa

Duodenal ulcer (ulcus duodeni), duodenal ca)

Corresponding with the germ layer order, this SBS is almost identical with the superficial stomach mucosa (see p. 190).

Conflict	Territorial-anger conflict or, less often, an identity conflict (depending on sex, "handedness," hormone levels and age). One is upset, because their territory or their territorial boundaries are violated.
Examples	➜ *Boundary dispute with the neighbor.*
	➜ *A man's partner flirts with another man. He suspects that she is having an affair with him.*
	• *Following a prostate surgery, a man is impotent and can no longer satisfy his wife. Territorial-anger conflict > cell degradation in the active-phase, restoration in the repair phase. (Archive B. Eybl)*
	• *A now 53-year-old patient meets her husband while still at school. When she sees her future father-in-law for the first time, she is repulsed by the man = territorial-anger conflict and fear-revulsion conflict. She has suffered from bulimia for many years, dating back to this first encounter. Her relationship with her father-in-law is bad to this day. Whenever he comes to visit, he insists on taking her usual seat at the table. Moreover, he always seems aggravated and never says a word. The patient is also always aggravated that she has to give up her place because of his stubbornness = recurring territorial-anger conflict. Therapy: "reformat and reboot" - and don't invite him anymore. Drink raw potato juice. (Archive B. Eybl)*
Conflict-active	Increased sensibility, later, cell degradation of the affected mucous membrane, pain. The longer the conflict lasts, the deeper the defect in the tissue (ulcer) becomes. Usually a recurring conflict.
Bio. function	Through increased sensibility, one can better determine what is digestible or indigestible.
Repair phase	Bleeding of the healing ulcer (causing tarry stools), no pain.
Repair crisis	Severe colicky pain, heavy bleeding, possibly absence seizures, chills.
Therapy	Questions: see p. 190. Determine the conflicts and conditioning and, if possible, resolve them in real life if they are still active! See also therapy p. 193.

E
C
T
O

− +

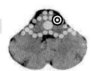

SBS of the Endodermal Duodenal Mucosa

Duodenal cancer (adeno-ca), duodenal polyps[1]

Conflict	Chunk conflict (see explanations p. 15, 16). Not being able to digest something.
Examples	→ *Aggravation with family members, fellow workers, friends.*
	→ *A woman must care for her mother day and night. She cannot enjoy the retirement she had been looking forward to for a long time.*
Conflict-active	Growth of a cauliflower-like tumor of secretory quality or a flat-growing adeno-ca of absorptive quality. Usually a recurring conflict.
Bio. function	With more intestinal cells, the lodged chunks (of anger) can be better digested or reabsorbed.
Repair phase	Tubercular, caseating, necrotizing degradation of the tumor via acid-resistant fungi and bacteria (mycobacteria). Fever, night sweats, duodenal inflammation or tuberculosis. If mycobacteria are not present: encapsulation of the tumor.
Questions	First, based on the symptoms, determine if the conflict is active or in the repair phase: If it is active or recurring: Diagnosed when? (Conflict probably significantly earlier). What happened during the time period in question? Which stress situations were there? Which chunk was I unable to digest? What put pressure on me? Which situations act as triggers for me? Which events related to this can I remember from my childhood? Is there further conditioning: pregnancy, parents'/ancestors' experiences?
Therapy	Identify the conflict or triggers and, if possible, resolve them if they are still active. Guiding principles: *"I will make peace with myself and my family." "Whatever has happened certainly had a purpose."* Possibly surgery, better sooner than later. See also: remedies for the colon, p. 209.

---

1   See Dr. Hamer, Charts p. 22

Duodenal bleeding, tarry stool

Possible causes

• **Duodenal ulcer** - Repair phase: the healing duodenal ulcers bleed. Pain and heavy bleeding in the repair phase crisis. Tarry stool.

• **Adeno-ca** - Repair phase: tubercular, caseating, necrotizing degradation of the tumor via acid-resistant fungi and bacteria (mycobacteria). Fever, night sweats, bleeding. Pain and severe bleeding in the repair phase crisis.

Note

Blood-thinning medication (anticoagulants) aggravate the bleeding.

Therapy

The conflict is resolved. Support the healing. With severe bleeding, monitor the blood count > possibly limited transfusions, see also p. 203.

Meckel's diverticulum (bulge in the small intestine)

This diverticulum is considered a remnant of the omphalomesenteric duct or yolk sac and thus, it is unclear as to whether it has a conflict cause.

SMALL INTESTINE - JEJUNUM AND ILEUM

The jejunum and the ileum together are about 3-5 m (10-17 ft) long. They follow the duodenum and together, the three sections form the small intestine.

The many folds, villi, and their threadlike cell extensions (microvilli) form a gigantic, metabolically active surface of about 60 m² (> 600 sq ft).

The jejunum and ileum are exclusively composed of endodermal tissue.

Note: Poisoning (antibiotics, etc.) may disrupt untold functions in the small intestine and contribute to many of the SBSs listed here.

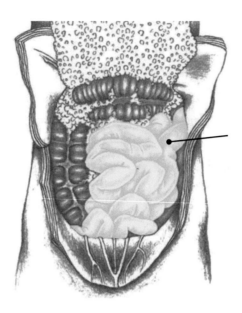

Small Intestine Mucosa
Not being able to digest something, often with a starvation aspect

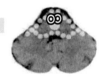

SBS of the Small Intestine Mucosa

Cancer of the small intestine (adeno-ca), polyps of the small intestine, tumorous thickening of the intestinal wall[1]

Conflict	Chunk conflict (see explanations p. 15, 16), not being able to digest something, often with a starvation aspect. Indigestible-anger. A project or something in which one has invested doesn't deliver the hoped for use/profit. *"One leaves empty-handed." "One has nothing to show for it." "One feels that fate is laughing at them."*
Examples	→ *A baby is weaned too suddenly. It believes it will starve since the baby food is unacceptable.*
	• *A 40-year-old, head secretary unexpectedly finds herself in a very unpleasant situation: She has to tell her boss that a coworker has divulged an important company secret. Afterward, she must face her colleague, as a "whistle-blower" = indigestible-anger conflict. Two days later, she seeks a clarifying discussion with the colleague = partial resolution of the conflict. However, she has to think of this unpleasant situation every time she sees her = trigger. Since then, the patient suffers from diarrhea and mild night sweats = persistent repair. Through a second conversation with her colleague, she can finally resolve the conflict. (Archive B. Eybl)*
	• *As the result of a stroke, a man is incapable of speaking. He cannot get used to the situation. He was a charismatic person, who was always at the center of things and everyone asked for his advice. Suddenly, he cannot say a word = indigestible-anger conflict > growth of a tumor in the active-phase - according to CM, a "malignant cancer of the intestine." (Archive B. Eybl)*

---

1   See Dr. Hamer Charts pp. 22, 27

Conflict-active	Increased function, growth of a cauliflower-like tumor of secretory quality or a flat-growing adeno-ca of absorptive quality. The cauliflower-like tumor can cause intestinal obstruction (ileus).
Repair phase	Tubercular, caseating, necrotizing degradation of the tumor via fungi and bacteria (mycobacteria). Fever, night sweats, bleeding, diarrhea, possibly with vomiting if the tumor is situated in the small intestine. If mycobacteria are not present: encapsulation of the tumor.
Repair crisis	Chills, heavy bleeding, intestinal spasms, colic due to involvement of the intestinal muscles.
Bio. function	Cell proliferation of secretory quality in order to produce more digestive juices to digest the lodged chunk more quickly. Cell proliferation of absorptive quality in order to better absorb the chunk (more efficient use of food).
Questions	First, based on the symptoms described, determine if the conflict is active or has been resolved (period without symptoms = active phase. Night sweats, pain, colics = repair phase. If these have lasted for longer than a half a year = recurring conflict. Diagnosed when? (Conflict probably long before this). What can't I digest/accept? Did I draw the short straw? Starvation situation? (Diagnosis shock, sympathy with someone dying, bankruptcy, theft, emergency situation)? Why did I react so sensitively? Who in the family has had something similar happen? (Research family history). Which beliefs are in the background of the conflict? (E.g., *"Those who have nothing have lost."*) Can I trust myself to leave the old behind me? Which new attitude would have a healing effect? Things that could hinder repair: Are there any advantages in having the disease that I am holding on to? (*"Everyone does everything for me now."*) Am I ready to take on the responsibility (with all its consequences)?
Therapy	Determine the conflict and conditioning and, if possible, resolve them in real life if they are still active. Guiding principles: *"I am at peace with those closest to me and everyone else." "We have enough to eat. I am well taken care of."* Surgery when the passage is obstructed or the polyp or tumor is too large. Better earlier than later, because today, small tumors are diagnosed as "benign" by CM. > This means less stress for the person concerned. See also: remedies for the colon, p. 209.

Acute enteritis (inflammation of the small intestine), bleeding - melena (tarry stool)

Same SBS as above.

Phase	**Repair phase** or repair phase crisis. Tubercular, caseating, necrotizing degradation of the tumor via acid-resistant fungi and bacteria (mycobacteria). Fever, night sweats, blood in (tarry) stool, usually diarrhea. Caution: blood-thinning medication (anticoagulants) increases the bleeding.
Therapy	The conflict is resolved. Support the healing and avoid recurrences. For very heavy bleeding, monitoring via hemogram (blood count) > if necessary, administer transfusions, OP. Schuessler Cell Salt: No. 13. See also: remedies for the colon, p. 209.

Gluten intolerance (celiac disease), lactose intolerance (lactose malabsorption)

SBS same as above, (see pp. 196f).

Phase	**Persistent repair**. Conflict-triggers gluten or lactose. By long-term degradation and degeneration of the intestinal villi > disrupted uptake of nourishment, causing chronic digestive problems, usually diarrhea, possibly nutritional deficiencies.
Example	• A six-year-old boy is sent on a six-week convalescence 400 miles from his parents. The, now, 49-year-old man describes the first two weeks there as "hell." The boy is forced to drink milk against his will. Due to this, he partly refuses to eat = conflict of not being able to digest something, indigestible-anger conflict with an aspect of starvation. Trigger = drinking milk. At home, he normally never drinks milk. For 43 years, the patient has suffered from diarrhea whenever he has consumed milk or milk products unknowingly = recurring conflict due to a milk trigger. When he becomes familiar with the 5 Biological Laws of Nature and understands the connection, the conflict is immediately resolved. Since then, the patient can drink a lot of milk without problems. (See www.germanische-heilkunde.at/index.php/erfahrungsberichte)
Therapy	Determine the conflict and conditioning and, if possible, resolve them in real life, so that the persistent repair can come to an end. If no resolution is possible, avoid the offending food (diet).

"Tromboembolism" (intestinal infarct)

Same SBS as above. (See pp. 196-197) According to CM theory, this is the blockage of a blood vessel, which leads to an intestinal infarction. Actually, our blood vessels have a net-like structure and everywhere in the body, there are parallel (collateral) vessels that guarantee the blood supply at all times. These symptoms are probably misinterpreted by CM. However, if a thrombus (clot) is actually found in the angiography, there is probably a tendency toward thromboses in the patient. An indication of this would be thromboses already having been diagnosed at earlier points in time.

Phase	In the case of an intestinal SBS: **repair phase crisis** in the context of a repair phase, thus bleeding. Severe edema by **syndrome**. If it is a blood SBS, see p. 137).
Therapy	The conflict is resolved. Support the healing and avoid recurrences! In the case of severe bleeding, monitor the blood count, if necessary, blood transfusions and/or surgery.

"Fungal infections" (mycoses) of the intestines (e.g., Candida albicans, aspergillus)

Same SBS as above. (See pp. 196-197)

Phase	**Repair phase.** Degradation of an adeno-ca via fungi or bacteria (mycobacteria). Flat-growing tumors are not recognized as such in CM because they are spread out widely.
Note	Fungi belong to the flora of a healthy human being. In intestinal repair phases, one finds even more of them - if they are verified with a stool analysis, they are called "fungal infections" in CM. Through the ingestion of sugar, the fungal population is also increased without conflict.
Therapy	The conflict is resolved. Support the healing and avoid recurrences. Colloidal silver. See also: remedies for the colon, p. 209.

"Bacterial infections," bacterial intestinal dysentery: typhus or paratyphus bacteria (without salmonella), cholera, Escherichia coli bacteria, campylobacter coli bacteria

In the case of a conflict: same SBS as described on pp. 196-197. Drinking dirty water, such as water that is contaminated with feces, does not mean getting infected but rather getting poisoned - the body's prompt response is one of expulsion: diarrhea, vomiting, sweating. In principle, poisoning does not fall into the area of the 5 Biological Laws of Nature.

Phase	**Repair phase.** The difference between poisoning and conflict is often unclear. However, even poisoning isn't a random event from a cosmic perspective. Everything in life has a reason and a purpose.
Therapy	The conflict is resolved. Support the healing and mitigate any conflicts caused by the poisoning. Colloidal silver, MMS. See also: remedies for the colon, p. 209.

"Viral infections" of the intestines: ECHO virus, Coxsackievirus, adenoviruses, rotavirus, Norwalk virus, parvovirus

Same SBS as above. (See pp. 196-197) In CM, the causes of most illnesses are unknown; therefore, pathogens have simply been invented. To this day, not a single virus has been conclusively proven.

Phase	**Repair phase**
Therapy	The conflict is resolved. Support the repair phase and avoid recurrences. See also: remedies for the colon, p. 209.

Amoebic dysentery and worm diseases, e.g., bilharziosis (schistosomiasis)

Do amorphous creatures (tape, round, and pinworms) have a specific task - a biological purpose? Is it possible that an "attack" by worms is no coincidence, and that it may even be beneficial? Does it only affect people who need it? At the University of Iowa, there was great success in the treatment of Crohn's disease patients with whipworms. It is possible that worms aid tubercle bacilli during repair phases in the degradation of excess intestinal mucosa. Regardless, doctors at the University of Iowa determined that bacterial flora improves under the influence of worms.

SBS of the Intestinal Muscles

HFs in the midbrain - topography still unknown

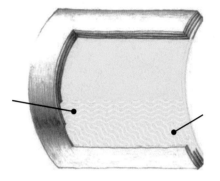

Smooth, Longitudinal Intestinal Muscle[1] (sympathetically innervated)
Motor conflict, not being able to move a chunk further

---

1   Master pattern for the involuntary (smooth), longitudinal muscle in the body

Smooth, Transverse Intestinal Muscle[2] (parasympathetically innervated)
Motor conflict, not being able to move a chunk further

---

2   Master pattern for the circular involuntary (smooth) muscle in the body.

Constipation, diarrhea, intussusception (one segment folding into another - invagination), twisting around itself (volvulus)

In cases where there is no poisoning with medication (e.g., with morphine):

Conflict	Motor chunk conflict (see explanations p. 15, 16), not being able to move something further (in real life or figuratively). Something does not come through. Topic standstill, stagnation or too many tasks simultaneously. Constipation: Something/a matter is not yet completely digested (awaiting a solution/resolution) or one wants to hold something back.
Example	➜ *"It won't budge." "I can't keep things moving forward." "Not that too!"* • *The 33-year-old son of a 70-year-old farmer still does not know if he wants to take over the farm. The farmer (our patient) postpones any decisions - the operation and the family are stagnating. = Conflict that nothing can be moved forward. Since this situation has come to a stand-still the farmer suffers from constipation and always has to burp. (Archive B. Eybl)* • *A 45-year-old construction foreman has to be at multiple construction sites at the same time he has "too many irons in the fire." On these days, he has to loosen his belt because his belly gets so fat. (Archive B. Eybl)*
Conflict-active	Increased tension in the longitudinal, intestinal muscle > limitation of the peristalsis, tense, swollen abdomen, stomach ache, constipation/diarrhea (see also: p 207ff). If nothing is happening or too much is happening at once, it is often accompanied by inner anxiety, restlessness or turmoil.
Repair crisis	Colic, sudden onset of diarrhea, pain or also the desire to be able to defecate.
Repair phase	Increased tension in the transverse muscles. Stomach back to normal, constipation/diarrhea.
Invagination	In this disease, a part of the intestine pushes into another. A segment remains in sympatheticotonia (extension), the other in parasympatheticotonia (narrowing). In healthy peristaltic contraction, waves flow through the whole intestine (longitudinal waves and transverse waves). The phase is unclear. OP if necessary. • *A young woman has a job as a pedicurist. Unfortunately, her hard work is not recognized by her boss. Often, she is paid late, which leads to disputes. = Conflict that things aren't moving forward professionally. At this time, she suffers an acute intestinal obstruction due to an intussusception, which isn't recognized immediately. The affected section of the intestine is removed surgically. (Archive B. Eybl).*
Volvulus	Slackening of the involuntary intestinal musculature and subsequent twisting of the intestine around its own axis > danger of intestinal occlusion or demise of the intestinal tissue (intestinal gangrene) caused by the blockage. OP if necessary.
Questions	Where am I stagnating? What isn't fully digested? What don't I want to give up? Why? Conditioning?
Therapy	Determine the conflict and conditioning and, if possible, resolve them in real life. See also: remedies for the colon p. 209.

E
N
D
O

(+−)

CECUM AND APPENDIX

The 9 cm (3 in) long appendix (cecal) is the blind-ended tube at the beginning of the large intestine (cecum). Its important function has not yet been discovered by CM and for this reason, up until recent years, many happily consented to having their appendix removed. (An ideal practice operation for young surgeons).

In the animal kingdom, herbivores have an extra-long appendix. This is where otherwise indigestible elements of their food (cellulose) are unlocked with the help of special bacteria.

Furthermore, this part of the intestine is a refuge/reserve storage for the intestinal bacteria in cases of diarrhea/poisoning. (Comparable to a sidearm of a river, which provides refuge for fish during floods and from where they can school out afterward).

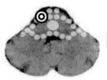

SBS of the Appendix Mucosa

Acute inflammation of the cecum, appendix (appendicitis), ruptured appendix

Conflict	Chunk conflict (see explanations p. 15, 16) of dipping into the reserves - one must suddenly do with less. The reserves/resources are in danger, the savings are gone.
Examples	→ *A child's spending money is cut off or something is taken away. "My reserves are gone."*
	• *A businessman trusts his cousin and integrates him into upper management. The cousin deceives him outrageously. Their dispute causes him great financial damage = Chunk conflict with regard to monetary reserves > growth of a tumor in the active-phase. When the patient cuts all contact with his cousin, an acute appendicitis is diagnosed = repair phase. (Archive B. Eybl)*
Conflict-active	Increased function, cell division in the endodermal appendix or mucous membrane.
Bio. function	Increase in the mucosa reserves to make room for more bacteria (more reserves).
Repair phase	Appendicitis, fever, night sweats, possible blood in the stool. Tubercular, caseating, necrotizing degradation of the tumor via acid-resistant fungi and bacteria (mycobacteria) or encapsulation.
Repair crisis	Chills, severe pain, colic.
Note	Relapses can cause chronic appendicitis, possibly with mucus collection (mucocele). In the repair phase, the extension of the appendix can also burst = "ruptured appendix." Nature is prepared for this case: the omentum spreads out over the perforation, thereby preventing the contents of the colon from getting into abdominal cavity. The inflammation is then limited to the immediate vicinity. With that said, an OP is nevertheless the sensible option for minimizing the risk in the case of a rupture.
Questions	Sudden pain? Yes > sudden conflict resolution. Pain came on gradually? Yes > drawn-out conflict resolution. Pain for a long time (over a half a year)? Yes > persistent conflict. Which positive event brought about the repair phase? (Which stress was there in relation to money before the repair phase? Did I feel like I was in danger, because the circumstances got so bad? (Extraordinary bills to pay, lost job, home, benefits)? Did I doubt that I was going to be able to make ends meed financially? In the case of a child: Is it experiencing a substitution conflict (look for it with the parents) or is it experiencing its own bottleneck? (Toy, spending money, no room of their own anymore)? Which conditioning has led me to this conflict? (Childhood, parental stress during the pregnancy, family tragedy)? Which new attitude could help me avoid recurrences?
Therapy	The conflict is resolved. Support the healing and avoid recurrences. If needed, antibiotics. In case of rupture, consider surgery.

LARGE INTESTINE: ASCENDING, TRANSVERSE & DESCENDING

The large intestine (colon) has a diameter of about 6 cm (2 in) and is about 1.5 m (5 ft) long. Unlike the small intestine, the colon has no villi. Nutritional elements and fluid are removed from the food pulp here.

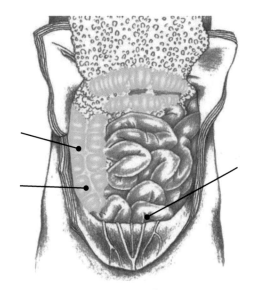

Appendix Mucosa
(not pictured)
**Chunk conflict of
the reserves being
in danger**

Sigmoid Colon Mucosa
(not pictured)
**Indigestible-anger,
not being able to
eliminate something**

Colon Mucosa
Indigestible-anger

SBS of the Colon Mucosa

Colon cancer, polyps[1]

Conflict	Chunk conflict (see explanations p. 15, 16): indigestible-anger. A situation that is ugly and hard to deal with.
Examples	→ *Something unpleasant, not being able to get rid of "crap."*
	→ *Not being able to cope with something vile, devious or mean.*

• *For many years, a man has been a founding member of an organization. A huge argument breaks out among the members because the man who owns the restaurant where they meet no longer wants the meetings to be held there. > Indigestible-anger. A few weeks later, the patient is diagnosed with colon cancer = active-phase. The tumor is surgically removed. Afterwards, he learns about the 5 Biological Laws of Nature. (Archive B. Eybl)*

• *A 43-year-old, married, department head uses a friendly approach with her colleagues. Four years ago, a new colleague joins the team. From the very beginning, she works against the department leader. A month ago, she learns that this colleague has been maligning her in the company behind her back. = Indigestible-anger conflict and an "attack-to-the-abdomen" conflict. A month later, the patient speaks of the matter, choosing two close colleagues and a girlfriend to confide in. She starts to feel better during the conversation = conflict resolution. Then, at night, she suffers an intestinal colic (= repair phase crisis) with a hard, swollen abdomen and sweating. It's so bad that she calls an ambulance. In the hospital, she is diagnosed with an inflammation of the colon and a thickening of the intestinal wall (= flat-growing tumor of absorptive quality). In addition to this, fluid has accumulated in the peritoneal (abdominal) cavity (ascites) and her blood sedimentation levels are high (indication of inflammation), which according to CM "cannot possibly come from the intestines alone" = peritonitis - resolved attack conflict. After a few days, everything is all right again. (Archive B. Eybl)*

• *An athletic, 50-year-old entrepreneur has a construction company and his business is booming. Suddenly, this good fortune abandons him: A major customer goes bankrupt and he loses a lot of money. Shortly thereafter, another customer refuses to pay 20% of the agreed fee. = Indigestible-anger con-*

flict. Since then, problems with business partners are always a trigger for him. The result is a chronic inflammation of the colon (ulcerative colitis). After retirement, the disease heals almost completely. (Archive B. Eybl)

Conflict-active	Increased function. Growth of a cauliflower-like adeno-ca of secretory quality with a conflict aspect of not being able to digest something or a flat-growing adeno-ca = "tumorous thickening of the intestinal wall" of absorptive quality with a conflict aspect of not being able to accept something.
Bio. function	With more cells in the colon, better ability to digest or absorb the lodged chunk of anger.
Repair phase	Normalization of function, tubercular, caseating, necrotizing degradation of the tumor via acid-resistant fungi and bacteria (mycobacteria), Fever, night sweats, colitis, ulcerous colitis. If bacteria not present: encapsulation. Bright-red blood and mucus in stool, diarrhea.
Repair crisis	Chills, heavy bleeding, and colicky pain.
Questions	First, determine if it is an active or a resolved conflict. (Questions about the symptoms, look at the inflammation levels in the blood). Estimate the length of the conflict based on the size. What was I unable to digest over the period in question? What has been pressuring me for a long time? What issue is hard for me to talk about (isolation)? What "crap" would I like to be rid of? Which conditioning is in the background of the conflict? Which new attitude and which external changes would heal me?
Therapy	Identify the conflict and conditioning and, if possible, resolve them in real life if they are still active. Guiding principles: *"Nobody profits from anger." "Everything has a purpose and I can only learn from this."* Surgery if the passage is obstructed or the polyp/tumor is too large. If you are going to have an OP, earlier is better than later, because small tumors are often diagnosed as "benign" by CM today CM. > I.e., less stress for the person concerned. See also: remedies for the colon, p. 209.

Intestinal obstruction (ileus)

This diagnosis can mean an obstruction due to a tumor or paralysis of the intestinal musculature (paralytic ileus). See SBS of the intestinal muscles p. 199. With paralytic ileus, no tumor is found during a colonoscopy. If a tumor is the cause: same SBS as above (see above).

Phase	**Conflict-active**: an intestinal occlusion occurs when the tumor is too big or often at the beginning of the repair phase due to the inflammation-swelling of the tumor.
Therapy	Determine the conflict and conditioning and, if possible, resolve them in real life if they are still active. Surgery if necessary.

Chronic inflammation of the intestines (Crohn's disease, colitis ulcerosa)[2]

Same SBS as above. (See pp. 201-202) In CM, the difference between Crohn's disease and colitis ulcerosa is vague; the differentiation is also unnecessary. If the small intestine is also affected, a starvation conflict is also underway (see p. 196).

Examples	• *A man is constantly angry and arguing with his wife = indigestible-anger. He would have separated from her long ago if it were not for their house, which he would lose in a divorce. The conflict has been growing now for two decades = recurring-conflict. The patient suffers from a severe case of Crohn's disease. (Archive B. Eybl)*
	• *The schoolboy feels he is being treated unfairly by his teacher. He thinks that she always grades him worse than he deserves. Diagnosis: Crohn's disease due to recurrences. (Archive B. Eybl)*
Phase	**Chronic-recurring process.** Active-phases alternate with repair phases. Flat-growing adeno-ca of resorptive quality, sometimes polyps as well (secretory quality). Blood, mucus in the stool. Diarrhea, constipation, and night sweats.
Therapy	Determine the conflict and triggers and, if possible, resolve them in real life, so that the SBS comes to an end. Questions: see above. Guiding principles: see above. Good chances of recovery, even with long-standing cases. See also: remedies for the colon, p. 209. The CM therapy with cortisone, immunosuppressants, and anti-TNF agents is not recommended over a prolonged period.

---

2   See Dr. Hamer, Charts p. 28

LARGE INTESTINE - SIGMOID COLON

The S-shaped, sigmoid section of the colon collects the indigestible remainder of what we eat from the descending part of the colon. Here, this content is further thickened by fluid removal and is "portioned."

SBS of the Sigmoid Colon Mucosa

Cancer of the sigmoid colon, polyps[1]

Conflict	Chunk conflict (see explanations p. 15, 16): indigestible-anger. Cannot eliminate (get rid of) something indigestible/burdensome/aggravating. E.g., denunciations, treason, bullying, insults.
Examples	→ *Not being able to get rid of unpleasantness, "crap" (e.g. accusations).* → *Not being able to tolerate "underhanded" behavior.* • *The marriage of a 54-year-old female patient is very chaotic. The couple has just moved into a new apartment. During the move, the husband - completely unexpectedly - announces that he is not moving in with her. He starts removing his things again. Later, as he asks for their marriage certificate in order to file for divorce, they have a terrible argument. = Indigestible-anger conflict. A cauliflower-like tumor that is several centimeters wide develops during the active-phase and is discovered during a physical examination 7 years later. It doesn't cause any problems. Nevertheless, the patient submits to chemotherapy. (Archive B. Eybl)* • *A young entrepreneur does not receive payment from an important client for a completed order.* (See Dr. Hamer, Goldenes Buch Bd. 2, p. 184) • *A man has been employed by a company for 15 years. He has a quarrel with a colleague. The boss takes the side of the colleague, which bitterly disappoints the patient. (Archive B. Eybl)*
Conflict-active	Increased function. Growth of a cauliflower-like tumor adeno-ca of secretory quality or a flat-growing adeno-ca (tumorous thickening of the intestinal wall) of absorptive quality. Usually a recurring conflict.
Bio. function	With more colon cells, the body is better able to "digest or absorb the anger."
Repair phase	Normalization of function, tubercular, caseating, necrotizing degradation of the tumor via acid-resistant fungi or bacteria (mycobacteria), fever, night sweats = inflammation of the sigmoid colon. Bright-red blood and mucus in the stool, diarrhea. Encapsulation of the tumor if no bacteria present.
Repair crisis	Chills, severe colicky pain and heavy bleeding, diarrhea.
Therapy	Determine the conflict and conditioning and resolve them in real life if still active. Questions: see previous page. Guiding principles: *"This situation has taken place so I can learn something from it." "I have brought it upon myself through my own thoughts and actions. I accept everything as it is and with God's help, I'll make the best of it."* See also: remedies for the colon, p. 209. According to my experience, polyp surgery is advised, because you do not know if they will continue to grow. In CM today, polyps that are about 3 cm (1 in) in diameter are referred to as "colorectal cancer" - with all its consequences.

Diverticulitis (colonic diverticula - inflammation of pouches in the colon)

Same SBS as above. The majority of intestinal diverticula are found in the sigmoid colon.

Phase	Excessive breakdown of tumors during **persistent repair** (diverticulitis) or after persistent repair (diverticulum/a). Thinning of the mucosa leads to a pouch bulging outwards = **recurring conflict**.
Therapy	Identify the conflict and conditioning and, if possible, resolve them in real life, if still active, so that no further diverticula develop. For chronic inflammation of the diverticula, consider surgery.

---

1   See Dr. Hamer, Charts p. 28

RECTUM - ANUS

In human beings, the rectum, including the anus, is about 15-30 cm (6-12 in) long. The last four centimeters (1.5 in) are considered the anus. This serves as a temporary storage area for feces. What is special about this last section of the intestine is that the old intestinal mucosa - from outside the body to about 12 cm into the rectum - is overgrown by ectodermal squamous epithelium. Thus, we find both superficial ectodermal and sub-endodermal tissue with two differing conflict contents.

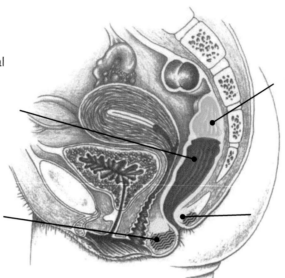

Superficial Rectal and Anal Mucosa (extodermal)
Identity conflict

External Anal Sphincter (striated muscle)
Identity conflict

Deep-lying Rectal and Anal Mucosa (endodermal)
Indigestible-anger, not being able to eliminate something

Internal Anal Sphincter (smooth muscle)
Not being able to hold back/eliminate the feces

SBS of the Rectum Submucosa

Rectal cancer (adeno-ca)

Conflict	Chunk conflict (see explanations p. 15, 16): indigestible-anger, not being able to get rid of something unpleasant, "crap."
Examples	→ *Somebody is unjustly accused or put at a terrible disadvantage.* → *Somebody is betrayed by a friend.* • *The patient's son has taken up with a bad crowd. Together with his friends, he ends up in court. The patient is sure that her son has been caught in a trap and that is why he is being prosecuted = indigestible-anger > growth of a rectal cancer in the active-phase. Half a year later, this is diagnosed by CM. (Archive B. Eybl)*
Conflict-active	Increased function, growth of a cauliflower-like tumor of secretory quality by a conflict aspect of not being able to get rid of something or a flat-growing adeno-ca of absorptive quality, through a conflict aspect of not being able to assimilate something.
Bio. function	To better be able to digest or resorb the anger chunk with more intestinal cells.
Repair phase	Inflammation of the rectum, possibly also diagnosed as "anorectal abscess" (see below). Tubercular, caseating, necrotizing degradation of the tumor via acid-resistant fungi and bacteria (mycobacteria), fever, night sweats, bright-red blood and mucus in the stool, diarrhea. If bacteria are not present: encapsulation.
Therapy	Identify the conflict and conditioning and, if possible, resolve them in real life if still active. Guiding principle: *"I accept the situation and will resolve it with God's help."* Surgery if tumor is too large. Better earlier than later, because today, small tumors are diagnosed as "benign" by CM. > Less stress for the person concerned. See also: p. 203.

Hemorrhoids (internal, rare), anorectal abscess[1]

Same SBS as above.

Example	• A 46-year-old, right-handed woman sweats for the last four nights. On the toilet, she has pain when she presses and when she wipes herself, she finds blood on the toilet paper. Conflict history: five weeks ago, the patient spoke with her mother-in-law on the phone. During the conversation, they talked about dividing up the inheritance they received from the recently deceased grandmother. (The patient is legally no heiress, but her husband is.) On the phone, the mother-in-law said to her, "Anyway, it only concerns the children." With this, the patient assumed that she is not invited to this meeting. On the day before the first symptoms appeared, her mother-in-law comes to visit and is very kind to her = conflict resolution > bleeding removal of the tumor in the following days = repair phase. (Archive B. Eybl)
Phase	**Repair phase**: A small tumor usually develops unnoticed under the epithelium layer during the conflict-active phase. It is not noticed until the repair phase, when it breaks open = CM: "hemorrhoids," "rectal abscess" > night sweats, pus, bright-red blood. Usually a **recurring-conflict.**
Note	The most important difference between this and the more common, superficial hemorrhoids is the fever and night sweats in the repair phase.
Therapy	The conflict is resolved. Support the healing. If recurring, find out the conflict and conditioning and resolve them. Questions: see p. 202. See also remedies for the rectum/hemorrhoids p. 207.

---

1 See Dr. Hamer, Charts p. 28

SBS of the Superficial Anal Mucosa

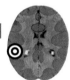

Hemorrhoids (superficial, common)[1]

Conflict	Identity conflict - not knowing where one belongs, not knowing which decision to make, not knowing which partner to choose. Often, the conflict has something to do with the mother (mother = identity). Less often, territorial-anger conflict.
Examples	• A seven-year-old boy loses his father. After that, his mother has various partners, who treat the boy very badly; they even abuse him = identity conflict. (See Dr. Hamer, Goldenes Buch Bd. 2, p. 397)
	• A 69-year-old patient lets himself undergo chemotherapy for cancer of the prostate gland. However, he becomes doubtful as to whether he is doing the right thing. "Should I continue the treatment?" = identity conflict. (See Dr. Hamer, Celler Dokumentation, p. 61)
	• A married women falls in love with another man. She doesn't know whether she should divorce her husband for the sake of the other man = identity conflict. Cell degradation in the anal epithelium. Restoration with bleeding in the repair phase. (Archive B. Eybl)
Conflict-active	Reduced sensibility of the anal mucosa, simultaneous slackening of the anal sphincter muscles. Later, degradation of epithelium = ulcer; tearing of the anal epithelium (anal fissures) are possible > no pain, no bleeding, numbness. One seeks belonging, wrangles with decisions.
Bio. function	Widening of the anus to insure better removal of feces. In nature, feces and urine serve to mark territory. The place of defecation defines one's living space and the location of the individual. With additional feces, the location can be defined better and the identity is emphasized. Feces-marking takes urine-marking to the next level.

---

1 See Dr. Hamer, Charts p. 129

Repair phase	Restoration of the degraded substance, pain, swelling, bright-red blood = "hemorrhoids," aggravated by syndrome. Usually a recurring-conflict.
Repair crisis	Heavy bleeding, possibly chills; if the voluntary anus muscle is also affected, rectal cramps (see below for 2nd possibility) and painful rectal tenesmus (feeling of having to defecate when one doesn't).
Questions	Irritation, bleeding since when? (When it bleeds, the conflict must have been resolved). First time bleeding? (No > also examine the first episodes. Yes > only examine this episode). Which problem did I solve the day before or on the same day? (Good conversation, personal decision, good news, the weekend, vacation)? When this is determined, one automatically knows the conflict. Has the conflict always dealt with certain people or is it about an inner dilemma, having nothing to do with people? (Specify the conflict). What are my earliest experiences with regard to this? (Childhood)? Were my parents also involved in the issue? (> Also, examine the issue in the family and heal through conversation/meditation/forgiveness/prayer). What has conditioned me additionally? Which beliefs nourish this conflict? Am I ready to make a new start?
Therapy	Identify the conflict and conditioning and, if possible, resolve them in real life if still active. Guiding principle: *"I will make a definite decision. Then, I will know where I belong."* See also: remedies for the rectum/hemorrhoids below. OP if necessary.

Fissures of the anal epithelium (anal fissures)

Same SBS as above.

Phase	**Conflict-active phase,** pain later in the repair phase when the fissures are healing.
Therapy	Identify the conflict and conditioning and, if possible, resolve them in real life if still active.

SBS of the Inner Rectal Sphincter   HFs in the midbrain - topography still unknown

Rectal cramps (sphincter spasms, tenesmus)

Conflict	Chunk conflict (see explanations p. 15, 16), not being able to sufficiently retain the feces. In the figurative sense: One is trying desperately no to bother anyone/not to be intrusive. One always shows great reserve. One would rather sacrifice their territory than become unliked.
Example	• *A woman is in the hospital for a hemorrhoid surgery. She is given an enema to cleanse the colon, and she becomes terribly nauseated. At the last second, she runs to the washbasin where she vomits and at the same time loses control of her bowels: she stands in a puddle of water and excrement. At that very moment, the doctor comes in and tells her to lie down in bed immediately because they want to give her an infusion. Fully soiled, she must lay herself in bed = conflict of not being able to hold back the feces. Since then, the patient suffers from intense rectal spasms. Sixteen years later, at a lecture by Helmut Pilhar, she goes behind the curtain and can resolve the conflict by means of meditation. (See www.germanische-heilkunde.at/index.php/erfahrungsberichte)*
Conflict-active	Increased muscle tension (hypertony), problems with bowel movement. When the stool is hard, it can only be pressed out with extreme effort, because the inner sphincter does not open completely.
Bio. function	Increased tension so that the feces can be held back. Harder feces stink less.
Repair phase	Normalization of the muscle tension; in the repair phase crisis: attacks of painful anal cramps.
Questions	Was there a real situation where I was not allowed to defecate? Was there a time when I experienced stress during defecation? Am I always reserved? (If yes: to remain well-liked)? Did the mother have to hold her child back during the birth? What are the parents like with regard to letting things out? What still conditions me? (Experiences during childhood).
Therapy	Determine the conflict and conditioning and, if possible, resolve them in real life. Transdermal magnesium.

Encopresis (paradoxical diarrhea) - voluntary or involuntary fecal soiling

By the age of three, children should be toilet trained. If not, the following conflict may come into question:

Conflict	According to Frauenkron-Hoffmann: The child feels neglected and draws attention to itself through the "scent." It is basically a call for the mother to take care of the child.
	According to Dr. Sabbah: The child "senses" a poisoning in ancestors (*"the poison must be expelled"*).
Phase	**Conflict activity** of the inner sphincter muscle > constant tension.
Questions	When did the symptoms begin? (Stress at school/family, divorce, fight, disharmony)? Does the child feel neglected? Was/is there a poisoning among ancestors or parents? (Also consider drugs/medications).
Therapy	Determine and resolve the conflict, causal conditioning and beliefs (of the family).

E
N
D
O

+ −

Remedies for the rectum/hemorrhoids

- Tea/hip bath: fenugreek, oak, mullein, horse chestnut leaves, yarrow, plantain
- Cayce: Gymnastic exercise - both arms over the head, lift heels and stretch upwards, then bend forwards with the hands to the ground - in the mornings and evenings for two to three minutes

- Schuessler Cell Salts: No. 1, 11; Kanne Bread Drink
- Colloidal silver internally and externally
- Comfrey or propolis salve - externally
- Zeolite powder
- Magnesium chloride ($MgCl_2$) foot bath

Diarrhea

Possible causes

- **Poisoning:** Spoiled or contaminated food, side effect of medication, especially antibiotics and psychopharmaceuticals as well as poisoning with the artificial sweetener, aspartame, etc. Diarrhea function = elimination of toxin.
- **Incorrect diet:** Ingesting the wrong combination of foods can promote diarrhea (e.g.: fruit - sugar - grain).
- **General sympatheticotonia and anticipatory anxiety:** = stress diarrhea (CM: diarrhea-dominant irritable bowel). This affects approximately one in five people worldwide. In anticipation of stress (= sympatheticotonia), the involuntary sphincter muscles of the body open: anal and bladder sphincter for "ballast-shedding," gastric sphincter for a speedy passage, pupillary sphincter for easier viewing, etc. Gaunt, thin, emaciated people are predominantly sympathicotonic, i.e., they are predominantly under stress. Peace and serenity are missing, little fat can accumulate = athletic or leptosomic people according to Kretschmer. These individuals tend to be "crapping their pants" at every opportunity. > Loose stools, diarrhea.
  Example: *a 16-year-old student is an amateur ski racer. On the day of the competition, specifically immediately before the start, he must go to the toilet constantly due to the diarrhea. = General sympatheticotonia, anticipatory anxiety. Later in life, he suffers from diarrhea before important appointments as well. (Archive B. Eybl). The opposite is the comfortable endomorph (vagotonic), who is a good eater with tendency toward constipation.*
- **Intestinal muscles:** If an indigestible-anger chunk gets lodged

in the intestines, two SBSs are usually triggered: An SBS of secretory quality (cauliflower-like tumor), so as to dissolve the chunk with gastric juices and one of motor quality (peristalsis), so as to expel it (conflict of not being able to dislodge something or move it forward). Diarrhea in the repair phase crisis during the repair phase or in persistent repair, e.g., Crohn's disease, colitis, ulcerative colitis.
- **Liver - gallbladder:** Recurring territorial-anger conflict. This type of diarrhea accompanies fat intolerance. Endodermal liver parenchyma or the ectodermal gallbladder ducts can be affected. Due to a shortage of bile, fat cannot be digested > pulpy, fatty stools that float in the toilet. Territorial-anger or identity conflict - starvation or existence conflict. (See p. 218ff)
- **Pancreas (rarer):** Recurring-conflict. After many bouts of pancreatitis, the glands that produce pancreatic juices deteriorate. Enzymes for the digestion of proteins, fats and starches are then lacking > pulpy, bright, malodorous stools that float. Conflict: trouble with family members, the battle for the chunk, inheritance conflicts. (See p. 226f)
- **Thyroid (rarer):** the thyroid hormone thyroxin makes the body sympathicotonic. It increases metabolism and promotes the emptying of the bowels. Diarrhea in the conflict-active phase. Conflict: not being able to grasp or get rid of something, because one is too slow. (See p. 119f).

Therapy for diarrhea
Depending on the cause:
- Centering exercises such as tai chi or strength training

• Foods: blueberries, barley, oats, honey
• Tea: elecampane, blackberry (dried fruits leaves), oak bark, chamomile, bistort, plantain.
• Zeolite powder internally, possibly Tannalbin tablets.

Bloating, flatulence

Every digestive process results in the production of intestinal gas. However, most of it diffuses into the circulatory system and is expelled through the lungs. Flatulence denotes an excess of intestinal gas exceeding 0.5 to 1.5 liters per day.

Possible causes

• **Improper nutrition**: A high percentage of high-fiber foods or an unfavorable combination of foods (e.g., fruit - sugar - grain) can promote flatulence. Legumes (with the sugar molecules rhamnose and stachyose) cause a definite rise in gas production.
• **Poisoning** due to antibiotics and other chemo-therapeutics: damage of the intestinal flora > incomplete digestion > fermentation > flatulence.
• **General sympathicotonia**: Gas in combination with diarrhea: signs of a general sympathicotonia. The passage of food is accelerated > incomplete digestion, incomplete air resorption.
• **Impaired functioning of the small intestine or colon**: Not enough air-resorption due to degeneration of the intestinal mucosa (low resorption capacity). According to Dr. Hamer, intestinal gases help to expand the intestine so that a lodged chunk can be moved onward. Histamine or lactose intolerance can cause strong flatulence, sometimes together with diarrhea. = Indigestible-anger (see above).
• **Pancreas or liver**: Too little pancreatic juices or bile > incomplete digestion > fermentation > flatulence = anger conflict with family members, the battle for the chunk, inheritance or starvation-existence and territorial-anger or identity conflict respectively.

Therapy for flatulence

Depending on the cause (e.g., diet change).
• Movement/gymnastics
• Deep breathing, so that the gases can be released.
• Hot, full baths, possibly with whole salt or magnesium chloride.
• Tea: anise, fennel, melissa, parsley, linden blossoms
• Hildegard of Bingen: bay leaf cookie powder special recipe
• Build-up of symbionts with OMNi-BiOTiC®,
• Symbioflor 2, EM.
• Swallow 1 tsp. whole mustard seeds with water regiment.
• Zeolite powder internally.

Constipation

Possible causes

• **Poisoning with medication**: Misuse of laxatives, sleeping pills, tranquilizers, antacids, iron preparations, diuretics, blood pressure medication, anti-Parkinson's disease medication, antiepileptic drugs, medications for bladder incontinence and morphine (paralyzes the colon due to a permanent contraction of the longitudinal muscles in the intestines).
• **Diets that are low in fiber, low in vital substances** (cheap, industrial foods).
• **Active kidney collecting tubules**: Water is collected for when one is on the run (i.e., on a trip) or feels abandoned, so that a shortage of fluids can be survived. The colon thoroughly removes water from the food pulp or feces > hard stool, tendency to constipation. = Refugee and abandonment conflicts. (See p. 230ff)
• **Too little exercise**: A well-functioning intestinal peristaltic is dependent on sufficient exercise. This is not just based on the mechanism of the colon itself; rather, it is linked to the 11th brain nerve (nervus accessorius). Lack of exercise > neglected breathing > under-functioning of the diaphragm (as a muscle aiding digestion).
• **General vagotonia**: During general parasympatheticotonia, it is common for all of the sphincter muscles of the body, including that of the anus, to be closed tight. Feces is only reluctantly released. People who are primarily vagotonic tend to be constipated. These corpulent, rotund, comfortable endomorphs (according to Kretschmer) are excellent eaters. Food (like life) is enjoyed and digested at leisure. Therapy: look for challenges.
• **Intestinal musculature**: Constipation in the conflict-active stage:
  1. Nothing can help (moving forward) (stagnation).
  2. Something is not yet finished, something takes forever and is waiting to be finished.
  3. The fear of leaving the old (e.g., traditions, values, home) behind.
  Often in combination with indigestible-anger.
• **Thyroid**: persistent repair, condition following persistent repair. Too little of the thyroid hormone thyroxin results in a lack of drive and slow metabolism > sluggish colon = conflict of not being able to grasp or expel something because of being too slow. (See p. 120)
• **Parathyroid gland**: Conflict-active phase of a persistent conflict. An overly high parathyroid hormone level can cause constipation.
• **Ileus (blockage)** by a tumor or twisted intestine (volvulus). Conflict-active phase or repair phase. Acute constipation, possibly with pain, vomiting of feces = indigestible-anger conflict (see above)

Therapy for constipation

Depending on the cause:
• Physical exercise/sport in order to stimulate the colon. Espe-

cially effective: endurance running and after that, gymnastics.

- Making a sharp distinction between resting and active-phases, so that both sympathicus and vagus come to fruition. For example, first exercise and then be really lazy.
- Regular massage of the trapezius and sternocleidomastoid muscle. These two muscles are innervated by the 11th brain nerve and correspond directly to the intestinal muscles.
- In the morning, drink lots of pure water.
- Foods: raw fruits and vegetables, flaxseed, dried fruits, figs, apples, garlic, onions, raw sauerkraut, raw red beets, lettuce.

Remedies for the colon

- For acute inflammation: colloidal silver, MMS
- Do not take unnecessary medications!
- Tea: centaury, agrimony, fennel, peppermint, yarrow, and others.
- Chew food thoroughly - enjoy your food!
- For symbionts: OMNi-BiOTiC®, EM, Symbioflor 2, kombucha, yogurt, Kanne Bread Drink.
- Cayce: Eat an almond every day, colon cleansing (water colon cleansing), and enemas for detoxification.
- Hildegard of Bingen: Season with fennel seeds, peppermint. Gentian-powder wine special recipe, absinthe elixir special recipe, sanicle (Sanicula europaea) powder- or elixir special recipe.
- Castor oil compress treatments.

- Breathing exercises.
- Tea: agrimony, centaury, vermouth, absinthe, common polypody, St. John's wort.
- Improve the intestinal flora: OMNi-BiOTiC®, Symbioflor 2, EM, Kanne Bread Drink.
- Enemas/colon cleansing therapy for purging and colon reboot. Such treatments should not activate/trigger conflict, otherwise, don't do them! Be cautious, especially with children (invasion of privacy can cause conflicts).

- Warm abdominal compresses with salt water
- Fasting - the oldest therapy for digestive disturbances. When fasting, we should follow our instincts and feelings, like when animals refuse to eat. Fasting under pressure or coercion triggers new conflicts and new illnesses.
- Willfort: Three-week health cure of drinking 0.5-1 l (16-32 oz) of freshly-squeezed white cabbage juice, distributed throughout the day.
- Zeolite powder, natural borax, internally.
- Treatment: Swallow mustard seed without chewing + medicinal clay + water. Linseed oil.

DIAPHRAGM

The diaphragm is a 3-5 mm thick, dome-shaped sheet of striated muscle separating the chest cavity from the abdominal cavity. Although the diaphragm is made up of purely voluntary (striated) muscle, it also receives impulses from the brainstem for the involuntary functioning of breathing and blood circulation (similar to the heart's ventricles).

Functions of the diaphragm:

- As a breathing assistant, the diaphragm usually works involuntarily, but it can be tensed up voluntarily, for example, when taking deep breaths or holding one's breath.

- As an auxiliary muscle for blood circulation, the diaphragm operates entirely involuntarily. It supports the right heart chamber in aspirating venous blood from the body's circulatory system (= pressure-suction-pump). The left half of the diaphragm is more important for this. The right half of the diaphragm has only limited movement, possibly due to the liver, which is located directly under the diaphragm.
- We tense up the diaphragm voluntarily when giving birth, defecating or emptying the bladder = abdominal press.

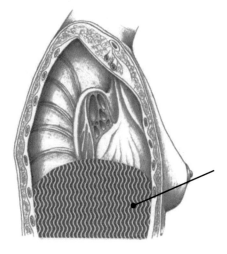

Diaphragm coupled with
the Heart Muscle
**Conflict of being overwhelmed
or outsmarted**

Diaphragm independent of
the Heart Muscle
**Not getting enough air,
not being able to inhale or exhale**

SBS of the Diaphragm Muscles

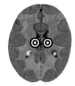

Sleep apnea, diaphragm cramps

Conflict	1. Conflict of being overwhelmed: With this conflict, the diaphragm is functionally coupled with the heart muscle, i.e., the diaphragm reacts along with the heart (see p. 126ff).
	2. Conflict for the diaphragm alone: not getting enough air, not being able to breathe and not being able to press out air, this also in a figurative sense: *"It took my breath away." "It knocked the wind out of me." "I need to take a deep breath now." "I can't breathe."*

Examples:
• *A four-year-old boy falls from a bench while playing. Shocked, he begins to cry = conflict of not getting enough air. Throughout the following night and day, the patient comes into healing. As he is sleeping on the sofa, his parents notice he is turning blue = cessation of breathing due to a repair phase crisis of the diaphragm - diaphragm cramp. His left leg twitches and his whole body cramps up = repair phase crisis of a motor conflict due to falling from a bench. The next day, everything is all right again. (See www.germanische-heilkunde.at/index.php/erfahrungsberichte)*

• *A 53-year-old, right-handed patient, a kindergarten teacher, is married for the second time and has two children, aged 33 and 31. For 25 years, she has suffered from an unusual symptom, CM cannot understand it at all. Several times a week when resting, especially at night, she gets a violent cramp-like pain that goes through the abdomen into the thoracic spine. During these attacks, the patient must stand up in order to breathe reasonably. The patient also describes that she can't urinate and defecate during and after the seizures, that she can't build pressure in the abdomen.*

Conflict history: The birth of her son is difficult, but thanks to an experienced doctor, everything goes well. During the press phase of her labor pains, she runs out of air - the doctor then kneels on her abdomen and presses the baby out - a healthy child is born.

During the birth of her daughter, the scenario is similar: The last phase of labor is too weak to expel the baby. The child remains lodged in the birth canal. The patient is told to press harder but she is too weak and gives up: "I cannot press any more. I cannot push the baby out." > Conflict of not being able to push out the child. The patient wishes that the doctor from her first birth was there but he is not. An episiotomy is performed, albeit too late, and the baby is pulled out by force. The child is permanently handicapped. Six years later, as the mother learns to accept what has happened, the nightly epileptic, diaphragm cramp attacks begin. Whenever she sees her daughter, she thinks of the birth. Finally, after 25 years of suffering, a therapist who works with the 5 Biological Laws of Nature sees the causal relationship between the two. The birth is replayed as therapy: The therapist kneels on the patient's belly and imaginarily presses the child down and out. The patient's subconscious should now realize that "everything is all right now," especially since her now 31-year-old, slightly-handicapped daughter is the "apple of her eye." Guiding principle: "It's wonderful that I have such a sweet daughter. Everything is fine the way it is and the birth was fine." After the treatment, the patient has especially violent cramp attacks for 5 days = closing repair phase crisis during the repair phase. After that, she is released from her 25-year-long ordeal. (Archive B. Eybl)

Conflict-active	Paralysis, weakness, reduction of innervation or function > diaphragm elevation due to a lack of muscle tension. Weakness during physical exertions, because the diaphragm cannot help as much with breathing (most important muscle assisting breathing), pressing (lifting). Everything usually unnoticed.
Bio. function	Play-dead reflex. Predators lose interest when the prey doesn't move or breathe.
Repair phase	Restoration of the nerve supply
Repair crisis	Epilepsy of the diaphragm = diaphragm cramp usually occurring at night or during periods of rest and piercing pain or twitching throughout the abdominal cavity. Due to the cramp in the diaphragm, breathing is restricted > acute shortness of breath, insufficient oxygen, turning blue (cyanosis).
Note	Through the functional coupling to the heart muscle (overwhelmed conflict), this may lead to sleep apnea or shortness of breath during the repair phase crisis of the heart muscle. This fact is confirmed by a French study, which installed pacemakers into apnea patients. The result was a surprising and serious improvement in symptoms in the group. (Source: N Engl J Med 346 2002 444)

E
C
T
O

−+

Questions	First, determine if the heart is involved, which is usually the case: Cardiac arrhythmia without pain when relaxed? (Yes > heart SBS - overwhelmed conflict, see questions p. 127f. No > diaphragm SBS alone). When did the symptoms begin? (Conflict shortly before). Did I have real problems with breathing, getting air or pressing out? In the figurative sense: What knocked the wind out of me? (A fright, unforeseeable stress, an argument)? Why couldn't I deal with the situation? (Determine the core of the conflict). Were there similar situations in my childhood that conditioned me? (Question parents, awaken memories). Did my parents or ancestors experience anything similar? (Question parents and relatives). These types of conversations should be carried out with the express (inner) intention of bringing healing/love to the family.
Therapy	Should the cramps reappear, identify the conflict or tracks and resolve them. Find out where the love is - there you'll find the solution.
	Breathing exercises, rhythmic sports (hiking, walking, cross-country skiing, dancing).
	See also heart-strengthening remedies p. 133.

Hiccups (singultus)

Same SBS as above. Hiccups are a sudden and uncoordinated tensing of the diaphragm. The unexpected rush of air through the pharynx causes the glottis to close with the resulting "hiccup."

Examples	➜ *Someone drinks so greedily that he "forgets" to breathe, causing an oxygen insufficiency.*
	➜ *Someone talks to his sports buddy, while they are running = conflict of not getting enough air.*
	• *The 47-year-old woman is planning a big celebration with relatives for her father's 80th birthday. She needs to coordinate everything with her two siblings, which costs her a lot of effort and nerves. Finally, everything is settled and she is looking forward to the party, which is to occur in 6 weeks. One day, the patient phones her father. In passing, he mentions that he doesn't want a party and that it shouldn't take place. The patient is completely taken aback - her breath is taken away (= conflict). Fortunately, she immediately has a heart-to-heart talk with her partner about the matter. Half an hour later, as the two laugh about the stubborn old man, the woman gets a case of the hiccups, stronger than she has ever had before. (Archive B. Eybl)*
Phase	**Repair phase crisis** in the context of the repair phase - diaphragm cramp = hiccups.
Therapy	Identify the conflict and conditioning and, if possible, resolve them in real life should they reoccur. Questions: see above.
	Breathe in deeply several times and hold the breath (hyperventilation) or cough, in order to bring the hiccups into "the right rhythm" again. Swallow a teaspoon of cumin seeds with water. Drink several sips of cold water, or lemon water or take a spoonful of sugar.
	Inhale with stimulating etheric oils (camphor, peppermint, etc.). These measures bring about a vegetative changeover, a "reboot" for the diaphragm contractions.

Side stitches

Same SBS as above. (See pp. 210-211)

Example	➜ *Someone eats a meal just before playing a sport.*
Phase	**Repair phase crisis** in the context of the repair phase - diaphragm cramps = side stitches.
Note	The main trigger is eating before physical exercise. Since the stomach and intestines are partly anchored to the diaphragm, the diaphragm is pulled down by full visceral organs > limitation of the diaphragm's breathing assistance mechanism > start of an SBS of the diaphragm. People, who have weak muscles and weak connective tissue, probably also have a weak diaphragm, which soon reaches its performance limits.
Therapy	Identify the conflict and conditioning and, if possible, resolve them in real life, should they reoccur. Questions: see above. Strength training, especially for the muscles of the trunk of the body. Pay attention to posture and body tension. Breathing exercises (possibly in the form of yoga) or alternative respiration.
	Do not eat before sport sessions. During sport sessions, breathe deeply and calmly. Do not talk.

Diaphragmatic hernia, hiatus hernia

Same SBS as above - hard to distinguish from an injury, accident. Due to a hole in the diaphragm, the stomach, intestines or other abdominal organs can protrude into the chest cavity. The most frequently affected organ is the stomach (hiatus hernia).

Phase	**Conflict-active phase:** reduction of transverse muscle fibers > thinning of the diaphragm > tendency for hernia, for instance, when lifting heavy objects or doing "crunches."
Therapy	Determine the conflict and conditioning and, if possible, resolve them in real life should they still be active. Questions: see previous page. Breathing training (possibly yoga); strength training, especially for the trunk of the body, surgery if necessary.

PERITONEUM, NAVEL, GREATER OMENTUM & ABDOMINAL WALL

The abdominal cavity is lined with the peritoneum, which is entirely composed of mesodermal tissue.
There are two layers:
The outer (parietal) layer is attached to the abdominal wall, the inner (visceral) layer forms the outer cover of the organs.
There is a lubricating fluid in the wafer-thin space between the two layers, which allows the organs to slide about.

The greater omentum is an apron-shaped fold of the peritoneum that is attached to the stomach and colon and hangs forward over the winding small intestines.
It can move around on its own, so that it can purposefully lay itself around centers of inflammation in order to isolate them. For example, it folds itself over a ruptured appendix to keep the contents of the intestine from entering the abdominal cavity.

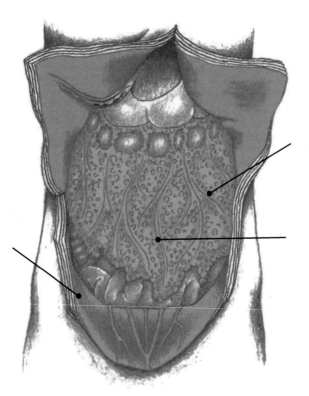

Greater Omentum
Conflict related to the abdomen

Peritoneum
Attack against the abdomen

Abdominal Wall
Self-esteem conflict, issues: pushing/pressing

SBS of the Peritoneum

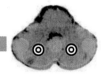

Cancer of the peritoneum (peritoneal cancer, peritoneal mesothelioma)[1]

Conflict	Attack-to-the-abdomen. Actual attack, threat, or perception of an attack. Fear that something is wrong with the abdomen (intestines, stomach, liver, pancreas).
Examples	➜ *Very often due to brutal diagnoses like: "You have a lung tumor," or "You have a malignant breast cancer. We will have to operate at once."* ➜ *Evil words, insults, or verbal abuse, can be felt as blows or injuries.* ➜ *Intense abdominal pain, regardless of where it comes from (colic, poisoning, etc.) can also be felt as attack conflict > cell proliferation in the active-phase, cell degradation in the repair phase.* • *A colon cancer tumor, 17 cm (6.7 in) in diameter, is diagnosed in a 69-year-old woman. Considering the size of the growth, the prognosis is very unfavorable = attack against the abdomen. The patient feels threatened by the gigantic tumor in her abdomen > growth of cells in the peritoneum = peritoneal cancer. Three weeks later, as the tumor is removed, the surgeons find a number of stipple-shaped mesotheliomas. (Archive B. Eybl)*
Conflict-active	Cell proliferation in the peritoneum, growth of small or flat mesotheliomas, depending on whether the person feels attacked over the whole abdomen or only at a certain spot.
Bio. function	Strengthening and thickening of the peritoneum to fend off attacks better.
Repair phase	Tubercular-caseating degradation along with fever, night sweats or encapsulation of the tumor if no suitable bacteria are present, development of abdominal fluid (ascites), especially with syndrome. Repair phase doesn't automatically mean that "everything's okay," because the conflict may be persistent and the repair phase pain could become problematic due to its intensity. After the healing is complete, calcium deposits and scarring may remain.
Repair crisis	Chills, intense pain.
Questions	First determine if it is conflict-active or in the repair phase. Real attack to the abdomen? (Accident, blow/punch, OP, severe abdominal pain like a bilious attack)? Imagined attack? (Diagnosis, thoughts about if one may have an intestinal tumor or not)? Substitute conflict? (E.g., sympathy with a loved one who has an abdominal disease). Why does it affect me so much? Which family conditioning plays a role?
Therapy	Identify the conflict and conditioning and, if possible, resolve them in real life should they still be active. Understand the connections. Guiding principles: *"I am safe. I am protected." "Everything is going to be all right again." "I know the connections, so this diagnosis cannot shake me."* In CM, this condition is treated with an OP, chemotherapy and radiation for about three months of life extension. Right after the surgery, mesothelioma usually grow back in the surgery wound. In our view (and "from the perspective of the peritoneum"), this is understandable, because the surgery represents a renewed attack. > Due to their low chances of success, these CM therapies are not recommended.

Inflammation of the peritoneum (peritonitis)

CM distinguishes between primary (the peritoneum is the source of the inflammation) and secondary (surrounding organs, e.g., intestines are the source of the inflammation) peritonitis. If primary peritonitis: Same SBS as above.

Example	• *A 35-year-old, right-handed man is sitting in the passenger seat next to his girlfriend, as she drives through an intersection with a green light. At this moment, a vehicle coming from the right crashes into the passenger side of the small car. The patient feels an impact from the side against his abdomen. The side airbag opens = attack conflict against the abdomen. He is brought to the hospital in an ambulance. Twenty-four hours after the accident, he experiences a strong pain. His abdomen is very hard and very sensitive to pressure = peritonitis. Forty-eight hours after the accident (the second day in the hospital), the abdomen of the athletic patient swells up into a big hard ball. The patient: "It was as if I were pregnant." = repair phase - ascites - exsudative peritoneal effusion. His swollen belly remains with him for two days and then he slowly urinates the fluid away and his pain subsides. (Archive B. Eybl)*
Phase	**Repair phase:** Inflammation of the peritoneum, tumor-degradation via bacteria, fever, night sweats.

---

1   See Dr. Hamer, Charts pp. 48, 53

The acute peritonitis has a serious set of symptoms: abdominal pain, "hard as a board" peritoneum, acute pain in the repair phase crisis.

Therapy   The conflict is resolved. Support the healing process. Slight inflammation: Cannabis oil, cold brine or curd cheese compresses, enzyme preparations, Schuessler Cell Salts: No. 3, lymph drainage massages. If severe, generalized peritonitis, CM does the following: surgical removal of inflamed tissue and pus. They then rinse the abdominal cavity (peritoneal lavage). Subsequently, the patient needs intensive care with antibiotics and pain-killers. Whether these drastic measures are actually necessary, I do not know. Decide on a case-by-case basis.

Ascites (exsudative ascites)

Ascites is when there is fluid in the peritoneal cavity. Ascites can form during the inflammation (repair phases) of any abdominal organ, even the bones, in conjunction with syndrome (= transudative ascites). A swelling of the liver can mimic ascites. Pronounced ascites occur in a peritoneum SBS + syndrome (= exudative ascites).
The Same SBS as above (see pp. 213-214), but with syndrome as well:

Example   • A patient is diagnosed with cancer of the liver and a surgery date is set = attack-to-the-abdomen conflict. The surgery is postponed 4-6 weeks in order to carry out pre-operative examinations. During the surgery, the abdomen is found to be "full of metastases" = cell proliferation in the peritoneum (peritoneal mesothelioma). (See Dr. Hamer, Goldenes Buch Bd. 1, p. 348)
               • A 55-year-old patient decides to have liposuction on her abdomen, because her husband has been criticizing her fat belly. When she sees the long needle poking around in her abdomen, she feels like she is being attacked. Mesotheliomas develop on the four spots where the needle was inserted. (See Claudio Trupiano, thanks to Dr. Hamer, p. 207)

Phase   **Repair phase**: A reduction of the mesothelioma goes hand-in-hand with the production of fluid. This prevents adhesions, since everything is "swimming" in ascites > enlarged abdomen with weight gain, severe ascites with syndrome. Possibly recurring-conflict.

Therapy   The attack conflict is resolved. Support the healing. Resolve any refugee conflict (kidney collecting tubules). Tea: nettle, horsetail, goldenrod, sage. Normal drinking, little salt (whole salt), no pork. Lymphatic drainage, saltwater baths, enzyme preparation. Breathing exercises. If necessary: pain medication. Avoid punctures if possible or slowly lengthen the intervals between treatments. For chronic ascites, possibly implant a self-operated catheter. For treating loss of protein due to puncture > intake of biologically valuable proteins, such as eggs, curd cheese, protein 88, possibly also albumin infusions.

SBS of the Navel

Cancer of the inner navel[1]

In our developmental history, the inner part of the navel arose from the so-called cloaca. Birds and reptiles have no separate exits for feces and urine like most mammals; rather, they have a joint opening for everything. Even their sex organs open into the cloaca.

Conflict   Chunk conflict (see explanations p. 15, 16), not being able to get something out (= elimination conflict).

Examples   • A woman notices that her husband is drunk again. = Conflict, not able to eliminate the alcohol.
                   • An 11-year-old boy has a 9-year-old sister. His conflict is that his sister still wets her bed = substitution conflict, not eliminating (correctly). When his sister is finally "dry," his navel begins to leak fluid = repair phase, degradation of the navel tumor. (See Ursula Homm, Lebensmittelheilkunde, p. 44)

Conflict-active   Increase in function or growth of a compact cauliflower-shaped tumor (adeno-ca) of secretory quality or a flat-growing cancer of absorptive quality.

Bio. function   Improvement of excretion.

Repair phase   Normalization of function, tubercular-caseating degradation of the tumor via fungi or bacteria.

---

1   See Dr. Hamer, Charts p. 28

Questions	What can't I eliminate? What do I want to be rid of? (For me or perceived as a substitute for someone else). Why did that appear in my life? Was it a message for me? Which familial conditioning sensitized me for the conflict?
Therapy	Identify the conflict and conditioning and, if possible, resolve them in real life if still active. OP if necessary.

SBS of the Greater Omentum

Cancer of greater omentum (omentum majus), cold abscess in abdominal cavity[1]

Tumors of the greater omentum are largely unknown in CM. Again, Dr. Hamer discovered something new.

Conflict	Conflict relating to the abdomen.
Example	➔ *A large tumor is discovered in someone's abdomen.*
Conflict-active	Cell proliferation in the greater omentum, growth of a mesothelioma.
Bio. function	1. Providing more fluid for a good lubrication of the abdominal viscera. 2. "Wrapping up" of the inflamed abdominal organs through the intrinsically mobile greater omentum.
Repair phase	Tubercular-caseating degradation of the tumor, often along with adhesions. The encapsulation of centers of inflammation in the abdomen are also known as "cold abscesses" in CM.
Questions	Determine if the conflict is active or in the repair phase based on the symptoms. What happened with my own abdomen or the abdomen of a loved one? (OP, injury, bad diagnosis or fear thereof)? Am I carrying something from the family (familial solidarity)? Are there unresolved issues in the family with relation to the abdomen/digestion?
Therapy	Determine the conflict and conditioning and, if possible, resolve them in real life if still active.

O L D M E S O +−

---

1 See Dr. Hamer, Charts pp. 48, 53

SBS of the Abdominal Wall

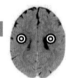

Abdominal wall hernia, inguinal hernia, umbilical hernia

90% of hernias occur in men. This is because, in the large inguinal canal, there is a weak spot in the male abdominal wall. This canal can become a hernial orifice and abdominal contents (intestinal loop) can force its way out.

Conflict	Self-esteem conflict: too much pressure, having to carry too much, always pushing and pressing. In the case of children, it is always a substitution conflict (check the parents).
Conflict-active	Unnoticed cell depletion in tendon sheets or in connective tissue of the abdominal wall. Prolonged conflict activity can cause tendons to be pushed to the side through increased abdominal pressure (long-term expansion of intestine from gas, straining during bowel movements, lifting, coughing) and a hernial orifice or a hernial sac develops.
Repair phase	Recovery only when the hernial orifice rests, closed, for a few months.
Bio. function	Strengthening the abdominal wall in order to be able to withstand more pressure.
Questions	When was the hernia noticed? (Conflict-active phase at least some weeks before). Which pressure from outside was I unable to withstand? Did I put myself under pressure? Tendency toward hernias in the family? (Yes > work out the family tendency) When did everything become so difficult?
Therapy	Identify the conflict and conditioning and, if possible, resolve them in real life. Guiding principle: *"I let it flow and it's easy going."* Comfrey, sanicle internally and externally. Improve nutrition so that no intestinal gases develop and the intestine isn't burdened. Wear an athletic supporter for a few months. The hernial sac must never fill during this time. OP if all else fails.

N E W M E S O −+

LIVER AND GALLBLADDER

The liver (hepar) is the largest internal organ of the human body. It is the central organ for metabolism and the "chemical laboratory." Venous blood enters the liver through the portal vein carrying nutrients from the intestines and through worn-out blood cells from the spleen. The primal, endodermal tissue of the liver (liver parenchyma) serves to take up nutrition (absorptive function) and produce bile (secretory function). Some of the bile ducts lie within the liver (intrahepatic), while others lie outside the liver (extrahepatic). The bile flows through the bile ducts over the dead-end-like gallbladder into the duodenum. The bile ducts and gallbladder are muscular tubes lined with ectodermal squamous epithelium. The liver is regarded as the bodily organ that is most capable of regenerating.

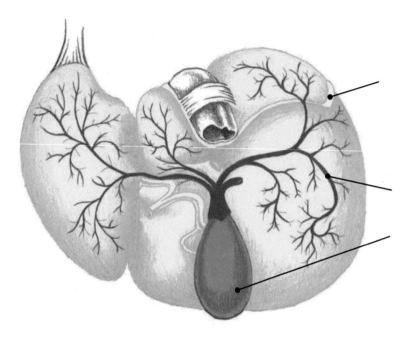

Liver Parenchyma
(basic tissue)
**Starvation conflict,
existential conflict**

Gallbladder
and Bile Ducts
**Territorial-anger
conflict**

SBS of the Liver Parenchyma

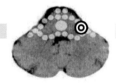

Liver adeno-ca, round liver lesions (hepatocellular cancer)[1]

Conflict	Existential or starvation conflict, fear for one's own existence because of hardship, poverty and food shortage, fear of starving (e.g., crop failure, unemployment). A lack of love, money, attention, recognition that is perceived as an existential threat.
Examples	→ *This conflict is often the result of a diagnosis of colon cancer. Many patients believe that they will starve because of colon cancer > growth of circular hepatic lesions in the active-phase, tubercular degradation in the repair phase.*

• *A mother during World War II told her six-year-old daughter: "You have to eat your milk soup or we can just order a casket right now." = Existential or starvation conflict. As with most starving war children, the little ones develop liver cysts (recurring-conflict) in the repair phase. (See Dr. Hamer, Goldenes Buch, Band 2, p. 314)*

• *The mother of a baby must often drive long distances because of her job. It often happens that the infant is alone for long periods. This causes him to suffer an existential or starvation conflict. (Archive B. Eybl)*

---

1 See Dr. Hamer, Charts p. 22

• *A rich patient hires a cook for her household. Since the patient is always interfering with her cooking, the cook quits her job. The next cook also quits after just a short time. One day - just before a big dinner party - another cook quits. "Who's going to cook now for all these people?"* = Starvation conflict (See Dr. Hamer, Goldenes Buch, Bd. 1, p. 254)

• *A patient, a small entrepreneur, is lying in the hospital and learns that the rent on her shop is to be raised, contrary to the rental agreement. This causes her to suffer an existential or starvation conflict.* (See Dr. Hamer, Goldenes Buch, Bd. 1, p. 608)

Conflict-active	Increase in function and growth of a tumor adeno-ca of secretory or absorptive quality = hepatic circular foci, rise of the enzyme cholinesterase level in the blood due to increased liver metabolism. A single (solitary) circular lesion appears, when an existential or starvation conflict is a substitution conflict for another person; a number of round liver lesions appear if the conflict affects oneself.
	<u>Fatty liver</u> (hepar adiposum): An SBS of the alpha cells of the pancreatic islets can probably cause fat storage in the hepatic cells, which would reflect the biological meaning of an existential threat. Possibly though, it is just the sugar relay that is responsible for the fatty liver.
Bio. function	With more liver cells of absorptive quality, the food can be "sucked up" (utilized) better. With more liver cells of secretory quality, more bile can be produced, with which the food can be better digested > both tumors help to avoid starvation or, in other words, ensure existence.
Repair phase	Normalization of function, tubercular-caseating degradation of the tumor via fungi or bacteria (mycobacteria), hepatitis, swelling of the liver, pain, night sweats, fever.
	If no bacteria are present: encapsulation and disconnection from the metabolism.
Repair crisis	Chills, severe liver pain.
Note	Nowadays, hepatic adeno-ca is most common in the famine regions of Africa (real starvation) - in the well-fed West, it is usually the consequence of a cancer diagnosis (iotrogenic). Typical sequence of early childhood starvation conflict: never getting the feeling that one is full.
	Caution: In cancer patients, very old liver cysts are often interpreted as "liver metastases."
Questions	First, determine if there is actually a relevant SBS of the liver running (look at the cholinesterase level). With cancer patients, a "metastasis" is often diagnosed from a harmless spot on the liver (hyper/ hypodense lesion). When did the symptoms begin? (Determine if they are repair phase symptoms or conflict-active symptoms). Was there a starvation conflict in recent months? Take a look at the career status, financial emergency, money problems due to a divorce, bankruptcy, etc.). Substitution conflict? (E.g., sympathy with a suffering child)? What was the infancy/childhood like? How did the parents live? Is there a history of liver disease in the family/ancestors? (Determine the causal conditioning - work out similar conflict situations). How am I dealing with the diagnosis? Am I able to see and understand the connections?
Therapy	Determine the conflict and conditioning and, if possible, resolve them in real life. Guiding principles: *"I will live." "My existence is secure." "I have enough to eat." "God guides me through all my difficulties."* Possibly surgery - of course, without chemo and radiation.
	See also: remedies for the liver on p. 221.

Liver tuberculosis, collection of pus in the liver (liver abscess)

Same SBS as above.

Phase	**Repair phase:** With the help of bacteria there is a tubercular, necrotizing degradation of the round lesions of the liver (= liver tuberculosis).
Note	If the conflict recurs, connective-tissue capsules of pus appear (liver abscess). Both situations are accompanied by swelling of the liver, pain, night sweats and fever. When the tuberculosis has run its course, calcium deposits can remain = CM's "calcification of the liver."
Therapy	The conflict is resolved. Support the healing. Possibly, pain relievers and antibiotics. See also: remedies for the liver p. 221.

■ SBS of the Gallbladder Bile Ducts ■

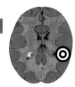

Gallbladder inflammation (cholecystitis), hepatitis (ectodermal), acute or chronic hepatitis types, autoimmune hepatitis, cancer of the bile ducts (cholangiocarcinoma)[1]

Conflict	Territorial-anger conflict or identity conflict (dependent on "handedness," hormone levels and previous conflicts). One is angry because the territory or territorial boundaries are not respected.
	According to Frauenkron-Hoffmann: Resentful, one can't forgive, always making accusations.
Examples	For territorial-anger conflict (see p. 205 for examples of identity conflicts):

→ *Most of the time, aggression plays a role either from oneself or from another.*

→ *Trouble with work colleagues or family members, boundary violations or encroachments by the neighbors. Fights over territory or money. One is livid with anger.*

→ *A person is irritated or provoked. They is drawn out of their normal reserve. One is "bilious."*

• *A family man and former police officer has been retired for years. For some time, his liver has been bothering him but he hasn't paid much attention to it. The problem originated from past anger at work. Adherence to law and order has always been his highest duty and this has led to territorial-anger conflicts. One day, he draws the last straw: He learns that his sister has misappropriated a large sum of money from his mother's estate = large, recurring, territorial-anger conflict. He breaks contact with his sister, but that cannot alleviate his anger. The patient dies of a hepatic coma (= repair phase crisis of the liver and bile ducts) and syndrome. (See Claudio Trupiano, thanks to Dr. Hamer, p. 333).*

• *A 71-year-old married, right-handed woman has a 41-year-old, mentally-ill daughter (seven suicide attempts), who often phones in the middle of the night and threatens to kill herself. The mother then immediately gets into her car and drives the 40 km (25 mi) to her daughter = 26 years of chronic-active territorial-anger conflict with regard to the bile ducts. A year ago, she began to draw the line strictly. She hangs up the phone immediately if her daughter is rude to her = beginning of the repair phase: increase in GGT to 144 and GOT to 68, nausea, swollen liver, side pain. Findings of the sonogram: "liver metastasis." Thanks to her trust in God and her knowledge of the 5 Biological Laws of Nature, she survives it all. (Archive B. Eybl)*

Conflict-active	Increase in sensibility of the bile duct mucosa, simultaneous slackening of the smooth ring musculature. Later, cell degradation (ulcer) in the gallbladder or in the bile ducts, within or outside of the liver (intra- or extrahepatic), moderate pain (side pain). Often furious, angry, aggressive. Typical for a recurring (chronic) conflict is fat and alcohol intolerance. Increased gamma-GT (most important value), GOT, GPT, AP (all or singularly, see p. 39).
Bio. function	Through an enlargement of the gallbladder or bile ducts, the lumen increases > bile can be sent to the duodenum better and quicker (to better vent one's anger).
Repair phase	Restoration of the squamous epithelium of the bile ducts or gallbladder caused by increased metabolism, repair of lost substance = inflamed gallbladder, gallbladder cancer; healing swelling or inflammation of the bile ducts (cholangitis).
	The flow of bile can be reduced or stopped (cholestasis). If the majority of the bile ducts are affected, jaundice (icterus) ensues. Possibly a **recurring-conflict.**
Repair crisis	Severe pain, chills, colic due to involvement of the bile duct muscles.
Questions	In the case that it is recurring: Which territorial situation is upsetting? (Coworkers, boss, partner, neighbor, siblings)? Are the symptoms better on vacation (Yes > indication of a conflict in daily life, e.g., workplace). When did the complaints begin? What changed in my life at that point? (Move or new workplace, separation, new partner, etc.)? Which childhood situations does the conflict bring to mind? (Aggressive father, teacher, a fight with siblings, parents fighting)? Aggressive tendencies in the family? Which side? Does the issue have a life-lesson to teach me? How will I deal with it in the future? Which new attitude would be healing? Which old resentment or reproaches are holding me back? Which out-

E
C
T
O

(–+)

---

1   See Dr. Hamer, Charts p. 116

ward changes could help?

| Therapy | The conflict is resolved. Support the healing process. If recurrent: Determine and resolve the conflict, causal conditioning and beliefs. Guiding principles: *"My anger lies behind me." "The next time I will remain calm from the beginning."* Enzyme preparations, Schuessler Cell Salts No. 3, 4 and 9. See also: remedies for the liver. p. 221. If necessary, pain relievers, anti-inflammatory medications, surgery. |

Jaundice (icterus)

Same SBS as above. The life cycle of the red-blood cells ends after about 120 days. After that, they are broken down into bilirubin in the bone marrow, spleen and liver and eliminated through the gallbladder. If the bile ducts are blocked, the concentration of bilirubin in the blood rises. If the concentration exceeds 2 mg/dl, jaundice (yellow skin) sets in.

Phase	**Repair phase:** healing swelling of the bile ducts with temporary occlusion > the bilirubin cannot be discarded > the level of bilirubin in the blood rises > yellowing of the skin and the whites of the eyes, as well as a brown-coloring of the urine; the stool remains light in color for lack of bile coloring.
Note	However, jaundice can also come from an accelerated degradation of red-blood cells (hemolysis). This can be caused by blood transfusions, poisons, medication, heavy losses of blood (bruises, contusions, etc.) and malaria.
Therapy	The conflict is resolved. Support the healing process, prevent recurrences. See also: remedies for the liver p. 221.

Jaundice in newborn babies (newborn icterus, kernicterus)

Same SBS as above (see p. 218). A large percentage of newborn babies are affected by a yellow coloring of the skin during the first two weeks of life. In CM, this is considered normal, except in severe cases. The jaundice is explained by a shortened life span (70 instead 120 days) of the red-blood cells, an immature liver and an increased reabsorption of bilirubin in the intestines of constipated newborns.

It would be interesting to know how common newborn jaundice is among indigenous peoples. If infants were not subjected to ultrasound and amniocentesis and if mother and child were not exposed to so much hectic rush and stress, newborn jaundice would certainly be less common.

The unfortunately, very-widespread ultrasound examinations pose a real risk to the embryo or fetus. The amniotic fluid is heated by the noise of the ultrasound and even forms little bubbles (cavitation). Noise = danger > fear.

Some newborns get through this excitement undamaged, but others are seized with panic and become ill.

From the viewpoint of the 5 Biological Laws of Nature, jaundice in newborns is not normal but rather the result of a territorial-anger conflict during the pregnancy and/or birth. The proof of this, as with all illnesses, can be found with a CT scan. However, in infants/toddlers a CT is not appropriate due to the radiation exposure and the need for anesthesia.

Conflict	Territorial-anger or, less often, an identity conflict (see above).
Examples	→ *A difficult birth takes place.*
	→ *An ultrasound test disturbs the newborn in its territory.*
	→ *The unborn registers the nearness of the needle used for testing the amniotic fluid. At the same time he feels his mother's fear of a gene defect.*
	→ *During pregnancy, the mother bumps her belly into the edge of a table.*
	→ *In the womb, the child hears his parents' quarreling.*
Phase	**Repair phase:** Healing swelling of the bile ducts with temporary occlusion > increased bilirubin in the blood and yellowing of the skin.
Therapy	The conflict is resolved. Support the healing process, prevent recurrences. The most important "treatment" is that the child can (more or less permanently) stay with their mother, undisturbed and feels harmony and love (the love for the child, but also the love between the parents). See remedies for the liver p. 221.

Gallstones (cholelithiasis), biliary microlithiasis, biliary colic

Same SBS as above. (See pp. 218-219.) 10-25% of adults have gallstones. They begin with a tiny condensation nucleus, around which layer after layer of additional material collects. They are made up of 98% cholesterol - the rest is calcium and bile pigment. Usually they are found in the gallbladder and remain unnoticed. However, if a gallstone slips into a bile duct, the fun's over > severe pain, colic due to irritation of the sensitive epithelial mucous membrane. The blockage causes a rise in the bilirubin level (> jaundice). In esoteric teaching, gallstones represent crystallized (not free-flowing) aggression.

Phase	**Recurring-conflict:** A long period of conflict activity is followed by scarred shrinkage of the bile ducts and/or gallbladder, inflammation (repair phase) indicates that there is a more or less pronounced blockage of bile flow > reduced "turnover" of bile > thickening, formation of condensation nucleus > growth of stones.
Repair crisis	Colic of the gallbladder, pain in the sides, chills: the body tries to expel the stone with peristaltic contractions of the bile duct. This works to remove biliary "sludge" and small gallstones, but not larger stones. For these, a CM intervention makes sense.
Note	Low-fat foods ("light" products) and foods without bitter-tasting compounds promote the formation of gallstones because the body responds by producing less bile > the bile thickens > formation of stones. (Comparison: A river's sediment load is a function of its capacity = less flow > less transport).
	An existential or starvation conflict (see above), in persistent repair, can probably lead to gallstones because of the low production of bile.
	Syndrome favors gall stone formation due to narrowed bile ducts. (This is most often seen in overweight people with high cholesterol levels).
Therapy	Determine the conflict and conditioning and, if possible, resolve them in real life so that the SBS comes to an end. Questions: see p. 218. Guiding principle: *"Lord, give me the strength to change what I can change, the serenity to accept what I cannot change and the wisdom to know the difference"* (Niebuhr). Liver cleansing according to Moritz[2]. Stone dissolution by "Lithosol" (mineral mixture, prescription).
	If necessary, surgery or treatments to break up or dissolve the gallstones. Beware: Gallbladders are removed too often (a nice, well-paid, beginner's surgery). Gallstones rarely cause problems. Colic: painkilling and anticonvulsant medication. See also: remedies for the liver p. 221.

Acute liver failure (hepatic coma, hepatic encephalopathy)

Same SBS as above. (See pp. 218-220) The symptoms range from an increased need for sleep to unconsciousness (coma). According to CM, these symptoms indicate that the end is approaching (insufficient detoxification). Unfortunately the repair phase crisis is not known by CM, for one would then realize that although the coma is dangerous, it is part of the repair phase. > For this reason, do not give up too early!

Phase	**Repair phase crisis:** A hepatic coma occurs when the gamma-glutamyltransferase (GGT) levels begin to drop. Dr. Hamer discovered that it is not only the non-functioning of the liver (ammonia and other nitrogen compounds find their way into the bloodstream) that is dangerous; the impact of the repair phase crisis on the brain is dangerous as well: a liver coma is a kind of "brain coma" = unconsciousness due to a build-up of pressure and severe hypoglycemia (low blood sugar levels).
Note	The enzyme gamma-glutamyltransferase, also known as gamma-GT, is the most significant laboratory value for us with regard to the bile ducts. Values of up to 40 units per liter for women and 70 units per liter for men are considered to be normal. The critical phase begins when the gamma-GT value is already beginning to rise. At values of up to 400, the repair phase crisis normally proceeds without complications; from 400-800, it becomes problematic. At such high levels, there is almost always a syndrome involved.
Therapy	The conflict is resolved. Support the repair phase. Prevent recurrences. Resolve any refugee conflict if active. During the repair phase crisis, the brain is operating "at its limit" and needs a lot of glucose > administer glucose through the mouth or with a feeding tube. Glucose infusions have the disadvantage of binding fluids in the body. Important: hospital treatments should be kind and humane because of a possible refugee conflict (syndrome). See also: therapy for symptoms of pressure on the brain (p. 56).

---

2   Andreas Moritz, Die wundersame Leber- & Gallenblasenreinigung, voxverlag.de, Bad Lausick 2008. Caution: This is a good way to cleanse the bile ducts, but the conglomerate excreted is not gallstones as Moritz contends, rather saponified oil.

Liver cysts (PLD - polycystic liver disease)

Cysts can form in the liver's functional, endodermal tissue as well as in its ectodermal squamous epithelium. Both kinds of cysts can grow up to several centimeters.

Active kidney collecting tubules SBS can strengthen the effect by "pumping up" old cavities with fluid.

- **Cyst(s) in the liver parenchyma** (cyst adeno-ca, solitary liver cyst): existential or starvation conflict; condition following round liver lesion ca (See liver adeno-ca).

- **Cyst(s) in the bile ducts** (squamous epithelium): territorial-anger conflict or identity conflict. (See section on hepatitis for examples and course of illness). Conditions following recurrences and persistent repair: If the blockage of a bile duct is protracted, the flow of bile begins to flow backwards > bile duct proliferation and formation of cysts. The backflow can also cause the liver parenchyma to die off (CM: necrosis of the omentum).

Liver cirrhosis

Possible causes

- **Bile ducts:** The bile ducts, with their finely branching structure, reach just about every corner of the liver. Recurring territorial-anger conflicts lead to a scarring shrinkage of the bile ducts. The epithelium is gradually replaced by inferior connective tissue. CM: "primary biliary cirrhosis." The liver parenchyma also dies off, because the transportation of bile from the gallbladder is disturbed > liver cirrhosis.

- **Liver Parenchyma:** Recurring existential or starvation conflicts lead to an alteration or death of the liver tissue (liver parenchyma necrosis). Condition after frequent liver tuberculosis = cirrhosis of the liver; note: reduced levels of cholinesterase.

- **Poisoning:** There is hardly a medication that does NOT harm the liver - from hormone preparations to simple pain medicine: every chemical must be neutralized and removed by the liver. Chronic misuse of medication, drugs and alcohol damages the liver and in the end, this leads to liver cirrhosis. Dr. Hamer rightly points out that most alcoholics are members of the lower level of society and are more conflict-endangered than others. *"Cancer doesn't come from alcohol - alcoholism and cancer come from anger and worry."* Liver cirrhosis usually leads to high blood pressure (intrahepatic portal hypertension) and blockage of the portal veins.

Remedies for the liver

- Stop poisoning with medication, alcohol and drugs; eat only small amounts in the evening so that no alcohol arises in the intestines due to fermentation.
- Pay attention to food combinations: do not combine starches (grain, bread) with sugar; possibly follow the Hay diet.
- Cleanse the bile ducts by drinking vegetable oil as described by Moritz. (See footnote 2 on p. 220).
- Drink a lot of water in the morning for detoxification.
- Bach flowers: beech, chicory, gentian, gorse, willow.
- Teas: blessed milk thistle, fennel, burdock root, dandelion, agrimony, Chelidonium, centaury, yarrow, barberry, chicory, absinthe.
- Spices: turmeric, fennel, saffron, rosemary, juniper.
- Hildegard of Bingen: chestnut honey - mulberry wine special recipe, Swedish bitters.

- Segment massage on the right thoracic spine and sides, acupuncture and acupoint massage, foot reflex-zone massage.
- Cayce: Seven-day treatment with dehydrated castor oil - soak a 30 x 30 cm (12 x 12 in) cloth with dehydrated castor oil and place it on the right flank. Place a piece of plastic and a warm hot-water bottle over it. Wrap it in the blanket and let it work for one hour. Take a small dose of olive oil after that.
- Kanne Bread Drink, internally.
- Eat fresh nasturtium and black radish often.
- Hot-moist liver compress.
- Linseed oil (omega 3 fatty acid).
- If emaciated, 2 tbsp cod liver oil daily.

PANCREAS

The fishhook-shaped pancreas lies transversely behind the stomach in the upper abdominal cavity. Its endodermal glandular tissue produces 1 to 1½ liters of digestive juice daily, which contains enzymes to break down fats, proteins and carbohydrates. The ectodermal excretory ducts collect the juice and lead it into the duodenum (= exocrine gland function).

Embedded in the glandular tissue and strewn "like raisins in a cake" are two kinds of ectodermal hormone glands (= the so-called pancreatic islets or islets of Langerhans) with two main types of cells:

• The alpha cells produce the hormone glucagon, which raises the blood sugar.

• The beta cells produce insulin, which lowers the blood sugar. Both hormones are fed directly into the blood (endocrine gland function).

As we see below, the two sugar SBSs provided by nature should only function as short-term programs - in preparation for a fight or for flight.

In this context, they are both meaningful and helpful. Unfortunately, thanks to our habit of continuously lugging conflicts around throughout our modern lives, this meaning is totally lost.

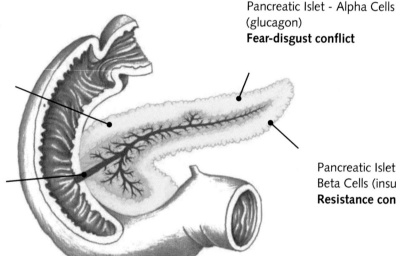

Pancreas - Parenchyma
Chunk conflict, not being able to utilize something

Pancreatic Islet - Alpha Cells (glucagon)
Fear-disgust conflict

Pancreatic Ducts
Territorial-anger conflict

Pancreatic Islet - Beta Cells (insulin)
Resistance conflict

SBS of the Pancreatic Islet Beta Cells

Chronic hyperglycemia (CM's diabetes mellitus type 1)[1]

The hormone insulin sinks the blood sugar level and opens the floodgates to the muscles. With this SBS, the insulin production in the beta cells is uniformly lowered and thus, the level of sugar in the blood rises. In the muscles, however, the sugar level is reduced - a consequence of the decreased insulin production.

When glucose levels are high, sugar is also eliminated through the urine. (This explains the name: diabetes mellitus = honey-sweet flow). The beta cells are controlled by the right (male) side of the cerebral cortex.

Conflict	Resistance conflict - pre-fight phase: One defends themselves against someone or something, but believes that they are not strong enough. One refuses someone (usually an authority) or a task (e.g., a certain job/work). One believes they have to fighting against something. One is forced to do something or completes something against their will. Less often, this is a female fear-disgust conflict (dependent on "handedness," hormone levels, or previous conflicts).
	Explanation: The masculine reaction to adversity is defend, resist and then strike.
	Frauenkron-Hoffmann: cold conflict (ancestors froze to death, existential emergency due to cold, etc.

E
C
T
O

−+

---

1 See Dr. Hamer, Charts p. 138

ECTO **−+**	
Examples	→ *A person must do something he doesn't want to do (for example, go to kindergarten or to school).* → *One is or feels compelled or coerced into something.* • *At the end of his political career, the former Italian Prime Minister Bettino Craxi was proven to have personal connections to the mafia. He was forced to face every imaginable kind of attack, while finding it difficult to justify himself = resistance conflict of not being able to defend oneself from accusations. As the pressure became too great, he fled to Tunisia but he found no peace there either, because he was constantly forced to defend himself in interviews = persistent-active conflict: reduced insulin production > increase in blood sugar = diabetes. Being on the run, caused him to suffer a refugee conflict (kidney collecting tubules). Massive fluid collection together with the diabetes then lead to his death in the year 2000. (See Claudio Trupiano, thanks to Dr. Hamer, p. 430)* • *Following the separation from her partner, a young, left-handed woman has difficulties getting him to provide financial support for their two children. She doesn't know what she can do other than threaten him with a lawsuit. However internally, she resists having to settle the matter in such an unpleasant manner = resistance conflict. (Archive B. Eybl)*
Conflict-active	In the pre-fight phase, one resists something = conflict activity. Now the insulin-producing beta-islet cells reduce their function > less insulin is released > increase in blood sugar levels (hyperglycemia, diabetes). However, the sugar is not yet brought to the muscles. - This is in preparation for its imminent discharge (use in the fight). In practice, though, we are usually dealing with a persistent conflict here. Main symptoms: terrible thirst, increased urge to urinate, fatigue, weakness, problems concentrating.
Repair phase	Discharge = fight, flight or both: secretion of insulin > drop in blood sugar because the floodgates open into the muscles. > Large supply of glucose to the muscles for a fight - at least until the increased blood sugar level is depleted. In the second part of the repair phase it can come to the opposite reaction, i.e., a sugar level that is too low (hypoglycemia).
Bio. function	"Damming up" the sugar in the blood (temporary reserve) for the coming fight.
Repair crisis	Attacks of extreme hyperglycemia.
Questions	When did the symptoms begin? (Conflict/trigger shortly before). What was I resisting against? (Bad situation, rebuke, being coerced)? What did I do even though I didn't want to do it? Was I forced/pressured to do something? (Sexual, school, duty)? Blood sugar measurements: After/during which situations is the sugar high/low? (Indication of conflict activity, triggers and the solution respectively). Diabetes in the family? Yes > work out the family issue: Which parallels are there between the ones affected? (Similar fates)? What was the earliest conditioning? What sensitized me to this conflict? (Childhood, parental stress during the pregnancy, ancestral experiences)? Children: Likelihood of a substitution conflict. (Parent's stress > child develops symptoms). Which advantages does the child have due to the difficulties the illness/convalescence presents? (Parents are worried, pay attention to the child because of the illness, the child is in the focus, receives privileges, has a special status at school)? What do I definitely want to change?
Therapy	Determine the conflict and/or trigger(s) and resolve them in real life if they are still active. If all else fails: CM insulin replacement therapy. However, one doesn't have to get carried away here, because increased glucose levels only have negative effects over the long term. The insulin therapy leads to the body producing even less. A few weeks with a fasting blood glucose level of 300 mg/dl (normal value 100) is not a problem. Long-term, there is a need for treatment if values remain over 200 mg/dl. See also: remedies for diabetes p. 225.

Hyperglycemia - other causes

• **Stress without subsequent energy release:** During periods of stress, the sugar level is raised through insulin reduction so that we can fight, flee or react optimally energetically. This is how it functions in humans and animals. The animal actually fights or flees and consumes the newly available sugar. Civilized human beings don't do the same. Sitting in our cars, we become angry and we only, at most, "flip the bird" or raise a fist - and that's it. No action and no energy consumption. At our desks, it is the same; it is also the same at home in front of the television set. Hyperglycemia is a typical civilization conflict > stress without movement or exercise makes the blood sugar level rise.

- **Overeating:** The energy balance between intake and output does not add up correctly > overweight and hyperglycemia. This is not always the case, as not every overweight person has hyperglycemia; there is a tendency, however.
- **Medications:** Taking many different medications makes a person sympathicotonic and raises the blood sugar levels indirectly. Especially unfavorable are cortisones, catecholamines, antibiotics, etc.
- **Vaccinations:** Conflictive by vaccination process + poisoning.

SBS of the Pancreatic Islet Alpha Cells

Reduced blood sugar (hypoglycemia, hyperinsulinanemia)[1]

The hormone glucagon brings the sugar from the liver into the bloodstream and raises blood sugar levels.

With this SBS, glucagon production is reduced. > The sugar is not retrieved from the liver and therefore does not enter the bloodstream > low blood sugar levels. As opposed to the SBS of the beta cells, this SBS remains largely unrecognized. A low blood sugar level is rightly considered as not requiring treatment.

Conflict	Fear-disgust conflict, towards someone or of something - one experiences something disgusting. Less often, this is a resistance conflict (dependent on "handedness," hormone levels and previous conflicts). Explanation: The female response to adversity is fear and disgust. Traditionally, the male takes the way forward, opting to attack; the female behaves passively at first. The alpha cells are controlled by the left (female) cerebral cortex. Women usually react with fear, disgust or revulsion.
Examples	→ *Somebody feels disgust or revulsion or is seized by sheer horror.* → *"To shudder with horror." "To pull back with disgust." "That's revolting!"* → *Horror of chemotherapy, a putrid wound, a badly injured person or disgust at one's own disfigurement (e.g., following an accident).* → *Fear of certain animals: for example, spiders, beetles, snakes, mice, rats.* → *A cleaning woman has to clean the filthy men's toilets = fear-revulsion conflict. Due to hypoglycemia, she is always hungry and becomes obese.* • *A 53-year-old mother of two grown sons has known her husband since her school days. At 16, she meets the father of her present husband. The encounter is a negative one because the patient finds the man repulsive from the beginning. At the same time, she suffers a territorial-anger conflict affecting the mucosa of the stomach. For years, she suffers from bulimia. Note: bulimia-constellation = fear-revulsion conflict + territorial-anger conflict affecting the mucosa of the stomach (see p. 190f).* (Archive B. Eybl)
Conflict-active	Reduced functioning of the alpha cells (CM's "glucagon insufficiency"), hypoglycemia, ravenous appetite, cold sweat, shivering, pale skin, feeling of walking on air, concentration and consciousness disturbances, possibly headache. With permanent conflict activity: weight problems (constant hunger). Psychological tendency: defensive attitude, one keeps things or people at a distance, compulsive cleanliness (cleaning mania).
Repair phase	Fear, disgust or rejection is overcome > production of glucagon is ramped up > release of sugar from the liver > normalization of blood sugar. Usually a recurring-conflict.
Bio. function	1. Through increased sugar intake (sugar cravings) and the storage of sugar in the liver during the conflict-active phase, the sugar depot is well stocked. This provides a lot of energy for subsequent action (escape or retreat). 2. Loss of consciousness is the most extreme form of passivity ("playing dead"). The individual withdraws itself from reality.
Repair crisis	Brief, sharp drop of the blood sugar level, afterwards, there can be a slow rise in blood sugar.
Questions	When did the symptoms begin? What disgusts me from the time in question until today? (Adverse living conditions, job, being pressured by one's partner)? Which beliefs and conditioning are the cause?
Therapy	Identify the conflict and conditioning and, if possible, resolve them in real life. Find out where the love is, you will find the solution there. In acute cases inject glucagon intravenously. It is better, however, to supply sugar orally (dextrose, fruit juice). See also: remedy for diabetes, next page.

[1] See Dr. Hamer, Charts p. 143

Binge eating disorder (BED)

Same SBS as above. In CM, bouts of binge eating are considered as purely a psychological disorder. Now, we understand the organic background (see above). It is nevertheless true that the binges express an inner deficiency (recognition, love).

Elevated, strongly fluctuating blood sugar (CM's diabetes mellitus type 1 or 2)

Conflict	Fear-disgust conflict of someone or something and at the same time a resistance conflict - to defend oneself against someone or something. = Combination of hyper- and hypoglycemia. Both SBSs described above are active.
Example	• *From an early age, the youngest of three children fully notices the daily quarrels of his parents. The father "explodes" regularly because the mother "irritates" him. At such times, the father sometimes becomes violent = resistance and fear-disgust conflict according to a CT. The, now, 41-year-old is diagnosed with diabetes at the age of 12. Even now, the blood sugar rises sharply when there is an argument between people who are close to one another (= trigger). The patient stubbornly refuses insulin therapy. However, he finds that his wounds heal badly when his sugar is high = indication of the damaging effects of hyperglycemia. In the last two years, he has been able to keep his blood sugar levels between 140 and 100 through weight reduction, physical exercise, and altered diet. The old wounds have healed.* (Archive B. Eybl)
Phase	**Switching of the conflicts and phases.** A combination of both SBSs, depending on which conflict is stronger at a given time, hyper- or hypoglycemia results, fluctuating values due to a "mixing" of the two conflicts.
Therapy	Identify the conflict and conditioning and, if possible, resolve them in real life. See also remedies for diabetes. When all else fails: CM insulin replacement therapy.

ECTO

−+

Adult-onset diabetes mellitus (diabetes mellitus type 2)

• It can come to adult-onset diabetes when the fear-disgust conflict of the alpha cells switches to the other side of the brain due to changes in hormones and activates the relay of the beta cells. (See the map of the cerebral cortex p. 17). A problem of low blood sugar suddenly turns into one of high blood sugar. This also explains why overweight people are consistently diagnosed with adult-onset diabetes. Many overweight people are actually overweight because of constant low blood sugar and the constant hunger they have as a result. The constant hunger is a habit that accompanies the switch and for this reason, diabetes mellitus type 2 can be diagnosed (see p. 222f).

• The second possibility of contracting adult-onset diabetes is when one suffers a resistance conflict at an older age that remains active. > Raised blood sugar levels (see p. 224).

Summary of blood sugar and diabetes

As a rule, diabetes is a persistent, active conflict.
CM claims that diabetes causes vascular damage (retinal vessels, diabetic foot). The fact of the matter is that glucose not reaching tissue is what causes damage. Regardless - in cases of long-term, elevated blood sugar, there is a need for treatment, to lower the glucose levels through conflict resolution, changes in lifestyle and diet or with medication (insulin). The last measure needs to be considered very carefully: The longer one receives insulin therapy, the more dependent one becomes on it - the islet cells' function decreases with time > insulin dependence increases. If insulin therapy is necessary, try to work with as small a dose as possible.

Remedies for diabetes

• Guiding principles: *"Either I do it right or I don't do it at all." "I'll do it my own way and the decision is mine alone." "Stress cannot touch me."*
• The most important remedy is **regular exercise**, preferably moderate endurance sports outdoors. In this way, the biological purpose is fulfilled and the muscle burns sugar. However, if the resistance conflict has to do with sport itself, then sport is not good because it would lead to conflict-activity, which would make the blood sugar go up.

• Avoidance of simple starches such as white flour, sugar etc.
• Biologically complete foods, such as all kinds of beans, lentils, strawberries, oats, potatoes, carrots, Jerusalem artichokes, asparagus, horseradish, Kanne Bread Drink; supplement vitamin D, chromium.
• Cod liver and flaxseed oil, hydrogen peroxide (H_2O_2).
• Cayce: Eat Jerusalem artichoke often (contains insulin).
• Teas: fenugreek, burdock root, elderberry, golden cinquefoil.
• Possibly petroleum-cure, learn deep breathing.

SBS of the Pancreatic Glandular Tissue

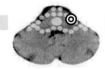

Pancreatic cancer (pancreatic adeno-ca, serous cystademona, acinar cell ca)[1]

According to CM, this is one of the deadliest cancers. This negative prognosis, coupled with CM treatment, leads to the death of the vast majority of patients. This is not necessary.

Conflict	Chunk conflict (see explanations p. 15, 16), a gain or income cannot be realized, inheritance or property conflict, disagreement among family members, fight over money or possessions.
	According to Frauenkron-Hoffmann: Something monstrous has taken place. Outrage/indignation of others about one's own behavior or one's own outrage/indignation about the behavior of others (e.g., caused by a family feud).
Examples	→ *Someone cannot incorporate something that they would like to have.*
	→ *Something is taken away from someone or somebody loses something that means a lot to him.*
	→ *One cannot realize or accept something unexpectedly, often in connection with their family.*
	• *In his book, "Was Gesund Macht" (see bibliography), Johannes F. Mandt describes his battle with pancreatic cancer and the cause of the conflict: "...I had been separated (from his wife) for eight years. In March 2002, I filed for divorce. At the end of October 2002, I received a letter from my wife's lawyer. It contained - among other things - two demands, which completely surprised me. I was caught completely off guard. From that moment on, I could think of nothing other than these new demands. By November, I always had cold hands and feet...the cold was always there, even in bed at night. I lost my appetite." (= Conflict-active phase. Mr. Mandt recovered well from it all).*
	• *The manager of a wellness spa appoints a substitute. Unfortunately, she turns out to be unsuitable. She talks a lot and leaves her work undone. The patient gets angry every time she walks past this woman's workspace = anger conflict with family members. (The manager considers her employees to be her family). On her colleague's last day, the patient says to herself, "Thank God. Tomorrow I won't have to look at her any more." = Conflict resolution and beginning of the repair phase. This is followed by vomiting and chills (repair phase crisis). The patient overcomes it all well, thanks to her knowledge of how everything is connected. (See Gisela Hompesch, Meine Heilung von Krebs durch das Goldene Buch von Dr. Hamer).*
Conflict-active	Increase in function or growth of a cauliflower-like tumor of secretory quality - usually unnoticed. Slight increase in amylase, lipase and CA 19-9, CA 50 and CEA in the blood (see p. 42).
Bio. function	With more pancreatic tissue, more pancreatic enzymes can be produced in order to digest food better. When we do not get something (for example an inheritance) that we had been counting on, nature sees that what we have is better utilized by producing additional cells.
Repair phase	Normalization of function, tubercular, caseating degradation of the tumor, empty spaces (caverns) or calcium deposits can remain in the tissue; pain, fever, night sweats, possibly diarrhea; if no suitable bacteria are present, the tumor is encapsulated with connective tissue and isolated from participating in metabolic functions. Usually a recurring conflict.
Repair crisis	Chills, severe pain
Questions	Which issue could/can I not digest? From what was I unable to extract the benefit I expected? What outraged me? What conditioned me in this direction? (Childhood, the way the parents think, experiences of my ancestors)? Which beliefs enabled this conflict? (E.g., *"I am entitled to my inheritance,"* fanatical righteousness)? What meaning might the diagnosis have for my direction in life? (Reorientation, contemplation about the meaning of life)? Am I ready to make a new start?
Therapy	Identify the conflict and/or trigger(s) and, if possible, resolve them in real life if they are still active. Absolute bed rest, so that the tuberculosis can heal. Surgery if necessary - if the tumor has grown too large - without chemo or radiation of course. Unfortunately, a surgeon rarely dares to operate under these conditions. See also: remedies for the pancreas.

---

1   See Dr. Hamer, Charts p. 23

Inflammation of the pancreas (pancreatitis, exocrine pancreas insufficiency)

Same SBS as above.

Phase	**Recurring-conflict** or persistent repair: excessive degradation of the glandular tissue, under-production of enzymes > digestive problems such as bloating/flatulence, fatty stool and diarrhea due to enzyme deficiency - moderate pain, bloated abdomen.
Therapy	Identify the conflict and/or trigger(s) and, if possible, resolve them in real life if they are still active. Low-fat diet, possibly substitute enzyme with pancreatin or enzyme-rich diet. See also: remedies for the pancreas.

SBS of the Pancreatic Excretory Ducts

Cancer of the pancreatic ducts (pancreatic ductal/intraductal cancer)[1]

Conflict	Territorial-anger conflict or, less often, identity conflict (dependent on "handedness," hormone levels and previous conflicts). One is angry that the boundaries of the territory are disrespected.
Examples	→ *Often, conflict arising either from oneself or from an opponent.* → *Conflict with colleagues or family members, overstepping of the boundaries by the neighbor, arguing over money.* • *Twenty-five years ago, a now 50-year-old manager married a woman who always made it clear to him that he was not the one she actually loved . The woman has always excluded him from the raising of their daughter, now 20 years old. He feels like a 5th wheel = territorial-anger conflict affecting the pancreatic duct > widening of the duct in the active-phase. Two years ago, he divorced his wife. The mother and daughter accused him of having deserted them. Luckily, he soon met another woman, who gave him the love he always longed for. Two months ago, his daughter suddenly approached him. She told him that her relationship with her mother was like a prison for her = conflict resolution > the abdomen swells up and is sensitive to pressure = cancer of the pancreatic duct. One weekend, he is admitted to the hospital because of colicky pains = repair phase crisis. His amylase and lipase levels are far above the norm. His gallbladder is unnecessarily removed. (Archive B. Eybl)*
Conflict-active	Increase in the sensibility of the great pancreatic duct (ductus pancreaticus) or its small branches, simultaneous slackening of the smooth ring musculature. Later, cell degradation (ulcer). Moderate pain.
Bio. function	Through the widening of the pancreatic ducts (= lumen enlargement) the pancreatic fluids can reach the duodenum quicker and easier.
Repair phase	Restoration of the "thinned out" passageways due to increased metabolism = inflammation, repair of the lost substance = inflammation of the pancreas (pancreatitis). Healing swelling can temporarily block the flow > rise in the levels of the pancreatic enzymes (amylase and lipase) in the blood; syndrome aggravates the symptoms. At the end of the repair phase, the ducts open up again > normalization of values, the pancreatic ducts can remain altered by scarring (fibrosis), bulges and/or narrowing and possibly pancreatic stones. Often a recurring-conflict.
Repair crisis	Painful pancreas colic = cramp attack of the duct muscles, chills.
Questions	First, based on the symptoms, determine if the SBS is in the repair phase, is active or recurring. When did the repair symptoms begin? (Usually at the point of conflict resolution). What was I unable to endure before this? Which territorial stress was there? What pressured me? What are the deeper causes of the conflict? (Conditioning in childhood, parents' experiences)? What beliefs/belief systems should I throw overboard?
Therapy	In the case it is recurring: Determine and resolve the conflict, causal conditioning and beliefs. Find out where the love is - there you'll find the solution. Possibly anti-inflammatory or antipyretic medications. See also: remedies for the pancreas below.

---

1   See Dr. Hamer, Charts p. 117

Acute inflammation of the pancreas (pancreatitis)

Possible causes

- **Inflammation of the glandular tissue of the pancreas:** Repair phase: tubercular, caseating degradation of tumor tissue (pancreas tuberculosis), belt-like abdominal pain, swollen, pressure sensitive "rubber belly," flatulence, nausea, vomiting, elevation of the pancreatic enzymes amylase and lipase in the blood and urine, fever, night sweats.
- **Inflammation of the pancreatic ducts:** Repair phase: repair of the squamous epithelium, colicky pain in the repair phase crisis (p. 227).

How to tell the difference

- Strong smelling, possibly stinking night-sweats only with pancre-as-tuberculosis. Due to inflammation of the pancreatic glandular tissue, pain from the beginning to the end of the repair phase.
- In the case of an SBS of the pancreatic duct, pulling pain in the conflict-active phase without signs of inflammation, colicky pains in the repair phase crisis.

Therapy

The conflict is resolved. Support the repair phase, avoid recurrences. Depending on the intensity of the inflammation: painkillers, infusions etc.

Remedies for the Pancreas

- Eat organic food, especially Jerusalem artichoke.
- Teas: mistletoe, centaury, fennel, peppermint.
- Cayce: treatment with dehydrated castor oil.
- Bach flowers: chicory, heather.

- Pancreatin enzyme supplement therapy, if necessary.
- Zeolite powder internally.
- Kanne Bread Drink.
- Cod liver oil.

KIDNEYS AND URETERS

The two bean-shaped kidneys, weighing approximately 120-200 g (4-7 oz) each, lie to the right and left of the spine behind the diaphragm. Their purpose is to filter blood plasma and make urine out of the residue. The kidneys regulate the body's water balance and acid-alkaline balance.

The actual filtering process takes place in the mesodermal kidney parenchyma. The renal cells (glomeruli) create 180-200 l (50 gal) of primary urine a day. Of this, 80-90% is reabsorbed in the renal tubules, which also belong to the kidney parenchyma.

Water is further removed in the endodermal kidney collecting tubules, so that only about 1% of the primary urine remains. This amount, about 1.5 l (3 pt) per day, passes through the ectodermal renal pelvis, the ureter and the bladder (vesica urinaria) before being excreted.

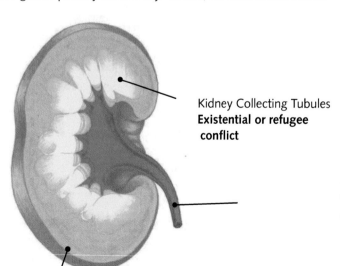

Kidney Collecting Tubules
Existential or refugee conflict

Kidney Parenchyma
Water/liquid conflicts

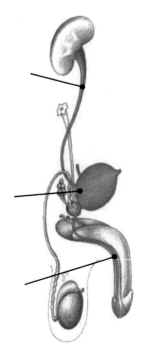

Renal Pelvis/Ureter
Territory-marking conflict

Bladder
Territory-marking conflict

Urethra
Territory-marking conflict

SBS of the Kidney Parenchyma

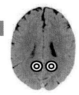

Kidney tumor (Wilms' tumor, nephroblastoma), kidney cavity (kidney cyst)[1]

Conflict	Liquid conflict, conflict due to too much water or liquid, conflict when liquids or water becomes dangerous, "non-swimmer-in-the-sea" conflict.
Examples	• *A man comes home and discovers, to his dismay, that the basement is full of water, because the washing machine's intake hose burst. = Liquid conflict > cell degradation in the parenchyma of the kidneys during the active-phase, restoration or growth of a tumor in the repair phase.* (Archive B. Eybl) • *A woman's beloved cat drowns in the swimming pool. She finds the animal floating lifeless in the water. = Liquid conflict. Three years later, a nephroblastoma is discovered by chance. She is advised to have chemotherapy at once. The woman dies.* (Archive B. Eybl) • *A woman suffers from severe incontinence = too-much-liquid conflict.* (Archive B. Eybl) • *A woman, now 40+, is five years old when she suffers a liquid conflict while playing with other children on the bank of a river. Suddenly, she slips into the water and is carried away by the current. Fortunately, an older playmate pulls her onto land again, but she remembers those terrible moments to this day. In the active-phase, a "hole" forms in her kidney; in the subsequent repair phase, a 10 cm (3 in) cyst forms, which hadn't caused her any problems for 40 years. Note: the patient is "sensitized" to the liquid conflict, because as an unborn child she came into danger in high water "with her mother." Since the water had already flooded the whole lower floor of the house, the pregnant mother had to flee to the attic = liquid conflict.* (See Claudio Trupiano, thanks to Dr. Hamer, p. 420)
Conflict-active	Cell degradation (necrosis) in one or more places > loss of kidney parenchymal (basic) tissue > in order that the filtering function continues unchanged, the organism raises the blood pressure = "compensatory hypertonia." The necroses are otherwise not noticed.
Repair phase	Out of the holes resulting from cell destruction, one or more fluid-filled kidney cysts develop (CM: "polycystic nephropathy" or "renal dysplasia"). In the course of time, the cysts are gradually filled out with functional kidney tissue. After nine months, an "additional" kidney has formed, with its own arteries and veins, etc. Connections to the neighboring organs (CM = "invasive growth"), having been necessary for the cyst's own blood supply, dissolve when the cyst's own circulatory connection is complete. In this "additional kidney," blood is filtered just like in the rest of the parenchymal tissue. The increased blood pressure is then superfluous > normalization of the blood pressure toward the end of the repair phase.
Bio. function	Increase in the filtering and urine-making capacity; in the future, an excess of water can be handled better (luxury group).
Note	There is no need to differentiate between the mother/child and partner side. "Handedness" is immaterial.
Questions	Determine the phase based on the symptoms (blood pressure, ultrasound, x-rays, general indicators). Which stress was experienced with water or other liquids? (Seaside vacation, water sports, kitchen/bath or work accident, sympathy with drowning victim(s))? What has conditioned me with regard to water? (E.g., childhood experiences - shoved into water, ancestors)? How could I come to terms with/reconcile this conditioning? How can I change the situation in real life?
Therapy	The conflict is resolved. No measures need to be taken, except to prevent recurrences. If the nephroblastoma is so large that it disturbs other organs, surgery is recommended - preferably after nine months, so that the tumor has had time to form its own circulatory system and has detached from its neighboring organs. In the case of complications due to lack of space, one should only continue to "wait it out" if they are absolutely sure that the conflict has been permanently resolved.

---

1   See Dr. Hamer, Charts pp. 69, 81

SBS of the Kidney Collecting Tubules

Fluid retention in the body, uremia, cancer of the kidney-collecting tubules (adeno-ca)[1]

At a certain moments, every SBS is important, but if we had to name the most important SBS, then this is the one. The significance of these little kidney tubules extends far beyond the kidneys themselves. All of the body's other SBS are negatively influenced by an active SBS of the kidney collecting tubules and this is very important when it comes to therapy.

The repair phase of any SBS worsens if a kidney collecting tubules SBS is conflict-active, because of the increased accumulation of fluids. For instance, a repair phase crisis of the heart - a heart attack - can have dramatic consequences. In the case of a bone SBS (e.g., of the spine), this can lead to excruciating pain. In the brain too, the pressure can become problematic if the healing Hamer focus is "pumped up" due to an active kidney collecting tubules SBS.

The term "**syndrome:**" Dr. Hamer came to call the simultaneous existence of an active kidney collecting tubules SBS along with another SBS in the repair phase a "syndrome." For instance, lower back pain (= repair phase of a central self-esteem conflict) + active kidney collecting tubules SBS = severe lower back pain, possibly a slipped disk.
When it comes to therapy for any syndrome, the resolution of the refugee conflict takes absolute priority.

Conflict	Existential or refugee conflict (e.g., losing one's home), having too little water, conflict of feeling abandoned or isolated. One feels like they have been left with no resources, abandoned, defenceless or forsaken. Usually a chronic, persistent conflict as a result of conditioning (childhood, family).
Examples	• *A woman is checked into the hospital. Nobody really has time for her. The doctors hardly check on her = refugee conflict. Note: This occurs frequently when a person goes to the hospital > growth of a tumor of the kidney collecting tubules in the active-phase, tubercular degradation in the repair phase.* (Archive B. Eybl)
	• *A man is told he has cancer of the prostate gland = existential conflict.* (Archive B. Eybl)
	• *A 15-year-old girl is placed in a boarding school against her will. The parents mean well - they want to put an end to her poor school performance. However, the girl feels terribly abandoned in the strange surroundings = refugee conflict. During this year, she becomes overweight.* (Archive B. Eybl)
	• *A 10-year-old boy has to move 700 miles away with his parents. He misses his friends and the familiar surroundings; he feels abandoned. At his new school, things go badly as well. Within two months, he becomes fat. Although he drinks a lot, he urinates only 2-3 times a day. Whenever he visits his old friends during vacation, he urinates more often and loses weight every time.* (See gnm-forum.eu).
	• *Somebody has an outstanding loan from the bank. Due to a loss of collateral, the bank accelerates the loan repayment = existential conflict - conflict of not being "liquid."* (Archive B. Eybl)
	• *A 41-year-old patient feels unloved by his mother. It begins at birth: For her third child, she wants a girl. A girl's name had been picked out and she is disappointed when a boy is born (and to make matters worse, with red hair). His hair is shaved by his mother three times. She hopes that brown hair will grow in its place. The patient explains that he never felt loved or cared for by his parents because of their constant fighting, only by his father later on = refugee conflict. Over the years, he gains up to 110 kg (240 lbs), and then, he loses weight again. He sometimes sweats at night due to repair phases.* (Archive B. Eybl)
	• *An older cat from the animal shelter has found a nice new home. When a second cat is taken in by the family, the older cat believes she will be abandoned again. Within a short time, she gains half a kilo (1 lb) = existential conflict.* (Archive B. Eybl)
	• *A 58-year-old mother of two finds out that her husband is being unfaithful and files for divorce. Within a year, she gains 10 kilograms = active refugee conflict.* (Archive B. Eybl)
Conflict-active	Increase in function; growth of a cauliflower-like adeno-ca of secretory quality or a flat-growing adeno-ca of absorptive quality (CM: "kidney cell cancer"); additional fluid retention > water, urine and other materials are retained by the body instead of being eliminated. In "good times" these materials would be discarded; however, during an existential conflict ("bad times") they are "recycled" when possible

---

[1] See Dr. Hamer, Charts p. 25

> raised uric acid and creatinine levels > decreased urine volume and high concentration (dark urine).

The body can eliminate all of the waste products normally destined for the urine with up to 150-200 ml (5-7 oz) of urine per day (oliguria, anuria). The creatinine value then climbs to 12-14 mg/dl (CM: "uremia"). One or both kidneys can be affected, each with three renal calyx levels. A creatinine value of 12 mg/dl indicates that both kidneys are affected. Until the creatinine reaches this value, performing dialysis does not make sense according to the 5 Biological Laws of Nature. CM: often begins dialysis at 4 mg/dl.

In summary: The most important diagnostic indications for an active kidney collecting tubules SBS: fluid retention in the body (for instance: under the eyes in the morning, swollen knuckles, creatinine and urea or uric acid is (usually but not always) increased in the blood), inexplicable weight gain (acute conflict-active) or being overweight (chronic conflict-active), soft, rounded body shape. Sometimes, however, thin people are also affected.

Endomorphs, craven people, collectors and people with messy tendencies, bargain shoppers, profit-oriented and possessive people, stockpilers (e.g., of food, money) and people who tend to cling or like sitting.

Bio. function	Retaining water and urea and other valuable substances, so that the individual can survive longer during a life-and-death emergency, when abandoned or when fleeing (seeking refuge).
Repair phase	Decrease or normalization of function. When preceded by long-lasting conflict activity: caseating, necrotizing degradation of the tumor = kidney tuberculosis, inflammation of the kidneys (nephritis) > increased elimination of fluids, drop in creatinine values, blood in the urine (hematuria), protein in the urine (proteinuria), heavy nighttime sweating, fever. If no fungi or bacteria are present, the renal pelvic outlets can become blocked (CM: "silent kidney"), despite conflict resolution.
Repair crisis	Chills, severe kidney pain
Note	There has always been a certain correlation between the moon and fluids. People with active kidney collecting tubules SBS "perceive" the moon more intensely than others > increased fluid collection by waxing moon and full moon. Changes in the weather (just before precipitation) are also felt more intensely. Following recurrences, one can find heavily clumped renal calices ("medullary sponge kidney," "sponge kidney") or calcium deposits in the kidney collecting tubules (CM: "nephro-calcinosis").
Questions	Symptoms (weight gain, creatinine, etc.) since when? What happened? (Left by partner, death, fight, loss of employment, moving house, money problems, pain, worries about children)? There must be a conflict to be found here. However, the original conflict or the conditioning often took place much earlier. What conditioned me in this regard during my childhood? (Too little parental affection, deprivation, divorce, moving house, death of a family member)? Is this SBS also currently running in a parent? (Yes > work out the conditioning in the family: What did the ancestors experience)? The ancestors' experiences should be equated with one's own. How far back in the family tree does the conditioning reach? Questions for the grandparents: these conversations are enlightening, but also a part of the therapy - especially when one is searching for the love. With which meditation(s) could I help the family and myself? Which new thoughts should become my daily companions?
Therapy	• **For nearly every illness, resolving an SBS of the kidney collecting tubules is the most important task.** • Determine the conflict, conditioning and beliefs and, if possible, resolve them in real life if still active. • Guiding principles: *"I am provided for." "I am sheltered and secure." "Even when I feel that I am all alone, there is always somebody there." "God protects me."* • Salt baths with at least 0.9% salt (the sea - our original home). A concentration of 0.9% salt is called the "physiological salt solution" because this is the concentration in blood plasma. Salt baths of over 0.9% are also good because they draw more water out of the body, which is the goal of the treatment. > Add about 2 kg (4-5 lbs) to a full bath tub. Cheaper variation: saltwater wraps. • Water treatments of all kinds, for example: sea vacations, thermal baths. • Regular sweating, sauna, infrared cabin, steam baths, or sweat-generating (aerobic) sports. • Drink enough clean and vital/structured water. Amount: follow your instincts. • No cortisone, that makes the kidney collecting tubules more sympathicotonic, which leads to even more water collection and a worsening of the symptoms (full moon face). • Make sure your home is cozy and comforting (nice furniture).

- Wool underwear, soft comfy bed, possibly with wool padding.
- Eat unrefined salt with your food, but do not salt too much.
- Alkaline diet, no pork (binds water).
- Lymph drainage massages to promote the elimination of water.
- Colloidal silver internally: silver, the moon and the kidneys resonate with one another.
- Therapy according to Professor Kopp: Professor Kopp accidentally administered an overdose of sodium bicarbonate to a patient who was critically ill with acute kidney failure. To his surprise, the patient's condition improved significantly, although she had hardly been given a chance of survival. In the following years, Prof. Kopp (b. 1935) was able to save over 300 patients from dialysis, with the help of his sodium bicarbonate therapy. The therapy is based on the pH-value of the urine.
  Step 1 - Measure the pH of the urine. Several times a day, hold a testing strip in the urine flow. For this, I use Uralyt-U from Madaus. The ideal biochemical milieu for kidney elimination is a urine pH-value of 6.5 - 7.5. Thus, this is the goal for the kidney collecting tubules SBS patient.
  Step 2 - Therapy: Take as many tablets of sodium bicarbonate as needed to reach the goal. Begin with 3 tablets of 1 g daily; afterwards, the dosage is raised or lowered according to the urine's pH-value. According to Dr. Kopp, if this does not bring about the desired water loss, one can also consume a diuretic, such as Lasix (available by prescription only). Along with the dose of sodium bicarbonate (with regular checking of the urine's pH-value), the diuretic remains effective - even when taken for years. Nonetheless, it is important to regularly check the blood's potassium level.
  Contraindications are metabolic and respiratory alkalosis and cardiopulmonary insufficiency.

Inflammation of the renal corpuscles ("nephrotic syndrome," "glomerulonephritis," "IgA nephropathy"), multiple spaces (cystic kidney)

Same SBS as above (see p. 230ff). The primary symptom for the conventional diagnosis is an excess of protein in the urine (proteinuria) or a protein deficit in the urine (hypoproteinuria) and fluid collection (edema). It is said that with the so-called nephrotic syndrome, there is too little protein in the blood because the kidney's cell filtering apparatus is defective.

According to CM, this is why there is protein in the urine. In fact, this "illness" is not an inflammation of the renal corpuscles but an inflammation, (i.e., the repair phase) of the kidney collecting tubules SBS.

Phase	Repair phase or **persistent repair**: when the illness is chronic, there are repeating tubercular degradation phases - lots of small empty spaces in the kidneys (cystic kidney).
Note	Protein in the urine: During the repair phase, the kidney collecting tubules tumor is broken down . The protein removed is washed out in the urine through the bladder and ureter > protein in the urine (proteinuria).
	Too little protein in the blood: If the conflict comes back, the cell buildup and cell degradation phases in the kidney collecting tubules alternate. During tumor buildup, the body takes in protein (mainly albumin) from the blood. In the repair phase, it eliminates this tumor-protein again. Night sweats contains large amounts of protein > sinking of the blood protein levels (hypoproteinemia) > lower blood protein levels promote edema in the body due to a lessening of the colloid osmotic pressure.
Therapy	Determine the conflict and conditioning and if possibly resolve them in real life. Questions: see previous page. Protein-rich diet and, if necessary, albumin infusions. The CM treatment, with drugs that lower the blood pressure, immunosuppressive drugs and cortisone, is not recommended. See also above.

Acute kidney failure, shock kidney (acute ischemic tubulopathy)

Same SBS as above. (See p. 230ff)

Phase	**Sudden strong existential conflict**: extreme water and urea storage > strong rise in creatinine and urea values, very little urine (oliguria or anuria).
Note	Usually caused by extreme pain, diagnostic shock or forced admission to a hospital.
Therapy	Identify the conflict and conditioning and, if possible, resolve them in real life. For measures, see above, especially Prof. Kopp's therapy.

SBS of the Renal Pelvis

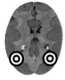

Inflammation of the renal pelvis (pyelonephritis), cancer of the renal pelvis[1]

E C T O

− +

Conflict	Territorial-marking conflict. The territorial borders are not being respected, one cannot mark them. Explanation: Not being able to distance oneself from someone/thing or delineate one's territory. Not knowing where one's territory (place) is. Not having the confidence to make a decision or not being allowed to make a decision oneself.

In nature, the male wolves mark the outer and the females mark the inner borders of the territory. With men, it is usually about the "outer" territory (the job, car, club, etc.). With women, it is usually about the "inner" territory (partner, child, friend, home, etc.).

In *Lexikon der Neuen Medizin*, Horst Köhler points out that the woman's most intimate territory is her own body. Gynecological examinations, involuntary or "tolerated" sexual intercourse could be one reason why women suffer from urinary illnesses more often than men. The right renal pelvis or ureter > "feminine" side = conflict of not being able to mark the inner territory. The left renal pelvis or ureter > "masculine" side = conflict of not being able to mark the outer territory.

Examples	→ *Not knowing where one should draw the line, not knowing how to define oneself.*

→ *A child doesn't have his own room.*

• *A woman is cheated on by her husband = territorial-marking conflict > unnoticed cell degradation in the renal pelvis. As she finally decides to leave him, she comes into the repair phase > restoration of the squamous epithelium of the renal pelvis = pyelonephritis.* (Archive B. Eybl)

• *A woman marries into a family in which she does not feel right. She doesn't know where her place is. She no longer has her "own realm" = territorial-marking conflict.* (Archive B. Eybl)

• *A salesman has a part of his sales area taken away, because he is not making enough sales = territorial-marking conflict.* (Archive B. Eybl)

Conflict-active	Degradation (ulcer) of the mucosa in the renal pelvis, renal calyxes or ureter (urothelium). Increased urge to urinate. No pain; therefore, usually unnoticed.
Bio. function	Through the relaxed ring musculature, the cross-section increases. > Improved elimination of urine so that the territory can be marked better.
Repair phase	Restoration of the urothelium, inflammation of the renal pelvis (possibly "cancer" of the renal pelvis as defined by CM), swelling, and blood in the urine (hematuria). With syndrome, the flow of urine can be impeded by repair swelling.
Repair crisis	Cramps, kidney colic, severe pain, chills, blood in the urine; during the colic (contractions of the ureter muscles) kidney gravel or calyx stones are pressed through the neck of the renal calyx into the renal pelvis or through the ureter, if they are present.
Questions	Inflammation/pain since when? (Conflict resolution shortly before) Which territory was I unable to mark before? Did someone overstep the boundaries? (Partner, family member, place of employment, superior)? Was I unable to bring someone into my territory? (With women, this usually concerns their partner). Was my "No!" ignored/overruled? Why do I react so sensitively? (Determine the precise conditioning). Do I react similarly to my ancestors? Which new attitude could help?
Therapy	The conflict is resolved. Support the healing. If it returns, identify the conflict and/or trigger(s) and resolve them. Guiding principle (if recurring): "*I have decided. Now I know what I want.*" "*My territory is my realm.*" "*I define the borders and they will be respected.*" Teas: sage, cranberry leaves, rose hip, lovage, horsetail. Colloidal silver internally. Drink a lot, e.g., natural beer. Antibiotics if necessary, if the repair phase is too intense. See also: remedies for the kidneys p. 235.

---

1 See Dr. Hamer, Charts pp. 117, 130

E
C
T
O

Enlargement of the renal pelvis, sacculated kidney (pyelectasis, hydronephrosis)

Same SBS as above.

−+

Phase	**Persistent repair:** Enlargement of the renal pelvis or the ureter, usually in connection with kidney stones > necrosis of the parenchymal tissue of the kidneys (narrowed parenchyma-seam) caused by blocked urine flow.
Therapy	Identify the conflict and conditioning and, if possible, resolve them in real life, so that the persistent repair can come to an end. Questions: see previous page. See also: remedies for the kidneys next page.

SBS of the Kidney Arteries

N
E
W

M
E
S
O

Renal artery stenosis (increased blood pressure from narrowed kidney arteries)

The narrowing of the main vessels leading to the kidneys means less blood reaches the kidneys. > Erroneously, the blood pressure receptors in the kidneys register low blood pressure > impulse to increase blood pressure (RAS) > increase in blood pressure (possibly acute), dizziness, morning headaches, possible lung edemas (shortness of breath).

−+

Conflict	According to Dr. Sabbah: One is boiling with anger on the inside and can't let off the steam.
Phase	**Recurring-conflict.** Alternating phases of depletion and restoration of the renal arteries results in the formation of a fatty-protein material > CM: "renal arterial sclerosis/stenosis."
Bio. function	Strengthening of the renal arteries. Persistent conflict and the resulting narrowing of the arteries doesn't make any biological sense - nature is always assuming that conflicts will be resolved quickly.
Questions	Why am I angry? Why don't I let it out? Which conditioning is responsible?
Therapy	Determine and resolve the conflict, causal conditioning and beliefs. OP if necessary.

Kidney stones (nephroliths), kidney gravel

Possible causes

- **Kidney collecting tubules** - Recurring refugee conflict: calcium oxalate stones and/or gravel as mineral deposits from tubercular caseation = the most common kind of kidney stones.
- **Ureter and/or mucosa of the renal pelvis** - Recurring territorial-marking conflict: uric acid stones and other stone types; healing swelling of the ureter > occlusion or flow blockage > damming of urine leading to sediment deposits and the forma-

tion of stones. In the course of a repair phase crisis, the stones are forced out through the ureter or urethra.

Therapy
Identify the conflict and/or trigger(s) so that no new stones form. Dissolution by "Lithosol" (minerals, by prescription). If necessary, surgical stone removal or lithotripsy. Drink sufficient, pure, "soft" water. See also: remedies for the kidneys next page.

Cirrhotic kidney

Possible causes

- **Kidney parenchyma:** Recurring (= persistent) liquid conflict. Demise of the basic tissue of the kidney - converts to connective tissue (fibrosis). > Reactionary increase in blood pressure due to lack of filter surface.

- **Kidney collecting tubules** - Recurring refugee conflict - nephrotic syndrome > scarred shrinkage.
- **Renal pelvis** - Recurring territorial-marking conflict > chronic inflammation of the renal pelvis > scarred shrinkage.

Kidney poisoning (acute toxic tubulopathy)

This is not a conflict; rather, it is a poisoning by chemicals, metals (e.g., aluminum, mercury and other metals e.g., in vaccinations, chemtrails) and/or medications (antibiotics, painkillers, antirheumatics, antihypertensives, contrast agents, chemotherapeutic

drugs, etc.). > Damage to the renal cells and tubules.

Therapy
Eliminate exposure to toxic substances. Also, see remedies for the kidneys - next page.

Remedies for the kidneys

- Renal colic: warmth, physical exercise, muscle relaxing agents, painkillers; drink sufficient pure, "soft" water.
- Food: alkaline diet, especially celery, carrots, cucumbers, squash, asparagus, strawberries, beans.
- Teas: nettle, goldenrod, birch leaf, fennel, speedwell, raspberry leaves, elderberry, lady's bedstraw, agrimony.
- Juniper berry treatment according to Kneipp: Begin with four berries per day; afterwards, for nine days, take one more each day. Then go back to four.
- Hildegard: elixir of absinthe, fennel mixed powder.

- Massage the kidney area with camphor oil; reflex, zone massage.
- Hot baths, sauna treatments.
- Always be sure to keep the feet warm; possibly hot foot baths.
- Natural borax.
- MMS (the better antibiotic) for chronic conditions.
- Kanne Bread Drink, zeolite powder internally.
- The best time for kidney treatments: 5 to 7 p.m.

BLADDER AND URETHRA

The bladder (vesica urinaria) as a hollow organ composed of smooth muscle. (According to Dr. Hamer, striated). The bladder collects the urine produced in the kidneys via both ureter and stores it until it is emptied over the urethra. The greater part of the bladder is lined with ectodermal tissue, so-called urothelium (transitional cells). Below it lies the endodermal bladder mucousa. The one exception: in the "bladder triangle" (Trigonum vesicae), a small island of endodermal mucosa protrudes from beneath the urothelium.

The bladder has two sphincter muscles at its transition to the urethra: the inner one (M. sphincter urethrae) is smooth and involuntary and the outer one (M. sphincter vesicae) is striated and voluntary.
The discharge of urine is proceeds in the form of a repair phase crisis of the bladder muscles. (The repair phase crisis as a functional building block of nature.)

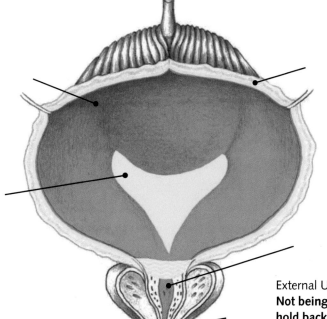

Superficial Bladder Mucosa
Territory-marking conflict

Deep-Lying Bladder Mucosa, Trigone
Hardly digestible, ugly situation

Bladder Musculature
Can't expel the urine

Internal Urethral Sphincter
Not being able to hold back the urine/chunk

External Urethral Sphincter
Not being able to hold back the urine

SBS of the Bladder Mucosa

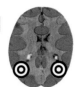

Inflammation of the bladder (urocystitis), cancer of the transitional epithelium of the bladder (urothelium cancer, urothelium papilloma, inverted papilloma)[1]

E C T O

− +

Conflict	Territory marking conflict; the borders of the territory are not respected, one is not able to mark the borders of the territory. Conflict explained under renal pelvis SBS, p. 233 (with more examples).
Examples	• *A patient can perfectly remember one of the most horrible experiences of her youth: She is 13 years old and her father, whom she describes as a "tyrant and sadist," deliberately kills her beloved rabbit for no reason. She wanted to "go crazy." Her father also overstepped her boundaries in other situations as well. She cannot defend her boundaries or mark them = territory-marking conflict. In the repair phase, she contracts an inflammation of the bladder. Since then, whenever she is nervous, she suffers from an urgent need to empty her bladder (= irritable bladder).* (Archive B. Eybl)
	• *One evening, the mother storms into her daughter's bedroom because she is "endlessly" talking on the telephone. The daughter cannot believe that her mother shamelessly barged into her "space" > cell degradation in the mucosa of the bladder, restoration in the repair phase. She repeatedly gets a "bladder infection" (= repair phase) when her mother interferes in her life = trigger.* (See www.germanische-heilkunde.at/index.php/erfahrungsberichte).
	→ *Term "honeymoon cystitis" (cystitis during their honeymoon). Conflict resolution of a female territorial-marking conflict by the exhilaration from their time together.*
Conflict-active	Decrease in sensibility of the bladder's mucosa, the ureter or urethra. Simultaneous slackening of the bladder's ring and/or sphincter muscles respectively. Later, cell degradation (ulcer). No pain, no bleeding. The need to distance oneself; one pays strict attention to the territorial boundaries, is irritated, hypersensitive.
Bio. function	With relaxed ring and/or sphincter muscles, the territory can be marked extensively.
Repair phase	Restoration of the mucosa = inflammation of the bladder, ureter, or urethra = bladder ca (urothelium ca), swelling of the mucous membrane, pain, burning sensation by urination, frequent urge to urinate (pollakiuria), possibly blood in the urine (hematuria) and occasional loss of urine. Due to the healing-swelling, the flow can be blocked, especially with syndrome > urinary retention, incomplete emptying of the bladder.
Repair crisis	Pain, blood in the urine, bladder cramps caused by the involvement of the bladder muscles; possibly chills, absence seizures.
Note	90% of bladder tumors are urothelium ca. Chronic bladder infection, recurring-conflict > scarred thickening of the mucosa (urothelium metaplasia) > "irritable bladder."
Therapy	Questions: see SBS of the renal pelvis p. 233. In the case of an individual bladder infection: The conflict is resolved. Support the repair phase. If recurring, identify the conflict, trigger(s), conditioning and resolve them. Guiding principles (if recurring): *"I know what I want." "My space is my space." "I define the borders and they will be respected."* For bladder remedies, see below.

Bed wetting (Enuresis nocturna)

Same SBS.

Conflict	Territory-marking conflict: No space of one's own (room). Neglect of the child's needs. May indicate sexual abuse in extreme cases. Sometimes also the opposite situation: the territorial borders are lacking (anti-authoritarian upbringing). Since the child doesn't have any territory, they mark the only territory available - their bed.
Examples	→ Birth of a sibling (perceived neglect).

---

1   See Dr. Hamer, Charts pp. 117, 130

E C T O

−+

→ Divorce of the parents, moving house.

→ No room of their own.

Phase	**Repair phase crisis**: Participation of the bladder musculature.
Questions	Is the child reflecting something for the parents? Mother/father under pressure? (Fighting in the relationship, divorce, overwhelming work environments, financial pressure)? Does the child have their own space? (Room, preschool)? Conflict/jealousy due to siblings? Do they long for attention?
Therapy	Determine and resolve the conflict, trigger(s) and conditioning.

SBS of the Bladder - Trigon Mucosa

Purulent bladder infection, bladder cancer (adeno-ca)[1]

E N D O

+−

Conflict	Hardly digestible, ugly situation.
Examples	• *A 45-year-old human resources manager of a company is informed, in front of her whole team, that from now on, she will be an assistant in the HR office and her office, which was "her living room," will be given to the new manager. Years later, the patient is still talking about this outrage. Shortly afterwards, she is diagnosed with bladder cancer, which is then abraded. However, it keeps coming back because she cannot overcome what happened. (Archive of Antje Scherret)*
	• *A civil servant is promised he will be appointed as the head of his agency within a year. He is preparing himself for this; however, he is suddenly confronted with the fact that a colleague, who he absolutely cannot stand, will get the post = hardly digestible, ugly situation > cell division in the deep-lying mucosa of the bladder in the active-phase, purulent bladder inflammation in the repair phase. (Archive B. Eybl)*
Tissue	Bladder - trigon mucosa - brainstem - endoderm; usually the "bladder triangle" (the region between the mouths of the ureters and the outflow of the urethra) is affected and also the regions under the superficial urothelium mucosa (submucosa). Approximately 10% of bladder tumors are of this type.
Conflict-active	Increase in function, growth of a cauliflower-like tumor of secretory quality or a flat-growing tumor of absorptive quality = endodermal bladder cancer.
Bio. function	Secretory type: "digestion" of the outrage; absorptive type: absorption of urine analog to the kidney collecting tubules SBS "absorption" of the ugly situation.
Repair phase	Degradation of the tumor = purulent bladder infection, pus, blood in the urine, pain, night sweats.
Repair crisis	Chills, severe pain, blood in the urine.
Questions	Which ugly situation was I unable to tolerate? (Conflict, betrayal, disappointment, deceit in a partnership, at the workplace, between family members)? Why am I still preoccupied by this matter? What from my childhood reminds me of the issue? What has conditioned me additionally? Do my parents act in the same way? Which beliefs should I get rid of? (E.g., too many expectations)? Which new inner attitude would help? (E.g., total forgiveness, see the good in those involved).
Therapy	With inflammation: the conflict is resolved. Support the healing process. Colloidal silver internally.
	Tumor without inflammation: Identify the conflict, triggers and conditioning and resolve them in real life if necessary. MMS (the better antibiotic) in chronic cases. Surgery, if the tumor is too large. See also: remedies for the bladder p. 240.

---

1   See Dr. Hamer, Charts p. 29

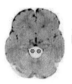

SBS of the Bladder - Smooth Muscles HFs in the midbrain - topography still unknown

Irritable/overactive bladder, imperative urinary incontinence

Constant urge to urinate, frequent urination with only small amounts of urine, is called an overactive bladder.

Conflict	A person's borders are not respected by others because they have not marked them clearly. One feels or puts themselves under pressure. One is unsure and easily influenced regarding one's own decisions.
Examples	• *A man must share an apartment with his son and his son's family. He doesn't like the situation and suffers greatly. Just to get to his own room, he has to walk through the others' living area. The man starts suffering from "irritable bladder," a conflict of not being able to mark his territory clearly. He wants to mark it, but cannot because he doesn't want to upset the family. (Archive B. Eybl)*
	• *A 64-year-old, divorced retiree has to get up seven or more times in the night and then urinates only small amounts of urine. The doctors tell him his prostate is fine. Conflict: following his failed marriage, the patient cannot bear to think about marrying for a second time. However, his girlfriend of many years wants to marry = territorial-marking conflict affecting the involuntary bladder muscu-lature. Often, when she comes home from work in the evening, she starts with the same unpleasant topic = recurrence. The evenings and nights at home have become "triggers" for the patient. Con-flict activity in the evenings and nights; thus, he has massive sleep disturbances. During vacations, the problem is reduced. (Archive B. Eybl)*
	• *An 8-year-old girl has to share her room with her sister. After a big fight over the toys, she wets the bed. = Territorial-boundary conflict. (Archive B. Eybl)*
Conflict-active	Heightened tension (hypertonia) of the bladder muscle, muscle thickening (hypertrophy) = so-called irritable bladder.
Bio. function	Strengthening of the bladder muscle so that the urine can be eliminated in a stronger stream in order to better mark one's territory.
Repair phase	Normalization of tension; the muscle remains thickened.
Repair crisis	Tonic-clonic bladder cramps, immediate urge to empty the bladder, "imperative."
Note	The symptoms are much like those of a recurring inflammation of the bladder's mucous membrane. The two are difficult to tell apart - they are possibly connected. The conflict contents are similar as well.
Questions	Imperative during which situations? (Indication of the trigger). Why do I allow myself to be put under pressure? Which personality structure makes this possible? Do I want to have good relations with every-one at any price? How do I deal with authority? Do I feel weak in comparison? What conditioned me? (Childhood, pregnancy, parental style, ancestors)? Which new attitude do I want to cultivate?
Therapy	Identify the conflict and conditioning and resolve them, so that the tension in the bladder lets up. Guiding principles: *"I make my decisions with confidence." "I won't let myself be put under pressure."* With children, create visible and practical solutions! See also: remedies for the bladder p. 240. Pelvic floor training, pubococcygeus muscle training - practice voluntary tensing up and relaxing.

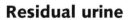

SBS of the Inner Bladder Sphincter

Residual urine

Conflict	Not being able to sufficiently hold back one's urine.
Examples	➜ *Occurs frequently after prostate surgeries.*
	• *Eight years ago, a now 64-year-old patient was still not familiar with the 5 Biological Laws of Nature and agreed to prostate surgery. Since then, he is impotent and incontinent. When he carries some-thing heavy, a few drops always spill into his pants = conflict of not being to hold back one's urine > strengthening of the inner sphincter muscle of the bladder. Years of conflict activity have made his urine stream weak, and he always has to press. (Archive B. Eybl)*

- *A patient, now 62-years-old, remembers his terrible experience as a three-year-old, as if it was yesterday: his very dominant mother goes shopping, leaving him at home alone. Before going out she threatens the boy: "You'd better not wet your pants, while I'm gone." As the child's urge to urinate becomes greater, he hops about, constantly losing urine and dreading the consequences > increased tension in the inner sphincter muscles. Since then he must always be alone to urinate and always has residual urine.* (Archive B. Eybl)

E
N
D
O

+ −

Conflict-active	Increased muscle tension (hypertonia), problems when urinating, weak stream, residual urine because the inner sphincter muscle does not open completely. Usually a recurring-conflict.
Bio. function	Strengthening of the inner sphincter so that the urine can be withheld better.
Repair phase	Normalization of muscle tension; in the repair phase crisis, periods of incontinence and cramps.
Questions	First, determine if the symptoms come from the prostate. If no: residual urine since when? (OP, anesthesia, accident, embarrassing situation)? Substitution conflict? (Sympathy with others)? Which conditioning could play a role? (Parents, birth, pregnancy, early childhood)? Which thought(s) give relief? Which traditional belief do I want to throw overboard?
Therapy	Determine and resolve the conflict and conditioning in real life. Pelvic floor training, pubococcygeus muscle training - tensing up and relaxing exercises.

SBS of the External Bladder Sphincter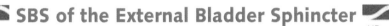

HFs motor function in top of cerebral cortex

Urine loss - stress incontinence

E
C
T
O

− +

Conflict	Self-esteem conflict of wanting or not being able to retain the urine (special territory marking conflict).
Examples	➜ *An elderly woman contracts a bladder infection and cannot control her urge to urinate = self-esteem conflict: "Now I am probably incontinent."* ➜ *A man doesn't dare to put his mother-in-law in her place because he is afraid of causing a family argument > he wants to "draw the line" but cannot for family reasons = self-esteem conflict.*
Conflict-active	Degradation of cells or limited innervation of the external bladder sphincter > the urine cannot be fully retained voluntarily = "weak bladder," stress incontinence. Loss of a small amount of urine when lifting, coughing, sneezing, laughing, etc. Usually a recurring-conflict.
Repair phase	Restoration (sphincter-hyperplasia) > recovery of innervation, possibly residual urine.
Repair crisis	Loss of urine because the sphincter muscle opens in an uncoordinated manner > incontinence.
Bio. function	Strengthening of the external sphincter muscle so that the urine can be retained better.
Note	During old age, this can also occur without a conflict: diminishing physical and muscular tension can lead to a slackening of the sphincter apparatus.
Therapy	Identify the conflict, conditioning and resolve them in real life. Exercises for the pelvic floor and for breathing; buildup of body tension, regulate body weight. If necessary, bladder ligament or bladder lift surgery. (See also p. 236)

Residual urine - other possible causes

- **Prostate excretory ducts or prostate gland** in healing: Swelling of the prostate excretory ducts is causing a backup in the bladder. This is probably the most common cause of residual urine in men. (See p. 258ff)
- **Urethritis:** Temporary residual urine for the duration of the inflammation: the urethral squamous epithelium swells up, resulting in obstruction and residual urine. (See p. 236f)
- **External bladder sphincter** in persistent repair: high tension in the bladder sphincter during the repair phase > residual urine (see stress incontinence above).

Bladder stones, urinary stones

- **"Primary urinary stones"** form in the bladder. Here, either SBS is possible (see p. 236 and 237).
- **"Secondary urinary stones"** come from the kidneys and are triggered either by an SBS of the kidney collecting tubules or an SBS of the renal pelvis (see p. 230ff and 233f).

Therapy:
Identify the conflict, trigger(s) and conditioning, so that no new stones appear. Drink enough fluids, "soft" water if possible and eat low-protein foods. If necessary, surgical removal of the stones.

Bladder remedies

- Teas: sage (also recommended by Hildegard), fennel, club moss, chamomile, horsetail, common daisy (Bellis perennis), speedwell, oak, etc. Kanne Bread Drink.
- For acute infections: drink plenty of fluids, especially beer.
- Massages for lower back, buttocks and legs.
- Foot reflex massage, acupoint massage.
- Keep the feet warm, take hot foot baths.
- Full hot baths, possibly with tea added.
- MMS or antibiotics help with bladder and kidney pain. It makes sense for persistent repair.
- Pelvic floor exercises, pubococcygeus muscle training - promote a strong bladder and vigor; for general energy - this body region is the basis of the life-energy (root chakra).
- Best time for bladder treatments according to the organ clock: 4 pm.

OVARIES

The ovaries have the size and shape of two small plums and lie in the pelvis on either side of the uterus. Except for the corpus luteum, they are made up of mesodermal tissue. The immature egg cells (follicles) are available in limited numbers. At the appropriate time, a small number of them mature to be ova. The female hormone estrogen is mainly produced in the stroma cell tissue of the ovaries. The corpus luteum produces progestogen, the "pregnancy hormone."

Ovarian Parenchyma
Loss conflict

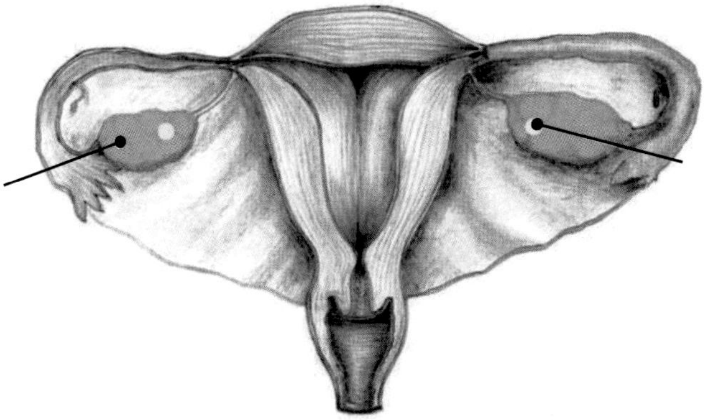

Corpus Luteum
Severe-loss conflict

SBS of the Ovaries

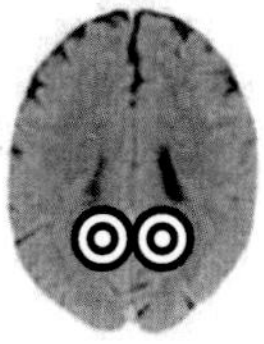

Ovarian cysts, ovarian cancer[1]

NEW MESO

Conflict: Loss or fear of loss of close relatives, friends or animals. In my experience, also an unfulfilled wish to have a child (for oneself or substituted for a daughter/granddaughter). One doesn't feel like they are able to take care of their offspring. Doubts about fertility/ability to procreate.

Examples:
➜ *Loss of child, husband, partner, parent, friend, or animal, through death or separation.*
➜ *A child moves far away to another city; the partner dies or turns away.*
• *A 26-year-old, right-handed woman is diagnosed with a 7 x 6 cm (2.5 x 2 in) cyst on the left (mother/child) ovary via ultrasound. Conflict history: Ten months ago, the patient learns that her married mother is having an affair. This comes as a great shock to her, for she believes in the ideal of marital fidelity. She suffers a traumatic-loss conflict, for the affair puts her mother at a distance. Six months ago, her mother ends the affair and the patient can forgive her at once. Their good relationship is restored*

1 See Dr. Hamer, Charts pp. 68 ff, 80

and the patient is fully confident that her mother will not do such a thing again = beginning of the repair phase, growth of a cyst. Against the advice of her gynecologist, the patient decides against the removal of the cyst, which would have ended her chances of having children. (Archive B. Eybl)

• *A 70-year-old, retired woman has just made friends with a man she admires. Upon meeting at their first date, he has a stroke and sinks to the floor = traumatic-loss conflict affecting the right (partner) ovary. In the repair phase, a 700 g (25 oz), malignant ovarian tumor develops. CM classifies it as a "colon metastasis."* (Archive B. Eybl)

Conflict-active	Cell degradation (ovarian necrosis) = "holes" in the ovarian tissue - generally unnoticed > reduced hormone levels > irregular menstruation, absence or withdrawal of menstruation; with a traumatic-loss conflict before puberty, the first monthly period (menarche) can be delayed.
Repair phase	Restoration, inflammation of the ovaries (adnexitis), swelling, pain; one or more cysts grow out of the "holes," which begin to fill up with functioning tissue. Along with the histological findings, the size is of primary importance to the diagnosis of ovarian cysts or ovarian cancer. Increased estrogen production. At the beginning of the repair phase, the cysts attach themselves to neighboring organs, which is often mistaken as "invasive growth." The cysts detach themselves as soon as they have developed their own blood supply. One should wait and make sure that the conflict is permanently resolved before opting for surgical removal. Possibly also a recurring conflict.
Bio. function	Additional ovarian tissue (= tumor) produces more estrogen. This gives the woman more sexual drive (libido). She looks younger and ovulates better > increased chance of becoming pregnant > loss compensation.
Note	An ovarian cyst, with its additional estrogen, keeps a woman young. Consider side + handedness
Questions	Diagnosed when? Were the ovaries normal at the time of the last examination? (Yes > conflict resolution afterward, because cysts first begins growing in the repair phase). Which loss affected me during the time period in question? (Death, a loved one (or pet) going away)? Wishing for a child for oneself or for someone else? Doubts about fertility/ability to procreate? (Self or substitute/sympathy)? Was there a death that affected me or was a tragic experience during my childhood? (Examine for conditioning). Did a family member die before or during the pregnancy? (Examine for conditioning). What are my thoughts about my own death? Am I at peace/can I deal with this concept? What do my parents think about it? Did ancestors have trouble/a hard time dealing with death/dying? Which new attitude would be helpful/healing?
Therapy	The conflict is resolved, support the healing process. In the case of continued growth: Determine and resolve the conflict, causal conditioning and beliefs. Meditate about death and transience. Recognize that the soul is immortal and that death is a harmless transition into another world. OP, when the ovarian tumor is too large or continues to grow.

Congenital female underdevelopment (Turner syndrome)

According to CM, Turner syndrome is a congenital, hereditary disease with the following primary symptoms: underdeveloped, non-functioning ovaries, small or no breasts and short stature. Life expectancy, however, is not limited. As always with hereditary diseases, we must turn our attention to the ancestors - in this case, the female ancestors.

Conflict	It is dangerous to be a woman; at least nobody may see that one is a developed/sexually mature woman.
Examples	→ *The great-grandmother of a girl was raped during the war under dramatic circumstances.*
Conflict-active	Limitation of the sexual development in particular and the physiological development in general. Multiple organs and tissue types are affected.
Bio. function	The underdevelopment protects against sexual assault. To remain as a child is safer.
Repair phase	A certain amount of post-maturing is realistic.
Questions	Are the female ancestors fully developed? Dramas in the family? (Rapes, humiliations; unforgiving, embittered women with regard to men)? How do I feel about my own femininity?
Therapy	Determine the conflict and conditioning of the female ancestors and attempt resolution. Conversations with the grandparents and aunts, a healing regression meditation for the women in the family. View the trauma again, dignify it and illuminate it with love. See also: remedies for the ovaries p. 243.

SBS of the Endodermal Portions of the Ovaries

Germ cell tumor (teratoma), ovarian abscess, dermoid cysts[1]

In this "special" tumor, one not only finds endodermal tissue, but also skin and hair at times. For this reason, it is often called a "monster" growth. According to Dr. Hamer, this originates in the corpus luteum in women. The teratoma represents a primitive attempt of duplication. This kind of reproduction is found in the simplest forms of life such as in bacteria. Here, the cell division takes place in the sympathicotonic, old brain schema.

Conflict	Severe-loss conflict
Example	→ *Loss of a beloved person or animal, loss of a dear relative, friend or partner (death, moving away, quarrel, coma, marriage).*
Conflict-active	Growth of a teratoma in women originating from the corpus luteum.
Bio. function	Reproduction by means of duplication so that the loss can be quickly compensated.
Repair phase	Stops growing quickly because of "embryonic growth spurt," ovarian abscess: degradation of the tumor via fungi or bacteria, dermoid cysts: empty spaces after completed repair.
Therapy	Determine the conflict, trigger(s) and conditioning and resolve them. OP if necessary.

1 See Dr. Hamer, Charts p. 24

Infertility in women, absence of menstruation (amenorrhea), irregular menstruation, reduced sexual drive

Possible causes

- **Poisoning** by chemotherapy, radiation, vaccinations (e.g., HPV), gene technology, environmental poisons, etc.
- **General sympathicotonia:** Generally, humans and animals only engage in sexual activity during states of relaxation. Conception and stress are polar opposites. She, who conceives, is the "passive" receiver (-). He, who impregnates, is the "active" giver (+). Hunters know that deer only copulate when the forest is very quiet. Too many pathways, cyclists and dogs prevent conception.
- **Female sexual loss-of-territory conflict** in the active-phase: > a territorial conflict on the left, "female" side blocks the "female" territorial areas. > The "female" in her becomes "male-brained," because it switches over to the right side of the brain. > Masculinization, ("dynamization," possibly homosexuality, etc.) > drop in estrogen level > absence of ovulation (= secondary amenorrhea) > infertility. (See the literature of Dr. Hamer.)

- **Under-functioning of the ovaries** - active-phase: degradation of ovarian tissue (necrosis) > "holes" in the parenchyma tissue > shrinking of the ovaries > lowered estrogen level > irregular menstruation, lack of periods (= primary amenorrhea) > infertility or reduced fertility.
- **Low levels of body fat:** Estrogen is produced in the body fat. Fat women and men have an increased level of estrogen. The minimum amount of fat needed for pregnancy is 24%. At less than 16% ovulation ceases.
- **Blocked fallopian tubes**: adhesions, tightening, scarring of the fallopian tubes due to recurring-conflicts > infertility (see p. 244f).
- **Pituitary gland** - active-phase: increased production of prolactin (see p. 113).

Therapy corresponding with the cause.

Lack of sexual desire (frigidity)

In our current "obsession with youth," which is now coming to an end - a lack of sexual desire is seen as an illness. From a biological viewpoint, this is only possible during the fertile years, but not for the long period we now experinece afterwards. Nature's will seems to be that sexual desire fades with age. As estrogen and testosterone levels come into balance, a woman starts tending towards the male, a man towards the female. I think we should welcome this and be glad to leave Eros and his desires behind

us. As we depart from a dependence on sex, the door opens up to new experiences and broader horizons. Women and men who have curbed their lust, even before the age of menopause, should be celebrating their freedom. The last thing we should be doing is believing that something is wrong with us and that we are suffering from "problems."

Still, if one feels the need to look for a cause, any of the points above can be considered, excepting blocked fallopian tubes.

Menopausal complaints

Between the ages of 45 to 55, women enter into menopause: Estrogen levels sink until ovulation no longer takes place and menstruation ceases. For some women, this change is accompanied by hot flashes, sweating, mood swings, sleep disturbances, dizziness and osteoporosis.

In our view, menopause is also significant with regard to the changes in the brain: right-handed women normally "work" more with the left (feminine) brain-side. A sinking estrogen level, when seen in the balance between estrogen and testosterone, means a rise in the relative testosterone level > "masculinization" due to the menopausal switch to the right (male) brain-side. > Certain feminine conflicts lose their significance, because the woman feels that she is a "man." Active conflicts centered in the feminine side of the brain become irrelevant; i.e., they are resolved due to the hormone change.

- Sweating: repair phase symptom - due to the hormonal change, certain sex-specific conflicts lose their meaning.

- Osteoporosis: women are often unable to accept their loss of attractiveness (conditioning) = generalized self-esteem conflict > degradation of bone substance.

Just as adolescents blaze a new trail when hormones begin surging inside them, women in menopause also enter uncharted territory. Mood swings, depression, sleep disturbances due to the switch to the other brain-side, lung embolisms and heart attacks or strokes due to the resolution of years of conflict activity.

Menopause is also problematic for their partner, who suddenly has to deal with a "man," or at least is no longer dealing with "the woman she once was."

Men experience a change (drop in testosterone level > feminization) later than women. This period - from menopause until the man has "changed" - is especially critical for the partnership (divorces).

After this change, both the emotional state and general health become stable again ("the serenity of age").

Therapy
- Welcoming the new stage of life.
- Guiding principle: *"My conflicts are resolving themselves now - the complaints will pass. A new time is beginning!"*
- Bioidentical hormones according to the findings of Dr. Lee, Dr. Platt, Dr. Lenard and Dr. Rimkus.
- Natural borax.
- 2 tbsp of cod liver oil daily.

Remedies for the ovaries
- Bioidentical hormones according to the findings of Dr. Lee, Dr. Platt, Dr. Lenard and Dr. Rimkus.
- Natural hormones in yam roots (important source), maca roots, beer (hops), blossom pollen.
- Moor mud - internally and externally; moor mud contains a high concentration of natural estrogen.
- Teas: hops blossoms, yarrow, chaste tree seeds.
- Segment massages, foot reflex massages.
- Sacroiliac joint mobilization.
- Natural borax internally.

FALLOPIAN TUBES AND UTERUS

The uterus (womb) is a pear-shaped, hollow muscle (myometrium) made up of the corpus uteri (body) and the cervix uteri (neck). The uterus and the fallopian tubes are lined with an endodermal mucosa (endometrium). It is covered with an ectodermal layer in the area around the cervix.

The fallopian tube takes the egg from the corpus luteum and leads it into the uterus, where, if fertilized, it settles into the mucosa and develops, over several stages, into a baby.

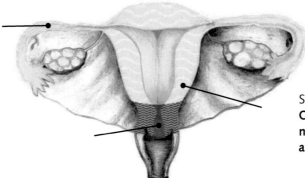

Uterus and Fallopian Tube Mucosa
Conflicts related to sexuality

Cervical Mucosa
Female sexual-frustration conflict, female loss-of-territory conflict

Smooth Uterine Musculature
Conflict, unwanted pregnancy, not being able to get pregnant and/or bear children

SBS of the Uterus and Fallopian Tubes Mucosa

Cancer of the uterine mucosa (uterine adeno-ca, uterine cancer, endometrial cancer), thickening (hyperplasia) of the endometrium[1]

Conflict	Sexual conflict, one feels disregarded, dishonored, dirtied, or offended as a woman. Conflict regarding femininity. Themes: procreation, partnership, men, sexuality. Conflict with relation to the "obligations of a woman" (satisfying a man, having children, etc.). According to Dr. Hamer: "ugly, half-genital conflict."
Examples	• *During the last few years, a 52-year-old married woman has become increasingly less interested in sex. Her husband, however, still has a strong desire to sleep with her. Although he is not demanding, she suffers from a sexual conflict with regard to the uterus. Repair phase: In summer, she goes off on vacation with two girlfriends for three weeks. The three get along well and have wonderful conversations. Suddenly, the patient gets an "inexplicable," heavy discharge lasting two weeks and sweats at night. (Archive B. Eybl)*
	• *A 41-year-old woman and her partner have been living together for 12 years. She suffers from the fact that he doesn't want to marry her. On the occasion of a family jubilee, the family publishes a family chronicle with a family tree, in which she does not appear. The patient is shocked and feels "so cheap" = sexual conflict > thickening of the mucosa due to cell division. The patient comes into healing when her partner proposes marriage > the thickened mucosa is discharged with a very heavy menstrual period. The patient sweats at night and is very weak. (Archive B. Eybl)*
	• *After separating from her alcoholic husband, a 60-year-old, retired woman finds a very nice partner, whom she likes very much. However, he leaves her - without warning and without telling her of his intention > sexual conflict. When she has gotten over this, she begins bleeding, although she no longer menstruates = repair phase. The gynecologist does a curettage. A histological examination reveals "malignant cells" and her uterus is removed in a surgery, along with the ovaries. (Archive B. Eybl)*
	• *A 36-year-old woman has been living with a man for 10 years. He has promised to marry her. Suddenly, he disappears with another woman = sexual conflict. (See Dr. Hamer, Goldenes Buch, 2, p. 122)*
Conflict-active	Increase in function; a cauliflower-like tumor of secretory quality or a flat-growing tumor of absorptive

---

1   See Dr. Hamer, Charts pp. 24, 35

quality develops in the uterine cavity, flat-growing tumor = "thickening of the mucous membrane" (endometrial hyperplasia). Often, a recurring conflict.

Bio. function	Thickening of the mucosa so that the ovum can embed itself better. Nature builds an especially thick and soft nest (flat-growing tumor). More secretion, so that the unwanted, sexual "problem" can be eliminated better (cauliflower-like tumor).
Repair phase	Inflammation of the uterine wall (endometritis), removal during the monthly period: very heavy bleeding, shedding of the thickened mucosa or a tumor with bits of mucosa (decidua) in the blood; or removal outside of menstruation: stinking discharge (fluor vaginalis), possibly with light bleeding; in both cases, night sweats and pain. Afterwards function normalization.
Repair crisis	Chills or feeling cold, strong abdominal pain, excessive bleeding.
Questions	First, determine if it is in the repair phase or the active phase. (Night sweats, bleeding and pain are signs of repair). If still active: What happened during the time period in question? What did I suffer as a woman? (Disappointment, separation, abuse, unfulfilled desire to have a child)? Why did this issue enter my life? (Find the deep-seated cause). Did my ancestors have similar symptoms? (Indication of a family issue). Do we have spiritual/emotional similarities? How do/did my ancestors live out/experience their femininity? Which beliefs do I want to leave behind me? Am I ready to start anew? What do I want to change externally?
Therapy	Determine the conflict and conditioning and, if possible, resolve them in real life if still active. Guiding principles: "What I experienced was unpleasant. Nevertheless, I look forward to the future with confidence!" "What has happened has a meaning. Now I can begin anew, leaving it all behind me!"
	Ritual cleansing, e.g., in the form of a bath. Natural identical hormones (progesterone, estradiol, etc.). If necessary, surgery. See also: remedies for the uterus p. 251.

Fallopian tube cancer, inflammations (salpingitis, adnexitis)

In principle, the same SBS as above (see above). In a fallopian tube is were the decisive union takes place, i.e., the fusion of the gametes. According to Daniel Stoica, this results in the following, additional conflict aspects: Conflict that the conception did not happen. > In a further sense, conflict that one will not become pregnant and will not have a child.

Example	• A 15-year-old schoolgirl is forced to sleep with a man = sexual conflict. She comes into healing with the help of a therapist, who helps her recover from the shock > now she gets a fever and abdominal pain. An inflammation of the fallopian tubes is treated in the hospital with a heavy dose of antibiotics. (Archive B. Eybl)
Conflict-active	Increase in function, cell division in the mucosa of the fallopian tubes > thickening of the mucosa (adeno-ca) > increased secretions. Long-term conflict may result in fallopian tube cancer (tubal cancer).
Bio. function	With more mucus, the sperm can move along the tubes more easily. After conception, the fertilized ovum can be transported toward the uterus better.
Repair phase	Inflammation of the fallopian tubes - tubercular-caseating degradation of the thickened mucosa via fungi and bacteria. At the beginning of the repair phase, the fallopian tube can close up due to healing swelling (especially with syndrome), purulent discharge from the vagina (fluor vaginalis) or discharge into the abdominal cavity, fever, pain, night sweats.
Note	After several recurrences, the passage can be impeded by scar tissue > possible infertility.
Therapy	The conflict is resolved. Support the repair phase. Determine the conflict and conditioning and, if possible, resolve them in real life if still active. Questions: see above. Colloidal silver internally. Possibly, antibiotics or OP, if the repair phase is too intense. See remedies for the uterus p. 251.

Pus collection in the ovary/fallopian tube area (tubo-ovarian abscess)

Same SBS as above.

Example	• An 18-year-old Catholic woman falls in love with an attractive young man - her first love. From one day to the next, he leaves her. Contrary to his promises, he never broke up with his previous girlriend and has gone back to her. The girl feels dishonored as a woman > cell-growth in the mucosa of the fallopian tubes. When she gets over him, she becomes feverish (= repair phase: inflammation of the

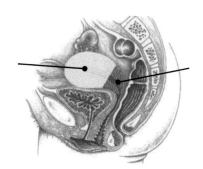

Smooth Uterine Musculature
**Conflict, unwanted pregnancy,
Not being able to get pregnant
and/or bear children**

Cervix Mucosa
**Female sexual-frustration
conflict, female loss-of-
territory conflict**

*fallopian tubes). Due to the quantity of pus in the abdomen, the doctors decide to operate imme-
diately. Due to another affair with this man, she relapses and after a few weeks: she gets the symptoms again (= repair phase). Adhesions in the fallopian tubes are diagnosed. (Archive B. Eybl)*

Phase	**Recurring-conflict** or persistent repair: purulent dissolution of tissue where the fallopian tubes meets the ovary (fimbria ovarica), encapsulation and adhesions as a result of recurrences, possible outcome: infertility.
Therapy	Determine the conflict and conditioning and, if possible, resolve them in real life so that the healing can complete. Questions: see previous page. Colloidal silver internally. Possibly, antibiotics and surgery when the repair phase is too intense. See cancer of the uterine mucosa above and remedies for the uterus on p. 251.

Ectopic pregnancy (tubal pregnancy)

Same SBS as above (see p. 244-246). Where there is an absence of menstruation, a positive pregnancy test and unusual abdominal pain, there could be a tubal pregnancy.

Phase	**Conflict recurrences** can lead to adhesions, narrowings, and bulges in the fallopian tubes > every inflammation leaves scar tissue behind > prevention or delayed movement of the ovum into the uterus, the ovum embeds itself in the place it is located on the 6th to 7th day following fertilization > tubal pregnancy.
Therapy	Surgery to end the pregnancy.

Endometriosis

One speaks of endometriosis when uterine mucosa cells grow outside of the uterine cavity and act according to the menstrual cycle in this location (regular monthly bleeding). Endometriosis is most often found on the outer wall of the uterus, the ovaries, peritoneum or intestines.

Conflict	According to Frauenkron-Hoffmann: Conflict of believing that one cannot offer a good home to their child. Often, this affects women who have had bad childhoods and wished that they would have had different parents or a different home. Belief pattern: It would be better to have no child than to raise one where it would have to be raised. Always keep the ancestors or a substitution conflict in mind (see example below).
Example	• *An endometriosis was diagnosed in the abdomen of a 40-year-old mother of one. Cause: Her grandmother was a gorgeous woman and as a maid, was impregnated four times by four different men. She died while trying to abort the last child herself. (Archive B. Eybl)*
Phase	**Persistent, active conflict.** Growth of endometriosis foci outside of the uterine cavity. Cyclical build-up and break-down of mucosa. Often, fertility is limited by growths on the fallopian tubes or ovaries. Menstrual pain, possibly abdominal, back or pelvic pain.
Bio. function	Creation of an emergency nest, because one feels their actual home (uterine cavity) is unsuitable.
Questions	Actual hardship with regard to having a good nest? Stress during pregnancy/birth with regard to the future home? Substitution conflict? Which of these dramas did my female ancestors experience? (Pregnant/giving birth as a refugee, disowned by the family, adoption, rape)? Which meaning does "home" have for me/for my family?
Therapy	Determine the conflict, triggers and causal family conditioning and resolve. Healing meditation for the ancestors/family. Warm wraps, infrared cabin. Possibly OP. See also: remedies for the uterus p. 251.

SBS of the Cervix Mucosa

Cervical cancer

The areas for the cervix and the coronary veins are located very close to one another the left side of the left in the cerebrum. - For this reason, these two important SBS are usually synchronized. This area represents the center of the female territorial area and has great significance, not just biologically. (For more explanation and case examples, see p. 165f).

Conflict | Female sexual-frustration or loss-of-territory conflict.

Examples | ➜ *Not being mated with, being abandoned, rejected.*

➜ *Being impregnated against one's will or at the wrong time (with force/rape).*

• *After the birth of a child, the husband of a 27-year-old woman has an affair. She can handle that relatively easily, but after he repeats his offense, she gets a female loss-of-territory conflict > no menstruation for a month (conflict-active phase). A gynecological examination results in an increased pap-value. Previously, it was always normal. (Archive B. Eybl)*

• *In kindergarten, a girl is "sexually molested" by a boy of the same age = female loss-of-territory conflict. Cell degradation in the cervical mucosa in the active-phase, restoration in the active-phase. (Archive B. Eybl) Conflicts often arise when children "play doctor."*

• *Following a broken marriage, a midwife lives alone without a partner. One day, she meets a man and decides that he is "Mr. Right." Within a short period of time, the two move in together. However, a few days later, the man disappears suddenly, without any reason = female loss-of-territory conflict. Six months later, she meets another man and a stable relationship develops = healing of the female loss-of-territory conflict. Shortly afterwards, she notices bleeding. The gynecologist diagnoses cervical cancer and schedules a surgery to perform a cervical conization or a hysterectomy. However, the patient changes her mind and begins to study the 5 Biological Laws of Nature. After she recovers from the repair phase crisis with a minor lung embolism, she enjoys perfect health. (See Claudio Trupiano, Thanks Dr. Hamer, p. 325)*

Conflict-active | Increased sensibility of the cervical squamous epithelium mucosa, slackening of the ring-musculature of the cervix. Later, local cell degradation, usually unnoticed. Due to involvement of the coronary arteries, possible mild angina pectoris. Reinforced sex drive, jealousy, tendency to hysteria (uterus = greek "hysterika").

Bio. function | Through increased sensibility, the woman can sense more. The relaxed cervix makes penile penetration easier > favorable conditions for conception > solution of the conflict.

Repair phase | Restoration of the mucosa via cell growth = cervical cancer, pain, inflammation (cervicitis), temporary healing swelling of the mucous membrane, bleeding outside the menstrual periods and/or severe and lengthy menstruation. Often, a recurring conflict.

Repair crisis | 3-6 weeks after the beginning of the repair phase: strong bleeding and abdominal pain, pulmonary embolism (often noticed as a difficulty in breathing), raised resting and active pulses, chills.

Pap smear | The pap smear for women is like the PSA value for men: an unnecessary, fear-loaded cancer test, often with fatal psychic and therapeutic consequences. From the point of view of the 5 Biological Laws of Nature, a positive pap test means that an SBS is running; it doesn't indicate which phase the patient is in. This would be the information that is actually worth knowing. (I.e., pap values can be elevated during conflict-active and during repair phases. In my experience, it is usually the repair phase. One can only be warned against having pap smears, especially without knowledge of the connections. During pregnancy, breast-feeding or with the flu, a pap smear can appear worse than usual. From our view, this is logical, because these phases are vagotonic.

Questions | Diagnosed when? Were the findings okay the last time? (Indication of event leading to conflict or repair in the meantime). Absent/shortened/irregular menstruation? (Indication of active conflict). Menstruation heavier than normal? (Indication of repair). General signs of repair phase or conflict activity? Partner: separation/thoughts of separation, fighting? Spurned love? Force/pressure? Too much or too little sex? Was that the first love? (Find the original conflict). Mother/female ancestors also affected? (Family issue)? What was my earliest sexual experience that I can remember? Which conditioning plays a role? (Divorce of the parents, similarity with the mother/grandmother, ancestors' dramas)? What should I change on the inside? What should I change on the outside?

E
C
T
O

−+

Therapy | Determine the conflict and/or trigger(s) and, if possible, resolve them in real life, if they are still active. Guiding principles: *"Even thought it didn't go as I wanted, I love and accept myself fully and wholly!"* *"As a woman I am lovable, courageous, and strong!"* CM: cone biopsy or hysterectomy are, from the perspective of the 5 Biological Laws of Nature, sometimes necessary.
Caution: In CM, pulmonary embolisms are treated with blood-thinning medication. This can cause extreme cervical bleeding > do not give any blood-thinning medication.
The HPV vaccination is, like all vaccinations, damaging and ineffective, i.e., it doesn't protect you.
After a cervical or ovarian surgery, the patient should replace the missing hormones with an external source, so that she can remain a "woman." Bioidentical hormones following the findings of Dr. Lee, Dr. Platt, Dr. Lenard, and Dr. Rimkus. See also remedies for the uterus p. 251.

Thickening of the cervical mucosa (epithelial metaplasia) and genital warts in the cervix (condylomata)

Same SBS as above.

Phase | **Persistent repair** - excessive restoration of the epithelium > thickening of the mucosa or local growths (condylomata).

Therapy | Determine the conflict and conditioning and, if possible, resolve them in real life, so that the healing completes. Questions: see above. Surgical removal of the condylomata, if required. See also remedies for the uterus p. 251.

SBS of the Uterus Muscle (Myometrium) HFs in midbrain - topography unknown

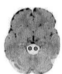

Tumors of the uterine muscles (myoma, leiomyoma)[1]

The uterine muscles are made up of three layers. The innermost layer, like the intestinal wall, is made up of transverse-running fibers, in the outer layers, the fibers run lengthwise. Approximately one in four women develop myomas.

E
N
D
O

+−

Conflict | Conflict of unwanted pregnancy or not being able to get pregnant or bear a child, not being able to retain the "fruit" - in a broader sense: unfulfilled wish to have a child. Failure having children or not being able to have enough. Can also be experienced as a substitute conflict (e.g., for the daughter).

Examples | • *A woman wants children but her partner is against having any = conflict of not being pregnant > in the active-phase, benign myomas develop.* (Archive B. Eybl)
• *A woman already has two children. When she becomes pregnant for the third time, she has an abortion. Myomas develop.* (Archive B. Eybl)

Conflict-active | Growth of a myoma, locally increased tension of the involuntary (smooth) muscle.

Bio. function | Strengthening of the muscle so that the "fruit" can be held better and the baby can be easily delivered.

Repair phase | Normalization of the muscle tension: the myomas remain and are usually harmless; possibly, but rarely, heavy bleeding could be a problem. Consider surgery.

Questions | Myoma since when? Desire to have children, abortion, premature or stillbirth, handicapped child? (Possibly substituted for daughter). What is the family's attitude about having children? Is it necessary? Is one only then appreciated? Ancestral dramas at birth? (Abortion, bleeding to death)?

Therapy | Determine the conflict and conditioning and, if possible, resolve them in real life if the myoma is still growing. If it stops growing, the conflict is resolved. The simplest therapy would be pregnancy. Guiding principles: *"God knows exactly what plans he has for me!"* *"I take the opportunity offered by a life without children."* *"I open my mind for other experiences."* *"I will dedicate my life to others who need me."* Surgery, if the myoma grows too large. There is no reason not to become pregnant if the myomas are small.

---

1   See Dr. Hamer, Charts pp. 37, 38

SBS of the Uterine Suspensory Apparatus

Uterine and pelvic organ prolapse

Conflict	Self-esteem conflict: A load is hard to bear (children, partners, parents, caring for family members). One carries something that is too heavy (according to Frauenkron-Hoffmann). Often related to the house (uterus stands for the house/home). The base feeling is passive endurance and silent suffering.
Examples	→ *The mother takes on all her children's worries and believes she has to bear everything herself.* • *Along with her three children, a woman has to take care of her senile father-in-law. Everything is simply too much for her.* (Archive B. Eybl).
Conflict-active	Weakening of the collagen fibers in ligaments and the musculature > lowering of the uterus.
Repair phase	Recovery the ligamentous apparatus, if the conflict can be solved at an early age. Even in an advanced age, a certain amount of regeneration is possible.
Therapy	Determine and resolve conflict and conditioning in real life. Consistent pelvic floor muscle training exercises (PFMT) (PC muscle). Ensure good body tension (while walking, sitting), deep diaphragmatic breathing. Optimize nutrition with silica (horsetail, millet) and quality proteins. If necessary, OP.

SBS of the Kidney Collecting Tubules

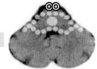

Poisoning in pregnancy (pre-eclampsia (PE), eclampsia, late gestosis)

The symptoms are protein in the urine, reduced urination, edema, headache, dizziness, and vision problems.

Conflict	Existential conflict, refugee conflict, conflict of not having enough water, conflict of feeling abandoned, conflict of not feeling cared for (see pp. 230ff).
Examples	→ *"How will I pay for this child?" "Who will look after us?"* • *The 33-year-old pregnant woman is under a lot of pressure from her boyfriend to have an abortion. However, the patient is determined to have the child. Existential conflict, conflict of not feeling cared for - affecting the kidney collecting tubules SBS. In the fourth month, her body begins to collect fluids - she gains more than 30 kg (65 lbs). Since she continues to be triggered by an existential conflict, she hardly loses weight, even after the delivery. Her general practitioner prescribes magnesium, which eases the edema somewhat. Now, she can at least put on her shoes.* (Archive B. Eybl)
Phase	**Conflict-active phase.** It is interesting how often this occurs among overweight, very young, first-time mothers = indication of an active existential or refugee conflict.
Therapy	Determine the conflict and conditioning and resolve it if possible. Avoid recurrences. Possibly anticonvulsants; if necessary, terminate the pregnancy. See also: remedies for the uterus p. 251.

Abnormally heavy menstruation (hypermenorrhea)

Possible causes

• **Uterus mucosa** in the repair phase: degradation of cells from the thickened mucosa (= flat growing tumor), leading to heavy, possibly stinking bleeding; possibly mucosa scraps (decidua) in the blood, pain, and night sweats. If the bleeding is very heavy every month: recurring-conflict, which comes into healing every month (triggers).

• **Cervix mucosa** in the repair phase: restoration of the epithelium, pain, inflammation (cervicitis), very heavy, long-lasting bleeding, also outside of the menstrual period, usually accompanied by increased pulse and breathing difficulties (see p. 247f).

• **Ovarian cysts or endometriosis** in the time after the repair phase (see pp. 240f and 246).

• **Uterine myoma:** bleeding in the repair phase or in the repair phase crisis (see p. 248).

Note

Intensification of the bleeding with syndrome or strong vagotonia, for example, resolved self-esteem conflict (pain in the loco-motor system) > liquefaction of the blood.

Therapy

Bioidentical hormones. Measures for kidney collecting tubules SBS p. 230ff. See also: remedies for the uterus below.

Menstrual pains (menstrual distress, premenstrual syndrome)

During the days before menstruation, estrogen drops sharply in favor of progesterone. Common concerns are: abdominal cramps, tenderness, nausea, headache = unique character of a **repair phase crisis**. The striated cervical muscles are affected; possibly, the smooth uterine muscles are also affected. The subject of conflict, in the broadest sense, has to do with femininity, sexuality, and womanhood (see pp. 244ff, 247f).

The biochemical dimension of being a woman is reflected in the estrogen levels. Therefore, it is not surprising that the conflict dissolves when estrogen levels drop. One is not strictly a woman anymore (biochemically speaking) and, as such, "is withdrawn from the conflict." The control takes place in the brain: the woman has her cerebral side switched for her. Most women with menstrual complaints are, therefore, "in constellation" (see p. 314f) and they switch sides every month during their period. This also explains the psychological changes (mood swings in the direc-tion of depression or mania). From this perspective: premenstrual syndrome is like the "little sister" of menopause.

- The most frequent conflict: A young woman had sexual intercourse and is afraid of being pregnant. Sexual intercourse or ovulation become a trigger for the conflict, even if she used protection. During the decrease of estrogen, she comes into the repair phase > therefore menstrual complaints.

Therapy

Determine conflict and resolve. Often, through pregnancy and maternity, the conflict is resolved.

Magnesium chloride ($MgCl_2$) foot baths.

In the background, a kidney collecting tubules SBS is often involved. > Therapeutic interventions p. 231f (salt baths, etc.). Breathing exercises, as recommended. Linseed oil. See also: remedies for the uterus on p. 251.

Miscarriage, premature birth

There are surely many causes for miscarriage or premature birth. Above all, there are spiritual/karmic causes. It is rarely possible to see behind the scenes of life; thus, the causes for this often remain hidden to us. However, we do know, thanks to the 5 Biological Laws of Nature, that conflicts during pregnancy harm the unborn and in the worst case, they can cause the pregnancy to terminate prematurely. In the first three months, the pregnant woman and embryo are mildly sympathicotonic (stressed). During this time, it doesn't take much to make the pot boil over, i.e., a conflict *"strikes."* A strong conflict can lead to cramped vessels in the placenta > blocked supply of nutrition and oxygen. In the last two-thirds of pregnancy, the so-called *"happy time,"* the danger is not so great, since the mother and child are vagotonic. A powerful conflict is needed to unseat the two. Nature tries by all means to bring the pregnancy to a successful conclusion; in the first three months, the "way back" is left open.

The unborn child can experience conflicts by itself (loud noises, screaming, shaking, ultrasound, tests of the amniotic fluid, etc.) or together with the mother. For instance, the mother suffers from fear or anger or she is quarreling with her partner. It is interesting to note that the frequency of Caesarians births increases along with the number of prenatal examinations. Children, born by Caesarian section, are 4 times more likely to suffer from respiratory illnesses than those who are delivered normally[1] (due to territorial-fear or fear-of-death-conflicts during birth). Breech presentation: the child wants to stay inside or tries "to turn back."

Phase   The miscarriage is preceded by a **conflict-active phase**: the dead fruit is ejected in the course of a repair phase crisis.

Therapy   Pregnant women need to be shielded from conflict and stress. They should lead a quiet and harmonious life. The mother and father should be aware that the structure of their own psyche and perceptions lay the foundation for their child. Knowing this, some character and spiritual maturity on the part of both parents would seem desirable. Of course, this does not mean that mature parents are immune to such tragedies.

---

1   From: faktor-L Neue Medizin 7, Monika Berger-Lenz & Christopher Ray, Faktuell Verlag, Görlitz 2009

Remedies for the uterus

- Moor Mud treatments; Moor Mud contains a high concentration of natural estrogen.
- Trinkmoor products, for instance SonnenMoor.
- Bioidentical hormones following the findings of Lee, Platt, Lenard.
- Keep the lower abdomen and feet warm.
- Bach flowers: crab apple, perhaps holly.

- Teas: melissa, yarrow, lady's mantle, linden blossoms, sanicle (Sanicula europaea), fennel.
- Bee pollen, royal jelly.
- Natural borax internally for hormone regulation.
- Osteopathy, segment massage, foot reflex-zone massage.
- Cod liver oil.

EXTERNAL FEMALE SEX ORGANS (VULVA)

The vulva is made up of the larger, outer lips (labia majora) and the smaller inner lips (labia minor), the clitoris, the pudendal cleft, the entrance to the vagina (vaginal vestibule) and the vagina itself. The outer lips belong to the epidermis and have dermis under the epithelium. The inner lips belong to the urogenital tract and, like the vagina, they have endodermal sub-mucosa under the ectodermal mucosa.

The vagina is a muscle tract that is about 10 cm (4 in) long, and it joins the outer genitalia with the uterus.

Located in the vaginal vestibule are endodermal glands, called Bartholin's glands, which secrete a lubricant upon sexual arousal.

Dermis, Epidermis and Outer Lips
Attitude/perception and/or a defilement conflict

Superficial Mucosa, Epidermis in the Genital Area
Separation conflict

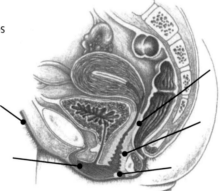

Vaginal Musculature
Not being able to prevent penetration or not being able to hold on to the penis

Vaginal Submucosa (yellow group)
Wanting/not wanting the penis

Bartholin's Glands
Conflict of vaginal lubrication/dryness

SBS of the Vaginal Muscles

HFs in the midbrain - topography still unknown

Vaginal cramps (vaginismus)

The vagina is a muscular tube of smooth (involuntary) muscle. As in the intestine, the muscles run longitudinally or ring-like. A vaginal cramp causes the ring-like muscles to tighten, so that entry is made very difficult if not impossible.

Conflict	Chunk conflict (see p. 15, 16): being unable to prevent penetration or not being able to hold onto the penis.
Example	→ *A woman is forced to have sex against her will or she wants to, but cannot.*
Conflict-active	A tensing-up of the involuntary vaginal ring musculature, vaginal muscle strengthening, narrowing of the vagina, vaginal tension.
Bio. function	With increased tension of the vaginal ring muscles, a undesired penetration can be better prevented, or the penis (desired) can be better retained.
Repair phase	Easing of the tension.
Repair crisis	Vaginal cramps (tonic-clonic seizures).
Note	If the subject of sexuality has a negative connotation (parental conditioning), small events or complications (e.g., the first sexual contact) are probably enough to set this SBS in motion.
Therapy	Determine the conflict, trigger(s) and conditioning and resolve them in real life, so the tension eases. See also remedies for the genitalia.

SBS of the Vaginal Epidermis or Mucosa

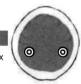

HFs sensory function in top of cerebral cortex

ECTO

−+

Inflammation of the outer genital area (vulvitis), vaginal inflammation (colpitis), vaginal epithelial cancer (squamous cell cancer, papillomas), genital warts (condyloma, condylomata acuminata, HPV-induced cell proliferation)

Conflict	Separation conflict, wanting or not wanting to be touched on the vulva or vagina, wanting or not wanting to have sexual intercourse.
Examples	→ *A woman would rather just cuddle. Her husband wants sex = conflict of not wanting sexual intercourse.*
	• *Following two bitter disappointments, a woman longs for a genuine partner, not just somebody who wants sex = separation conflict of not having the desired skin contact > degradation of epithelial tissue in the active-phase. When she finds a real partner, she suffers from itching in the outer genital area for one year = repair phase, restoration of the lost substance; false diagnosis by conventional doctors: "vaginal fungus."* (Archive B. Eybl)
	• *A woman was raped by a man when she was a young girl. Since then, she has a sexual trigger with inflammation and itching of the external genitals in the repair phase after sexual intercourse.* (Archive B. Eybl)
Conflict-active	Mostly unnoticed degradation of squamous cells of the labia, vagina or clitoris (= ulcer-cancer). No pain, possibly numbness.
Bio. function	The numbness (reduced sensitivity) allows the lacking or unwanted skin contact to be forgotten temporarily.
Repair phase	Restoration of the epithelium - inflammation of the labia, vagina, clitoris (squamous cell cancer), itching, pain, reddening, swelling; in CM, usually mistakenly diagnosed as "fungal infection" or "herpes vulvitis," genital warts in persistent repair: excessive local repair of the epithelium.
Questions	Inflammation since when? (The conflict must have been resolved immediately before - i.e., one enjoyed the sexual activity or being left alone). First inflammation? (No > find the original conflict. Often, the first partner is decisive). Does upbringing and/or religious dogmas play a role? (Sexual intercourse is something bad)? Did my mother also have symptoms of the sort? (Conditioning through the mother's emotional environment)? Which (family) religious beliefs play a role? (E.g. *"Sex is something dirty." "The drive is something negative." "Men only ever want just one thing." "I always find the wrong one." "One has to simply be available for the man."*) With which new attitude do I want to approach the issue of sexuality? Which old behavior pattern(s) do I want to get rid of? Which meditation would be helpful?
Therapy	The conflict is resolved. Support the healing process. In case of a relapse, determine the conflict and conditioning. If possible, resolve the conflict in real life. For instance, choose a sexually compatible partner, who is willing to fulfill one's sexual wishes. Guiding principles: *"I don't have to if I don't want to." "I'll do it when I feel like it." "Sex is nice, but true friendship and satisfaction lie outside the physical sphere."* Colloidal silver. CM: antibiotics and/or cortisone if necessary in intensive repair phases. Possibly surgery. See also: remedies for the genitalia p. 254.

Chancroid (ulcus molle) in women

Same SBS as above. (See above). Both women and men can suffer from "soft chancres." Small nodes form on the external genitals that develop into round, painful ulcers.

Phase	**Active-phase** - painless cell degradation from the epithelium: local loss of substance = skin ulcer.
	Repair phase - restoration of the epithelium with pain.
Therapy	Determine the conflict and conditioning and, if possible, resolve them in real life if still active. Questions: see above. Possibly CM: antibiotics for intensive repair phases. See also: remedies for the genitalia p. 254.

SBS of the Vaginal Submucosa

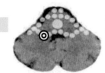

Fungal "infection" of the inner labia or vagina (soor vulvitis, vaginal mycosis)

A reddening and itching of the female genitals is usually diagnosed as a "fungal infection." Most diagnoses of this nature are usually inaccurate because these symptoms are usually related to a separation conflict. But, as in the mouth, thrush is also possible in the genital area, because underneath the superficial mucosa of the inner labia and the vagina there lies a layer of endodermal (intestinal) mucous membrane.

Conflict	Chunk conflict (see explanations p. 15, 16): not getting or not being able to take away the penis. Simply: Wanting or not wanting sexual contact.
Examples	→ *A woman doesn't want to have intercourse with her partner.*
	→ *A woman longs for a reunion with her beloved partner.*
Conflict-active	Increased function, thickening of the mucosa lying under the epithelium (submucosa).
Bio. function	Increased mucus production so that the penis can be better received or removed.
Repair phase	Tubercular caseating - white residue, intense itching, white, stinking discharge.
Note	During an SBS of the intestines with intestinal fungi in the repair phase, the vaginal or labial submucosa often reacts accordingly > vaginal mycosis without separation conflict, with intestinal symptoms.
Therapy	The conflict is resolved, support the repair phase. Should it recur, determine the conflict, trigger(s) and conditioning and resolve them.
	Cream mixture: aloe vera gel + natural skin cream.
	Colloidal silver, Hydrogen peroxide (H_2O_2), DMSO externally.
	Possibly CM: antibiotics in intensive repair phases. See also: remedies for the genitalia p. 254.

SBS of the Bartholin Glands

Inflammation of the vaginal glands (bartholinitis, Bartholin's cyst)

Conflict	Chunk conflict (see explanations p. 15, 16): dry vagina, not producing enough vaginal mucus to facilitate sexual intercourse. Conflict related to sexuality.
Examples	→ *A man is too careless and wants to penetrate his partner although she is not ready.*
	→ *A young woman from a strict religious upbringing sleeps with a man even though she isn't married. She now thinks she has committed a mortal sin.*
Conflict-active	Cell growth in the vaginal vestibule glands (Bartholin glands) = tumor of the vaginal glands (adeno-ca) with increased mucus production.
Bio. function	Increase in the mucus production so that the penis can enter more easily.
Repair phase	Tubercular-caseating degradation of the tumor > purulent stinking discharge, possibly mild night sweats, recurring-conflict: Bartholin's cysts.
Note	If the Bartholin gland ducts are swollen (syndrome) a collection of pus, up to the size of a chicken egg, can develop (= Bartholin's cyst or abscess), which empties spontaneously.
Therapy	The conflict is resolved. Support the healing. Should it recur, determine the conflict or trigger(s) and, if possible, resolve them in real life. Possibly CM: antibiotics in intensive repair phases. Possibly abscess surgery. Perform intercourse only if desired or use a lubricant. See remedies for the genitalia p. 254.

SBS of the Dermis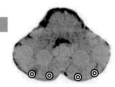

HFs in the cerebellum - topography still unknown

Vaginal "yeast infection" of the outer labia and externally

Beneath the squamous epithelium of the outer labia lies a layer of dermis.

Conflict	Feeling defiled or dirtied in the genital region, violation of integrity.
Example	→ *Coarse, unwanted practices, being called foul names, unwanted sexual intercourse.*
Conflict-active	Local cell division in the dermis > thickening.
Bio. function	Strengthening of the dermis in order to be protected from disfigurement or harm to the integrity.
Repair phase	Tubercular, caseating degradation via fungi, bacteria or bacteria, swelling, reddening, itching.
Therapy	Should it recur, determine the conflict, trigger(s) and conditioning and resolve them. Questions: see p. 252. Colloidal silver externally. CM: antibiotics if necessary in intensive repair phases. See also below.

Vaginal discharge (fluor genitalis), gonorrhea (colloquially called "the clap")

A small amount of clear discharge is normal in women of child-bearing age. Yellowish, whitish, brownish or bad-smelling discharge can be caused by any of the following:

- **Inflammation the uterus or fallopian tubes mucosa** in the repair phase (see p. 244ff).
- **Inflammation of the Bartholin glands** in the repair phase, stinking tubercular degradation of the glandular tissue (see above).

- **Inflammation of the vaginal mucosa or submucosa** in the repair phase (see pp. 253-254).
- **Purulent bladder infection** in the repair phase: tubercular, caseating degradation of endodermal bladder mucosa from the trigone > not actually a discharge, but stinking, opaque urine (see p. 237).

Therapy: according to the cause.

Remedies for the genitalia

- Bach flowers: crab apple, centaury, cerato.
- Teas: melissa, yarrow, lady's mantle, linden blossom, sanicle, fennel.
- Colloidal silver applied externally.

- Full or half bath with hydrogen peroxide, healing earth, EM, MMS or a decoction of yarrow, chamomile.
- Cream mixture: aloe vera gel and natural skin lotion.

TESTICLES

The two male testicles (testes) are contained in a sack called the scrotum. They produce testosterone (male sex hormone) and male germ cells (sperm).

The tubes that lead from the testicles, i.e., the epididymis and the deferent ducts (vas deferens), are used for the maturation and temporary storage of sperm.

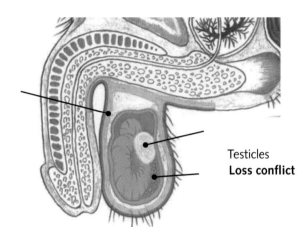

Peritoneum
of the Scrotum
**Attack against
the testicles**

Teratoma
"Special Tumor"
Severe-loss conflict

Testicles
Loss conflict

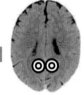

SBS of the Testicles

Testicular tumor (testicular cancer, seminoma, Leydig cell tumor)[1]

Conflict	Loss conflict, loss or fear of losing a loved one or a loved animal. Conflict with regard to one's manhood.
Examples	➔ *A beloved family member or pet dies.* ➔ *A person is abandoned by his or her partner.*
	➔ *A child moves away from home.* ➔ *A person is suddenly alone after a divorce.*
	• *A boy's mother dies when he is 13 years old, thus he experiences a loss conflict. When he is 58 his wife dies, triggering the loss conflict. When the pain of her death lets up, he feels a pulling in the testicles for a long time = repair phase, with a restoration of testicular cells. In a brain CT, it can be seen that the original conflict (the death of his mother) was a long time ago.* (Archive B. Eybl)
	• *The now 60-year-old, right-handed man suffers a loss conflict when he is 38 years old: His girlfriend abandons him one day and he does not recover for another two years, until he meets a new partner. During this time, an inflammation of the testicles is diagnosed (= repair phase).* (Archive B. Eybl) *Note: this could have just as well been diagnosed as testicular cancer.*
	• *The patient's partner has a bad epileptic seizure, during which she turns blue in the face. The patient fears she will "die in his arms" = loss conflict.* (Report from a forum).
	• *A man unexpectedly finds his beloved cat lying dead in a light shaft = loss conflict.* (Archive B. Eybl)
Conflict-active	Degradation of testicular tissue ("holes" = testicular necrosis) > gonadal insufficiency (see below) > drop in testosterone levels, usually unnoticed.
Repair phase	Restoration of the tissue, inflammation of the testicles (orchitis), swelling, pain. Where the "holes" were, a cyst develops, which gradually becomes filled with functioning tissue; CM: "testicular tumor."
Bio. function	Additional testicular tissue produces more testosterone and more sperm > strengthening of sexual drive and increase in fertility - in this way, a loss suffered can quickly be replaced again or one's manliness can be proven.
Questions	If a recurring conflict: Enlargement of the testicles since when? (A conflict must have been resolved beforehand). Clap test: mother/child or partner side? Which loss have I suffered? (Death, moving away, accident, separation from a beloved person or pet, substitution conflict for a child, grandchild)? Was

N
E
W

M
E
S
O

– +

---

1   See Dr. Hamer, Charts pp. 69, 80

my manhood in question? (Impotence, fatherhood)? What conditioned me in this regard in my child-hood/during the pregnancy? (Loss in early childhood, death of a young sibling, stillbirth and parental grieving, loss of a twin sibling before/during/directly after birth)? Which of my beliefs are out of date? (E.g., a man must always be able. Regular sex is important). What do I want to change on the inside and on the outside?

Therapy	The conflict is resolved. Support the healing process. Should it recur, determine the conflict, trigger(s) and conditioning and resolve them. Horsetail wrap according to Treben, poultice with steamed onions. Agrimony internally and externally. Surgery is better performed earlier than later.

Inadequate functioning of the gonads (testicular hypogonadism, Klinefelter syndrome)

Same SBS as above.

Phase	**Conflict-active phase:** degradation of testicular tissue (necrosis) > drop in testosterone levels > reduction of fertility due to lower production of sperm cells (oligospermia). Usually inadequate functioning is linked to smaller testicles (testicular hypoplasia) = persistent, active conflict.
Note	In the repair phase, one can expect a smaller or larger tumor. The poor functioning can also come from a deficiency or excess of another hormone, for instance a deficiency of gonadotropin or excess of estrogen or cortisone. (Perform a blood-hormone test).
Therapy	Determine the conflict or trigger(s) and resolve them in real life if possible. Questions: see above. Guiding principles: *"I know there is a reason for my loss." "I will make the best of it and carry on in peace."* Strength training or martial arts. High-quality proteins, e.g., eggs, honey, flower pollen, royal jelly. For testosterone levels, consider nature-identical progesterone and perhaps testosterone, taken short-term. Caution by younger patients: The goal is to stimulate the body's own hormone production; dependency on hormone replacements is harmful > short-term therapy only. Bioidentical hormones following the findings of Dr. Lee, Dr. Platt, Dr. Lenard and Dr. Rimkus. Natural testosterone in ginseng root, damiana (Turnera diffusa) (tea, tablets), maca (Lepidium meyenii) (powder), yohimbe. Borax internally. Cod liver oil. These suggestions are also valid for lack of drive due to testosterone shortage.

Undescended testicles, sliding, rocking, walking testicles

The testicles are formed in the abdomen during embryonic development and usually migrate down into the scrotum in the seventh month of pregnancy. If they do not, the condition is called undescended testicles. In 75% of cases, the testicles descend, during the first year of life by themselves. Undescended testicles is, along with other symptoms such as not fully developed lungs, a sign of immaturity in infants. If the testicles do not come down after more than a year and the child is otherwise developing normally, the following conflict may exist:

Conflict	According to Frauenkron-Hoffmann: this is often a proxy conflict for someone from their own family who may not be allowed to act out or show masculinity. May not be manly or want to be a man (similar to phimosis (inability to retract foreskin)).
Examples	➜ *An ancestor was raped and now she hates all men.*
	➜ *A man in the family has not resolved the issue of his gender in general or sexual orientation (e.g. forbidden or concealed homosexuality).*
Bio. function	One doesn't want to be a man, the genitalia (testicles) remain hidden, are not shown outwardly. Reduced ability to reproduce. "If male, then at least infertile."
Questions	Who does the child reflect? Who doesn't want to be/isn't allowed to be a man? (Usually a male ancestor). Why is this particular child carrying this conflict? Did ancestors also have undescended testicles/phimosis? (Indication of generational issue). Which specific changes do we want to achieve? (On the inside and outside).
Therapy	Find out who the child reflects. Then, try to heal the issue within the family. If necessary, use the therapy proposals above. If necessary, CM: hormone therapy or surgery.

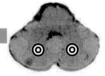

SBS of the Peritoneum

Hydrocele (fluid in the testicular pouch) with closed inguinal canal

Before or after birth, the testicles move down from the abdominal cavity through the inguinal canal into the scrotum. Normally, the inguinal canal closes thereafter.

Conflict	Attack on the testicles + syndrome. Most common attack: sterilization (vasectomy) or OP.
Examples	→ *A boy receives a blow to the testicles.*
	→ *Verbal or perceived attack: "I'll have your balls!" "A kick in the nuts!"*
	• *Hydrocele was diagnosed in a 4-year-old boy - the doctors wanted to operate. It came to light that the parents were having a disagreement over the last few months. The mother wanted the father to have a vasectomy. = Substitute attack to the testicles conflict. As therapy, the parents should come to an agreement, thank the child and explain to him that he doesn't need to carry this problem for them anymore. Two days after this explanation and gratitude, the testicles became inflamed and swelled even more (= repair phase). The parents again refused an OP. 10 days later, the hydrocele was completely gone without any surgical procedure. (Archive B. Eybl)*
Conflict-active	Cell proliferation (mesothelium).
Bio. function	Thickening of the testicular peritoneum, in order to better protect the testicles from attack.
Repair phase	Caseating, tubercular degradation of the tumor, accumulation of fluid = hydrocele. This usually occurs due to chronic conflict activity, but only in conjunction with syndrome.
Note	A hydrocele can also come from an injury (blow, contusion) or an inflammation of the testicles. See testicular tumor.
Therapy	See pp. 213ff and 230ff. The attack conflict is resolved. Support the healing. Avoid recurrences. Resolve any active refugee conflict. Avoid punctures due to conflict potential. Lymph drainages. OP if necessary.

O L D
M E S O
+ −

Hydrocele (fluid in the testicular pouch) with open inguinal canal

If the closure of the inguinal canal is incomplete, fluid from the pelvic cavity can leak into the scrotum.

Possible causes
- Peritoneum: "attack to the abdomen" in the repair phase: collection of abdominal fluid (ascites) that flows into the scrotum (see p. 213).
- Scrotum - peritoneum "attack to the testicles" in the repair phase: the fluid arises in the scrotum itself (see above).
- Abdominal organs such as the intestines, liver or pancreas in healing: fluid is produced by every inflammation, but if the inguinal canal is open, the fluid can leak into the scrotum.

Note: Because this illness usually affects newborns, CM calls it "congenital hydrocele;" always in combination with **syndrome**.

Therapy
Determine and resolve the conflict and the causal conditioning (also refugee conflict). Children: substitution conflict. Lymph drainages. Hydrocele usually resolves spontaneously. > OP if necessary after first waiting and observing.

Germ cell tumor (teratoma)

Conflict	Painful loss of a person or animal. Similar to teratoma of the ovaries (see p. 242).

PROSTATE GLAND

The prostate gland is partly attached to the base of the bladder and is made up of a muscle complex embedded with endodermal glands. It produces an alkaline secretion. The urethra goes through the middle of this chestnut-sized organ. The deferent duct (vas deferens) also leads to the urethra in the prostate gland. The ectodermal, urothelium-lined prostatic ductules (ductuli prostatici) discharge the prostatic secretion from the prostate gland into the urethra. Seminal fluid is made up of 40% prostatic secretion. Upon the release of seminal fluid (ejaculation), it is mixed with prostatic secretion, and with the help of involuntary muscle activity is pushed out through the urinary-seminal tract. The prostatic secretion gives the seminal fluid its typical musk - a chestnut-blossom odor. The smell of musk is an aphrodisiac and thus, sexually arousing.

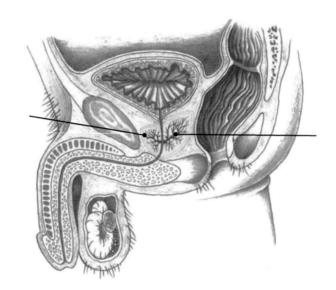

Prostate Parenchyma
**Sexual conflict,
conflict with regard
to the man's duties**

Prostate Ducts
**Territory marking
conflict with
sexual aspect**

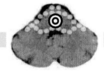

SBS of the Prostate Parenchyma

Enlargement of the prostate (prostatic hyperplasia), prostate cancer (adeno-ca)[1]

Conflict
1. Sexual conflict, problems with regard to procreation. One does not feel manly (potent) enough. One doubts his own manliness or erectile function. Stress due to "abnormal" sexual perception (e.g., not married in a Catholic family, homosexuality). According to Dr. Hamer: "ugly-genital conflict" most often found in older men, who no longer react to territorial conflicts.

2. Conflict with regard to the "man's duties" (satisfying a woman, having children, etc.).

3. According to Frauenkron-Hoffmann: A belief that one has not passed on the right impulses or enough maturity to his child for its life (e.g., motivation, ambition, education, behavior).

Examples
➜ *A man wants to but cannot (potency problem) or he wants to but may not (the woman doesn't want to or would prefer a different man).*

• *In the midst of divorcing his wife, the patient meets a young woman, who offers him everything that he could want sexually. During the divorce proceedings, he finds out that this woman is passing important information to his wife's lawyer - she is betraying the patient = sexual conflict. In the active-phase, his PSA value climbs to just over 4. Although the patient shows no symptoms, a prostate puncture (cell sample) is taken. After 18 punctures, a few proliferating cells are found and a diagnosis of testicular cancer is made. After the prostate gland has been removed, the patient finds*

---

1   See Dr. Hamer, Charts pp. 24, 35

himself impotent and partly incontinent. During the course of chemotherapy, he begins seeking an alternative and gets to know the 5 Biological Laws of Nature. Impotence is another sexual conflict for the man > cell division in the area of the sphincter > urine retention > OP > radiation... (Archive B. Eybl)

• *A 46-year-old executive employee has an extra-marital relationship. When he decides to end the affair, his mistress threatens to destroy his family = sexual conflict. In the active stage, his PSA value soars to 46. The patient knows about the 5 Biological Laws of Nature and refuses conventional therapy. He confesses to his wife and she forgives him = conflict resolution. During the repair phase, the patient suffers for several days from severe urine retention. The PSA value drops back to 2. As a result of the affair, the patient suffers from gingival atrophy (see p. 184). (Archive B. Eybl)*

• *A patient notices that his wife is being unfaithful. He remains conflict-active for 15 years, because he cannot let go of the situation. (Archive B. Eybl)*

• *A father learns that his grown daughter is regularly being forced to have sex with her partner = substituting for his daughter, he feels a sexual conflict. (Archive B. Eybl)*

Conflict-active	Increase in function, growth of a cauliflower-like prostate (adeno-ca) tumor = cell growth in the prostate gland, rise in the PSA value. With prolonged conflict activity, swelling pressure > restricted fluid flow > difficulty urinating.
Bio. function	Production of more prostatic secretion > stronger musk odor in the urine and sperm signals potency and the readiness to mate to the female, furthermore, with more sperm, he can be more impressive > older man shows females that he is not yet "over the hill" and can keep up with the younger men. More prostatic secretion also increases motility, lifespan and the protection of genetic material in sperm.
Repair phase	Normalization of function, tubercular, caseating necrotic degradation of the tumor = stinking, murky, possibly bloody urine; pain, inflammation (prostatitis), swelling, night sweats; if no bacteria is present: symptom-free encapsulation of the tumor.
	Often, urine retention, but not always, because the prostate gland has enough space to expand out wards. Usually, a recurring conflict.
PSA value	The enzyme PSA is produced primarily in the prostate gland and is a rough parameter for the size of the prostate gland or tumor. Unfortunately, it is a fact that the more often PSA values are measured, the more men die of prostate cancer. Regular checks of the PSA value and follow-up biopsies are, from the viewpoint of the 5 Biological Laws of Nature, unwise.
	For patients that do not know the 5 Laws, just being told that something is wrong with their prostate gland can trigger a further conflict. This is especially the case with diagnoses of *"prostate cancer"* (usually based on a biopsy).
Questions	When did the symptoms begin? (Usually a few months/years lead time). Which conflict is there with regard to manliness, sexual intercourse, eroticism? I want to, my partner doesn't? I am unable? Do I feel as old as the hills? Do I think that I am perverse? Do I believe that I'm not a good/real man? Do I condemn my sexual uniqueness? Am I worried about the development of my child? Do I feel like I failed as a parent? What conditioned me? (E.g., religious upbringing, father's style with regard to women/sexuality)? Did ancestors also have issues with their prostate? (Yes > work out the family issue) Do I identify too strongly with my gender? Who am I? What is the meaning of life?
Therapy	Determine the conflict, trigger(s) and conditioning and resolve it.
	Guiding principles: *"There are more important things than sex and sexual potency!" "I will no longer base my identity on that." "I will let go of this dependency." "I enjoy my freedom and my new quality of life." "What will count when it's all over?" "Bless you my child, in whichever direction your life develops."*
	CM: transurethral resection, (TUR) or prostate surgery (prostatectomy) often leads to impotence and incontinence. = New prostate conflict and possibly a worsening of the conflict. Local self-esteem conflicts affecting the pelvis. CM: "bone metastases."
	5 Biological Laws of Nature: TUR or surgery should never be performed due to elevated PSA levels or test-biopsy, but only if it is necessary to reduce symptoms (prolonged urinary retention).
	Prior to that, use natural resources (see p. 260f) and, if necessary, try CM, alpha blockers.
	Chemotherapy, radiation, and hormonal blockade therapy are not recommended.

Gonorrhea in men

Same SBS as above. Symptom is purulent discharge in the morning, some pus comes out before the first urine (= so-called "bonjour drip").

Phase	**Repair phase** or persistent repair: degradation of prostate tumor tissue, presence of pus in the urine; odorous, murky, possibly bloody urine, "bonjour drips," night sweats.
Note	Gonorrhea is only rarely diagnosed nowadays. This is due to effective prostate tumor treatments becoming more and more available. Thus, symptoms do not progress past prostatitis with purulent discharge. After a long, active, territorial-marking conflict, pus can be discharged during the repair phase if the connective tissue under the mucosa is also affected.
Therapy	The conflict is resolved. Support the healing. Colloidal silver internally. MMS or antibiotics if the repair phase is too intense. See remedies for the prostate below.

SBS of the Prostate Ducts

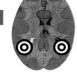

Urine retention without significantly high PSA values (intraductal prostatic cancer, prostatic intraepithelial neoplasia = PIN)

Conflict	Territorial-marking conflict with sexual aspect (= combination of prostate and bladder conflict).
Examples	• *A 60-year-old employee has a wife, who has never had much interest in sex. After the birth of their second child, she no longer wants sex at all = territorial-marking conflict with sexual aspect. Over the years, he suffers from worsening complications with urination = recurring-conflict in persistent repair > chronic repair-swelling of the prostatic excretory ducts. (Archive B. Eybl)* • *A patient's disapproves of the man his daughter married. However, the couple has a child to whom the patient feels very attached. Every time he and his wife want to visit their grandchild, their son-in-law thwarts their plans by taking the child away. Since then, he has suffered from urine retention = territorial-marking conflict with sexual aspect. (Archive B. Eybl)* • *A farmer's wife is 10 years younger than he is. Because he doesn't allow her to smoke in the house, she regularly visits the neighbor to smoke and drink coffee. During a visit to check on his wife, the farmer sees his wife sitting between the neighbor and his child all arm-in-arm. Although the situation was just an innocent coincidence, the farmer becomes suspicious and begins having problems urinating. When the couple is told what the cause is, the wife stops visiting the neighbor = territorial-marking conflict with sexual aspect. (See: Berger-Lenz, Ray, faktor-L, Neue Medizin, Band 1).*
Conflict-active	Slackening of the smooth ring-formed musculature in the prostatic excretory ducts. Later, cell degradation, usually unnoticed > widening of the lumen.
Bio. function	Increase in the diameter through broadening of the ring musculature > better flow > better discharge of prostatic secretions for territorial marking and for "courting." For the female, the musk odor is a sign of potency and readiness to mate.
Repair phase	Restoration of the urothelium, healing swelling, leading to urine retention, residual urine, for CM: "intraductal prostatic carcinoma (PIN)," = excessive degradation of urothelium. Most important indication: hardly or slightly raised PSA value. Often, a **recurring conflict.**
Therapy	If the condition does not improve, determine the conflict, trigger(s) and conditioning and resolve. See remedies for the prostate below.

Remedies for the prostate gland

• In the case of total blockage of the urethra with a backlog of urine, a catheter can bring relief until the swelling decreases. Urine retention will cease when the conflict has been definitely and permanently resolved.

• Yam roots (natural progesterone), linseed oil, pomegranate, saw palmetto, frankincense, stinging nettle preparations.

- For inflammation: enzyme preparations (for example "Wobenzym"), Schuessler Cell Salt no. 3.
- Hildegard of Bingen: mugwort (Tanecetum vulgaris) elixir special recipe.
- Cod liver oil.
- Selenium, zinc, coenzyme Q10, vitamin B6, C, E.
- Cayce: regular classic massage of the pelvis and legs with peanut oil and olive oil, mixed 1:1, chiropractic.
- Alkaline foods, especially pumpkin/squash, pumpkin seeds, asparagus, oysters, soy, tomatoes (ingredient: lycopene).
- Tea: boxberry (Gaultheria procumbens), fireweed, bearberry, stinging nettle leaf and root, green tea.
- Anti-inflammatory, muscle-relaxing medication (alpha blocker), if needed.

- A transurethral resection of the prostate (TURP) should only be considered if the urethra is permanently blocked due to a backlog of residual urine in the bladder or renal pelvis = recurring-conflict or persistent repair.
- The conventional practice of administering hormone blocking drugs to inhibit testosterone after an surgery is senseless and has many side effects > not recommended. This practice is based on the false assumption that a high testosterone level contributes to carcinoma growth. The fact is that only the PSA value correlates with the testosterone level.
It is advisable to have a blood-hormone analysis done a few weeks after the surgery. If there is a hormone deficiency, the intake of natural progesterone and possibly testosterone would make sense (bioidentical hormones).

PENIS

Basically, the penis can be divided into root, penile shaft and the glans penis. The mesodermal cavernous bodies (two larger ones on the side and a smaller one below containing the urethra) cause erection.
The foreskin (preputium) constitutes a doubling of the shaft skin in the form of two leaves of skin. The inner leaf holds endodermal glands, which produce a sebaceous lubricant (smegma). The penile shaft and glans penis are covered with ectodermal squamous epithelium, as well as the urethra (urothelium).

Penile, Glans Epidermis
Separation conflict

Cavernous Body,
Subcutis,
Penile Frenulum
Local self-esteem conflict

Penile Dermis
Disfigurement or defilement conflict

Sebaceous Glands
Conflict, that the vagina is too dry

Urethra
Territorial-marking conflict

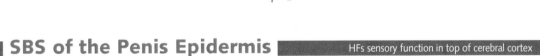

SBS of the Penis Epidermis

HFs sensory function in top of cerebral cortex

ECTO

Genital herpes (herpes on the penis or testicles), inflammation of the foreskin (posthitis), inflammation of the glans penis (balanitis), genital warts (Condylomata acuminata), pearly penile papules (hirsuties coronae glandis)

Conflict	Separation conflict - wanting or not wanting contact with/on the penis.
Examples	➜ *A man wants to have sexual intercourse several times a week. However, his wife doesn't cooperate = separation conflict of not getting the skin contact one wants.*
	➜ *A man wants oral gratification from his partner but she is against it out of principle = separation conflict.*
	➜ *A man does not want sexual intercourse or he wants another kind of sex = separation conflict - not wanting to have skin contact with the penis.*

-+

	Conflict-active	Local cell degradation from the epithelium of the prepuce or glans penis; pale and possibly numb skin (usually unnoticed).
	Bio. function	Reduced sensibility that temporarily leads to a lack of desire for direct contact.
	Repair phase	Restoration of the epithelial tissue = "genital herpes," actually penile epithelial cancer, inflammation of the prepuce and glans penis, pain, reddening, swelling. **Persistent repair** or **recurring conflict**: Genital warts on the penile shaft or on the prepuce or "pearly penile papules" on the lower edge of the penis = local excessive growth of epithelium.
	Questions	When did the inflammation/symptoms begin? (The conflict must have been resolved before that). Warts since when? (Conflict before, this continues to this day it "recurs"). With what am I sexually unsatisfied? (Too little contact, too much contact, another woman, other practices)? How was the first sexual relationship? Did it work or not? What conditioned me aside from that? (Try to get a sense/ask about the sexual needs of the ancestors) Did a religious upbringing play a role? (Negative connotation to sexuality)? Have I spoken about it with my partner? (Resolution through vocalizing the taboo issue).
	Therapy	In case of inflammation: the conflict is resolved. Support the healing process. For genital warts, "pearly penile papules:" determine the conflict and/or trigger(s) and, if possible resolve them in real life, so that the persistent repair comes to an end. Open your heart and discuss the conflict honestly. Meditate on the meaning of eroticism. Colloidal silver, DMSO externally. Under certain circumstances, surgical removal.

Chancroid (ulcus molle) in men

Same SBS as above. Symptom: small, sometimes painful skin ulcers on the penis.

Conflict-active   Degradation of epithelium, local loss of substance without pain = ulcer.

Repair phase   Restoration of the epithelial tissue with pain.

Therapy   Questions: see above. Determine the conflicts and/or trigger(s) and, if possible, resolve them in real life if they are still active.

Syphilis (lues)

Same SBS as above. In CM, syphilis is seen as an infectious disease that advances in three stages (lues I-III). As a matter of fact, the different lues stages are a collection of various SBS: pain in the head and limbs, swollen lymph nodes, hair loss, diseases of the stomach, liver, spleen, kidney, nerves, etc. First-stage of syphilis symptoms: Painless ulcer on the outer genitals. The tissue defects heal leaving hardened scars, which leads to the term "hard chancre".

Phase   **Recurring-conflict,** thus hard scars.

Therapy   Determine the conflict and/or trigger(s) and, if possible, resolve them in real life so that the persistent repair comes to an end. Questions: see above.

SBS of the Penis Dermis   HFs in the cerebellum - topography still unknown

Penile melanoma

	Conflict	Disfigurement/attack/defilement, violation of integrity with regard to the penis.
	Examples	→ *A man finds sexual intercourse or certain sexual practices disgusting.*
		→ *Can also be experienced as a substitute for another person: a father is disgusted by the thought of the sexual practices of his homosexual son.*
		→ *Verbal attack on the penis or on a man's qualities as a lover.*
	Conflict-active	Cell proliferation local to the penis, growth of a melanoma.
	Bio. function	Strengthening and thickening of the dermis so that the individual is protected better from disfigurement and deformation.
	Repair phase	Caseating degradation of the melanoma.

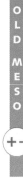

Therapy	If the melanoma bleeds, the conflict is at least partially or temporarily resolved. If it grows imperceptibly, the conflict is active. Determine the conflict and conditioning and, if possible, resolve them. Hydrogen peroxide (H_2O_2) externally. If necessary, black salve or surgery. See also: chapter on skin, p. 278ff.

SBS of the Penile Connective Tissue

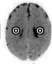

N
E
W

M
E
S
O

−+

Constriction of the foreskin (phimosis), short frenulum (frenulum breve)

Conflict	Self-esteem conflict with relation to the foreskin or penis. Deeper cause: This symptom is usually worn by children on behalf of someone in the family to hide their masculinity. May not be or want to be a man. (For example, in the family, men are rejected or vilified). Similar conflict as with undescended testicles > often both symptoms occur at the same time.
	According to Frauenkron-Hoffmann: "Sex may not be pleasurable," or a woman did not want to become pregnant.
Examples	• *A grandmother and her daughter are single parents and resent men, blaming them for all their ills. The only son has a constriction of the foreskin. = Substitution conflict: To be loved he "holds his manhood back."* (Archive B. Eybl)
• *The father of a boy, who is affected by a constricted foreskin, lived in a family dominated by women: his father (the grandfather) died young and he had a domineering mother and dominant sister. = The boy carries the conflict for his father: "I am not allowed to be a man."* (Archive B. Eybl)
Conflict-active	Degradation of cells from the collagenous and elastic fibers. Shrinkage due to a persistent conflict. > Constriction of the foreskin, shortening of the frenulum.
Bio. function	Reflecting the family energy outward to bring the issue to the attention of the family.
Repair phase	Restoration, i.e., dilation of the foreskin without surgery is realistic if the conflict is resolved.
Questions	What is the manhood situation in the family? Do the women dominate? Where is the man? Does he influence family life? (Time, interest)? Does he lack the will to make his presence felt?
Therapy	Determine the conflict and conditioning and, if possible, resolve them. Man! Don't be a coward! Mars meditation. Any surgery should be delayed as long as possible (is more tolerable later). This also increases the chances that the constriction of the foreskin repairs itself through conflict resolution.

Peyronie's disease (induratio penis plastica), deformation of the penis (penis deviation)

Conflict	Self-esteem conflict regarding the penis.
Examples	→ *A late-developing boy is teased about his penis.* → *A man has potency problems.*
→ *A man suffers a painful and embarrassing kinking of the penis during sexual intercourse.*
Conflict-active	Cell degradation from the cavernous bodies or other mesodermal part(s) of the penis.
Phase	**Persistent repair or condition thereafter:** restoration of the lost substance, possibly with excessive tissue growth; formation of flat, longish plaques; shrinkage; hardening; hour-glass-shaped constrictions; bottle-shaped narrowings in the area of the cavernous bodies, as well as penis deformations.
Bio. function	Strengthening of the affected structures. (Deformations indicate an unnaturally long conflict duration).
Note	According to the literature, patients with this disease pattern are at an increased risk of developing a prostate carcinoma. This is understandable from the point of view of the 5 Biological Laws of Nature, because a malformed penis brings ugly-genital conflicts along with it.
Questions	Did something happen during intercourse? A disparaging remark? Self-doubt? Why do I identify myself so strongly with my penis? (The fact of the matter is: For women, the penis is usually a secondary attribute at best. Being a good partner is more important to women). Is there a background of insecurity? What were my ancestors like?
Therapy	Determine the conflict and conditioning and, if possible, resolve them. OP if necessary.

SBS of the Sebaceous Glands

Inflammation of the prepuce II (inflammation of the smegma-producing glands)[1]

The smegma-producing glands lie on the inner side of the prepuce (foreskin) and secrete a whitish-yellow sebaceous substance (= lubricant and scent).

Conflict	Chunk conflict (p. 15, 16), that the vagina one wants to penetrate is too dry. Problems during intercourse.
Examples	→ *A man cannot enjoy sexual intercourse, because the vagina is too dry.* → *Wanting to have sex with a woman, but not being allowed to.*
Conflict-active	Increase in function, growth of the preputial glands and increased smegma production.
Bio. function	Increased lubrication facilitates the penis' entry into the vagina.
Repair phase	Tubercular-caseating degradation of excess cellular material, glandular inflammation of the prepuce, pain, swelling, reddening, probably often diagnosed as "inflammation of the foreskin."
Questions	Inflammation since when? (A related stress must have been resolved before this). First occurrence of symptoms? (No > find the first conflict). How was the first sexual contact? (Complications, disappointment)? Does sexuality have a negative connotation? (Something indecent, forbidden)? In a child: Did the father have difficulties during intercourse or problems related to sexuality? > Schedule/include parents in the therapy.
Therapy	The conflict is resolved. Support the healing. If it recurs, determine the conflict and/or trigger(s) and resolve them. Pay attention to the needs and desires of the woman, so that she also feels pleasure. If needed, use a lubricant. Colloidal silver internally and externally. If applicable, MMS or antibiotics.

1   See Dr. Hamer, Charts p. 29

Potency disturbances (erectile dysfunction), reduced sex drive, male sterility

Possible causes

- **Medication poisoning:** Antihypertensives, psychopharmaceuticals, anti-cholesterol medications and many more particularly disturb the interaction of the autonomic nervous system > potency problems.
- **Continuous-sympatheticotonia** due to stress (one or more active conflicts or tracks): Sexual desire is pre-requisite to having an erection. Desire only comes during relaxation (vagotonia).
- **Territory conflict or constellation:** "Feminization" due to the switch from the right "masculine" side of the brain to the "feminine" left side of the brain > potency problems or homosexuality (see p. 124f).
- **Testicles** in persistent-conflict activity > reduced production of testosterone > reduced sex drive > potency problems (see p. 255f).
- **Self-esteem conflict** in the conflict-active phase: reduced self-esteem, low energy levels > potency problems (see p. 287ff).
- **Pituitary gland** in the conflict-active phase: increased production of prolactin > potency problems (see p. 113).

Undersized penis (micropenis)

Possible causes (if not just imagined)

- **Self-esteem conflict with regard to the penis** in adolescence (CM: "idiopathic micropenis"). For example, derogatory notes about the appearance or size of the penis, possibly perceived vicariously = local self-esteem conflict: *"I am not worth anything here!"* > persistent conflict activity - cell degradation or ceased growth in the mesenchymal penis tissue.
- **Cerebral cortex constellation** during adolescence > general developmental delay with postponed and inadequate development of the reproductive organs (see p. 314f).
- **Testicles** in persistent repair during adolescence > reduced production of testosterone > underdevelopment of the male sex organs (see p. 255f).
- **Not enough growth hormone** (somatotropin) during the growth phase (see p. 114).
- **In the case of children, always think of the family**: Possibly men are despised in the family or treated badly. In this case, the child is carrying the symptom for the family. *"If I must be a man, then only with a small penis."* If the adults change, reconcile > the child no longer needs to carry anything, can change naturally and return to "normal."

BREAST

The female breast is, in principle, a protrusion of the skin over the pectoral muscles. Old-mesodermal mammary glands are found embedded in fatty tissue. These evolved from the sweat glands over the course of our developmental history.

The milk (lactiferous) ducts are lined with ectodermal epithelium, which migrated from the outer skin. They guide milk from the lobe of the breast to the nipple.

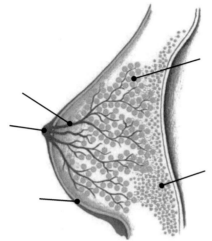

Mammary Gland
Excretory Ducts
Separation conflict

Mammary Glands
**Worry, fight or
nest conflict**

Epidermis, Nipples
Separation conflict

Lymph Nodes
Self-esteem conflict

Dermis
**Disfigurement
conflict**

Breast cancer (mammary carcinoma, inflammatory breast cancer = IBC)

There are two different types of breast cancer. The name "breast cancer" says nothing about which type is meant. About 80% of the time, the milk ducts are affected; in the other 20% the mammary glands are.

SBS of the Mammary Glands

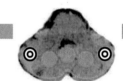

Cancer of the mammary glands (adeno-ca, lobular breast cancer, lobular carcinoma in situ = LCIS)[1]

Conflict	Right-handed woman, left breast: worry or fight conflict with regard to the mother-child or "nest"; right breast: worry or fight conflict with regard to the partner. Left-handed woman: inverse. Further possibilities: Conflict in relation to being able to feed, give, be there for someone. Nest conflict: The home is in danger, one fears for one's house or apartment, fighting in or about the house or apartment.
Examples	• A 43-year-old, left-handed woman is blamed by her daughter for having destroyed her marriage = mother-child fight conflict. A tumor of the right breast develops. (Archive B. Eybl)
• A right-handed woman embarks on a week-long vacation with friends, while her ex-husband cares for their epileptic daughter. On the very first day of the vacation, she receives a phone call from home: her ex-husband reports that their daughter has had a severe epileptic fit and is currently in the hospital. He blames his ex-wife (the patient) for not being there. She wants to fly back to her daughter right away but is unable to book a flight = mother-child worry conflict - one week of very strong conflict activity. A breast-gland tumor develops in the left breast. In the following years, the patient remains mildly conflict-active because she is expecting another fit at any time. Not until the daughter has been stable for several years does she come into healing: the patient sweats at night, the breast reddens, swells up and after six weeks breaks open and gives off stinking pus. (Archive B. Eybl)
• A woman moves to a large city in a colder climate for her education where she has to accept living

---

1   See Dr. Hamer, Charts pp. 45 ff, 50 ff

O L D M E S O

(+−)

in a dark, inner-courtyard apartment. Accustomed to a sunny climate, she is unhappy in the apartment and longs for life-giving sunlight. She comes to the conclusion that "everything is so dark in this land" = nest conflict. To relieve her distress, she moves her bed right up to the window so she can "catch" a little light. Subsequently, she is diagnosed with breast gland cancer. (Archive Antje Scherret)
• *A 44-year-old has a pubescent daughter who is driving her crazy. They are constantly arguing - it has even gotten to the point where they avoid each other = mother-child fight conflict. A tumor develops in a breast gland. As their relationship suddenly improves, the tumor comes into healing.* (Archive B. Eybl)
• *A 65-year-old, right-handed patient takes care of her granddaughter during the day. One summer day, she holds a children's party in the garden and the patient's dog joins in. In their excitement, the children come up with the idea of riding the dog. The dog does not like the idea and bites one of the children. The wound is not serious, but at the hospital, charges are brought against the dog's owner. The patient is afraid that she will have to give up her beloved dog = mother-child worry conflict involving a dog. A breast gland tumor develops. When the charges are dropped, she comes into healing and is diagnosed with a mammary gland cancer.* (Archive B. Eybl)

Conflict-active	Cell division in the mammary gland tissue, growth of one or more nodes (= adeno-ca); the longer and more intense the conflict is, the larger the tumor grows. If a tissue sample is taken during the growth, medicinal practitioners will speak of *"malignant cancer."* If one does not find an above average rate of cell division (= resolved conflict) under the microscope, the diagnosis may be "benign." In the conflict active phase, there is a tendency to be over-caring/over-protective and to "hover." Often a recurring-conflict.
Bio. function	With more mammary gland tissue, more milk can be produced. With the extra food supply, the child or family member can heal faster. One can feed and give more.
Repair phase	Caseating, tubercular degradation if bacteria are present; the cell remnants are eliminated over the lymph system. Although the tumor is no longer growing, the breast swells up at the beginning of the repair phase because of the increased metabolism. Pain, night sweats, possibly slight fever; only later in the process do the nodes and breast feel smaller. Especially strong swelling caused by syndrome > danger of panic, if no bacteria are available, the tumor will be encapsulated and separated from the body's metabolism (CM: "benign"); the tumor remains but is no longer malignant.
Repair crisis	Chills or a feeling of being cold, severe pain.
Note	The tumor can break open externally if, due to the tumor or puncture, the woman has also suffered a disfigurement conflict affecting the dermis or in the case of a superficially located tumor, the skin no longer can hold up to the pressure > bloody, oozing, stinking, degradation of the tumor outwardly (= open breast tuberculosis). An external eruption may cause a vicious conflict circle. Consider "handedness" (right or left) and side (mother/child or partner) or local conflict.
Questions	First, determine if the mammary glands or lactiferous ducts are affected. (Medical history, touch and visual findings, x-ray, CT, biopsy). Study the findings, but keep in mind that CM often misses the mark. (Absurd diagnoses like "ductal-adenoidal mammary carcinoma" are not so rare). Was/is the nipple drawn-in? (Yes > sure indication for lactiferous ducts. No > indication for mammary glands). "Micro calcifications" in the findings? (Indication of lactiferous ducts). The nearer the nodes are to the nipple, the more likely that it is the lactiferous ducts. Reddening of the skin or nipple? (Yes > indication for lactiferous ducts) Are the nodes painful/hot/reddened? (Yes > indication of the repair phase of both SBSs). When was the last examination? (Good possibility that the conflict is located within this time frame). Open ulcerations on the breast? (Yes > persistent conflict, both SBSs come into question). Nodes tangible since when? (Conflict considerably earlier - take the development time into account). General sign of conflict activity during the growth of the node(s)? (Waking up early in the morning, poor sleep, weight loss, stress, no night sweats)? Yes > indication for mammary glands. General repair phase signs during the node-growth phase? (Good sleep, cheerful emotionally, good appetite, light night sweats? Yes > Indication for lactiferous ducts). If we now know that we are dealing with an SBS of the mammary glands, perform the clap test. Which worry, fight or nest conflict was there? Who was I unable to feed anymore? What stressed me? What was I constantly thinking about? Why can't I deal with the issue? What has conditioned me? Did ancestors suffer from breast cancer? (Yes > work out any similar character traits/family issues). Which beliefs fed the conflict? (Beliefs that kept me from dealing with/resolving the conflict = disease-causing beliefs)? Would a conversation/discussion to clarify the issue be helpful? (E.g., with the person the conflict is centered around)? Which new inner attitudes would ease my mind? What can I change on the outside?

Therapy	Determine the conflict and conditioning and, if possible, resolve them in real life should they still be active. Guiding principles: *"Don't worry, live!" "My worries won't help anyone!" "I am not responsible for everyone. Destiny knows what's best." "Life is too precious to spend it bickering over trifles."* Surgery - yes or no? If the tumor is too large, it is doubtful whether the patient will be able to survive a long-lasting breast-tuberculosis. For this reason, surgery is recommended. The doctor should use care, to only remove the tumor, leaving the lymph nodes in place.
	Caution: After the OP (disfigurement of the breast), the patient often suffers from a self-esteem conflict in the repair phase. > Growth of breast-lymph nodes > danger of a vicious circle if an understanding of the correlations is lacking. Here too, surgery may be advisable.
	If applicable, instead of surgery, black salve is an option for people who have a high tolerance for pain and very strong nerves (order at www.cernamast.eu).
	CM: chemotherapy and anti-hormone therapy (anti-estrogen or aromatase inhibitors) are not recommended, because of adverse side effects. See also: remedies for the breast on p. 270.

Side bar: O L D · M E S O · +−

Adhesions on the breast glands (sclerosing adenosis, fibroadenoma)

Same SBS as above.

Phase	**Condition following the repair phase** or following reoccurrences = scarred remnant of a healed breast gland tumor.
Therapy	The conflict is resolved. If the breast continues to change, this means that the conflict has not been conclusively resolved. > Need for therapy: questions, conflict resolution (see above), OP as necessary.
	Gentle massages or lymph drainage massages with marigold salve, so that the tissue becomes smooth and supple again. Daily morning ritual by Anton Styger (see p. 68).

SBS of the Lactiferous Ducts   HFs sensory function in top of cerebral cortex

Intraductal cancer (ductal carcinoma in situ = DCIS, lobular cancer in situ = LCIS, invasive lobular cancer, ductal hyperplasia, papillary adenoma, Paget's disease)[1]

Conflict	1. Right-handed woman, left breast: separation conflict related to mother/child; right breast: separation conflict related to partner. Left-handed woman: inverse, i.e., conflicts are reversed. Mother/child or partner has pulled away from the breast. 2. One feels "sucked dry." Mother/child or partner is too demanding - one's own energies are dwindling. One can't go on anymore. Note: This conflict possibility corresponds with the separation conflict of undesired skin contact (wanting to be separated from someone).
Examples	➔ A woman's daughter moves to a city far away. ➔ A woman finds out that her partner is unfaithful.
	• A left-handed, happily-married woman has a son, whom she loves above all else. At the beginning of his studies, he is still living at home with his parents. She is severely affected by his announcement that he plans to move into his own apartment. She never imagined that he would leave so quickly. For her, he was always her "little boy" = conflict that her son is being pulled away from her breast > unnoticed cell degradation in the lactiferous ducts in the active-phase. One day, after the patient has accepted that her son's leaving is a positive and normal development, she notices a lump in her right mother-child breast. CM: invasive ductal carcinoma. (See Claudio Trupiano, thanks to Dr. Hamer, p. 298)
	• A 39-year-old, right-handed patient has a number of fierce disagreements with her husband about his ex-wife. In her opinion, he is too friendly and cooperative toward her = partner-separation conflict affecting the lactiferous ducts of the right breast > cell degradation in the active-phase, restoration (= intraductal cancer) in the repair phase. (Archive B. Eybl)
	• A 41-year-old, childless, right-handed patient has a dog named Benni whom she loves very much. She makes it clear to her mother, who lives on a farm, that she mustn't lay out any rat poison because

Side bar: E C T O · −+

---

1   See Dr. Hamer, Charts pp. 120, 133

that could endanger Benni. Her mother ignores her warnings and misfortune strikes: Benni eats the poison and dies. Her pet-child is "pulled away from the breast." She doesn't want to talk about it to anyone, because Benni was "just a dog" > cell degradation in the active-phase. Not until a year later, does the patient recover from the incident. In the repair phase, she notices a white lesion on the left nipple. A 2x2x4 cm lump develops in the lactiferous ducts. The patient is relieved as she learns about the causal relationships and refuses CM-treatment. Within a year, the lump is almost gone. (Archive B. Eybl)

• A 42-year-old, right-handed married patient, mother of two children, has a husband who is very much under his mother's influence. The patient's mother-in-law tries to pull the two children onto her side and this has nearly ruined their marriage. On Christmas, her husband takes the children "for a quick visit" to his parents. However, he and the children stay and celebrate with the mother-in-law = mother-child separation conflict - the children are "torn from her breast." (Archive B. Eybl)

Conflict-active	Limited sensibility = numbness (usually unnoticed). Simultaneous slackening of the lactiferous duct's ring musculature. Later, epithelial cell degradation in the lactiferous ducts (ulcer) > increase in lumen. With longer conflict activity, the lactiferous ducts shrink up painfully. The nipple or the affected spot is pulled inwards (so-called "inverted nipple," CM: cirrhotic lactiferous duct ulcer). After longer conflict activity and if many lactiferous ducts are affected, the breast can become smaller as a whole. Possibly a recurring conflict.
Bio. function	1. Through the numbness, the separation is easier to forget. It no longer feels so strong. 2. Expansion of the lactiferous ducts, so that the milk does not become blocked and can drip out by itself, because, due to the separation, the child or family member cannot drink the milk.
Repair phase	Restoration of the epithelial mucosa (= CM: "intraductal mammary cancer," periductal mastitis), swelling, itching, pain. In this SBS, the outer skin often reacts with a reddening of the breast in the repair phase. Secretions (bloody or clear) build up in the milk ducts due to increased metabolism. However, since the milk ducts are swollen closed, the fluid can back up behind the nipple, especially with an active kidney collecting tubules SBS = syndrome. After the completion of the repair phase, the breast shrinks, dimpling and hardenings and (micro) calcifications possibly remain. The nipple usually stays inverted.
Repair crisis	Feeling cold, possibly chills, and severe pain. Possibly blood/secretions leaking from the nipple.
Note	Cancer of the nipple is called "Paget's disease" in CM. Tissue-wise, they belong to the lactiferous ducts = same SBS. Consider "handedness" (right or left) and side (mother/child or partner) or local conflict.
Questions	Determine which breast SBS, see p. 265ff and 267f. Nipple inverted? (Yes > indication of an extended active conflict). Nodes since when? (= Start of the repair phase or the start of a chronic process). Has the breast changed unpleasantly? (= Indication of a recurring conflict). Clap test/handedness? Who was torn from my breast or from whom do I feel "sucked dry?" (E.g., by my child, partner)? Why do I react so sensitively? Who/what has conditioned me when it comes to separation/distance? (E.g., parents' divorce, death of a sibling)? How was my birth? Was I with my mother? Was I a planned child? Am I similar to one of my parents? (Work out family issue(s)). Breast cancer in the family? Which mediation/which guiding principle would be helpful? What else do I want to change inside? What outside?
Therapy	The conflict is resolved. Support the healing process. Determine the conflict and conditioning if still active. Guiding principles: *"I love you, and that is why I am letting you go." "I am setting you free."* For a blockage: Somebody (partner, child) should suck out the secretion orally, like a baby.
	Surgery if the tumor becomes too large due to recurrences. Remove only small areas (not too far into the healthy tissue). Caution: The surgery is often followed by a breast self-esteem conflict in healing > growth of breast-lymph nodes > danger of a vicious circle, if the interrelationships are not understood. Anti-hormone therapy (anti-estrogen or aromatase inhibitors) is not recommended because of the numerous side effects. See remedies for the breast p. 270.

Small calcifications in the breast (micro calcifications)

Same SBS as above. Calcifications, often only pin-sized, are sometimes found in the mammography and are seen as possible "signs of cancer." Calcifications also remain after breast gland tuberculosis.

Phase	Condition **after the repair phase**. Completed and finished or recurring lactiferous ducts SBS. In principle, after the healing swelling or scarring in the lactiferous ducts, this is "left-over," calcified milk.
Therapy	The conflict is resolved. No further measures needed, except - prevent recurrences!

SBS of the Breast Dermis

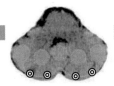

Melanoma on the breast

Conflict	Disfigurement conflict: the feeling that the breast is disfigured, violation of integrity.
Examples	• *A breast cancer patient feels disfigured because of the tumor in her breast. A widespread melanoma develops. Note: very common follow-up conflict, interpreted by CM, as "metastases" > danger of a vicious circle. (Archive B. Eybl)* • *A woman has recently weaned her third child from the breast. One day, as she is sitting alone in bed, she notices her limp, drooping bosom and has feelings of anxiety = disfigurement conflict with regard to the dermis. At the spot she finds especially unattractive, she develops a 5 mm melanoma = growth in the conflict-active state. (Archive B. Eybl)*
Conflict-active	Cell division in the dermis, growth of a melanoma = common follow-up conflict to breast cancer.
Bio. function	Strengthening as protection from disfigurements or damages to integrity.
Repair phase	Caseating degradation via bacteria (mycobacteria), or bacteria.
Questions	In the case of small melanomas, one sometimes doesn't find the cause (minimal limit). Since when has it been growing? (Conflict time frame). Is it bleeding while degrading? (No > indication of an active conflict). By what do I feel attacked/injured? (Breast cancer, real blow, groped, harmful words)? Is this why I'm upset? (Yes > OP). Which new attitude would be helpful? (E.g., to develop a healthy robustness)?
Therapy	Determine the conflict and conditioning and, if possible, resolve them in real life if still active. Doing nothing is possible with small melanomas when the patient has no fear whatsoever. If the patient thinks about it constantly, one should have it removed for the purpose of minimizing risk. If necessary, black salve or surgery (see p. 278).

O L D M E S O
+−

SBS of the Microvascular Musculature

Vasospasm of the arterioles (Raynaud's phenomenon of the nipple)

Symptoms: Severe, pulling-stabbing pains in the nipple, most often in breast-feeding mothers, but also often continuing after breast-feeding has ended. The nipple is pale/blue and sensitive to cold. Most of the affected also suffer from Raynaud symptoms somewhere else on their body (see p. 142). At the beginning of the illness, the symptoms are often difficult to differentiate from a nipple inflammation (thelitis, mastitis).

Conflict	Not wanting to come in contact with/get close to death or a dead body. The situation must have a connection to conception, pregnancy, nursing, offspring or the family.
Example	• The breast-feeding mother suffers from Raynaud's phenomenon of the nipples. *During the pregnancy, a close relative died, but the young woman didn't want to hear anything about it. She repressed the death itself and didn't go to the funeral. Conflict that she doesn't want to come into contact with the death. (Archive B. Eybl)*
Phase	Persistent **active conflict.** Tension in the vascular musculature > insufficient oxygen supply to the nipple > white discoloration, pain during sympathicotonia.
Questions	When did the symptoms begin? Experience with dead people/animals during or before the pregnancy? How did I deal with it? Are there repressed corpse experiences among the ancestors? (Ask the parents, look for conditioning). Beliefs with regard to death/dying? (E.g., "death is something dreadful").
Therapy	Determine and resolve the conflict, beliefs and conditioning. Heat treatments (hot showers/baths, hot water bottles, warm wraps). Guiding principle: *"I acknowledge what was and I make my peace with it completely."* Healing conversation. Farewell ritual. Come to terms with death.

E N D O
+−

Inflammation of the breast glands (mastitis), inflammation of the nipple (thelitis)

Both SBSs come into question. The condition usually appears during the postpartum period (mastitis puerperalis). Both inflammation of the mammary glands, as well as inflammation of the nipples or milk ducts, are called mastitis by CM.

Example	→ *The baby is born healthy and is nursing well. The worries of pregnancy have all been forgotten = beginning of the repair phase > inflamed breast gland or nipple.*
Phase	**Repair phase** of both SBSs in question.
Note	An inflamed nipple can also have a mechanical cause, e.g., if the infant sucks too vigorously.
Therapy	The conflict is resolved. Support the healing. Avoid recurrences. See remedies for the breast below.

Shape changes of the breast

Lumps
- Milk glands in the active-phase or repair phase.
- Excretory ducts in the repair phase.
- Active kidney collecting tubules SBS can cause old lumps to be "pumped up" again, giving the false impression that a new SBS of the breast is underway.

Skin indentations or inverted nipples
- Mammary ducts in active-conflict or following recurrences.

Sagging breasts
- In women with generally weak connective tissue, the breasts drop in early years, because the collagenous fibers are soon thinned out = indication of reduced self-confidence (mild general self-esteem conflict). Usually the low self-esteem and "weak connective tissue" is passed down over several generations.

- In women with normal to good connective tissue, sagging breasts can come from an SBS of the lactiferous ducts, if previously full lumps collapse after dissolving.
- If a woman has firm breasts due to an active refugee conflict, the breasts will collapse after the resolution of the conflict > Good sign! Indicated by fluid loss, weight loss, night sweats.

Firm breasts
- Active kidney collecting tubules SBS can provide attractively firm breasts. Disadvantages: This is usually accompanied by becoming overweight, edema, and fat deposits due to a refugee conflict. If the conflict is resolved, the breasts usually shrink and appear relatively less attractive.

Remedies for the breasts
- Bach flowers: red chestnut, chicory, willow.
- Teas: tea or tea compresses: marigold, yarrow, fennel, chamomile, comfrey, yellow meliot.
- Schuessler Cell Salts: No. 3, 11, 12.
- Enzyme preparations for inflamed breasts.
- Lymph drainage massages, gentle massages.
- For an open wound on the breast: Apply honey, change wound compresses regularly.
- Beat curly-leaf cabbage and white cabbage until soft and apply regularly.
- A silver activated charcoal bandage is useful against the unpleasant odors of tuberculosis.
- Hydrogen peroxide (H_2O_2) internally and externally.

SKIN, HAIR AND NAILS

The skin (cutis) connects us with our surroundings and protects us from them at the same time. The ectodermal outer-skin (epidermis), including hair, has a connecting function. The mesodermal dermis (corium) of the cerebellum has a protective function. Under the dermis, lies the mesodermal, subcutaneous tissue = connective tissue and fat layer.

From the viewpoint of the 5 Biological Laws of Nature, the skin is a very "forgiving" organ if one works precisely.
The location of any skin problem always plays a role. Nothing appears where it does by chance - it is important to find out exactly what happened at the location.

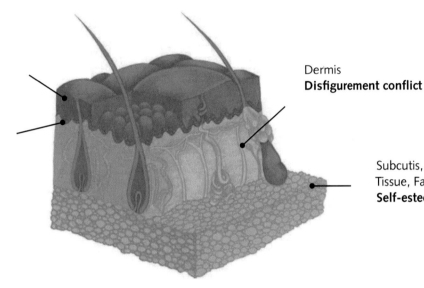

Epidermis, Hair
Separation conflict

Deep Epidermis
(dermis side)
Intense-separation conflict

Dermis
Disfigurement conflict

Subcutis, Connective Tissue, Fatty Tissue
Self-esteem conflict

SBS of the Skin Epidermis

HFs sensory function (foot) - top of cerebral cortex

Skin rash (exanthema), inflammation of the epidermis (neurodermatitis), eczema, efflorescence, erythema, hives (urticaria), pemphigus, erysipelas, lupus erythematodes, squamous cell cancer, basal cell cancer (basalioma)[1]

Conflict	Separation conflict - wanting or not wanting to have skin contact. 1. Separation conflict in the sense of "wanting to have contact": contact is broken off or one loses contact with a beloved person or pet, being abandoned; sometimes also not noticing a danger, not being able to feel something. Affected are the inner surfaces of body parts (yin meridian): the inner sides of the belly, breast, arm, leg. We embrace with the inner sides of the arms and legs. We make skin contact with the belly or breast if we like someone. 2. Separation conflict in the sense of "not-wanting-contact": Someone is closer than they have the right to be. Affected are the outer surfaces (yang meridian) of the back, buttocks, arms and legs, as well as the elbows, wrists, knee joints and the outer sides of the ankle joints. With the elbow, fist, shinbone, or knee, we shove away unwanted persons or things. Separation conflicts with regard to the head or face are related to missing the caresses of mother or father (typical mother-child touching). Also consider local conflicts: Many skin symptoms have no mother/child or partner reference, but are located precisely where something conflictive/unpleasant happened.
Examples	• *At 19, a, now, 53-year-old patient lost her "partner of a lifetime," a musician who left to travel. Instead of leaving with him, she stayed at home to help take care of her three young siblings because her mother was gravely-ill and unable to take care of them herself = separation conflict. Epidermal cell degradation in the active-phase. Not until some years later does she come into healing.*

ECTO

---

1 See Dr. Hamer, Charts pp. 118, 131

A neurodermatitis appears all over her body (restoration of the epidermis) = two separation conflicts simultaneously: one affecting the inner surfaces as a result of coping with the loss of this loved one and one affecting the outer surfaces as a result of her desire to abandon her siblings and pursue the boyfriend. (Archive B. Eybl)

• *A child suffers a separation conflict because his single mother has found a new partner and he may no longer sleep in the same bed with his mother. (Archive B. Eybl)*

• *At a patient's workplace, coworkers greet one another by shaking hands. However, one employee does not wash his hands and due to this, the patient refuses to make contact with him = separation conflict in the sense of "not wanting to have contact." As he changes jobs and is no longer obligated to shake the colleague's hand, he comes into healing (= skin rash). The affected area is the back of the right hand, which he uses to shake hands. (See www.germanische-heilkunde)*

• *A mother, with a 4-year-old daughter, returns to work after six-months of maternity leave. She works 20 hours a week, and the child spends two and a half days a week with her grandmother. The child misses her mother = separation conflict that causes her to suffer from neurodermatitis. The whole family, including the grandmother, then spend a week on vacation. For the first few days, the rash is worse than ever before = repair phase. Towards the end of the vacation, however, the daughter's skin becomes wonderfully smooth and healthy = complete healing. Unfortunately, the mother returns to work after the vacation and cycle repeats. (Archive B. Eybl)*

• *Three weeks ago, an intelligent, right-handed, 16-year-old schoolgirl contracts a rash, first on her left ankle, then on the right. When she is asked whether she has had a separation conflict with her mother, her two pet cats or with somebody else, she says no. When asked if something related to her shoes or feet had occurred, she immediately remembers the following: three weeks ago she wore high-heeled shoes for the first time for an outing, which she enjoyed = separation conflict in healing. Recommended therapy: Do not take such events seriously. If that doesn't work, she should wear high heels as often as she pleases. (Archive B. Eybl)*

• *In her childhood, a 39-year-old, childless, right-handed patient was beaten by her mother, and her relationship with her mother has not improved. At 25, she broke off contact with her mother in order to protect herself. Recently, her mother contacts her and they meet for the first time in years. The patient considers reconciliation, but struggles with feelings of resentment = separation conflict of not wanting to have contact. A specific incident: She is sitting on a park bench when her mother happens to walk by - she hides her face so that her mother will not recognize her. She is in persistent repair and within a year, three epithelial cancers (CM: "superficially spreading cancer") develop on the outer sides of her lower leg, thigh and upper arm. The patient is relieved as she hears about the 5 Biological Laws of Nature and learns these "melanomas" were in principle "warts" of little significance, which had been operated on unnecessarily. She decides to break off contact with her mother so that she can end the persistent repair. (Archive B. Eybl)*

Conflict-active	Cell degradation (ulcer) from the ectodermal, epidermal epithelium - usually unnoticed; at the affected location, the skin feels somewhat cold and rough; it is pale and insufficiently supplied with blood, sensation is limited (numbness). Short-term memory problems in the case of having two active separation conflicts at the same time, left and right (constellation); longer lasting separation conflicts can lead to symptoms of dementia. Also, the sensory paralysis that often goes along with MS (multiple sclerosis) is nothing but an active-phase of a separation conflict. Separation conflicts form dependencies (child screams until mommy comes), one wants to be among people. One has trouble being alone or goes into isolation (injury prevention).
Bio. function	Through numbness (diminished sensitivity) the missing or unwanted skin contact is temporarily forgotten. Limitation of memory to reduce suffering.
Repair phase	Restoration of the epidermis, metabolic recovery, inflammation, reddening, swelling, itching, and sometimes burning pain. It looks like the skin is really diseased now but, in fact, it is under repair. If it was diseased at all, it was during the active-phase. Most common diagnoses: eczema, neurodermatitis.
Repair crisis	Feeling of being cold, possible chills, pain, blackouts (absence seizures).
Note	Consider "handedness" (right or left) and side (mother/child or partner) or local conflict. Syndrome can aggravate the symptoms. Not only people and animals can cause separation conflicts, but also shoes that are too tight or uncomfortable, hated clothing, bitter cold, etc.

E
C
T
O

−+

Erysipelas: repair phase with syndrome > intense reddening and swelling.

Lupus: CM: systemic lupus erythematosus: a subcutaneous SBS > self-esteem conflict. In practice, however, it is often an epidermal SBS with syndrome > separation conflict. In each individual case this must be clarified by examining the symptoms and conflict history.

Questions Symptoms for the first time? (Yes > separation conflict in resolution for the first time > only clarify this episode. No > clarify this episode, then go back and try to determine the first episode). On which body parts did it begin? Inner surfaces? (Indication of wanting contact). Outer surfaces? (Indication of wanting distance). Face? (Indication of wanting to be seen or getting recognition). Which separation happened? (E.g., fight with partner, divorce, workplace, child going away, grandchild)? Which situation from my childhood does this situation remind me of? (Find conditioning). Look for the earliest conditioning: Was I a planned child? (No > important, original conditioning should be definitely dealt with in therapy). How was the birth? (Difficult birth can be the initial separation event). Was I allowed to stay with my mother immediately after birth? (Common initial separation event). Was I breast-fed for long enough? When was I placed in a nursery/pre-school? Did I cry when I was dropped off there? Did my parents fight often? Separation/divorce? Moving house during childhood with hard separations? Are there similar symptoms in the family? (Yes > indication of family issue). Is my family situation similar to that of my ancestors? (Work out the separation situations). Which steps will I take to heal myself inside? (E.g., meditation regression, ritual)? Which external measures would be good? (E.g., conversation, definitive farewell)?

Therapy The conflict is resolved. Support the healing. If recurring, find and resolve the conflict and conditioning. Guiding principles: *"I accept the separation and look to the future." "I am bound to God. This tie is never broken."* If it's a family issue: *"I recognize everything now and shine the light of love upon it - now I don't need to carry it with me anymore." "I am allowed to start over."*

Friendship bracelets for a child's separation conflict from the mother or father: Together, they braid the two bracelets; the mother makes one for her child and vice versa. Then they have a ceremony of binding the bracelets around each other's wrists. Whenever the child looks at the bracelet, he or she is immediately reminded of the bond.

Touch and be touched: For example, let yourself be stroked or massaged to have skin contact. Pound cabbage leaves soft and apply regularly. Petroleum externally. Hildegard of Bingen: Bathe or wash with a decoction of mulberry leaves. See also: remedies for the skin on p. 285.

Numbness, tingling, sensitivity disorders (neuropathy, polyneuropathy)

Similar SBS as above, but without visible skin symptoms. Most often it is numbness in the fingers and toes, but other body parts can be affected (e.g., back, legs or arms).

Conflict Separation conflict (details see p. 271). One wants less contact with someone (e.g., unhappy couple relationship, problematic workplace) or contact is lacking (e.g., because of a divorce, a child moving away, etc.).

Example • *A 55-year-old is married to a very dominant woman and unhappy for this reason. Nevertheless, he doesn't want to get a divorce. In a quiet time of his career, this dilemma becomes painfully apparent to him. He experiences multiple toes that go numb on his right partner side. Note: Nature helps the patient so that he doesn't have to feel his partner so intensely. (Archive B. Eybl)*

• *An introverted farmer is suffering because of a wife who is continually cheating on him with another man. After several weeks, his lips become numb. Note: The lips stand for speaking, kissing or eating. His suffering (a lack of kissing, conversation) is reduced with this condition. Unfortunately this married couple is unable to resolve their problems. (Archive B. Eybl)*

Phase **Conflict-active:** Reduced sensibility of the afferent nerve fibres. Numbness, sensitivity disorders. In CM, this is designated as "neuropathy," possibly as "suspected MS" (if there are also motor symptoms).

Bio. function One senses less - in this way, the disturbing contact is mitigated or the lacking contact blocked out.

Further causes Side effects of medications (psychopharmaceuticals, antibiotics, chemo and much more). Slipped disc: Compression of the nerve canals in the repair phase (see pp. 296, 301).

Questions When did the symptoms begin? (Conflict continuing from then until now). Eliminate other causes (medications, slipped disc). Which part of the body is affected? (Inner surfaces: one misses someone; outer surfaces: one wants to be rid of someone. Toes, soles of the feet: location conflict). Which events have sensitized me? Find the conditioning - childhood, pregnancy, ancestors)? Which change in my perception would help? Which further measures could heal me? (E.g., talking it out, etc.).

Therapy	Further qestions: see p. 273. Determine the causal conflict and conditioning and resolve.

Allergic contact eczema, sun allergy

Same SBS as above. Allergies are not "systemic illnesses," but rather nature's warning signals. Allergies always function on the basis of triggers. Discovering the trigger takes a bit of exacting "detective work." The conflict always has something to do with cause of/trigger for the "allergy." Something dramatic/unpleasant happened while one was in contact with it.

Example	• *A girl is undertaking an apprenticeship to become a baker. Just as she is standing at a machine, the baker approaches her and grabs under her skirt. Since then, the patient has been allergic to flour.* (From the forum www.neue.mediz.in)
	• *During summer vacation, a 5-year-old girl falls asleep under a beach umbrella. When she wakes up, she goes into a panic because her mother is gone = generalized separation conflict. Triggers: sun, sand, and sea; for forty years the patient has suffered from a sun allergy, but only when she is at the beach in the summer.* (See Claudio Trupiano, thanks to Dr. Hamer, p. 371)
Phase	**Repair phase** - recurring-conflict caused by triggers.
Questions	Allergy since when? (Conflict immediately beforehand). When is it the worst? When is it best? (Indication of the conflict). What happened at the time? What has changed in my life? (Family, partner/relationship, workplace - review everything carefully). Why couldn't I deal with it? (Determine conditioning).
Therapy	Determine the conflict and conditioning and, if possible, resolve them in real life so that the SBS comes to an end. Vitamin D3 (cod liver oil), colloidal gold. If this does not work, avoid the "allergens." See also: remedies for the skin p. 285.

Basal-cell carcinoma (BCC)

Same SBS as above, whereby the deepest epidermal layer is affected. Basal cell cancer usually appears as a stubborn, itchy, outcropping of reddish skin. They often appear smaller than they actually are, because they become wider with depth.

Example	• A right-hander gets a slap on the right cheek. On the right cheek, a basal cell cancer develops = local separation conflict - unwanted skin contact. (Archive B. Eybl)
Phase	**Recurring-conflict**. The deepest part of the epidermal layer is affected.
Therapy	Questions: see previous page. Determine the conflict and conditioning and, if possible, resolve them so that the SBS comes to an end. Doing nothing is possible with basal cell cancers if the patient doesn't have any fear whatsoever and it doesn't grow any larger. If one is constantly thinking about it, one should have it removed for the purpose of minimizing risk. Vitamin D3. Colloidal Gold, DMSO. If necessary, black salve or OP (see p. 278).

Psoriasis[2]

Same SBS as above. (See pp. 271-274) A chronic skin disease with clearly demarcated red patches.

Examples	• Psoriasis since childhood (Report of a young woman in the faktor-l-forum): *I was born after just seven months - thus, I was too small and too light. Nevertheless, I braved through it all without noticeable damage. I was neither physically handicapped nor mentally retarded. But something tells me that this birth was too early for me personally, that for a long time I vegetated without protection and security. Nobody was with me during those hours. After about half a year, my mother put me in a children's home. In the meantime, I had a broken arm because my older sister pushed me from the sofa. Before that, she wanted to suffocate me with a pillow.*
	I wasn't in the home for long - I soon was adopted. My father was a very loving person; my mother was more the rational type. The marriage broke up after 5 or 6 years. I had to stay with my mother. It was all about her. Nobody paid any attention to me. My grandparents were only interested in my

---

2   See Dr. Hamer, Charts pp. 118, 131

mother. A single woman with a child - no, that can't work! Nobody cared that my heart was bleeding. Again, I was very much alone. Soon after that, my mother met a new man. They were together for one year and wanted to get married. He left her the day before the wedding. I had already started calling him "papa" (which wasn't easy for me). Then came the third man, the one I now call my father, because he acted as a father for the longest period of my life. And then, as it was bound to be, this marriage broke up too. I was already out of the house and had my own life but it still eats at me. Three months ago, I lost my baby in the 10th week. A moving story - separation conflict from the beginning onwards, some active, some in healing. (http://www.faktor-l.de/index.php?f=18&t=2251)
• A 64-year-old, right-handed, divorced patient has a grown daughter with whom he has a wonderful relationship. One day the daughter meets a man that the patient doesn't approve of at all. As such, the daughter distances herself from her father = separation conflict - wanting to get rid of the daughter's boyfriend > severe psoriasis on the outer sides of both lower legs due to relapses. (Archive B. Eybl)

Phase	Two separation conflicts overlap each other on the same area of the skin, one is in healing (= red skin) and the other is in conflict-activity (= scaling). In general, one can call this **persistent conflict activity**.
Note	Consider "handedness" (right or left) and side (mother/child or partner) or local conflicts. The unattractive places could have a disfigurement conflict as a consequence. Put away the mirror or at least try to ignore the affected areas of the skin as much as possible.
Therapy	Determine the conflict and conditioning and, if possible, resolve them in real life. Questions: see p. 273. See remedies for the skin on p. 285.

Measles (rubella), chicken pox (varicella)

Same SBS as above. (See pp. 271-275)

Conflict	Generalized separation conflict - wanting or not wanting skin contact. Proximity-distance conflict.
Examples	→ *The pupils in an elementary school love their teacher. In the middle of the school year, she becomes pregnant and she goes on maternity leave = collective separation conflict. As the children grow to love their new teacher, they come into healing > measles in the repair phase.*
	→ *For some of the children born in the same year, pre-school starts too early. They would rather stay at home with their mommies. As they become friends with the other children and begin seeing the kindergarten teacher as a mother-substitute, they all come down with the chicken pox or measles = repair phase.*
	• *A couple's three children, each born nearly two years apart, miss the skin contact with their mother and father when at school. During vacation, they enjoy staying home, being able to cuddle with their parents and playing. All three contract chicken pox at the same time = repair phase. (Archive B. Eybl)*
Phase	**Repair phase**, restoration of the epidermis in the form of small, red flecks (measles rash); chicken pox sometimes produces blisters.
Note	Why do several members of a family or school class become ill at the same time? Group members experience and feel certain situations together. A group feeling and field of thought develops (Rupert Sheldrake: "morphogenetic field"). The more homogenous the group is, the more similar the feelings are amongst its members. Similar feelings lead to similar conflicts.
	Nowadays, unlike in earlier times, there are no measles epidemics anymore because the bonds within school classes and families are breaking down (keyword "individualism").
	Usually, several organs suffering from the same conflict come into healing at the same time > inflammations of the throat, nose, connective tissue or lymph glands.
	The developmental leaps associated with childhood diseases are not due to the disease but happen before that. "Developmental leaps" = conflict resolution = starting signal for the repair phase. As adults we also make a "developmental shift" before we get "ill," otherwise we wouldn't become ill.
	Please do not confuse this developmental leap with the "maturity stop" associated with territorial conflicts. Separation conflicts are unlike territorial conflicts and do not cause a stop in maturation.
Therapy	The conflict is resolved. Support the healing. Avoid recurrences. Questions: see p. 273. If necessary use cortisone, only briefly and only for the lack of any other options. The measles vaccination does not protect against measles. Unfortunately, the vaccines often contain various toxins that permanently harm the child. See also: remedies for the skin p. 285.

Warts (verrucae), plantar warts, condyloma, molluscum contagiosum ("MC")

Conflict	Local separation conflict. In children, according to Frauenkron-Hoffmann: One feels inferior in a specific location due to disparaging looks from others, e.g., mother, teacher, "critical inspection."
Examples	➔ *A child senses his mother's stern gaze on his writing hand.*
	• *A schoolgirl loves her riding pony, Neptune, more than anything else. One day, the mother and daughter arrive at the pony farm and find the stall empty. Neptune is dead = partner separation conflict with regard to sitting on the pony. Several MC lesions develop on the right buttock. The pony was perceived as a "partner." New lesions keep appearing because the mother and child keep visiting the pony farm ("recurring-conflict"). When the correlations become clear thanks to the 5 Biological Laws of Nature, they drive to another farm where the girl soon finds another horse to give her heart to > the lesions disappear. (See www. germanische-heilkunde/erfahrungsberichte)*
	• *A 21-year-old reluctantly takes an apprenticeship as a postman. Warts develop on the insides of his fingers, just where he has to grip the letters. When he stops working, they disappear. (See www. gnm-forum.eu)*
Phase	**Persistent repair** - excessive local restoration of the squamous epithelium.
Questions	Warts since when? What happened at the location? (Unwanted/lack of skin/visual contact)? What conditioned me in this regard? (Early separation, perfectionist parents)? Which healing measures would be best?
Therapy	Determine the conflict and conditioning and if possible resolve them in real life, so that the SBS comes to an end. *"Turn-around"*: on the night of a full-moon, spread half of an onion on the warts then throw the onion behind yourself and say "goodbye" to the wart. Do not think of the conflict or the wart afterward. Dab the warts with celandine juice, lemon juice, vinegar, freshly cut onion or tea tree oil. Hildegard of Bingen: celandine salve. Surgical removal is rarely successful because the warts usually come back. In this case, the scars provide a reminder. Most of the time, warts disappear on their own anyway.

Age warts (seborrheic keratosis)

Same SBS as above (pp. 271-275).

Phase	**Persistent repair** - excessive local restoration of the squamous epithelium
Note	In natural medicine, it is thought that the warts come from the age-related waning of the body's capacity to eliminate wastes, causing waste to be excreted via the skin in the form of brown warts. I think that this could be partly true but probably in connection with the above-mentioned conflict. If aesthetically disturbing > surgical removal.

Excessive calluses on the feet (Hyperkeratosis)

When you walk around outside barefoot, you notice how much the ground can hurt. To adapt to this kind of mechanical irritation, the soles of our feet form a callus layer (e.g., in summer or on vacation). However, when calluses thicken and crack for no reason, the following conflicts may be present:

Conflict	That one has to protect oneself from the hard world (comparable to the hard ground). Conditioning: little love in childhood; life's hard from the beginning and one must make it on their own.
Example	• *The daughter of a business owner has to help out with the business as a child. When the company goes bankrupt in her youth, she even has to take care of unpleasant business with the bank. Hard, cracking calluses on the her heels and big toes. (Archive B. Eybl)*
Phase	**Persistent repair** - excessive formation of callused, squamous epithelium on the soles of the feet.
Bio. function	Thickening of the callus layer for protection against a hard life.
Therapy	Determine the conflict, causal beliefs and conditioning and resolve them. Use a pumice stone/callus shaver regularly. To prevent cracking, apply deer sebum, marigold ointment.

SBS of the Deep Epidermis

Pigmentation disturbances (vitiligo)[1]

Conflict	Intense or brutal separation conflict. Separation perceived as very painful, unjust or unpleasant. Severe proximity-distance conflict. According to Frauenkron-Hoffmann: Outwardly, one shows purity or "is clothed in white," while one sees oneself as being impure. Often found in children of problematic mixed-marriages: "Better not to have any skin color."
Examples	• *A woman has white patches all over her body. She no longer goes out in the sun anymore, because when she is tanned, the patches can hardly be seen. She lacks melanin almost everywhere. Conflict history: The patient is married to a drug addict. Even after the children arrive, he cannot stop his addiction. In spite of many attempts, the man cannot get a grip on his problems. After waiting for a long time, the patient finally decides to separate from her husband for the sake of the children. She is overcome by a feeling of helplessness and injustice in having to take this step. (See Claudio Trupiano, thanks to Dr. Hamer, p. 283)*
	• *A married woman goes to a therapist because of three white patches on the inside of both arms and both legs. When he asks about a separation from her husband, she denies this vigorously. However, the therapist doesn't give up and asks again whether she had suffered a separation she perceives as unjust. She begins to tell her story: A year ago she fell in love with a man who lives in another city. The relationship ends because her partner never bothers to come to her. She must always go to him = brutal, unfair separation conflict. Since the two are still exchanging text messages, the conflict remains active. (Claudio Trupiano, thanks to Dr. Hamer, p. 282)*
Conflict-active	Tissue degradation (ulcer) in the lowest layer of the epidermis - this layer contains the brown pigment melanin > white patches because the melanin is reduced.
Bio. function	Increase in sensitivity due to degradation of the lowest layer of the epidermis. The missing pigment makes the skin more transparent to sunlight. > More light and warmth can penetrate. > In this way, the separation conflict can be healed. "Comfort through the sun's radiance."
Repair phase	Restoration of the melanophore layer > retreat of the patches, usually starting at the edges. Consider "handedness" (right or left) and side (mother/child or partner) or local conflict.
Therapy	Determine the conflict and conditioning and, if possible, resolve them in real life. Questions: see p. 273. See skin remedies p. 285.

Scarlet fever

The "illness" - scarlet fever - consists of several symptoms, each of which must be examined separately. Primary symptom: "raspberry tongue" (see p. 173). Scarlatina rash: same SBS as above.

Examples	• *The older brother of a 4-year-old boy has a birthday. The family goes to a toy store and the birthday boy is allowed to choose a present. He decides he wants a pedal car. The little one sees the car, runs to it and wants to drive it. His mother holds him back: "No, that's for your brother's birthday!" The little one begins to cry = intense separation conflict from mother/brother. He then breaks out in scarlet fever in the repair phase = restoration of the epidermis. (See www.germanische-heilkunde.at/index.php/erfahrungsberichte)*
Phase	**Repair phase** - widespread restoration of the lowest levels of the epidermis = outbreak of scarlatina rash.
Therapy	The conflict is resolved. Support the healing. See also: remedies for the skin, p. 285.

---

1   See Dr. Hamer, Charts pp. 120, 132

SBS of the Dermis 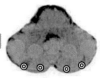 HFs in the cerebellum - topography still unknown

O L D M E S O

+ −

Skin cancer (melanoma, amelanotic melanoma, nodular malignant melanoma)[1]

Conflict	Disfigurement conflict: To feel injured, dirtied, defiled or attacked. Violation of the integrity. A real life injury (hit, push, slap) or defilement (dirt, feces, urine, etc.) or words that hurt, often due to arguments, cursing or doctors' diagnoses.
Examples	• *Due to bone cancer, a woman has surgery on her upper arm. Radiation leaves a brownish burn scar = disfigurement conflict. Instead of forgetting about the scar, she picks around at it and in doing so keeps the conflict-active. A melanoma grows = growth in the active-phase.* (Archive B. Eybl) • *A successful, right-handed businessman becomes president of a large soccer club. Unfortunately, right after he takes office a losing streak begins. The sports media blames the new president for this. The newspapers hit him with a barrage of criticism, which is "below the belt" = damage to his integrity. On the right side of his belly (the partner side) at about the level of his belt, appears a melanoma in the active-phase. Then when the soccer club starts winning again, it breaks up, bleeding = repair phase. CM: benign.* (Archive B. Eybl) • *A man is always arguing with his wife. She has the following habit: With the words, "You, my little friend…" she presses her fingernail against his chest. For the husband, this is anything but amusing = disfigurement conflict with dermal cell growth on this spot.* (See www.germanische-heilkunde).
Conflict-active	Local cell division in the dermis, growth of a melanoma. Often, a recurring conflict.
Bio. function	Strengthening of the dermis to be better protected from disfigurement.
Repair phase	Tubercular, caseating degradation via fungi, bacteria or bacteria; if the melanoma breaks open, this is called an "open skin tuberculosis." Nowadays this occurs very rarely because the melanoma is immediately cut out, often cutting *"deep into healthy tissue"* unnecessarily.
Note	Consider "handedness" (right or left) and side or local conflict. Often the result of a disfigurement conflict: One wants to have a good appearance, because they feel insecure > "wear a mask."
Questions	When did the melanoma appear and grow respectively? (Conflict in the time shortly before). What happened at this location on the body? (OP, punch/kick, injury)? Is this about an associated verbal attack instead? Clap test? Why do I react so sensitively? Am I already "damaged" by an OP? (Unsuccessful surgery)? What family conditioning do I have? Similar traumatic experience among ancestors? How am I dealing with the diagnosis? (Replace fear with knowledge).
Therapy	Determine the conflict and conditioning and, if possible, resolve them in real life if still active. Guiding principles: *"I am strong and well-protected." "A wall of crystal surrounds me." "I allow in the good, the rest bounces off."* Bach flowers: crab apple. Surgery: if the melanoma is felt to be mechanically or optically disturbing. Limited tissue removal. Black salve: Magnificent means for the immediate removal of melanoma with active cell division ("malignant") instead of surgery. Only suitable for people with a high tolerance for pain and with strong nerves (www.cernamast.eu.). See also: remedies for the skin, p. 285.

Shingles (herpes zoster)

Shingles is probably the combination of an SBS of the dermis (disfigurement conflict in healing), an SBS of the epidermis (separation conflict in healing) with the participation of peripheral nerve pathways.

Examples	• *A mother learns that her daughter is lesbian. She feels defiled when her daughter hugs her > dermal cell division in the active-phase. In the repair phase, shingles develop.* (See Dr. Hamer, Charts, p. 49) • *A 12-year-old, right-handed girl in puberty has a very dominant father. One evening her father takes hold of his daughter's breast. The girl knows that this is not a normal touch = disfigurement conflict. Even now, 40 years later, she experiences a "trigger" whenever she feels hurt by her father's loud voice or criticism. > In the repair phase, shingles develop on the left breast.* (Archive B. Eybl)
Conflict-active	Growth of small dermal tumors along the individual nerve segments - usually unnoticed.
Bio. function	Strengthening of the dermis for protection.
Repair phase	Painful tubercular, caseating degradation of the tumors; in the case of open shingles: painful, burning

---

1 See Dr. Hamer, Charts pp. 44, 49

blisters appear which gradually scab. Aggravated by syndrome. Consider mother/child, partner side or local conflict.

Therapy   Directly before the pain appeared, the conflict must have been resolved. Support the healing process. Avoid recurrences. Questions: see above. Alkaline diet, enzyme preparation, tenderize cabbage leaves and apply. Colloidal silver internally and externally. Hydrogen peroxide (H_2O_2) 3% strength internally/externally. Curd cheese poultice, St. John's wort flower oil externally. CM: treatment with antiviral drugs is not recommended because of the harm. For severe pain, non-steroidal anti-inflammatory drugs (NSAIDs) such as aspirin make sense. See also: remedies for the skin on p. 285.

Inflammation of the sebaceous and sweat glands (acne)

Same SBS as above. (See p. 278). Acne is THE skin disease of pubescence. As children, we are not very concerned about how we look or are perceived by others until we reach puberty, when it takes on utmost importance: "Do people like me?" "Am I attractive?" Being so self-conscious, young people are highly susceptible to disfigurement conflicts. The acne stage usually passes, when they realize that other things are more important than how they look, and that despite imperfections, they are liked nonetheless.

Examples   ➜ *A teenager is teased because his ears stick out.*
• *A girl, from a foreign country, is placed in an new middle school without knowing a word of the local language. She suffers because her classmates always talk about her behind her back and giggle because she is a foreigner and cannot speak the language = disfigurement conflict coming from behind > dermal cell growth in the active-phase. She has frequent relapses. In the subsequent repair phases, acne breaks out on her back. At the same time, she suffers from a moral-intellectual, self-esteem conflict with regard to the cervical spine. (Archive B. Eybl)*
• *A pretty, 15-year-old, high school girl has the feeling that at dance class, she is being excluded by her clique. Even more disturbing is that the older boy she has a crush on chooses another girl in the clique = disfigurement conflict with regard to her face and looks. As she recovers from this disappointment (= repair phase) her face breaks out in acne and a two-year vicious circle begins. (Archive B. Eybl)*

Phase   **Repair phase.** Usually a recurring-conflict, tubercular, caseating degradation of the dermis - sebaceous glands = acne. Acne makes a person feel even more disfigured = vicious circle.

Questions   Did one of my parents also suffer from acne? (Yes > family issue > work out the situation that the affected person was in at the time - what they were suffering from. Establish parallels to the patient. Explain to the adolescent that they are carrying on an pattern they have taken over and that they can leave it behind them).

Therapy   Determine the conflict and conditioning and, if possible, resolve them in real life so that the persistent repair comes to an end. Guiding principles: *"It's not important what others say and think about me. I think I'm okay." "I'm just fine the way I am!"* Get rid of mirrors in the house. Sunbathing; possibly use a solarium in winter. Bach flowers: crab apple. Cayce: Promote elimination through the intestines. Alkaline food, good cleaning and maintenance (olive oil soap). See also p. 285.

Athlete's foot, nail fungus (tinea, onychomycosis, dermatomycosis)

Same SBS as above (see p. 278).

Examples   • *Somebody's toenail turns blue because of a shoe that is too small = real disfigurement > the body strengthens the nail bed or nail so that the pressure can be withstood in the future. Nail fungus develops in the repair phase = cell degradation from the nail bed. (Archive B. Eybl)*
• *A young man, who is very conscientious about cleanliness has to wear the same pair of socks for three days, while he is on a train trip. He is repulsed by the smell of his sweaty feet and is embarrassed by this. Disfigurement conflict. Dermal cell proliferation in the repair phase. If he has to wear a pair of socks for more than one day, he experiences a trigger. If he changes his socks every day, there is no problem. (Archive B. Eybl)*
➜ *A child learns from his parents that the hairs found at public pools are something disgusting and that "You shouldn't step on them!" The child steps on a clump of hair = disfigurement conflict.*

Conflict-active   Strengthening and thickening of the nail bed or dermis of the foot.

Bio. function   Strengthening, so as to defend against disfigurement.

Repair phase	Stinking, caseating tissue degradation via fungi or bacteria (mycobacteria) = athlete's foot and/or nail fungus; this again results in disfigurement > often a life-long vicious circle.
Therapy	Determine the conflict and conditioning and, if possible, resolve them in real life so that the SBS comes to an end. Questions: see above. Good foot hygiene, so that you feel good about your feet again. Ignore the athlete's foot > break the vicious circle. Bathe or brush with liverwort extract. Bach-flowers: crab apple. Colloidal silver or MMS externally. Hydrogen peroxide (H_2O_2) 3% strength internally and externally. The CM antifungal drugs applied externally (antimycotic) do not help. The antifungal drugs for internal use are not recommended because of serious side effects.

Nail bed infection (paronychia)

Same SBS as above (see p. 278).

Example	• A 42-year-old, right-handed woman has a mother who is constantly interfering in the rearing of her son. She does this in a very pushy way. One day, they have a terrible argument because her mother oversteps her boundaries again. The patient has the feeling that her mother is "stepping on her toes." Disfigurement conflict with cell proliferation in the nail bed in the active-phase; in the repair phase, she gets an inflammation of the nail bed on the left mother-child side = tubercular, caseating cell degradation in the thickened nail bed. (Archive B. Eybl)
Phase	**Repair phase:** purulent, caseating cell degradation from the nail bed via fungi or bacteria.
Therapy	The conflict is resolved. Support the healing. Avoid recurrences. Wear open-toed shoes and keep your feet cool. Compresses with vinegar, clay, healing earth, curd cheese. Colloidal silver internally and externally. Hydrogen peroxide (H_2O_2) 3% strength internally and externally. Pound white cabbage leaves soft and wrap toes with them, put socks over it. If necessary, apply blistering ointment; release the enclosed pus by piercing (incision).

Excessive perspiration (hyperhidrosis)

Night sweats is a sign that you're in a repair phase. Sweating in the heat is used for cooling. Severely smelling armpit sweat during stress has a territory reference. Cold sweat may occur with low blood sugar. Sweating can also be promoted by drugs such as antidepressants, antibiotics, cortisone.

Here, the sweating from the rest of the body during stress will be described. A variant of a disfigurement conflict.

Conflict	One feels attacked, hurt, exposed or insecure.
Phase	Increase in function of the sweat glands in the dermis during the **conflict-active phase**.
Bio. function	When an individual is sweaty, they are slippery and "slick as an eel" and can thus escape the attacker or the uncomfortable situation. One is no longer "graspable" (according to David Münnich).
Questions	Why does one generally feel that they are often attacked or embarrassed? Lack of self-confidence? Paranoia/persecution complex? Who in the family behaves similarly? (An open discussion with this person would be sensible - for understanding and for healing). Am I ready to leave this behavior pattern behind me? What is the source of self-confidence? (The divine aspect inside me). Do I want to awake this source?
Therapy	Danger of a vicious circle, because one becomes even more insecure or "caught" due to the sweating. Find the conflict or triggers and solve them in real life, if possible. Practice serenity. Unity with God.

Leprosy, bubonic plague

Same SBS as above (see p. 278). During the Middle Ages and in developing countries today, these are the "illnesses" of the poor > miserable hygienic conditions (urine, feces, sweat, stench), injuries, brutal and coarse manners = "ideal" for disfigurement conflicts:

Leprosy	Tubercular-caseating cell degradation from the dermis via "mycobacteria leprae" = healing- phase.
Bubonic plague	Direct contact with, or even the sight of a stinking bubonic plague sufferer, was enough to make a person feel disfigured or defiled. The belief in and fear of "infection" did the rest > more and more people fell ill (tubercular dermis degradation), vicious circle caused by the stigma. With the improvement of living conditions, these "illnesses" disappeared.

"Fungal infection" of the skin (dermatomycosis, candidiasis, epidermomycosis)

One must assume that the majority of these diagnoses are mistaken, because usually no cells are cultured. They are most probably the result of separation conflicts (see inflammation of the epidermis), possibly with syndrome. However, if a laboratory culture comes back positive and there really is a fungus, we have an SBS of the dermis.

Phase	**Repair phase:** caseating degradation of dermal tissue via fungi.
Therapy	The conflict is resolved. Support the healing. Colloidal silver internally and externally. See also: remedies for skin p. 285.

Preliminary stages of skin cancer (pre-cancer): e.g., moles, pigment nevus, benign melanocytic nevus, lentigo maligna, light-damaged epidermis (actinic keratosis)

Whether these SBS belong to the epidermis or to the dermis must be determined on a case by case basis. We have to consider both possibilities and see whether the "thing" is seated on the surface (= separation conflict) or comes out of the depths (= disfigurement conflict).

Sunburn - skin cancer due to ultraviolet (UV) rays

For decades, the sun has been regarded as aggressive and damaging. This notion is incorrect, for sunlight is necessary for life. In fact, when enjoyed in reasonable amounts, it is the greatest source of healing for the body and soul. From a spiritual perspective, the sun is the largest consciousness in our solar system. We should welcome its rays as a **"sacred gift."**

There is no doubt that sunburns are harmful for the skin (aging), but they are not the absolute cause of skin cancer. It is interesting that melanomas often appear on parts of the body, which are hardly exposed to the sun (e.g., breast, buttocks).

Melanomas are more often diagnosed in "sun worshippers," because they are more often sought on these people.

Sunbathing becomes dangerous when a person is convinced that the sun is dangerous = self-fulfilling prophecy > conflict of feeling deformed or defiled > cell proliferation in the dermis > melanoma.

Corns (clavus)

A corn is a local thickening of the epidermis with a central cone reaching into the deeper skin. It usually appears where a shoe is too tight.
Possible causes ->

- The epidermis' adaptive reaction to an ill-fitting shoe > thickening of the horny layer.
- Separation conflict in persistent repair - wanting to be separated from the ill-fitting shoe.

"Leper"

Traditionally, "lepers" are not sick per se, this was a general term for those poor creatures who were banned from the city during the Middle Ages = "rejects/outcasts."

Beginning in the 11th century, the Holy Roman Empire held a health court headed by a priest. Based on a catalogue, including symptoms from "goose bumps from drafts" to "fever," it was decided whether the person under review could remain in the city or should be banished beyond the city walls (which was a basically a sentence of certain death at the time).

There is no question that those who were ostracized in this way, in addition to their material misery, suffered from every possible sort of conflict: for example, territorial conflicts, because they lost their home and families, existential conflicts because they didn't know how or why they should go on living, separation conflicts because skin contact with loved ones had been cut off and disfigurement conflicts because they felt dirty (spiritually unclean and/or poor hygiene) and many more.

▌SBS of the Subcutaneous Connective Tissue ▌

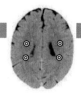

Stretch marks (striae cutis atrophicae)[1]

Conflict	Self-esteem conflict of feeling unaesthetic or unattractive on this part of the body.
Examples	• *A pretty, slender, nutrition-conscious woman of about 40 has very flat breasts and suffers because of it > local self-esteem conflict of feeling unaesthetic > cell degradation in the active-phase, restoration in the repair phase (reddish stripes), the breasts are scarred with stretch marks.* (Archive B. Eybl)
	• *An amateur bodybuilder works hard to build up his upper arms, but he thinks they are still too small = local self-esteem conflict with regard to the upper arms > stretch marks appear.* (Archive B. Eybl)
Conflict-active	Atrophy of the collagenous elastic fibers > weakening or atrophy of the net-like fiber structure of the subcutaneous connective tissue > distention. Consider "handedness" (right or left) and side (mother/child or partner) or local conflict.
Repair phase	Restoration of the fibers, the areas where distention has set in remain unchanged. On the lines where the tissue is torn, repairing, connective tissue is added. The stretch marks are red at the beginning, later they turn pale = condition **after the repair phase.** Usually a recurring conflict.
Bio. function	Strengthening of the connective tissue.
Questions	Do my ancestors also have stretch marks, cellulite or lipomas? (Yes > family issue). Why do I wrangle with my external appearance? Was I conditioned by my parents? (Mother struggled with her weight, father criticized mother for this reason)? Did mother have a problem with weight gain during the pregnancy? Are my parents body-oriented/fitness fanatics? (Endurance athletes, always physically fit)? Do I allow myself to be blinded by the beauty industry? Is one's body not just a shell? What is the meaning of my life? With which kind of a balance do I want to depart from this life one day?
Therapy	Determine the conflict and conditioning and, if possible, resolve them in real life if still active. Guiding principles: *"I feel good in my skin and am satisfied with my appearance." "My body is just a transitional shell. My soul is immortal."* Morning ritual according to Anton Styger (see p. 68). Alkaline diet, gymnastics, movement, exercises, cold-warm treatments (sauna, cold effusions). Vigorous massages with camphor, rosemary oil, cinnamon oil. Skin brushing. Bach-flowers: larch.

Lipoma

Conflict	Local self-esteem conflict, feeling not aesthetically beautiful at this part of the body. Conflict that the body is not sufficiently padded or protected (e.g., if one bumps into things often).
Example	• *The 45-year-old, right-handed man is usually very concerned about physical fitness. He goes running and trains at a fitness studio on a regular basis. Then, due to a project at work, he hardly has time for exercise and for two years he neglects his body. When he looks at his out-of-shape arms, he is unhappy about the "deterioration" = local self-esteem conflict of not finding himself aesthetically pleasing. When the project comes to an end, he decides: As of now, my body will be my first priority. In the following two weeks, a bean-sized lipoma appears on his right underarm = repair phase.* (Archive B. Eybl)
Phase	**Persistent repair** - local excessive buildup of new fat and connective tissue, emergence of lipomata and fibroma.
Therapy	The conflict is resolved. No measures need to be taken. If new growths appear, determine the conflict and/or trigger(s). Questions: see above. Resolve them with surgery, if visually disturbing.

Subcutaneous induration (localized scleroderma, morphea)

In this disease, the skin induration of the subcutaneous connective tissue (collagen) becomes hard and inelastic. Affected is usually only a small, coin-sized area. A larger induration, e.g., at joints, can limit movements drastically. The skin is transformed into a "suit of armor." If connective tissue in muscles, blood vessels and internal organs harden, then it is

---

1 See Dr. Hamer, Charts pp. 60, 71

called systemic scleroderma.

Conflicts	Self-esteem conflict: Life or a situation is unbearably hard. One feels defensive - and powerless.
Example	• *A 50-year-old worker in an underdeveloped country was fired by his company. He cannot find a job and the collapsing social system no longer supports him = unbearable hardship.* (Archive of B. Eybl)
Phase	Recurring, **persistent-active conflict**, degradation and restoration leads to hardening and scarred shrinking of collagenous and elastic fibers (subcutaneous connective tissue).
Bio. function	The dermal protection is not enough; the individual needs a suit of connective tissue armor to withstand a certain situation.
Questions	Hardening since when? (Conflict beforehand). Which hardship was/am I unable to cope with? What is changing in my life? What stresses me? Which location on the body was affected first? (Indication of the conflict). With what do I associate this body part? What does it represent? Clap test? Am I responsible for the situation? (Yes > take definite steps toward resolution). May I place the problem in God's hands? May I forgive myself? What has conditioned me in this respect? What were my ancestors like? Which inner changes would be helpful? What can I really/practically change? With whom could/should I speak about this?
Therapy	Determine the conflict and conditioning and, if possible, resolve them in real life, so that the SBS comes to an end. Find out where the love is, you will find the solution there. See also: remedies skin p. 285.

Cellulite ("orange peel syndrome"), lipedema

Conflicts	Aesthetic self-esteem conflict (see p. 282) and simultaneously a refugee conflict (= syndrome).
Examples	➜ *A woman has heavy legs and she thinks this is a problem.* ➜ *A man has the feeling he is being ridiculed in the sauna because of his belly.*
Conflict-active	Degradation of fatty tissue (fatty tissue necrosis).
Repair phase	Restoration of the fatty tissue, in **persistent repair**. Excessive buildup of new tissue; running in the background at the same time is an **active** kidney collecting tubules SBS (syndrome) > storage of fluid and fat = cellulite or lipedema. Usually, a recurring-conflict.
Bio. function	Proliferation of adipose tissue, reinforcing the layer of fat, because "fat is beautiful." A thick individual is beautiful - it is regarded as successful in procuring food. Animals can be thin doing nothing.
Therapy	Determine what the self-esteem and refugee conflicts are and, if possible, resolve them in real life so that the SBS comes to an end. Questions: see above. Morning ritual according to Anton Styger (see p. 68). Bach-flowers: larch, crab apple (see p. 54).

Scar proliferation (keloid)

Conflict	Local self-esteem conflict with regard to the injured or operated spot. Fear before/of an operation.
Example	• *A woman is very unhappy that her abdomen needs a surgical procedure - local self-esteem conflict. An ugly overgrowth of scar tissue forms = persistent repair.* (Archive of B. Eybl)
Conflict-active	Cell degradation in the subcutaneous connective tissue at the location of the scar.
Repair phase	**Persistent repair:** Restoration of the tissue, excessive, new formation of scar connective tissue; the keloid remains.
Bio. function	Strengthening of the scar.
Therapy	Prevent a keloid: If you are injured and/or are going to have an OP, go forward with full confidence. Get surgery on the injury. Do not argue with fate. Reconcile with what has happened. Do not doubt the recovery. Scar treatment with camphor, cinnamon oil. Energetic interference suppression by acupoint-massage. Cayce: Massage with peanut oil and camphor oil in equal parts. Using these measures, I may observe a significant improvement of keloids.

Abscesses, folliculitis (boils, carbuncles)

Abscesses or folliculitis usually develop in the dermis, sometimes in the subcutaneous tissue.

Conflict	Disfigurement conflict - "deep hurt" or a self-esteem conflict with regard to the location on the body.
Examples	• *The supermarket cashier repeatedly gets boils on her buttocks and on the inner sides of her thighs. Due to of a light case of incontinence, she always wears pads. When the store is very busy, she cannot change the pads at the usual time. This makes her feel "dirty" - disfigurement conflict, repair phase > boils.* (Archive B. Eybl)
Phase	**Repair phase**.
Therapy	The conflict is resolved. Support the healing process, avoid recurrences. Apply chopped onions. As necessary, lance to release the pressure. White cabbage leaf compresses, tea externally: arnica, club moss, fenugreek, chamomile, etc. DMSO externally.

■ SBS of the Epidermis
HFs sensory function in top of cerebral cortex

Dandruff, hair loss (alopecia totalis), spot baldness (alopecia areata)[1]

According to CM, hair loss in men is caused by a high testosterone level. Then, it must be young men (high testosterone), who are affected. However, from the point of view of the 5 Biological Laws of Nature, the frequent loss of hair in men is somewhat unclear: why should only men suffer from separation conflicts of the head, but not women?
Many kinds of medication can lead to hair loss: chemo, "the pill," painkillers, antirheumatics, blood thinners, cholesterol-lowering drugs, etc. Where medication is not involved, there is no doubt that patchy or sudden hair loss is caused by a conflict.

Conflict	Separation conflict with respect to the affected area (head). One does not feel accepted. According to Frauenkron-Hoffmann: We must show that we are smart. Many modern men identify themselves with their intellect - a modern ailment. Women don't seem to suffer from worries like these.
Example	• *The now 20-year-old, married, right-handed woman suffers her first separation conflict with her head, when she is just 8 years old, when her beloved grandmother dies suddenly. Her grandmother had the habit of pressing the child's head against her abdomen. She liked that a lot. A second, even stronger separation conflict happened a year ago, when her two very best friends suddenly turned away from her in a very distressing manner. All attempts to restore contact failed. She begins to lose her hair in patches - about 70% of her head is bald = conflict active-phase.* (Archive B. Eybl) • *A six-year-old girl is banned from her parents' bed. This causes a separation conflict with regard to the head. She loses hair.* (Archive B. Eybl)
Conflict-active	Reduced metabolism in the hair's roots in the epidermis. Hair loss, dry scalp with poor blood circulation, dandruff (= indication of conflict activity). Usually a recurring conflict.
Bio. function	Loss of sensitivity lets the missing or unwanted skin contact be forgotten. One shows their head.
Repair phase	Increased scalp metabolism, swelling, reddening, itching, new hair growth with a 2 - 3 month delay. The rest of the scaly skin falls away, no new dandruff forms.
Questions	Hair loss since when? (Conflict before that) Was there a separation, harsh rejection or another sort of shock? Why do I associate this with my head? (E.g., stroked, massaged, caressed or the opposite: struck/injured)? Otherwise, do I have to show my head/prove my intellect? (E.g., career training/performance). What value does intellect have in our family? Do I identify strongly with this? What am I if I'm not clever? Was there an event with relation to my head/hair that affected/moved me? Which change is needed in my consciousness? Which new attitude should I develop?
Therapy	Determine the conflict and conditioning and, if possible, resolve them in real life if still active. At least a 4-week course of treatment: Apply pounded, white cabbage leaves and drink the fresh juice. (See S. R. Knaak, Die kreisrunde Haarausfall, Ennsthaler 2010). Rub in tea from wormwood, nettle, burdock root, boxwood roots. Head massage with sesame oil and essential oils of thyme, rosemary, cedar. Cayce: Massage with "crude oil" (stone oil or petroleum), head massage, exercise, internal cleansing with alkaline nutrition. Eat brown millet regularly. Enemas. Schindele's Minerals.

E
C
T
O

– +

---

1   See Dr. Hamer, Charts pp. 119, 131

SBS of the Deep Epidermis

HFs sensory function in top of cerebral cortex

Gray hair

When pigment (melamine) production slows, the hair turns gray; a normal part of the aging process. However, unusually early or sudden graying is certainly related to a conflict.

Conflict	Brutal separation conflict, usually with a generational aspect (family, descendant issues).
Examples	• *The 49-year-old single mother of three children has to go to the hospital for an operation. She promises her children she will call right after the surgery. When she wakes up from the anesthesia, she is in the intensive care unit. She asks the nurse what time it is. She is told that the surgery was the day before = brutal separation conflict from her children. Within three days, her hair turns gray = active-phase.* (Archive B. Eybl)
	• *A 40-year-old woman who wants to have a child goes to her gynecologist for an examination. He tells her that she will never have children = strong separation conflict with a generational aspect. Overnight, her hair turns snow-white.* (Archive B. Eybl)
Conflict-active	Cell degradation, slowdown of metabolism in epidermis - lower layer (melanophore layer) > reduced melamine production > graying of the hair.
Bio. function	Increased sunlight transparency, so that more light (warmth, information, knowledge, wisdom) can penetrate. > "Comfort and wisdom through the rays of the sun." "The wisdom of age."
Repair phase	Restoration of the melanophore layer, restoration of hair color.
Questions	What happened when the hair suddenly went gray? (Event shortly before). Was there stress in the family? (E.g., fighting with children/relatives, accusations because of inheritance)? What should I change on the inside and outside to affect a resolution?
Therapy	Determine the conflict and conditioning and, if possible, resolve them in real life if still active.

E
C
T
O

− +

Remedies for the skin

- Natural stimulants like light (sunbathing in moderation), water, rain, wind.
- Vitamin B complex in yeast products (brewers yeast).
- Vitamins E and A in cold-pressed vegetable oils, especially linseed oil.
- Cod liver oil.
- Colloidal Gold.
- Cayce: alkaline diet, pay attention to elimination (colon) and circulation (gymnastics), eat two almonds a day, massages, rubbings with olive oil, olive oil soap for cleansing.
- Tea for the skin (internally or externally): barberry, birch leaves, blackberry leaves, sage, mullein, chamomile, speedwell, chicory.
- Baths and rubbings with effective microorganisms (EM see p. 59).
- Hydrogen peroxide (H_2O_2) 3% strength.
- Seawater full baths or alkaline baths.
- Natural borax, externally.
- Hildegard of Bingen: thyme, quince, red beets.
- Black salve: Great remedy for immediate removal of skin tumors with active cell division processes ("malignant") instead of surgery. Only for people with high tolerance for pain and steady nerves: order at www.cernamast.eu.

- For inflammations: chamomile, healing earth, clay, acetic acid/healing earth compresses, cooked potato compresses, Schuessler Cell Salts No. 1, 3, 11. Miracle Mineral Supplement from Jim Humble (MMS).
- Open sores, badly healing wounds: Spread with blossom honey, curly-leaf cabbage compresses, marigold salve, comfrey salve or propolis salve.
- Skin care: Olive oils and other oils from the kitchen, refined with a bit of ethereal oil, instead of expensive and unhealthy chemical cocktails from the cosmetics industry.
Olive oil would be ideal but its smell and short shelf life are problematic. Alternative: sunflower seed oil. The inexpensive, heat-extracted oils have the advantage over the cold-pressed oils (which are actually better) in that they keep well and don't become rancid so quickly.

BONES AND JOINTS

The human body's structure is composed of roughly 206 bones. The supportive part of the bone is the bone cortex (substantia corticalis), which surrounds the bone marrow (substantia spongiosa) and the exterior is covered by the substance periosteum. Except for the ectodermal periosteum, all of the structures of the musculoskeletal system, meaning the ligaments, tendons, muscles, intervertebral discs, menisci and bursae, are made up of mesodermal tissue.

When it comes to determining conflicts, the musculoskeletal system is certainly the most "rewarding" part of the body and when proceeding with care, even a beginner can experience "success" here.

The main conflict content is self-esteem, self-worth or inability conflicts. However, every part of the musculoskeletal system contains its own certain nuances.

For the psyche, self-confidence is also the structure-forming, load bearing element. The equivalent to this in the body is the musculoskeletal system.

Powerful self-esteem conflicts manifest themselves in the bones, the hardest tissue, while less serious conflicts are reflected in softer tissues, such as cartilage and ligaments.

If the muscles and tendons are affected, the self-esteem conflict has a mobility aspect.

The musculoskeletal system is controlled by the cerebral white matter. This part of the brain has a spongy structure in which the Hamer foci sometimes appear somewhat blurred. Dr. Hamer points out that self-esteem conflicts can be an exception due to the fact they do not necessarily have to be preceded by a conflict in the form of a dramatic shock.

In other words, self-esteem conflicts can also be initiated by "undramatic," nagging, insidious perceptions, *for example, as when a person sees themselves as the inferior partner or is convinced that they cannot endure something.*

In my opinion, not all problems of the musculoskeletal system are caused by a conflict. Too much of anything (e.g., extreme sports), too redundant or too little physical exercise (e.g., desk job all day and TV in the evening, in between driving the car) can also do damage. There is an old Germanic proverb, "A fool always wants, either too little or too much."

Our joints in particular thrive on movement - just not too much. Our bodies are not made for hours of sitting nor for years of kneeling (e.g., tile-laying).

The consequence: hardened muscles, abnormal metabolism in the joints > danger of injury and pain without conflict, but with a potential for subsequent conflicts: "My knees are ruined as well!" = local self-esteem conflict.

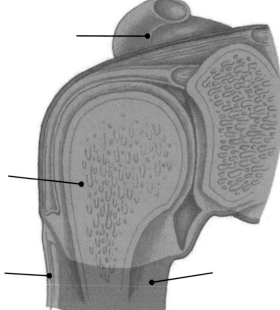

Cartilage,
Joint Capsule,
Bursa
**Self-esteem,
inability conflict**

Bones and Inner Periosteum
Self-esteem conflict

Tendons, Ligaments
**Self-esteem,
inability conflict**

Superficial Periosteum
**Brutal-separation
conflict**

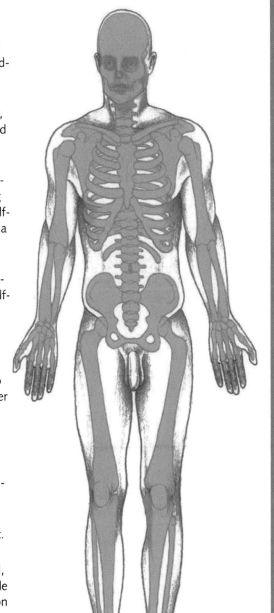

SELF-ESTEEM CONFLICTS IN DETAIL[1]

Skull, cranial bone and cervical spine
Moral-intellectual self-esteem conflict: perceived injustice, dissatisfaction, bondage, dishonesty, ingratitude, indecency, intolerance, feeling stupid or unintelligent. Saying: "To rack your brains (skull) over something!"

Eye socket (orbit): Self-esteem conflict with regard to the eye.

Upper and lower jaw
Self-esteem conflict of not being able to "bite" or a local self-esteem conflict with regard to the jaw or chin.

Shoulder
Self-esteem conflict to believe one is not a good parent or good child (right-handed, left shoulder) or not being a good partner (right-handed, right shoulder).

Elbow
Self-esteem conflict of not being able to embrace, hold, fend off, throw, shoot, push, hit. Elbow = equivalent to the knee. > Conflict of unsatisfied ambition (e.g., tennis players, golfers, craftsmen).

Hands and fingers
Clumsiness self-esteem conflict: one believes that he has treated somebody incorrectly, approached a task incorrectly, done something wrong or that his hands have failed (often found in perfectionists) or a local self-esteem conflict, for instance when a hand loses its resilience following a broken scaphoid bone.

Thoracic spine
Self-esteem conflict of being "a broken man" (or woman), feeling humiliated or defeated, conflict of feeling debased or degraded; or a local self-esteem conflict, as when something in the thorax is out of order.

Breastbone, ribs
Local self-esteem conflict, e.g., due to breast cancer.

Lumbar spine
Central self-esteem conflict: E.g., one believes that one is not able to withstand the pressure. Or local self-conflict, e.g., for colorectal cancer diagnosis or hemorrhoids "This is breaking my back!"

Tailbone, pubic bone, pelvic bones
Local self-esteem conflict, often regarding sexuality or potency.

Ischium bone
Self-esteem conflict of not being able to possess something or sit something out or a local self-esteem conflict.

Hipbone and femoral neck
Self-esteem conflict of not being able to persevere or a local self-esteem conflict.

Knee
Self-esteem conflict of not being athletic/mobile, not being recognized, unfulfilled ambition or a local self-esteem conflict due to not being able to run, jump, kick, etc. Also the issue of obedience, authority/religion (kneeling before a temporal/religious authority).

Ankle, feet, toes
Self-esteem conflict of not being able to put up with something or somebody, or not being able to run, balance, jump, kick or stop. Often a "location" issue.

N
E
W

M
E
S
O

– +

---

1   See Dr. Hamer, Charts pp. 63, 75

SBS of the Bones, Cartilage and Ligaments

BASIC SEQUENCE[1]

Conflict	Self-esteem conflict corresponding with the location in the body; see p. 287.
Tissue	Bones, cartilage, muscle, tendons and ligaments - new mesoderm/cerebral white matter.
Conflict-active	Cell degradation in the bones (osteolysis), joints or muscles. No pain, reduced metabolism, possible "feeling of being cold." Spontaneous fractures are rare because the periosteum acts as a *bandage*. Reduced production of new blood cells (hemato-poiesis) in the bone marrow > anemia (see p. 134).
Repair phase	Increased metabolism = inflammation; restoration of the tissue with the help of bacteria, swelling, reddening, pain (pain in the neck and lower spine, joint pain, etc.), expansion of the periosteum = bone cancer (osteosarcoma), excessive production of blood cells = CM: "blood cancer" (leukemia). Worsening of symptoms, while resting or sleeping; painkillers help.
Bio. function	Permanent conflict activity: The affected joint or the bone dissolves itself/becomes unusable. > The individual must find another field of activity (e.g., a different career), where they can make themselves useful again. The extreme: One dissolves from within, because the individual is of no more use to the "clan." In doing so, the chances of the clan's survival are increased. The repair phase: keeping the person still with pain in order to promote repair. After the course of a normal, brief SBS: strengthening of the bones, cartilage, ligaments, tendons, or muscles. After the SBS is complete, the affected spot (a healed bone, for instance), is stronger than before and remains somewhat thickened (luxury group).
Note	With joint or spinal pain, we are usually not sure whether the SBS is affecting the bones or other structures such as the cartilage or ligaments. Generally, this is merely of academic interest, because pain means that the conflict has been resolved and the patient is in the repair phase. The only exception here is the rarer "brutal-separation conflict," which affects the sensitivity of the periosteum and causes pain in the conflict-active phase (see rheumatism). Possible consequence of self-esteem conflict: one always want to be good/the best, one likes to compare oneself, one wants to accomplish monumental tasks (a drive for exceptional performance) > risk of burnout.

The following are listed by the disorders in general, the stages of disorders and then according to location from head to toe:

Degenerative joint disease (osteoarthritis)

Conflict	Self-esteem conflict according to location in the body (see p. 287).
Tissue	Cartilage, ligaments or menisci - new mesoderm.
Phase	**Persistent conflict activity** or **recurring-conflict**, usually longer conflict-active phases alternate with short repair phases > substitution of functional tissue with inferior soft scar tissue > reduced elasticity and resilience.
Note	Danger of vicious circle, for a painful joint causes a new self-esteem conflict - *"I can no longer go on long hikes. It's just too much for my hips." "My knee is worthless." Consider "handedness" (right or left) and side (mother/child or partner).*
Questions	First determine handedness (e.g., clap test). Which joint on which side is affected? When did I feel the complaint for the very first time? (Conflict since then). Do I have complaints more during the day or at night? (<u>During the day</u>: chronic, fatigued, no drive = more or less conflict active phase > requires warm measures (see next paragraph). <u>Night</u>: currently an acute phase, full of energy, inflammation = interim repair phase > requires cooling measures (see therapy for inflamed joints, p. 291) Complaints at night: Which conflict was resolved immediately before the night pains began? (> Clue toward the original conflict). Now we know if it is dealing with the mother/child or partner and if the conflict has at least been resolved for the meantime. Look for the original conflict: In which situation did I feel demeaned when it

---

1   See Dr. Hamer, Charts pp. 63, 75

began? What was my life like at the time? (Family relationships, educational level)? What stressed me, which emotions were dominant? Parallels to the current emotional state? How was the pregnancy/birth/infancy? (Look for conditioning). Was I planned? Am I similar to any ancestors? (Mother/father/grandparents/great-grandparents)? What behavioral patterns do I carry on from this person? How far back does this pattern go in the family? Which healing thoughts am I going to send my ancestors? (Healing the family affects a cure). Which new attitude do I want to adopt? Am I in harmony with the order of the family? (see pp. 24ff and 48f).

Therapy	Determine the conflict and conditioning and, if possible, resolve them in real life.
	Guiding principles: *"Pain = repair!" "I am full of self-confidence and look to the future hopefully." "I have faith in my divine guidance!"*
	Bach-flowers: larch, possibly elm, centaury, rock water.
	Morning ritual by Anton Styger (see p. 68).
	Whole, alkaline nutrition, brown millet, Kanne Bread Drink.
	Linseed oil (omega 3).
	3x/week eat soup with boiled bones of beef, fish, poultry. 1 teaspoon cod liver oil daily. Vitamin D3. Natural borax internally.
	For all physical measures, the principle is: Energize!
	Cayce: Regular massage with peanut and olive oil with a touch of camphor oil.
	Warm baths, sauna, steam bath, red light, infrared irradiation, skin brushing (dry or wet).
	Sunbathing, possibly, solarium.
	Vigorous massage with circulation-stimulating oils, such as rosemary, marjoram, thyme, coriander, cinnamon, camphor, among other things.
	Massage: accupoint, connective tissue, reflexology.
	Hot potatoes or mustard poultice. Cupping (dry), cantharides.
	Physiotherapy. Exercises, but not excessive, strength training - toning.
	Often helpful in the case of older patients are natural (or identical with natural) hormones (rejuvenating effects, also for the joints).

Decrease in bone mass and density (osteoporosis)

According to CM, this is an illness of old age, where loss of bone mass leads to diminished bone strength and bone fragility. Nearly half of those over 70 suffer from osteoporosis and women twice as often as men.

Conflict	More or less generalized self-esteem conflict.
Examples	➜ *"I am good for nothing anymore, I'm a burden for my family."*
	➜ *Somebody is forced into retirement and suddenly feels old: "I am ready for the scrap heap!"*
	• *Her children, the most important thing in her life, left the house: "I ask myself what I'm good for!"* *Self-esteem conflict in the active-phase = osteoporosis; restoration with pain in the repair phase, should it come to that.* (Archive B. Eybl)
Phase	**Conflict-active** phase, usually with short, intermittent repair phases > degradation of bone tissue > osteoporosis.
Note	It is interesting to note that in Asia, where old people are highly valued and held in high social esteem, osteoporosis was almost unknown. In large Asian families, the oldest family members have traditionally occupied a respected position and usually have the last word. The preservation of self-esteem and self-confidence in old age is a social and individual duty. However, this difference is already being labeled a "myth," as Asian cultures westernize and osteoporosis rates skyrocket.
Further causes	Lack of movement: If bones are not used, they are broken down to the bare essentials. Bone density can be increased by regular exercise (similar to muscle training). Regular exercise also promotes self-esteem, when not done under pressure to succeed and it is done in a relaxed atmosphere.
	Long-term use of cortisone: steroids inhibit the tissue development and promote bone loss.
	Poor diet: in particular, too much sugar damages the bone metabolism.
Questions	What do I think about getting/being "old?" Do I feel valued? What status do the elderly have in my family? Which goals do I still have? How can I reestablish myself on the inside? (New tasks, inner values)?
Therapy	Determine the conflict and conditioning and, if possible, resolve them in real life. Guiding principles:

"Goodbye to the obsession with youth!" *"Inner values are what count. I will strive for wisdom and strength of character!"* *"I am strong and courageous!"*

Movement: especially strength training, muscle building.

Vigorous massage with warm oils. Use comfrey oil or ointment.

Alkaline diet! Avoid: white flour, sugar, soft drinks, e.g., Coca-Cola (phosphoric acid). Natural vitamin D3 (cold pressed vegetable oils, cod liver oil, eggs, dairy products), calcium (sesame, millet, vegetables, nettle seeds, dairy products, etc.), linseed oil. Tea: horsetail, green oat, mugwort. Natural borax internally. Schindele's Minerals.

CM bisphosphonates are not recommended because of their uselessness and harmfulness. For further options see osteoarthritis p. 289.

Demise (necrosis) of marrow tissue, replacement of bone marrow with connective tissue (bone marrow fibrosis, myelofibrosis, osteomyelosclerosis)

Conflict	The most intense self-esteem conflict, corresponding to location (see p. 287). The bone marrow is the innermost part of the bone, this is why we are dealing with the pure substance here.
Phase	**Conflict-active phase** (marrow necrosis) or recurring-conflict (fibrosis), degradation of marrow tissue or its replacement by connective tissue.
Therapy	Determine the conflict and conditioning and, if possible, resolve them in real life if still active. Avoid recurrences. Questions, therapy see osteoarthritis p. 289.

Complex regional pain syndrome after injury (CRPS, Sudeck's dystrophy)

If after an accident, a bone fracture will not heal, chronic pain occurs and the affected joint possibly even atrophies, the diagnosis of "Sudeck's dystrophy" may follow.

Conflict	Local self-esteem conflict or, more precisely, devaluation because of the injury or restriction.
Example	→ *"My ankle is broken. Now I'm totally out of the race. Will it ever be as good again? "*
Phase	**Conflict-active phase or recurring-conflict:** degradation of bone tissue, hardly any formation of callus. In between optimistic phases with bone formation (callus formation), pain.
Questions	Why did the injury affect me so much? How did my ancestors deal with accidents/injuries? What can I learn from doing nothing? (E.g., practicing patience, questioning my mission/goals in life)? Which positive effects are there? (E.g., life will slow down again, more time for the family, etc.).
Therapy	Through unwavering optimism, break out of the vicious circle. Question the identification with one's own body > new orientation, reestablish priorities in life. See measures p. 289.

Brittle bone disease (osteogenesis imperfecta)

According to CM, this is an "inherited disease" marked by incomplete bone construction and extreme fragility.

Conflict	Generalized self-esteem conflict. Like all hereditary diseases, the cause lies with the ancestors or the pregnancy/birth.
Phase	**Conflict-active phase** - reduced cell division or degradation of bone tissue.
Therapy	Determine the conflict and conditioning and, if possible, resolve them in real life. (See also osteoarthritis p. 289)

Inflammatory thickening and deformation of the bones (Paget's disease)

This chronic disorder begins with an increase in the activity of bone degrading cells (osteoclasts). As the disease progresses, the bones become deformed and thickened.

Conflict	Self-esteem conflict according to location. (See p. 287)
Phase	At first, **persistent-active conflict** (cell degradation, softening of the bones). Then, **repair phases** (cell growth, stabilization of deformed bones) alternate with conflict-active phases.
Therapy	Determine the conflict and conditioning and, if possible, resolve them in real life, so that the persistent repair comes to an end. (See also osteoarthritis p. 289)

Inflammation of the joints (arthritis)[2]

Conflict	Self-esteem conflict according to body location (see p. 287).
Phase	**Repair phase** - Restoration of the tissue due to increased metabolism: pain, swelling, reddening; aggravated by syndrome. Consider "handedness" (right or left) and side (mother/child, or partner) or local conflict.
Questions	Did the inflammation begin suddenly? (Yes > a surprising, positive event resolved the conflict). This resolution event often doesn't have a direct relation to the conflict: e.g., one falls in love, the beginning of vacation or retirement, a wonderful party (where one really had a good time). Did the inflammation come on slowly? (Yes > slow, anti-climactic conflict resolution, e.g., through a healing attitude, positive developments in a relationship, etc.). What stressed me before? Which new attitude will I need to avoid recurrences?
Therapy	The conflict is resolved. Support the healing. Avoid recurrences.
	Rest, elevation, moderate movement, but only in the pain-free range.
	Principle for all physical measures: dissipating energy.
	Cold showers, cold compresses, cold salt wrap.
	Ice, ice pack (applied directly to the skin for max. 2 minutes, otherwise, it comes to so-called reactive hyperemia with warming effect).
	Compresses with curd cheese, clay or aluminum acetate (e.g., Pasta Cool), hay flowers.
	Colloidal silver internally and externally to the affected area. Schindele's Minerals internally.
	Natural borax internally/externally.
	Tenderize cabbage leaves and apply.
	Alcoholic rubbings with Swedish bitters, French brandy, spirit of melissa, tincture of frankincense or myrrh.
	Essential oils gently applied (diluted): lavender, mint, lemon balm, chamomile.
	Lymphatic drainage, acupuncture, reflexology massage.
	Cayce: rubbing with peanut oil and myrrh tincture or castor oil.
	Alkaline diet, no pork, even better no meat. Kanne Bread Drink.
	Vitamin D3 (cod liver oil). Linseed oil.
	Enzyme preparation (e.g., Wobenzym).
	Traumeel Ointment (Fa. Heel).
	Schuessler Cell Salts No. 3, 4, 9.
	Blue-light irradiation, consider leeches.
	Cannabis Oil.
	If necessary - CM, antirheumatic medications (see p. 62), cortisone (not recommended for long-term). All anti-inflammatory measures ease the healing symptoms but they can extend the repair phase somewhat. After relief of intensive pain - motion, strength training, muscle building.

Inflammation of the bursa (bursitis)

The bursae are sacs of lubricating fluid lying close to the joints where the muscles and ligaments glide over the bones or the skin is exposed to higher pressure (e.g., tip of the elbow). They help reduce friction and absorb pressure.

Conflict	Derived from the function: Self-esteem conflict, that too much pressure is being exerted from the outside according to location in the body (see p. 287).
Phase	**Repair phase**, inflammation of the bursa, swelling, pain, reddening.
Note	Aggravated by syndrome; take into account "handedness" (right or left) and side (mother/child or partner) or local conflict.
Therapy	The conflict is resolved. Support the healing. See also above.

Inflamed bone marrow (osteomyelitis)

According to CM, this is a "bacterial infection" caused by staphylococci. From the view of the New Medicine, naturally, this is not an infection.

Conflict	Self-esteem conflict according to body location (see p. 287).

---

2   See Dr. Hamer, Charts pp. 63, 75

Phase	**Intensive repair phase** > acute inflammation of the bone marrow, the exudate coming from the bone marrow stretches the periosteum > pain, bacteria optimize the healing.
Note	Aggravated by syndrome; if the inflammation is chronic (= recurring-conflict), cysts and abscesses can develop. Consider "handedness" (right or left) and side (mother/child or partner) or local conflict.
Therapy	Determine the conflict and conditioning and resolve them, if still active. See also: joint inflammation p. 291.

Bone marrow tumors (plasmacytoma, multiple myeloma, Kahler's disease)

Conflict	Intensive self-esteem conflict according to location in the body (see p. 287).
Phase	**Repair phase:** cell division, restoration of the bone marrow.
Note	The tumor is always preceded by a necrosis of bone marrow. If flat bones are affected, leukemia (excessive blood production) occurs. Consider "handedness" (right or left) and side (mother/child or partner) or local conflict.
Therapy	The conflict is resolved. Support the healing. Avoid recurrences. See also: arthritis p. 291. In our opinion, stem cell transplantation is not useful (because it is ineffective).

Bone tumor (osteoblastoma, osteoma, Ewing's sarcoma, osteosarcoma, etc.)

Conflict	Self-esteem conflict according to body location (see p. 287).
Conflict-active	Cell degradation from the bones (osteolysis), no pain.
Repair phase	Restoration of the bone substance = CM: "bone tumor." Often a recurring conflict.
Bio. function	Reinforcement of the bone. The affected area is stronger than before after the SBS is completed.
Note	According to CM, most bone tumors are metastases (= secondary tumors). The reason for this is that people suffer local self-esteem conflicts from cancer diagnoses or by debilitating therapies (surgery, chemotherapy). E.g., after a breast cancer diagnosis: "I am no longer a real woman! " = local self-esteem conflict with resulting cell division in the breast bone or ribs = CM's "bone cancer." Decreasing examination intervals/progressively better imaging technology ensure that these tumors are discovered sooner and more often.
	So-called primary bone tumors are usually discovered when a patient complains of pain. In earlier times, the patient was sent home for bed rest. Now they keep looking until they find something. In CT scans, not only are tissue-dense (hyper-dense) areas suspected of being carcinogenic but also areas with low density (hypo-dense) = CM's giant cell bone tumor or "osteoclastoma."
Osteosarcoma	Unfortunately, when cancer is suspected, a biopsy puncture is often performed. > Liquid bone (callus) runs out through the hole into the periosteum and "hardens" in the surrounding tissue. = Osteosarcoma = CM evidence of "malignancy." > Osteosarcomas mostly arise due to medical malpractice (puncture), sometimes they arise due to unfortunate injuries during a bone repair phase. If the hole does not close on its own, one can try to stop the callus from leaking out with irradiation or surgery.
Therapy	Determine the conflict and conditioning and, if possible, resolve them in real life if still active. The big problem is usually the pain. Thus, use CM antirheumatic drugs generously. If necessary, CBD oil. Of course, no chemo. Irradiation possible in exceptional cases, if the pain is unbearably intense. See also: arthritis.

Cartilaginous tumor (chondrosarcoma, chondroblastoma, osteochondroma, etc.)

Cartilaginous tumors are rarely diagnosed. Progression is similar to the above.

Conflict	Self-esteem conflict, matching the corresponding part of the body (see p. 287).
Example	• *A 40-year-old, married, left-handed woman has two daughters, ages 11 and 13. The first daughter is a "loud child" for the first two years, driving her mother to frustration. She finds it difficult to develop motherly feelings for the child and she often thinks about the time before she had children = central self-esteem conflict. While on vacation, she realizes for the first time that the children are fairly independent now = conflict resolution. At this point, severe, pain begins to radiate from the right side of the pelvis into the right mother/child leg = restoration phase. When the pain doesn't relent when she returns home, a neurosurgeon wishes to further investigate by performing a needle biopsy. The medical finding of "malignant" is confirmed during surgery. Due to the two openings, callus runs into the*

N
E
W
M
E
S
O

– +

pelvic cavity, where a 10.5 x 5.5 x 9 cm chondrosarcoma develops. The doctors want the patient to undergo lifelong chemotherapy. (Archive B. Eybl)

Phase	**Repair phase or recurring-conflict.** Restoration of the cartilaginous substance.
Therapy	Determine the conflict and conditioning and, if possible, resolve them in real life if still active. See also arthritis p. 291.

Ankylosing spondylitis (Bechterew's disease)

A "rheumatic" disease of the spine (see Rheumatism I), calcifications make movement progressively difficult > fusing of the vertebral bodies.

Conflict	Pressure from an authority. Self-esteem conflict affecting the spinal column (see p. 287).
Example	• *A now 52-year-old patient has suffered from the influence of his dominant father. Even during his childhood, the boy's father constantly found fault with his son. The patient vividly remembers the following accident and, as a result of his father's influence, he continues to blame himself: The boy knocks over a handicapped man with his bike and the man later dies as a result = self-esteem conflict of being battered by life and a central self-esteem conflict. The conflict is recurring > alternating destruction and restoration of the spine. > Calcification > diagnosis: ankylosing spondylitis.* (Archive B. Eybl)
Phase	**Persistent repair:** During every repair phase, more bone tissue is added (luxury group) > exaggerated calcification and stiffening of the spinal column. Consider "handedness" (right or left) and side (mother/child or partner) or local conflict.
Bio. meaning	Adding to the spine's hardness/strength so one can withstand the pressure (staying power).
Questions	From which person (authority) or situation do I feel overwhelmed? Are/were ancestors also affected? (Yes > family issue). What conditioned me? (Childhood, similar feelings of the parents, pregnancy)?
Therapy	Determine the conflict and conditioning and, if possible, resolve them in real life so that the persistent repair can come to an end.
	Hildegard of Bingen: Copper boiled in wine ("copper wine") special recipe. For remedies during acute phases, see arthritis. p. 291. In chronic quiet phases, see osteoarthritis p. 289.

Gout

According to CM, gout stems from high concentrations of acid in the body, with uric acid crystals responsible for inflammation in the joints. In our view, too much uric acid means that the kidney collecting tubules SBS is involved. Gout is a combined phenomenon of two SBS running at the same time, but in different phases.

Conflict/phase	**Resolved or persistent self-esteem conflict** according to body location (see p. 287) + **active refugee conflict** (kidney collecting tubules) = syndrome.
Note	Increase in uric acid, because the kidney collecting tubules SBS not only store water, they also stores protein in the form of uric acid. Fluid collection > swelling, severe pain = acute gout attack. Take into account "handedness" (right or left) and side (mother/child or partner) or local conflict. Often there is a family tendency toward hyperacidity.
Therapy	Determine the conflict and conditioning and, if possible, resolve them in real life if still active. Determine the refugee conflict and resolve it (see p. 230ff). Alkaline diet, plenty of exercise in fresh air, aerobic (sweaty) sports or sauna. These measures alone usually bring marked improvement. Hildegard of Bingen: Chew three cloves daily, drink centaury tea; parsley-rue-fat compress. Colloidal silver internally and externally. If necessary, CM medication for too much uric acid (uricosuric and uricostatics) and for those who are too comfortable to attempt conflict resolution and lifestyle change. See arthritis p. 291.

Rheumatism I (rheumatic spectrum disorder, chronic polyarthritis)[3]

CM labels rheumatism as a so-called auto-immune disease where, for an unknown reason, the body's own cells are said to turn against its own tissue and destroy it. An indication of this are "rheumatism factors" and rapid blood sedimentation and its primary factors are antibodies, which work against the body's own tissues. They are determined by observing the reaction of blood serum with other proteins in a test tube or plate. Various other tests are also used, such as the

---

3   See Dr. Hamer, Charts pp. 63, 75

so-called Waaler-Rose test or the ELISA test. For us, these tests and their results are meaningless. The term "antibodies" implies a fight between good and evil - from this erroneous notion come the terms "immunoglobulin," "antibodies" and "antigens." The truth is: we have not observed these processes anywhere in the human body to allow us to conclude that such activity occurs.

The term "immune system" is not used in the 5 Biological Laws of Nature, because there is no such thing, nor are there any "immunoglobulins" or "antibodies" or "antigens." Instead, we have "globulins," which increase after poisonings (inoculations, antibiotics, drugs, alcohol, etc.), injuries (bruises, contusions, etc.) or during repair phases.

Conflict	Self-esteem conflict, according to body location - see p. 287.
Example	• *"Rheumatism attack": A slim, 36-year-old teacher has suffered for years from polyarthritis of the arms and legs. The patient is very excited about her upcoming wedding, but her mother continuously meddles with the preparations. The bridal bouquet is the issue at hand: the mother wants to pick it out herself because the patient has not been able to. This frustrates the patient = self-esteem conflict, conflict trigger with regard to the mother. She finally decides to arrange the bouquet herself, and also decides on the music for the wedding = conflict resolution and beginning of the healing- phase; attack of rheumatism in her left, mother/child knee.* (Archive of B. Eybl)
Phase	**"Acute attack" = repair phase, symptom-free intervals = conflict activity**, more cells are removed with each inflammation > progressive thickening and deformation of the affected joint. Consider "handedness" (right or left) and side (mother/child or partner) or local conflict.
Therapy	Determine the conflict and conditioning and, if possible, resolve them in real life, so that the SBS comes to an end. Understand that rheumatism is not a progressive disease sent by fate, but that everything is dependent on the psyche. Guiding principles: *"I won't take it to heart!" "Enough of my high demands!" "Enough perfectionism!" "I trust myself." "I am strong."* Hildegard of Bingen: Centaury tea, curly leaf mint elixir, cedar fruit powder (internally), thyme paste special recipe. Measures in acute phase, see: arthritis p. 291. In chronic, quiet phase see joint deterioration, p.289. CBD oil. If necessary, CM-modifying antirheumatic drugs, possibly cortisone briefly. In exceptional cases and briefly - methotrexate.

SBS of the Superficial Periosteum

Rheumatism II[1]

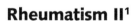

Symptoms	Pain during conflict activity, flowing pain in "cold" tissue.
Conflict	Intense or brutal-separation conflict. Suffering experienced oneself. Also, a separation conflict due to suffering inflicted on someone else.
Example	See pain at the back of the head, p. 45f.
Tissue	Periosteal surface - ectoderm. In the periosteum, we distinguish two layers: the deep-lying (interior) layer in direct contact with the bone is included in the bone SBS (self-esteem conflict) with pain in the repair phase (see above). The superficial (exterior) layer is responsible for rheumatism, pain in the active phase - during the day and under stress (= brutal-separation conflict).
Conflict-active	Migrating pain during the day, the area feels cold or actually is cold. There is no swelling or reddening, rather insufficient supply. Most important symptom: cold feet, possibly also cold calves and usually also cold hands. false sensations in the affected areas.
Repair phase	Reduced sensitivity to pain.
Note	Pain worsens during sympathicotonia (during the day) and eases at night and when resting. Painkillers hardly bring relief. Much rarer than a self-esteem conflict. (By self-esteem conflicts it is just the opposite). Consider "handedness" and side or local conflict.
Questions	With this SBS, the symptoms must have begun during stress, otherwise one is dealing with a self-esteem conflict. What was stressing me when it began? Which separation happened? What condi-

---

1   See Dr. Hamer, Charts pp. 142, 147

tioned me to this end? (Childhood, e.g., parents' divorce; pregnancy, e.g., unwanted child; birth, e.g., one wasn't allowed to be with the mother for whatever reason). Which new, inner attitude would be helpful? Which emotion(s) do I want to leave behind? What can I change on the outside?

Therapy	Determine the conflict and conditioning and, if possible, resolve them in real life. Hildegard of Bingen: cold feet - shoe inlays of badger fur, ash leaves compresses against pain. Kanne Bread Drink. Cod liver oil. If necessary: petroleum-cure. Additional therapeutic measures see p. 289 and above.

Bone fracture, fatigue fracture

Broken bones are acute injuries that are not governed by the 5 Biological Laws of Nature.

Nevertheless, from a broader (spiritual) perspective, accidents do not happen by chance. Thinking about the possible reasons is useful when one feels personal development is important.

From the perspective of the 5 Biological Laws of Nature, an SBS may be in play when a bone breaks: In the conflict-active phase of a bone SBS, the bone is weakened due to cell degradation > danger of fatigue fracture despite the "bandage effect" of the periosteum. (This encloses the bone tightly and gives it some, albeit limited, strength). In the repair phase, this bandaging effect is absent, because the periosteum is lifted off of the bone by edema. Furthermore, the bone tissue becomes sponge-like during the repair phase and is thus more susceptible to breaks > pain

makes the individual remain still, so that the bone can heal (= biological function).

For sprained or torn ligaments, tendons and muscles, it can be the same - in the active-phase of corresponding SBSs, they are weakened structurally. *One feels nothing and is "fit"* > danger of injury. In the repair phase, one is warned and slowed down by the pain.

Therapy

CM care, immobilization, but a brief cast is best.

Compresses of freshly crushed comfrey roots or a thick layer of comfrey ointment, if you have access to the place of injury.

Tea: comfrey root, horsetail.

Hildegard of Bingen: centaury, plantain internally and externally.

For after the cast removal, see arthritis p. 291.

THE MUSCULOSKELETAL SYSTEM FROM HEAD TO TOE

SBS of the Bones, Cartilage or Ligaments

Neck pain, cervical syndrome, falling asleep of the hands

Through demand for space in the area of the nerve roots, nerves and blood vessels in the arm can become compromised, causing hands to "fall asleep" in a resting state (greater pressure from edema). (Usually not a separate SBS of the hands).

Conflict	Moral-intellectual self-esteem conflict, perceived injustice, discord, bondage, dishonesty, ingratitude, indecency, intolerance, feeling stupid or unintelligent.
Examples	• *A retired woman leads an exercise class at the local senior-citizens' club. Without warning, the club president informs her that she is no longer needed for the class. She begins to recover when her students and coworkers insist that she continue = unjust self-esteem conflict, degradation of cells from the cervical spine in the active-phase and restoration in the repair phase with neck pain.* (Archive B. Eybl)
• *A patient is a student and is studying for his diploma exam. He is "running out of time" = intellectual self-esteem conflict. Since then, he experiences a trigger: whenever he has to study, he has neck pains.* (Archive B. Eybl)
• *A secretary is challenged past the limits of her intellectual abilities. Her boss is a perfectionist and insists that she finish everything punctually = intellectual self-esteem conflict. When her boss has to leave for health reasons (heart attack), the secretary comes into healing > CM: "cervical syndrome."* (Archive B. Eybl)
• *A 48-year-old, right-handed, athletic man is married for the second time and has two daughters. For a year and a half, the elder, 24-year-old daughter has been living with her boyfriend who, in the eyes of her father, doesn't suit her at all. "A big egoist!" = moral self-esteem conflict affecting the left*

N
E
W

M
E
S
O

− +

(mother/child side) of the cervical spine. After a lot of trouble, she finally separates from this man. The patient is relieved that the matter is over and his daughter has her peace again = beginning of the repair phase > for four months, his left arm always falls asleep at night. (Archive B. Eybl)

Phase	**Repair phase**, possibly persistent repair, usually recurring-conflict.
Note	Too little exercise (e.g., sitting for hours) increases the symptoms. Common attendant symptom: dizziness. Consider "handedness" (right or left) and side (mother/child or partner) or local conflict.
Questions	What brought me into the repair phase? (Weekend(s), vacation, vocalizing the problem)? What was making me feel devalued/demeaning to me before? Was that the first conflict of this type? Which conditioning lies behind the conflict? (Pregnancy, parents' feelings, school experience, upbringing, first partner)? Which internal and external changes could be helpful/healing for me? Which daily meditation would help? See also: questions p. 288f and p. 291.
Therapy	Determine the conflict and conditioning and, if chronic, resolve them in real life if possible. Guiding principles: *"I trust in my abilities." "I can't do everything at once. Easy does it - I've gotten this far and that's enough for now." "What I cannot change won't upset me."* For measures to take for acute pain, see arthritis, p. 291. In the chronic phase, see osteoarthritis, p. 289.

Cervical disk herniation (prolapsed cervical disc)

Same SBS as above .

Phase	**Intensive repair phase** - the space requirement becomes so great that the gelatinous mass at the disc core is pressed outwards. As soon as the edema retreats, the prolapsed disc corrects itself. Unless there are relapses, the matter is over at this point. May also be a recurring conflict.
Note	A disc herniation often occurs in conjunction with syndrome. The diagnosis "prolapsed disc," especially "prolapsed cervical disc" sounds threatening. Many patients believe that they will have to *"live with it"* and fear permanent paralysis > self-esteem conflict with regard to this spot = diagnosis shock. As a result, the SBS becomes self-perpetuating, much like with multiple sclerosis (MS). Naturally, the repair phase was preceded by a conflict-active phase with cell degradation in the adjacent spinal bodies or in the disc itself > this can cause the gelatinous core to become herniated (pressed out) in the repair phase or possibly in the active-phase, if the pressure is too strong. Consider "handedness" (right or left) and side (mother/child or partner), also which side is radiating pain or local conflict.
Therapy	The conflict is resolved. Support the repair phase and prevent recurrences. Always remember that a herniated disc is just temporary, i.e., after the completion of the repair phase, "it's over and done with." Measures see arthritis p. 291. For severe pain: rest (possibly for weeks). When the repair phase is too intense, one can try infiltration (syringe with painkillers and cortisone in the vicinity of the nerve root). Surgery as a last resort.

Tumor of the eye socket

Conflict	Self-esteem conflict with regard to the eye.
Example	→ *A person is confronted with the following statement: "Your eye looks so ugly that I could vomit!"*
Phase	**Repair phase**: Restoration of the eye socket = tumor.
Therapy	The conflict is resolved. Support the healing. Avoid recurrences. Do not perform a puncture.

Shoulder pain

Conflict	Self-esteem conflict, believing not to be a good mother/father (right-handed, left shoulder) or not a good partner (right-handed, right shoulder). Left-handed vice versa. In German, the word "shoulder" and "guilt" have the same root (Schulter/Schuld). In English, we say "shoulder the blame." When it comes to the shoulder, it's about a bad conscience, guilt, self-blame. Particularly common with women.
Examples	• *During her pregnancy, the patient considers having an abortion. She knows the child feels her thoughts = self-esteem conflict of believing she is not a good mother. The boy is born and is now 14 years old, but the patient is still plagued with feelings of guilt. At every opportunity, she doubts her motherly qualities = recurring-conflict with chronic pains in the mother/child shoulder. (Archive B. Eybl)* • *A patient's daughter complains that she never looks after her children, but she always has time for*

N E W M E S O

her other daughter's children > the patient thinks she's not a good mother/grandmother > the conflict is constantly recurring because she doesn't seem to be able to please her daughter > chronic shoulder pain. (Archive B. Eybl)

• *The patient cannot nurse her baby properly because her nipples are inverted. When she goes to the hospital, the doctors criticize her because the child is undernourished = self-esteem conflict of believing that she is not a good mother. The patient does not come into healing until three years later, when she is able to nurse the next child without problems > restoration of the tissue > shoulder pain.* (Archive B. Eybl)

• *The patient has an argument with her husband, loses her composure and screams at him. A short time later, she feels guilty about her behavior.* (Archive B. Eybl)

Phase	**Repair phase** or recurring conflict - restoration of bone, cartilage, ligament or muscle. Pain, inflammation. Consider "handedness" (right or left) and side (mother/child or partner) or local conflict.
Questions	Based on the symptoms, determine if it is in the repair phase or is a recurring conflict. (Over 6 months > persistent-recurring). Which event brought me into the current repair phase? (E.g., praise, a good conversation, forgiveness)? Why did I doubt before? (Determine the conflict). First instance of shoulder pain? (No > determine the original episode). Why do I always look for the fault in myself? Which conditioning lies behind it? (Lack of self-esteem based on upbringing, similarity to the parents, pregnancy)? Do I have a sufficient spiritual connection? Further questions: see p. 288f and p. 291.
Therapy	The conflict is resolved. If it is chronic, determine and resolve the conflict and/or trigger. Guiding principles: *"There's no use in feeling guilty." "I am doing my best today and now." "What's done is done." "From now on, I won't take everything so seriously."* Bach-flowers: pine, larch, scleranthus. After intense pain has subsided: targeted movement. For measures to take for acute pain: see arthritis, p. 291. In the chronic phase, see osteoarthritis, p. 289. When the repair phase is too intense, one can try an infiltration (syringe with painkillers and cortisone under the acromion). Surgery is sometimes useful but sometimes unsuccessful.

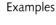

Calcium deposits in the shoulder joints

Same SBS as above

Phase	**Recurring-conflict -** persistent-repair. Local, excessive cell build-up (luxury group) > formation of calcium deposits in the articular space of the joint.
Therapy	Determine the conflict and conditioning and, if possible, resolve them in real life, so that the SBS comes to an end. Questions p. 288f and p. 291. The calcium deposits are usually not a problem. However, if they get too large and become lodged in the articular space of the joint, one can (after a period of observation with dietary changes, etc.) consider surgery. For measures to take for acute pain: see arthritis, p. 291. For the chronic phase, see osteoarthritis, p. 289.

Tennis elbow, golfer's elbow (epicondylitis)

Painful inflammation of the elbow tendons. Outside = tennis elbow. Inside = golf elbow.

Conflict	Local self-esteem conflict, inability conflict. Tennis elbow: not being able to press, push, beat, etc. something away. Golfer's elbow: not being able to hug, hold, etc. something (tightly). In my experience, the people most often affected are those who define themselves in terms of their arm performance (tennis and golf players, artisans, waiters, etc.), otherwise this type of conflict tends to manifest in the knee joint. The elbow can also react (as a "victim" or "perpetrator") to conflicts because of the "elbow technique."
Examples	• *A patient is 22-years-old and has a summer job at his relatives' restaurant. He commits himself to his work in order to show his relatives how capable he is. After two weeks of hard work, they pay him a meager salary, far below his expectations = self-esteem conflict due to lack of recognition for his work with his arms (waiting tables). He comes into healing when he gives the money back out of protest > acute tennis arm as sign of healing, strong swelling due to syndrome.* (Archive of B. Eybl) • *A semi-professional boxer is preparing for a big fight with his trainer. He loses the fight = self-esteem conflict of unsatisfied ambition with a local self-esteem conflict of not being able to hit hard enough. Nevertheless, under great pressure to succeed, he keeps on training. When he decides to box only for fun, the pain in both elbows begins = repair phase.* (Archive B. Eybl)

• A construction manager sacrifices himself for his company without receiving any special gratitude = self-esteem conflict due to lack of recognition. In a phase of total exhaustion, he decides not to take his job so seriously anymore and to reduce his efforts = conflict resolution. In the repair phase, a tennis elbow follows, which lasts for many months. (Archive B. Eybl)

• A 14-year-old, right-handed high school student is an avid practitioner of judo. Sixteen months ago, she sprained her elbow during a training accident. In the hospital she is given a cast = local self-esteem conflict. Even after her recovery, her elbow becomes inflamed after every training session. This has been occurring for 15 months and the patient begins to doubt her abilities. Before every session, she wonders whether the joint will hold = recurring local self-esteem conflict. Her therapist advises her to take a break from training and to take care of her elbow. It is not by mere chance that her mother/child elbow is the injured one, for the patient says that her mother's praise is very important to her, far more important than her father's or other people's. (Archive B. Eybl)

Phase	**Repair phase:** Restoration of the tendons = inflamed elbow, tennis elbow, golfer's elbow. Possibly a recurring-conflict.
Questions	Since when? Mother/child or partner side? What do I use my arms for the most? (Sport, work)? Which self-esteem problem was resolved at the time? Why did I identify with it so much at the time? Why do I have to prove my abilities? (Own insecurity)? What has conditioned me in terms of ambition? (E.g., ambitious parents, failure and the black sheep of the family)? Which new attitude could be helpful?
Therapy	The conflict is resolved. Support the healing. Avoid recurrences. After the intense pain is gone: stretching, movement and strength-training. For measures, see p. 291.

Osteoarthritis and polyarthritis of the finger joints

Conflict	Self-esteem conflict due to clumsiness. One believes they have treated someone wrong, to have gone about something wrong, to have done something wrong - for real or in the figurative sense. To have failed while doing and activity with their hands (perfectionism, *"my hand slipped"*). Also, local self-esteem conflict, e.g., hand is weak following a fractured wrist. The thumb represents "I," the ego. Index finger for accusations, rebukes, being right (*"with a raised index finger"*). Middle finger: expressions of contempt ("the finger"), sexuality. Ring finger: partnership/relationship, connection (wedding ring).
Examples	*• A young patient wants to learn a craft, but his mother begs and pleads with him to finish his high school diploma first. The boy acquiesces = self-esteem conflict of not being allowed to learn a craft, to work with his hands. Cell degradation in the wrist bone during the active-phase, arthritis is the repair phase. (Archive B. Eybl)* *• A woman constantly doubts whether she is doing everything right in everyday life. She was raised this way - even as a little girl, she was trained to please everybody. Her perfectionism has led to daily self-esteem conflicts with regard to her hands. The result is thickened joints. (Archive of B. Eybl)*
Phase	"Acute attack," polyarthritis - repair phase: arthrosis/osteoarthritis = **recurring-conflict**; thickened joints through recurring inflammation = danger of a vicious circle. Take into account "handedness" and side.
Therapy	Determine the conflict and conditioning and, if possible, resolve them in real life so that the SBS comes to an end. Guiding principles: *"Anybody can make mistakes." "I trust my abilities and don't take clumsy mistakes so seriously."* For measures to take for acute pain: see arthritis, p. 291. In the chronic phase, see osteoarthritis, p. 289.

Inflammation of the synovial membrane (tenosynovitis)

Same SBS as above. According to CM, caused by overuse, which is partially true, but conflicts can play a role.

Example	*• A young woman is just beginning to train as a masseur. She doubts whether this vocation suits her, because she has delicate hands = clumsiness self-esteem conflict. She comes into healing when many of her customers praise her. In the repair phase, she gets tenosynovitis. The result is a vicious circle because she sees her original doubts as confirmed and she must give up the profession. (Archive B. Eybl)*
Phase	**Repair phase:** Reconstruction of the tendon or tendon sheath. Inflammation, pain. Possibly a recurring conflict.
Bio. function	Reinforcement of the structure. Biological function of pain: immobilization, so that the body can strengthen the tendon and tendon sheath in peace. After the SBS, the tendon is stronger than before.
Therapy	The conflict is resolved. Support the healing. Avoid recurrences. For remedies, see arthritis, p. 291.

N E W   M E S O

Carpal tunnel Syndrome

Same SBS as above. The so-called carpal tunnel forms a passageway for the hand-flexing tendons and medial nerve of the hand. Chronic inflammation leads to tightening and friction.

Phase	**Persistent repair:** Excessive restoration of the carpal tunnel and/or hand-flexing tendons > strengthening of structure, tightening of the carpal tunnel, inflammation, pain = carpal tunnel syndrome.
Bio. function	Reinforcement of structures. Biological function of pain: immobilization.
Note	Frequently found in meat eaters with acidification tendency. The inability to hold onto something conflict may play a role (see below).
Therapy	Determine the conflict and conditioning and, if possible, resolve them in real life so that the persistent repair comes to an end. After the acute phase: stretching, gymnastics and flexibility exercises. For treatment measures: see arthritis, p. 291. In the chronic phase, see osteoarthritis, p. 289. Surgery if necessary.

Shortening of the flexor tendons (Dupuytren's contracture)

Conflict	Probably: Clumsiness self-esteem conflict, conflict of not being able to hold onto or keep something, not being able to "clutch/seize" something.
Examples	→ *Somebody believes that he has sold a piece of land too cheaply = conflict of not getting the money in their clutches.* • *A patient has lost his best friend because of a disagreement = conflict of not being able to hold onto his friend. Since they run into one another often, the conflict keeps recurring > Dupuytren's contracture.* (Archive B. Eybl)
Conflict-active	Cell degradation in the wrist flexor tendons.
Repair phase	Restoration, shortening of the tendons due to **recurring-conflict** > permanently scarred shortening and thickening of the tendons > the hand can no longer be opened and closed completely but the "claws" function better than ever (luxury group).
Bio. function	Strengthening of the tendons, so as to hold on better.
Note	Consider "handedness" (right or left) and side (mother/child or partner) or local conflict.
Questions	Since when? (Consider the run-up time). Who or what do I want to hold close to me? Is holding on tightly my general attitude? What were my ancestors like in this regard? Which events conditioned me? Which measures would resolve the present conflict? Which new letting-go attitude do I want to develop?
Therapy	Determine the conflict and conditioning and, if possible, resolve them in real life if still active. Guiding principle: "*I let go.*" Stretching and flexibility exercises, swimming, gymnastics. Surgery is usually not very successful - last resort. See osteoarthritis p. 289.

Sternum (breastbone) or rib pain

Conflict	Local self-esteem conflict: not being hugged or not being able to hug someone (ribs). Not being squeezed to the chest or not being able to squeeze someone to the chest (sternum) or conflict in relation to beauty (cleavage). Usually a follow-up conflict.
Examples	• *After a mastectomy, a patient no longer feels like a complete woman = local self-esteem conflict. In the repair phase she feels pain on the costal margin. CM interprets the edema as metastases.* (Archive B. Eybl) • *A doctor examines a patient's lungs during a check-up and says, "Something's not right with your lungs."* (Archive B. Eybl) • *Due to a diagnosis of breast cancer, a woman suffers a self-esteem conflict. She thinks: "Now I'm not worth anything here anymore." When the tumor is successfully removed, her ribs begin to hurt = repair phase.* (Archive B. Eybl)
Phase	**Repair phase:** reconstruction of sternum or ribs, pain. Possibly a recurring-conflict.
Therapy	The conflict is resolved. Support the repair phase. For measures, see osteoarthritis, p. 289.

Pain in the thoracic spine

Conflict	Self-esteem conflict of being battered by life, feeling humiliated or inferior; conflict of being a "loser." "He has no backbone!" Or local self-esteem conflict because something is wrong in the chest region.
Examples	• *A patient is a trainee and is happy that she has finally found a position. She thinks she has to accept the fact that her boss is always putting her down. She is unhappy but doesn't defend herself = self-esteem conflict of being a loser. During her two years as a trainee, she suffers intense pain in the thoracic spine = recurring-conflict. After that, she swears to herself that at her next job she will not be forced to put up with anything. Since then, the pain is gone.* (Archive B. Eybl)
	• *A woman has a complex, because she believes her breasts are too small = local self-esteem conflict.* (Archive B. Eybl)
Phase	**Repair phase** or recurring conflict. Restoration of the spinal body or cartilage, pain.
Note	Applies to the whole spinal column: Every individual vertebra has a connection to an internal organ, e.g., thoracic vertebrae 9 - 11 with the kidneys. > With complaints, consider a kidney conflict.
Questions	Do I submit? (Authority, independence, to elders or superiors)? Do ancestors have similar tendencies? (Indication of a family issue). What would happen if I didn't subordinate myself anymore? Which beliefs allowed me to become this way? (E.g., *"I'll only be loved if I'm a good child"*).
Therapy	The conflict is resolved. If it recurs, determine the conflict or trigger and resolve it in real life. Guiding principles: *"Nobody has the right to humiliate me." "I will walk straight and upright through life."* From an energetics point-of-view, thoracic spinal pains usually have to do with empty conditions. Hildegard of Bingen: rub with bay leaf oil. If necessary, antirheumatics when repair pain is too intense. For additional measures, see osteoarthritis, p. 289.

Scoliosis (side to side curvature of the spine), round back (juvenile kyphosis, Scheuermann's disease, wedge vertebrae)

Same SBS as above, if the thoracic vertebrae are affected. Curvatures of the spine, usually combined with twisted vertebrae, usually begin in childhood or youth.

Conflict-active	One-sided degeneration of the vertebrae, depending on the nature of the conflict (mother/child or partner side) > side to side curvature of that section of the spine; the body attempts to compensate by means of opposing curves above and below the affected vertebra > "S"-shaped spine > scoliosis; wedge-shaped vertebrae and a round back occur when the vertebrae degenerate on the "belly" side.
Repair phase	The degenerated, now asymmetrical spinal chord becomes fixed in this position - it all becomes "cemented." There is pain only while cells are being built up, but the spinal chord remains permanently curved.
Note	These curvatures mustn't necessarily cause trouble later. I know "completely crooked" patients, without the slightest difficulties and others with perfectly straight spinal cords with massive complaints > the body can usually deal with these differences quite well.
Questions	When the scoliosis began in childhood > work out the parental or family issue. > One can only help their child through their own conscious work. Issues/topics: honesty (uprightness), straightforwardness, bent out of shape for love, money, prestige. Do other family members have scoliosis? (Find similarities).
Therapy	Determine the conflict and conditioning and resolve them, if it is still active. Send good thoughts to the spine. Doubt and discord are neither appropriate nor relevant. Postural exercises, strength training, versatile sports.

Pain in the lumbar spine or coccyx, lower back pain (LBP), sciatica

Conflict	Central-personality self-esteem conflict. Explanation: A person is shaken to the core, the burden is too great - the pressure is unbearable; or a local self-esteem conflict, for instance, because of sexual desperation or a diagnosis of colon cancer or hemorrhoids.
Examples	• *A right-handed, married mother of a two-year-old, has suffered from LBP and sciatica on her left mother/child side, since the child was born. Conflict history: Her mother-in-law lives with them in the same house. The mother-in-law has no confidence in the patient's ability to care for the child.*

She consistently criticizes the patient for this = central loss of self-esteem with regard to the child. She feels inferior and has resigned herself to the situation = hanging-conflict > constant back pain. (Claudio Trupiano, thanks to Dr. Hamer, p. 261)

• *A now 41-year-old patient is treated extremely unfairly by his math teacher at a technical school. The sensitive young man takes this very personally = central-personality self-esteem conflict. After he finishes at the school, he completes an advanced degree under the motto: "I'll just show him." Since his days at the technical college, the patient has suffered regularly from severe lower back pain = recurring-conflict. Trigger: mathematical work under stress.* (Archive B. Eybl)

• *A man is diagnosed with an intestinal tumor = local self-esteem conflict.* (Archive B. Eybl)

• *A woman is abandoned by her partner, whom she loved very much. She believes that he has left her because she wasn't good in bed = local or central self-esteem conflict.* (Archive B. Eybl)

Phase	**Repair phase** or recurring conflict. Restoration of the tissue that was previously degraded, practically unnoticed; the healing bone or cartilage tissue swells up and presses against the spinal cord or nerve roots (sciatica). Consider "handedness" (right or left) and side (mother/child or partner) or local conflict. Into which leg does the pain radiate?
Note	The most common diagnosis by therapists, *"Your sacroiliac joint is blocked, you have unequal leg length,"* shouldn't be taken seriously, because it is a mechanical conception. I know people with perfect symmetry who have constant pain and others with very misaligned skeletal components (pelvic obliquity, scoliosis) without pain. Nevertheless, therapeutic procedures to unblock the SIJ make sense, because the pelvic organs also benefit from this.
Questions	Which conflict was resolved when the pain began? What brought me into healing? (E.g., praise, completion of a burdensome project, weekends, vacation, retirement)? Do I have a problem with sitting? (Yes > indication that the conflict was experienced while sitting - sitting trigger). Why couldn't I deal with the pressure? Did I put myself under pressure? Similar symptoms among ancestors? (Indication of a family issue. > Work out why people in the family put themselves under pressure and which beliefs are at play. E.g., *"All that counts is performance." "Only hard workers will be loved." "Only the sick have an excuse"*). Which inner and outer changes will I make?
Therapy	The conflict is resolved. If chronic, determine and resolve the conflict and conditioning. Guiding principles: *"Pressure exists in order to be shaken off." "I want to be free and happy - that makes life easier."* Hildegard of Bingen: galangal root wine. Possibly chiropractic, osteopathy, strength training, muscle building. If necessary, an antirheumatic agent. When the repair phase is too intense, one can try an infiltration (syringe with painkillers and cortisone in the vicinity of the nerve root). Measures to take for acute pain, see arthritis, p. 291. In the chronic phase, see osteoarthritis, p. 289.

Slipped (prolapsed) disc of the lumbar spine

Same SBS as above.

Example	• *A married patient is building his own house. At the same time, he has to "hold his own" at work = central-personality self-esteem conflict. When the house is finally finished and the family moves in, he suffers a slipped disc in his lower back = repair phase.* (Archive B. Eybl)
Phase	**Intensive repair phase,** a herniated disk only occurs along with syndrome. The repair phase was preceded by a conflict-active phase with cell degradation in the adjacent vertebral bodies or in the disc itself. > In the repair phase, this can cause the disc's gelatinous core to be squeezed out. If the burden is great, this could occur as early as the active-phase. As soon as the structure is repaired and the edema recedes, the disc corrects itself. This should be the end of the matter if there are no recurrences.
Note	A diagnosis of "herniated disc" can lead to a follow-up conflict. Many patients believe that *"they will have to live with it"* = diagnosis shock in the form of another self-esteem conflict with regard to this location > danger of a vicious circle. Earlier, slipped discs were also common. Fortunately, they were diagnosed much less often (when toes went numb), because there still weren't any CT and MRI machines.
Therapy	The self-esteem conflict is resolved. Resolve any refugee conflict. Guiding principle: *"I will leave all the pressure and doubt behind me."* Remember that the herniated disc is temporary, i.e., after completion of the repair phase, the problem is over and done with. For therapy, see arthritis, p. 291. If the repair phase is too intense, one can try an infiltration (syringe with painkillers and cortisone in the vicinity of the nerve root). Surgery should be the last resort for numbness.

Spinal stenosis

Same SBS as above. (See p. 300ff)

Phase	**Persistent repair** over a long period of time, excessive bone buildup leads to permanent stenosis (narrowing) of the spinal canal > compressed nerves with pain radiating into the leg.
Therapy	Determine the conflict and conditioning and, if possible, resolve them in real life so that the SBS comes to an end. Questions: see previous page. Do not magnify the diagnosis - the complaints often disappear completely. Stretching and other gymnastics. For measures, see arthritis p. 291. In the chronic phase, see osteoarthritis, p. 289. If necessary, anti-inflammatory drugs if the pain is too intense. After exhausting all measures, one may consider attempting the difficult surgery.

Slipped vertebrae (spondylolisthesis)

This diagnosis is rather uncertain (presumptive diagnosis). SBS same as above. (See p. 300ff)

Phase	Recurring-conflict - **persistent conflict activity**. Shrinking of the spinal cord or the space between the discs > individual discs can become loose and slide forward or backwards.
Therapy	Determine the conflict and conditioning and, if possible, resolve them in real life. Questions: see previous page. Strength training, muscle building (no stretching). For measures to take when the pain is acute, see arthritis, p. 291. In the chronic phase, see osteoarthritis, p. 289.

Pain in the pubic bone or pelvic bone

Conflict	Local self-esteem conflict. With men, this often has to do with sexuality or potency. Women react to a sexual self-esteem conflict with the pelvis, sacrum, or pubic bone.
Examples	→ *Somebody suffers from incontinence = local self-esteem conflict, degradation of bone substance in the active-phase, restoration and pain in the repair phase.* → *After prostate gland surgery, a man is impotent.* → *A husband suffers from premature ejaculation. For this reason, he cannot satisfy his wife.*
Phase	**Repair phase:** restoration of the pubic bone or pelvic bone substance. Possibly recurring conflict. Consider "handedness" (right or left) and side (mother/child or partner) or local conflict.
Therapy	The conflict is resolved. Support the healing. For therapeutic measures, see p. 291.

Fatigue fracture of the pelvic bone

Same SBS as above (see above).

Phase	**Persistent conflict activity:** Degradation of bone tissue > loss of stability, very little pain, possibly sensitivity to cold.
Therapy	Determine the conflict and conditioning and, if possible, resolve them in real life.

Ischium bone pain

Conflict	Self-esteem conflict of not being able to sit something out or a local self-esteem conflict. Also, sexuality issues.
Examples	→ *Someone believes he won't be able to endure something, such as a situation at work.* → *Someone has hemorrhoids = local self-esteem conflict.*
Repair phase	Restoration of the bone, pain. Possibly a recurring conflict
Therapy	The conflict is resolved. Support the healing. For measures, see arthritis, p. 291.

Hip pains

Conflict	Self-esteem conflict of not being able to endure something or a local self-esteem conflict. Also, sexuality issues.

Examples	• *A young, right-handed woman was born with a deformed pelvis, which does not cause her any problems. She would like to have a child with her partner and decides to consult the best doctor in the region, to see if there is any reason why she might not be able to have a child. The specialist looks at the undressed woman from all sides with a professional look. His commentary: "I hope you don't want to have children! If you do, we would have to perform surgery to widen your pelvis. To be exact, we would have to take a part of the pelvis out and temporarily plant it into the knee area. After the birth and nursing period, we would have to reverse the process!" = Local self-esteem conflict with regard to the pelvis and hips. The patient cries on her friend's shoulder and decides to get a second opinion. An experienced gynecologist then gives her the "green light." As a healthy child is born, the left (mother/child) hip comes into healing. The pain lasts for half a year and is so severe that the patient cannot even walk to the car. In the meantime, a second healthy baby boy has been born and the patient is completely free of symptoms. (Archive B. Eybl)* • *A patient's mother is constantly meddling in his marriage. The man does not know the solution to this dilemma. He's being pulled in two directions at once. He knows no way out of this situation. (Archive B. Eybl)* • *A 69-year-old, left-handed mother of two grown sons has a dog that she loves very much. He belongs to the family and is her "partner." The dog is becoming increasingly frail. The patient knows that in the end she will have to put him to sleep so that he will not suffer pain = self-esteem conflict - "I just won't be able to bear it, having to put the dog to sleep." The left (partner) hip is affected. Finally, her husband makes the difficult trip to the veterinarian. The patient is terribly sad, but glad to have it behind her. Ten days afterwards, in the course of the repair phase, pain in the left hip begins, which lasts for four weeks. (Archive B. Eybl)*
Phase	**Repair phase** or recurring-conflict. Reconstruction of hip joint or femoral neck > inflammation, limitation of movement, pain. Consider "handedness" and side or local conflict.
Questions	How long have the complaints been apparent? (Longer than 6 months > chronic, persistent conflict. Less than 6 months > repair phase or chronic, persistent conflict). Handedness - side? What am I unable to get through/withstand? What is my heavy burden? Which thing or person can I not endure? Hip problems among ancestors? (Indication of a family issue). Which emotions accompany the issue? What are the earliest childhood memories related to this issue? How was the pregnancy? The birth? Did the mother think that she wasn't going to be able to survive the birth? What do I want to change on the inside? What on the outside? With which new attitude will I be able to achieve relief?
Therapy	The conflict is resolved. If recurrent, determine and resolve the conflict, trigger(s) and conditioning. For measures, see arthritis, p. 291.

Hip joint arthrosis (coxarthrosis)

Same SBS as above.

Phase	**Recurring-conflict:** Constantly recurring phases of cell degradation and cell growth result in inferior scar tissue. > Roughening of the joint surface > progressive destruction of the cartilage, limited movement, pain.
Therapy	Determine the conflict and conditioning and, if possible, resolve them in real life. Guiding principles: *"Just when you start thinking it's no longer possible, a light suddenly appears from somewhere." "I know everything's going to be all right."* Bach-flowers: larch, sweet chestnut, willow. A hip replacement surgery is recommended when the joint surfaces are too damaged by recurring-conflicts. Most surgeries are successful, thanks to great surgeons and good techniques! For measures, see arthrosis, p. 289.

Necrosis of the femoral head (Legg-Calve-Perthe's disease)

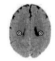

Same SBS as above. (See p. 302f)

Symptom	A part of the femoral head dies off (necrotizes) and in the worst case, disintegrates > sudden severe pain, limping; this disease is common among dogs and small children.
Phase	**Conflict-active phase:** destruction of bone tissue > loss of stability > crumbling of the femoral head.
Therapy	Consider individually. In children, always consider inheritance from parents/ancestors.

Knee pains, inflammation of the knee joint (arthritis), inflammation of the bursa (bursitis)

Conflict	Non-athletic self-esteem conflict, lack of recognition, unsatisfied ambition. From this, a feeling of humiliation can arise. Among those who define themselves through their legs (soccer players, runners, bikers, etc.), it is the knee that is affected.
Examples	• *A young, right-handed man marries into a family business where he always stands on the sidelines. His in-laws never praise him, although he takes great pains and works until the brink of exhaustion. When his in-laws step back from the business, he suddenly gets praise from all sides. Due to the great conflict mass, the right (partner) knee is inflamed and swollen for many years = repair phase. Finally, when his symptoms do not improve, he has an artificial knee implanted.* (Archive B. Eybl)
	• *A now 50-year-old, right-handed man has had a hard life. His parents rob him of every bit of self-esteem. His school years are a "catastrophe." He is kept back a year because he cannot keep up with the others. With much effort, his parents find him an apprenticeship with a hairdresser, where he muddles his way through: "I can't dress hair!" = Self-esteem conflict of being non-athletic with regard to the right partner-knee. He takes the final hair-dressers' exam, although he is convinced that he is incompetent and will fail. After three weeks, the results come ins: he passed. = The right knee begins to swell up = repair phase. The patient has unsuccessful surgery on his knee and is bedridden for two years. Then, things start to improve but only because of the many surgeries and recurrences he suffers from chronic, severe pain.* (Archive B. Eybl)
Phase	**Repair phase:** increased metabolism in the knee joint, cell growth, swelling, reddening, pain. Consider "handedness" (right or left) and side (mother/child or partner) or local conflict. Possibly a recurring-conflict.
Questions	Pain since when? (The conflict must have been resolved beforehand). Acute (nighttime) pain: sudden resolution. Pain beginning slowly: drawn-out conflict resolution or chronic conflict. Which conflict was resolved? Handedness - side? Who did I want to show (up)? (Clap test provides an indication). Why was I hungry for recognition/praise? (Which deeper need lies behind this - usually a need to be loved)? Why do I define myself through performance? (Upbringing, parental style, ancestors)? Did I feel humiliated or small? Which family member do I resemble? (Indication of conditioning > work out similar motivations). What am I worth without recognition? Which specific measures could resolve the conflict? Which new inner attitude do I want to take on? Which meditation would be helpful/healing?
Therapy	The conflict is resolved. Support the healing. When the repair phase is too intense, possibly anti-inflammatory drugs or infiltration (syringe with painkillers and cortisone). For measures, see arthritis, p. 291.

Knee: torn meniscus, damaged cartilage, ruptured cruciate or collateral ligament

Same SBS as above.

Examples	• *As a 23-year-old competitive windsurfer, I took a year off after taking part in the Los Angeles Olympic Games. Afterwards, I tried to make a comeback, so I could compete again in the next Olympics. However, things went badly for me during the trial races - I had "missed the boat" > self-esteem conflict of being non-athletic. Before the trials were over, I had torn the meniscus of my left partner-knee and had to undergo arthroscopic knee surgery = injury in the active-phase due to weakened tissue.* (Personal experience of B. Eybl)
Phase	**Recurring-conflict.** Torn meniscus and ruptured ligaments usually occur as accidents. We shouldn't classify them as "injuries" however, as the cause of damage is soft, weak tissue. Such injuries can occur in the active-phase or in the repair phase. Also, poor diet and lack of exercise may play a role. Repair phase tears would not be necessary if the pain message would be interpreted properly. When the knee hurts, move conservatively and gently.
Therapy	Determine the conflict and conditioning and, if possible, resolve them in real life. Guiding principles: *"I know what I am capable of, even if others don't notice." "True recognition comes from within. It is a good feeling to have done something good and to have given love."* For measures to take for acute pain, see arthritis p. 291. In the chronic phase, see osteoarthritis, p. 289. When the healing process is too intense, possibly anti-inflammatory drugs or infiltration (syringe with painkillers and cortisone directly into the joint). A knee replacement surgery is recommended when the joint surfaces are degraded by recurring-conflicts. Most surgeries are successful - a compliment to the surgeons!

Knee joint mouse (loose joint body), osteochondritis dissecans

Same SBS as above (see p. 304). A small foreign body, such as a small piece of bone or cartilage "swims" about in the joint and can cause sudden immobility or pain.

Phase	Condition after a complete SBS - **recurring-conflict,** possibly due to injury.
Therapy	Determine the conflict and conditioning and, if possible, resolve them in real life if still active. Should the "mouse" become lodged repeatedly > arthroscopic joint cleansing to prevent further inflammation (and prevent subsequent self-esteem conflicts). Moreover, in the case of a herniation, there is a risk of consequent self-esteem conflicts.

(Anterior) cruciate ligament or collateral ligament tear (partial/complete)

Conflict	Non-athletic self-esteem conflict. According to Frauenkron-Hoffmann, the cruciate ligaments - derived from their function - have to do with the inability to turn around, to change course, to start over.
Phase	**Recurring-conflict** through which the ligaments become brittle and prone to injury.
Therapy	Determine and resolve the conflict, causal conditioning and beliefs. Discuss an OP or a brace with your orthopedist.

Inflammation of the ankle or toe joints

Conflict	Cannot stand someone or a situation, self-esteem conflict: cannot run, jump, dance, kick, brake etc. or it's a local self-esteem conflict. Often, also a localization-theme: *"I wish I would be there and not here." "I am out of place here." "Unfortunately, I have to stay here."*
Example	• *A schoolboy cannot join go along on the school hiking week, which he had been looking forward to for so long, because he has a cold = self-esteem conflict of not being able to run, jump, etc. He comes into healing when the hiking week is over > inflamed ankle. (Archive B. Eybl)*
Phase	**Repair phase:** restoration of the bone or cartilage, pain, swelling. Metatarsophalangeal joint inflammation are often an indication of gout (= syndrome). Possibly a recurring conflict.
Questions	Complaints since when? (The preceding conflict entered the repair phase shortly before). First instance of pain? (No > find the first episode). Who or what couldn't I stand? Otherwise, am I unhappy with where I am? (Workplace, town, family)? Which emotions are affecting me? What does this remind me of from my childhood? Did any ancestors go through a similar experience? (Speak with parents). Which new emotions could be helpful/healing? What can I change externally?
Therapy	The conflict is resolved. Support the repair phase. If recurrent, find conflict, triggers, conditioning and resolve. Hildegard of Bingen: solanus special recipe. When the repair phase is too intense, possibly anti-inflammatory drugs or infiltration (syringe with painkillers and cortisone directly into the joint). For measures, see arthritis, p. 291.

Inflammation of the Achilles tendon

Conflict	Self-esteem conflict. Without the Achilles tendon, one cannot run or jump. This is the reason it's about upward and forward mobility. According to Frauenkron-Hoffmann: One is striving higher, wants to climb, but cannot achieve it.
Example	• *The patient is a soccer coach. He internalizes every little failure of his team = substitute self-esteem conflict of not being able to run fast enough. As his team finally racks up a series of victories, his Achilles tendon comes into painful healing. (Archive B. Eybl)*
Phase	**Repair phase:** restoration, strengthening of the Achilles tendon, pain when loaded; the tendon remains thick (luxury group). Possibly a recurring-conflict.
Questions	Which conflict was resolved when the pain began? Symptoms for the first time? (Examine the first episode if necessary). Is it about not being able to walk/make progress? Is is about not being able to move upward? Which emotions and conditioning are the cause? (Ambition, impatience)? Where do they come from?
Therapy	The conflict is resolved. Support the healing. Attention: Due to the danger of a rupture, be careful about putting weight on it. For measures, see arthritis p. 291.

Rupture of the Achilles tendon or collateral ligament

Same SBS as above.

Phase   Recurring-conflict, conflict activity or repair phase.

Note   The line between "injury" and SBS is often blurred. Soft, weak tissue is often the basis for injuries. Ruptures of the Achilles tendon in the repair phase happen to impatient athletes. (Full training, despite pain).

Therapy   Determine the conflict and conditioning and, if possible, resolve them in real life if still active. For treatment, see arthritis, p. 291, particularly alkaline diet. Surgery if necessary.

Heel spur (calcaneal spur)

Conflict   Self-esteem conflict: someone can't spur onward, can't spur someone onward.
Also, not flee fast enough/is unable to run away (take to one's heels).

Examples   • *A teacher is being bullied by her colleague, who tries to hinder every project she wants to undertake = self-esteem conflict, not being able to spur someone onward. As the patient finally succeeds in pushing a big project through, she gets a painful heel spur in the repair phase.* (Archive B. Eybl)
• *Due to the left-handed, adult patient's clumsiness, her mother has a gardening accident and breaks her ankle. The patient blames herself and suffers a self-esteem conflict substituting for her mother. When the cast is removed and her mother can walk about freely again, the patient comes into healing > severe pain in the right (mother/child) heel.* (www.germanische-heilkunde.at)

Phase   **Repair phase:** Excessive restoration of the calcaneus or fascia or Achilles tendon attachment (luxury group); although the spur still appears on an x-ray after the repair phase, the pain usually disappears completely.

Questions   Who couldn't I spur onward? (Aggressive moment)? Did I want to run away from someone? (E.g., mother-in-law, an arrogant boss)? What conditioned me? (Parents, childhood)?

Therapy   The conflict is resolved. Should it recur, determine the conflict and/or trigger(s) and conditioning. Guiding principles: *"I make peace in my heart. Whatever happens to me has a meaning. I can only learn from it."* Wear only comfortable and possibly open-heel footwear, e.g., an insert with a recess at the pressure point, so that the area can recuperate. Surgery is rarely necessary. > It is better to wait for a long time. Treatment, see arthritis, p. 291 and osteoarthritis, p. 289.

Bunion (hallus valgus - deformation of the big toe joint)

Conflict   Not being able to kick somebody away; self-esteem conflict of not being able to run, dance, balance, jump, kick, stop, etc. Sometimes its is a location conflict. According to Frauenkron-Hoffmann: direction conflict - the direction, in which one should go, is forced upon them. One wants to go in one direction, but is not allowed to. The doors are closed to someone.

Example   • *A 35-year-old mother of two sons developed bunions on both feet despite wearing flat shoes and eating a healthy diet. Her one big conflict is that both boys are constantly fighting with one another. = Self-esteem conflict. Most of all, she would like to give the older, aggressive son a good kick in the pants to get him to stop. It turns out that her children are reflecting her own behavior; she, herself, fought terribly with her brother their whole youth and doesn't have contact with him anymore.* (Archive B. Eybl)

Phase   **Recurring-conflict,** persistent repair: with every inflammation (= repair phase, cell growth) another layer is added > thickening, crookedness, deformation of the toe and toe joint.

Note   Shoes that are too tight or heels that are too high can destroy the toe joint mechanically (in this case, there is no conflict). Self-esteem - danger of vicious circle due to the unaesthetic bulging of the big toe. Consider "handedness" (right or left) and side (mother/child or partner) or local conflict.

Therapy   Find the conflict or trigger(s) and resolve them so that the SBS comes to an end. Flat, broad, possibly open footwear with enough free space for the toes. Measures, see arthritis p. 291. In an advanced stages, surgery may be an option.

MUSCULAR SYSTEM

There are two kinds of muscle tissue: the involuntary (smooth) muscles of the internal organs, which are controlled by the midbrain of the brainstem and the voluntary (striated) muscles of the of the musculoskeletal system, which are controlled by the cerebrum.

This chapter is about the voluntary (striated) muscles. These are controlled by two different parts of the brain:

1. The cerebral white matter - responsible for muscle nutrition.
2. The cerebral cortex - responsible for the muscle innervation/ transmission of neural stimulation.

In the SBS described below, they are usually coupled with each other; i.e., they often operate concurrently. However, most muscle symptoms, like paralysis, cramps, epilepsy and Parkinson's, stem from the SBS of the muscle-nerve supply (below).

SBS of the Muscle-Nerve Supply

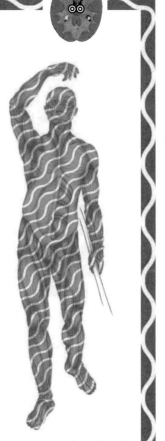

BASIC SEQUENCE[1]

The motor nerve impulses - i.e., the tensing and relaxing commands, come from the motor cortex of the cerebral cortex:

Conflict	Motor conflict, most often due to a real fall, accident, or injury. In a figurative sense: paralyzing fear = conflict, not being allowed, wanting or able to move. Not being able to escape a situation. One feels abandoned, unable to cope, doesn't know which way is up. Phrases: "Paralyzed with fear." "Frozen by the shock." "At a loss for what to do." Back muscles: Not being able to escape from someone or from something, inability to protect oneself. Shoulder musculature: Feelings of guilt, inability to embrace or bring someone closer. Leg and arm flexor and adductor muscles: Feeling unable to hold, bring closer or embrace someone or something. Leg and arm-extender and abductor muscles: Unable to push, punch, kick or shove someone or something away, fend off. Legs in general: Not being able to get away, escape, go with or catch up. Not being able to (fast enough) run, climb, go up or go down, dance, jump, balance, etc. "My knees go weak!"
Tissue	Voluntary (striated) muscles - cerebral cortex - ectoderm (nerve supply = innervation).
Conflict-active	Restriction of nerve function, less and less stimuli from the cortical motor center to the muscle. > Weakness, paralysis, depending on the intensity of the conflict. Possible restlessness, fidgeting.
Bio. function	Play-dead reflex: Many animals instinctively stop when they see a predator or are being chased and the situation seems hopeless. The predator, then, often can't spot the prey's movement (birds) or lets its prey be (e.g., cats are only interested in moving/living objects and not in motionless/dead prey). The motto: *"Don't move until the danger has passed!"*
Repair phase	Restoring innervation after initial deterioration.
Repair crisis	Uncoordinated twitching and convulsions = epileptic seizure. Local spasm = muscle spasm, muscle twitching. Feeling cold, cold chills. Possibly tics, restless legs.
Note	Warning: At the beginning of the repair phase and after the repair phase crisis, the paralyses can even be briefly stronger if edema causes the nerve connections in the brain to swell. While this is actually a good sign, it is often wrongly interpreted by the patient, which can lead to a fatal, vicious circle. Many muscle problems are caused by poisoning with medication. As such, they have no psychic cause. There is often a combination of conflict and poisoning. The usual suspects here are often blood pressure medication, cholesterol-lowering medication, psychotropic drugs and many more. > Read the information on the package. Take note of any link between when the medication was first taken and any symptoms.

E
C
T
O

− +

SBS of the Muscular Metabolism

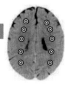

N E W M E S O

−+

BASIC SEQUENCE[1]

The metabolic control (nutrition, the growth and breakdown of tissue) originates in the cerebral white matter.

Conflict	Self-esteem conflict with regard to mobility (for conflict details, see p. 287).
Tissue	Voluntary (striated) muscle - new mesoderm - nutrition, metabolism.
Conflict-active	Limited nutrition, muscle deterioration in the affected muscle(s), muscle weakness (necrosis, atrophy).
Repair phase	Restoration of the muscles accompanied by pain, swelling, enlarged muscles (hypertrophy).
Bio. function	Strengthening beyond the original state (luxury group).

1   See Dr. Hamer, Charts pp. 61, 72

SBS of the Muscle Innervation

E C T O

−+

Muscle paralysis, multiple sclerosis (MS), polio, amyotrophic lateral sclerosis (ALS)[1]

In MS, the (myelin) nerve sheaths in the central nervous system become inflamed and cannot fulfil their task of quickly transmitting neural stimuli. Thus, this SBS is about command transmission.

Conflict	Motor conflict. Paralyzing fear. Conflict of not being able, or allowed to move. (See p. 307). According to Dr. Sabbah: Obedience conflict. One believes that they always have to carry out all commands. They resist, but wind up submitting nonetheless. The beginning of this conflict may lie in the childhood years: One is broken (tamed) during the defiant phase. Saying no is not allowed - authority must be obeyed mercilessly.
Examples	• *A 63-year-old is never bored, not even in retirement. He spends his time as an amateur athlete and handyman. One day, he has a skiing accident and breaks his hips. He must endure four months of complete bed rest = motor conflict of not being able to move. After the long, forced rest, he is sent to rehabilitation and makes excellent progress. He realizes that he is his old self again = conflict resolution. Then he starts having nighttime cramps in his lower legs. The cramps continue for weeks and keep getting stronger. He finds these spasms more painful than the broken hips = motor conflict because of the cramps = vicious circle. After many consultations with doctors, he is sent to the hospital where they do a lumbar puncture, an MRI and nerve conduction tests. Suddenly he sees the worried expressions on the doctors' faces: the diagnosis is ALS. He is told about the "progressive symptoms" ending in death via suffocation due to general paralysis = generalized motor conflict of knowing he is soon to be completely paralyzed. Within half a year, the disease advances so far that the one-time amateur athlete has to sit in a wheelchair all day and at night cannot even turn over in bed = vicious circle and fulfillment of the prognosis (= the self-fulfilling prophecy). A truly tragic case.* (Archive B. Eybl)
	• *A 50-year-old, right-handed woman goes to a neurologist with steady, acute pain in the face. He prescribes painkillers and anti-depressants. For both prescriptions, paralysis is mentioned as possible side effects. After several weeks, the patient notices light paralysis of the right leg. The facial pain remains. After several consultations with neurologists, along with a CT scan and lumbar puncture, the diagnosis is multiple sclerosis (MS) = motor conflict due to the diagnosis. The patient sees herself in a wheelchair and buys a cane, which she doesn't even need yet > the paralysis intensifies > the vicious downward spiral begins.* (Archive B. Eybl)
Phase	Active-phase, **persistent conflict activity.** > Weakness or paralysis of the muscle.

1   See Dr. Hamer, Charts pp. 138, 143

Note	Even for CM, the diagnosis for multiple sclerosis (MS) is imprecise. The proteins measured in the cerebrospinal fluid (CSF) also appear in healthy samples. In the CT and MRI, dubious "white flecks" are sought, which are also found in everyone. A diagnosis of MS usually triggers another motor conflict (which is worse) than the original one. Some patients see the wheelchair before their eyes (post-hypnotic engram). This conflict can often no longer be overcome = persistent-active conflict as a result of the doctors' diagnoses (iatrogenic). A small percentage of paraplegics also belong to this group of thusly damaged patients.
Further causes	1. Accidents or unsuccessful surgeries (mechanical paralysis - severing of the nerve). 2. Poisoning, e.g., with chemicals, medication (toxic paralysis), e.g., aspartame. 3. Brain pressure (edema) on the surrounding motor relays (usually a self-esteem conflict in healing).
Questions	When did the symptoms begin? (Conflict beforehand. Close to the time of a sudden onset of symptoms. With a disease that comes on slowly, the conflict could have happened years before). Only weakness/paralysis? (Yes > purely conflict-active). Cramps/spasms also? (Yes > intermittent repair phases). Which part of the body was affected first? (One can deduce the conflict from the affected muscle groups, see: p. 307 and also p. 287). Mother/child or partner side? (Clap test). Was there a fall or an accident? (Typical motor conflict). Was there an obedience conflict? Am I always obedient and conformist? Was my defiant spirit broken in childhood? Muscular diseases among ancestors? (Yes > indication of a family issue > work out the affected family member's exact issue/conflict). Which other conditioning comes into play? How was the pregnancy? (Accidents, obedience conflict for the mother)? How was the birth? (Often a reason for motor conflicts). Does the disease also provide me with benefits? (I receive love/care, don't have to struggle anymore, don't have to exert myself anymore, don't have to listen to orders anymore). Do the advantages outweigh the disadvantages? (If yes, this will be an impediment to getting better > one has to be honest with oneself about what one really wants). Which inner changes do I want to make? Would, e.g., a special healing-meditation make sense? Which measures to I want to use externally?
Therapy	Determine the conflict and conditioning and, if possible, resolve them in real life. Very important: understanding the interrelations. Guiding principles: *"Now I know what's going on and I will free myself from the spell!" "I will be able to move as before!"* Movement therapy, but without (self-applied) pressure to succeed. All of the stimulating treatments like classic, acupoint and reflex-zone massages. Cayce: Vigorous massage with peanut oil or olive oils with tincture of myrrh. If necessary, take petroleum. Swimming, gymnastics, yoga, etc. Magnesium chloride ($MgCl_2$) - foot baths. (Source: www.salzschwarzmann.de). Sunbathing - possibly solarium. Brushing and contrast baths. Vitamin B complex. Liniments with rosemary, cinnamon or camphor oil. If necessary, low-dose naltrexone (LDN). Cod liver oil. CM therapies with cortisone, beta-interferon and many more are not recommended because they are not effective. (See also: further measures, p. 287).

Muscle spasms

Motor conflict corresponding to the location (See p. 307 and also p. 287).

Examples	• *In winter, the patient is driving down a steep mountain road. Suddenly she realizes she is driving too fast and won't be able to make the next curve = motor conflict of not being able to brake. Thanks to a snow pile, the car comes to a stop just before the abyss. During the next three nights, she has severe cramps in her right ("brake") calf = healing- phase - repair phase crisis.* (Archive B. Eybl)
	• *An older mountain climber has trouble keeping up with a younger group = motor conflict of not being able to keep up. After the tour, she suffers severe thigh cramps = repair phase. This happens every time she goes hiking with this group. When she goes alone, she has no cramps afterwards.* (Archive B. Eybl)
Phase	**Repair phase crisis** (= epileptic crisis) in the course of the repair phase. Possibly a recurring-conflict.
Note	Cramps always arise during rest or after strain. The prior paralysis is, normally, not perceived. The cramp is a "local epilepsy." Generalized cramp = "real epilepsy" (see p. 310). Consider "handedness" (right or left) and side (mother/child or partner) or local conflict.
Questions	Which muscle group? (= Indication of the conflict. Which activity was I doing before the cramp appeared? (Conflict usually directly beforehand or the day before). Mother/child or partner related? (Clap test). Why couldn't I deal with the situation? Which emotions were in play? What has conditioned me in this regard?

Therapy	Determine the conflict or trigger(s) and resolve them in real life so that the conflict comes to an end. Nighttime cramps usually stop if one gets up out of bed (= end of the vagotonic repair phase crisis). Magnesium chloride (MgCl$_2$) - foot baths. Hildegard of Bingen: leg cramps: liniments with olive oil and some genuine rose oil, sage ointment - special recipe. Vitamin B complex in yeast products (e.g., brewer's yeast). Linseed oil, Vitamin D3, cod liver oil.

Spasticity

Motor conflict corresponding with the location. (See p. 307 and also p. 287).

Examples	• *During the last term of the pregnancy, the unborn child experiences its parents' countless, loud arguments = motor conflict of not being able to run away > in the active-phase - paralysis of the calf muscles; in the repair phase crisis - cramps; in persistent repair - permanent cramps > the child is born with talipes equinovarus (clubfoot). After the birth, the parents continue to argue. (See Dr. Hamer, Goldenes Buch, Bd. 2, p. 419).* → *Motor conflicts are often caused by ultrasound examinations and tests of the amniotic fluid during pregnancy or inoculations later in life if the child is restrained.*
Phase	**Persistent repair** with emphasis on the repair phase crisis - permanent tension in the affected muscles. The advantage of persistent repair is that the complaints can immediately improve after conflict resolution.
Questions	Which muscle group? (= Indication of the conflict. Most often, the arm flexing musculature is affected > conflict of not being able to hold on). Side mainly affected, handedness? Further questions: see p. 311.
Therapy	Determine the conflict and conditioning and, if possible, resolve them in real life so that the persistent repair can come to an end! Magnesium chloride (MgCl$_2$) - foot baths, physiotherapy, occupational therapy, hydrotherapy. Dance and music therapy, therapeutic riding. Cannabis oil, vitamin B complex in yeast products. Linseed oil, cod liver oil. Acupuncture, classic, acupoint and reflex-zone massages. Sunbathing, possibly solarium. If necessary, low-dose naltrexone (LDN).

Restless legs syndrome, motor neuropathy

Conflict	Motor conflict, not knowing the way in or out, not being able to escape or catch up, not being able to run (see p. 307).
Phase	<u>Restless legs:</u> **Repair phase crisis** (= epileptic crisis) during the repair phase, usually persistent repair: the symptoms appear during rest periods (vagotonia). The restless legs accomplish what one couldn't/wasn't allowed to do during the period of stress. <u>Motor neuropathy</u>: Can be diagnosed due to convulsions, paralysis, muscular atrophy, limited reflexes. Altogether an unnecessary disease classification. Mostly a **recurring-conflict**.
Therapy	Determine the conflict and conditioning and, if possible, resolve them in real life so that the persistent repair can come to an end. Magnesium chloride (MgCl$_2$) - foot baths, Cannabis oil. Classical massage, lymphatic drainage, acupuncture, reflexology. Swimming, gymnastics, yoga, etc.

Epilepsy

Motor conflict corresponding with the location (see p. 307). Patients who suffer from repeated, spontaneous convulsions, with or without loss of consciousness, are conventionally diagnosed with epilepsy.

Examples	• *A 30-year-old woman suffers the following motor conflict: She is sledding down a mountain when she suddenly realizes that she is going too fast. She crashes into an icy stream and fractures the spinous processes of two vertebrae. Immediately after the accident, she thinks she is paralyzed because she cannot move for a short time = motor conflict of not being able to brake and not being able to move. A few days later, she has an epileptic seizure with urine loss and a brief blackout. A few hours before the seizure, she had to weep with relief, realizing she could have been paralyzed. After the seizure, she feels peaceful and clear headed. (See www.gnm-forum.eu/board)* • *A man is hiking up a mountain and doubts whether he will be able to make it to the top. He can hardly keep up with the others = motor conflict of not being able to keep up, not being able to walk fast enough. Upon reaching the pass at the summit, he has an epileptic seizure. The seizures keep repeating, always in the same situation: during the ascent he is conflict-active (unnoticed paralysis*

of the legs) and at the top, he comes into healing with an epileptic seizure. (Archive B. Eybl)

• *A boy is born prematurely and is blind. As he wants to explore his surroundings, he suffers one motor conflict after the next, because he keeps bumping into things and falling down. During the resting phases he very often has epileptic seizures.* (Archive B. Eybl)

→ *A child sees a doctor coming toward him with a needle. He wants to run away but his mother holds him tight = motor conflict of not being able to run away, not being able to escape the needle > epilepsy in the repair phase (so-called inoculation-damage in this case is caused by the conflict). Note: The doctor's white coat, the hypodermic needle or the smell of the doctor's office can remain as triggers. Aside from the loss of trust, the mother sometimes becomes a trigger, since she was the one holding the child tight.*

Phase	**Repair phase crisis** = epileptic seizure. In principle, this is a more or less generalized muscle cramp (whole-body cramp). Muscle cramps and epileptic seizures only occur during states of rest (vagotonia). During the seizure, the patient sometimes relives the conflict in slow motion.
Note	The CM notion that cells die off during every epileptic seizure is wrong. The muscle groups that are mainly affected point the way to the conflict. An epileptic seizure with unconsciousness means that the person found the situation to be so unbearable, they would have rather left reality ("beamed away") during the conflict situation. Arms cramping inward is an indication that one wants to gather/hold onto someone or something, but can't. Cramping into the fetal position reveals the conflict aspect of defense/defenselessness. The opposite, cramping outwardly, indicates a conflict aspect of missing intimacy.
Questions	Seizures since when? (First conflict beforehand). What happened on the day before the last episode? (Indication of conflict recurrence). Then, examine the episode before that and so on. The affected muscle groups show the way to what happened in the conflict. In case one doesn't know the conflict/cause: get a description of which movements were made during the episode. When the seizures happen repeatedly, one has to look for the recurrence situations/triggers (e.g., dreams, memories of certain places, etc.). Which conditioning prepared the ground for the conflict? (Accidents or falls, also possibly by the mother during pregnancy or with ancestors). Which steps toward healing do I want to implement? Which new emotions/attitudes do I want to cultivate?
Therapy	Determine the conflict and, if possible, resolve it in real life. If the seizures continue, look for relapse situations or triggers (for example, dreams or memories). Guiding principles: *"I can do or not do whatever I want." "I am free." "With the help of God, I will break free of all my limitations."* Hildegard von Bingen: Wear agate stone and chrysoprase stone, put agate into drinking water. Magnesium chloride ($MgCl_2$) - foot baths. Vitamin B complex, Vitamin D3 (cod liver oil). Cannabis oil. Dancing, yoga. CM antiepileptic drugs: only recommended if the conflict resolution does not work. If taking drugs, keep trying to taper them off, because they may eventually no longer be necessary.

Parkinson's disease

According to CM, Parkinson's is a slow, progressive, degenerative disease of the brain. Typical symptoms: muscular trembling (tremor), muscle stiffness (rigidity) and slowness of movement (bradykinesia)

Conflict	According to Dr. Sabbah, motor conflict that the person is trembling in front of someone else or others tremble before the person. Also, according to my experience, that one absolutely (with force) wants to change others. It definitely has to do with the issues of aggression, authority, coercion and fear. Parkinson's trio: 1. Trembling: *"Shaking like a leaf."* Trembling means fear. 2. Muscle stiffness: *"Paralyzed by fear."* 3. Slowness of movement: When a cat (or human) wants to avoid a fight, they often slink away from the danger in "slow-motion" instead of bolting. Expression: *"Don't make any sudden moves!"*
Examples	• *A forty-year-old businessman has a major customer who he has delivered goods to for years. Due to a cost-reduction program, the customer takes bids from other providers. After a great deal of back and forth, the businessman loses his customer = motor conflict of not being able to hold onto the customer with his hands. For 20 years, the conflict has been persistently active = Parkinson's disease - trembling hands.* (Archive B. Eybl) • *A 70-year-old retiree started developing Parkinson's symptoms some months ago. In his childhood, his father hit him regularly, "usually even before dinner." He also raised his child with a similar strictness and he is sorry for it to this day. = Conflict that others tremble before him. During a meditation, he learns that the men in his family have been extremely strict for 6 generations.* (Archive B. Eybl)

• *The Parkinson's patient, Muhammad Ali, reported that he regularly dreamt of his fight with Joe Frazier. During this fight, he suffered his first and probably most painful defeat. In doing so, he suffered the following conflict: Trembling before someone > shaking hands. The tremors and paralysis represent the repair phase, or more exactly, the repair phase crisis that never ends (= persistent repair).*

Phase
Persistent repair - **Recurring healing crises**, tremor, muscle rigidity, slowing of movement (= Parkinson's disease); the conflict activity is only briefly touched by recurrences or triggers. The repair phase dominates but never comes to an end.

Note
According to my experience, Parkinson's can have a run-up time of years. Consider "handedness" (right or left) and side (mother/child or partner) or local conflict. The affected muscle group shows the way to the conflict. Much like MS, the diagnosis *"You have Parkinson's!"* can lead to a further motor conflict: the thought, of never being able to keep the hands still again, can become anchored in the subconscious.

Questions
With which muscle group did it begin? (Indication of the conflict, see p. 307 and also p. 287). Handedness, side? (Clap test). Did it start slowly? (Yes > indication of conflict that lies further back and still persists). Did I make people tremble or was I the victim? (Look for fear situations that still occupy me to this day). Was there a fall/accident that I couldn't get over? (Consequences until today)? Violent conditioning? (Beatings in childhood, strict parents, ancestors)? What will I change on the inside, on the outside?

Therapy
Determine the conflict and conditioning and, if possible, resolve them in real life so that the persistent repair can come to an end. Cannabis oil. Cod liver oil. Magnesium chloride ($MgCl_2$) - foot baths, Vitamin B complex. If necessary, low-dose naltrexone (LDN), possibly petroleum cure. The effectiveness of the CM drugs for Parkinson's - L-DOPA and dopamine agonists among others are questionable > not recommended.

SBS of the Muscle Metabolism

Muscle tension, myosclerosis, myogelosis[1]

Conflict
One is tense and believes they always have to do something. Lack of composure.

Self-esteem or incompetence conflict corresponding with the location. (Conflict details and examples see p. 287ff). For example, neck tension - moral-intellectual self-esteem conflict.

Phase
Constant tension of the striated musculature > **Recurring-conflict.**

Note
Unnatural lifestyle or forced position (constant desk-sitting) promotes muscle tension. Take into account "handedness" (right or left) and side (mother/child or partner) or local conflict.

Therapy
Determine the conflict and conditioning and, if possible, resolve them in real life if still active. Guiding principles: *"I take everything easy - no need for stress."* *"I trust in my abilities."* Reduce stress. Balance intensity (sport) with relaxation phase (nap). Motion variation in everyday life. Varied sports, especially gymnastics and physiotherapy. Yoga, dancing, swimming. Classical, acupoint and reflexology massages. Magnesium chloride ($MgCl_2$) - foot baths. Water treatments, mud wraps and baths, sauna, infrared cabin. Vitamin B complex in yeast products (e.g., brewing yeast), Cannabis oil.

Muscle distension, torn muscle fibers, ruptured muscles

Even in the case of an injury, an SBS can play a role. Same SBS as above.

Phase
Conflict-active phase or persistent conflict activity, possibly also repair phase: weakening of the muscle structure, less firmness, making the muscle is more susceptible to injury.

Therapy
Classic massage, lymph drainage massage, acupoint massage, reflex-zone massage, water therapy, mud packs and mud baths, sauna, infrared cabin, physiotherapy; if necessary surgery.

---

1   See Dr. Hamer, Charts pp. 61, 72

Muscular dystrophy, muscular atrophy, myasthenia

Possible causes (usually combined):
- **Physical inactivity** (e.g., being bedridden, handicapped).
- **Motor conflict** (paralyzed with fear conflict): active-phase or persistent-active: paralysis or weakness of the affected muscle > muscle atrophy (see p. 307 and also p. 287).

- **Self-esteem conflict:** active-phase or persistent-active: muscle degradation, cross-sectional reduction, weakness (see page 312).
- **Being underfed or malnourished** (e.g., fasting period).
Therapy: according to the cause. All stimulating measures.

CONSTELLATIONS

In the course of his research, Dr. Hamer discovered that most psychic illnesses are also linked to conflicts, or to be more precise, to conflict constellations.

In order to understand "psychoses" in their full depth, one would have to study Dr. Hamer's original literature, but without any great expectations with regard to therapy. After many years of practical experience, I must (unfortunately) say that the knowledge of constellations, albeit interesting, isn't as useful for patients as I'd hoped. In this context, I find Family Constellations as discovered by Hellinger (p. 48f) and the knowledge of conditioning (p. 24ff) much more important for aiding conflict resolution and bringing an end to patients' complaints.

By constellation, we mean the interplay between two or more active Hamer foci on the right and left sides of the brain.
We are all more or less affected by constellations, even when it is not always obvious. Where and in which order the conflicts affect the cerebrum depends on sex, handedness, hormone levels, age and previous conflicts.

Even if I always mention the right-handed when talking about cerebral constellations, that doesn't mean that the left-handed are not affected by constellations.

How the conflict is perceived and the order of conflicts is different for left-handed people, simply because they are, in principle, "operating" on the other side of the brain.

Constellations do not automatically cause physical illnesses, because when they come into alignment, the gathering of conflict mass (and its maturation) stops.

This is why, for example, when we find a Hamer focus in constellation in the bronchial relay, we often do not find any bronchial symptoms.

The following provides an overview of the currently known constellations:

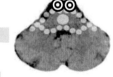

Constellation of the Brainstem

Confusion, bewilderment, Alzheimer's disease, vegetative state[1]

Characteristics	Frozen, spatially/temporally disoriented, unreactive, persisting, apathetic, lethargic, forgetful, inability of making decisions, "collector," "hoarder," Alzheimer's disease, in extreme cases - persistent vegetative state.
Conflict	Chunk-conflict left + right in the brainstem. (Image: kidney collecting tubules SBS)
Organ	Brainstem SBS, especially kidney collecting tubules SBS, both sides.
Bio. function	It is better to wait quietly, to get through the bad times (energy saving).

1   See Dr. Hamer, Charts p. 11

Constellation of the Cerebellum

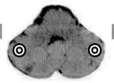

Emotionally "like dead/burned out," asocial or overly social[1]

Characteristics	Listless, empty and cold, one feels nothing, aloof, inaccessible, emotionally blunted and encapsulated, burnout. Inclination to unconventional or crazy acts.
Conflict	Attack, worries, quarrel conflicts. Left + right cerebellum conflict. (Image: breast glands)
Organ	Breast glands, peritoneum, pleura, left + right pericardium or dermis right + left.
Bio. function	Asocial: self-protection from becoming further "burned out." Overly social: One gives it all to be accepted back into the community/tribe.

1   See Dr. Hamer, Charts p. 43

Constellation of the Cerebral White Matter

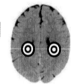

Delusions of grandeur (megalomania)[1]

Characteristics	The kind of megalomania depends on the conflict topics. Knee: physical megalomania. Testicular/ovarian: potency/sex megalomania. Heart muscle: "I-create-everything mania," helper syndrome. Cervical spine: "I-am-the-smartest mania."
Conflict/Brain area	Self-esteem conflict - cerebral white matter left + right. Musculoskeletal right + left.
Note	Exception: this constellation (megalomania) continues to the end of the repair phase.
Bio. function	The individual's self-esteem has been destroyed. By believing in his greatness, he gains courage and pulls himself up, out of the mud.

1   See Dr. Hamer, Charts p. 59

Constellation of the Cerebral Cortex

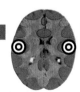

Mania and depression[1]

Whether a person is or becomes manic or depressed depends on whether the so-called territorial part of the left or right cerebral cortex is affected by conflicts and which side is accentuated (more affected).

The territorial area of the left (feminine) side: • coronary veins and cervical mucosa • rectal mucosa • laryngeal mucosa and muscles • right bladder mucous membrane.

The territorial area of the right (masculine) side: • coronary arteries and mucosa of the seminal vesicles • stomach mucous membrane-epithelium • bile ducts and pancreatic excretory ducts • bronchial mucosa and musculature • left bladder mucosa.

Summary: If the left side is affected more, the tendency is toward mania. If the right side is affected more, it is toward depression. If the conflicts switch between the two, the person is manic-depressive.

There are many different variations, according to which relays are specifically affected and how strongly. For example, there are depressive or manic autistic persons as well as manic-depressive mythomaniacs (compulsive liars). (See below)

1   See Dr. Hamer, Krebs und alle sog. Krankheiten (see resources) pp. 59. See also p. 70f Depression/Burnout-Syndrome.

Restless activity (mania)[2]

Characteristics	Exaggerated excitement, inner compulsion, *"lack of sensitivity,"* inability to pay attention (cannot listen), uncritical behavior, unwarranted good mood - *"Ants in his pants!"*
Label	Manic constellation.
Conflict	Territorial conflict - conflict emphasis on the left (feminine) side.

Despondency (depression)[2]

Characteristics	Lack of motivation, listlessness, one cannot look forward to anything enjoyable. Mild forms: *"sensitive person,"* shyness or introversion.
Label	Depressive constellation.
Conflict	Conflict emphasis on the right (masculine) side. We can become despondent, as soon as the conflict strikes us, however, we are usually in a safe constellation.
Organ	Cerebral cortex - territorial area. Normally, the relay of the coronary arteries is affected. Heart problems and heart-fear are common in depressive patients, but are not always the case, because in constellations, no conflict mass is built up - one is "protected."
Therapy	Find and resolve the conflicts and conditioning but be careful with conflicts that have long been "solo."

Postmortem constellation - afterlife constellation[2]

Characteristics	Feeling of being redundant. Familiar with the subject of death and afterlife. Interest in religion and esoteric subjects. Susceptibility to sects. Contact with the dead, angels, good connection to animals. Draws up a will. Questions: "What will everything here be like after I die?"
Conflict	Female loss-of-territory conflict + male loss-of-territory conflict.
Brain area	Cerebral cortex - peri-insular left + right, coronary veins and arteries.
Bio. function	In this world, everything is lost > The individual feels that their place is in the afterlife.

Nympho, and Casanova constellation, increased sex drive (nymphomania, satyriasis)[2]

Same constellation as above.

Characteristics	The focus is on the opposite sex. Chasing men/women but not capable of a relationship, because of the old wounds. Limited orgasm capability/frigid. Tendency to homo-, bisexuality, nymphomania. Common constellation of prostitutes, pimps, nuns & priests. An early constellation is also likely responsible for pedophilia because of the maturity stop.
Conflict	Female loss-of-territory conflict + male loss-of-territory conflict. Also in the male loss-of-territory conflict - sexual or partner-related content.
Brain area/Organ	Cerebral cortex - peri-insular left + right. Coronary veins + coronary arteries.
Bio. function	Strong sexual desire > quick mating choice > solution to the loss-of-territory conflict.

Compulsive stealing (kleptomania)[2]

Same constellation as above. In addition a motor conflict occurs.

Bio. function	The individual has lost his territory (= life support, source of food). In order to survive, he must take his food from foreign territory.

Autistic constellation - seclusion, introversion (autism)[3]

Characteristics	Depressive emphasized: little contact with the environment, brooding, loner, apathetic staring into space. Manic emphasized: thirst, may be extremely engrossed in work.

---

2   See Dr. Hamer, Charts p. 101

3   See Dr. Hamer, Charts p. 103

Conflict	Shock-fright or speechlessness conflict + territorial-anger conflict (in the right side). Brain area: cerebral cortex - left + right temporal lobes.
Bio. function	Hard working, "stays tuned" to the end - an important task in the pack.

Mythomaniac constellation (compulsive exaggeration/lying), extroversion[1]

Characteristics	Talks a lot and well, usually in a good mood, funny, not very reliable. Often politicians, journalists, writers, priests, communication coaches, presenters, comedians, used car salesmen.
Conflict	Identity conflict + territorial-fear conflict (in the right-handed).
Brain area	Cerebral cortex - left + right temporal lobes, rectal mucosa + bronchial mucosa.
Bio. function	According R. Körner: Through communication, the pack is held together and strengthened.

Bioaggressive constellation - aggression, mania, running amok[4]

Characteristics	Great thirst, high energy level, athletic (especially martial arts). Easily provoked, violent, thoughts of revenge. Emphasized depressiveness: piercing and cutting.
Conflict	Identity conflict + territorial-anger conflict (in the right-handed).
Brain area	Cerebral cortex - temporal lobes right + left.
Bio. function	The individual was driven into a corner. Renewed attacks are reached with increased aggressiveness - perceived: there's no more room.

Frontal-fear constellation - anxiety, fear of the future (anxiety neurosis)[4]

Characteristics	Fear of the future (e.g., before appointments). One imagines the worst.
Conflict	Powerlessness conflict + frontal-fear conflict (in the right-handed).
Brain area	Cerebral cortex - left + right frontal lobes, thyroid excretory ducts + branchial arches.
Bio. function	Extreme anxiety and cautiousness safeguards the individual from new disasters.

Territory marking constellation - claustrophobia, bed-wetting

Characteristics	Anxiety in crowds, tunnels, elevators, public places, etc.
Conflict	Territorial-marking conflict.
Brain area	Cerebral cortex - left + right temporal lobes.
Organ	Bladder mucosa, left + right.
Bio. function	Persons with claustrophobia avoid tight places = protection.

Occipital constellation - paranoia, hallucinations[4]

Characteristics	Unfounded fears, one suspects behind everything is a ruse or conspiracy. Always careful and suspicious. Sometimes clairvoyant, hunches.
Conflict	Fear-from-behind conflict.
Brain area	Cerebral cortex - left + right visual cortex, retina or right + left vitreous body.
Bio. function	Protection from further harm through caution and premonitions.

Fronto-occipital constellation - shocked solidification (catalepsy), anxiety[4]

Characteristics	Unpredictable - the individual feels trapped; panic, anxiety.
Conflict	Powerlessness or frontal-fear conflict + fear-from-behind conflict(s).
Brain area	Cerebral cortex - the frontal lobe left or right + left or right visual cortex.
Organ	Thyroid excretory ducts or branchial arches + retina or vitreous body.

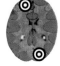

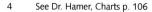

4   See Dr. Hamer, Charts p. 106

Bio. function	The individual is caught *"in a trap"* and danger is approaching from the front and back. In this case better not to move or to do something completely unexpected.

Floating constellation - withdrawn aloofness[5]

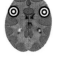

Characteristics	One floats above it all, is enlightened, sublime. Haughtiness, arrogance, flighty dreams, astral travel (manic), falling dreams (depressive), tendency toward sects, loves heights, not grounded, often pilots, parachutists and gurus.
Conflict	Shock-fright or speechlessness conflict + territorial-fear conflict (in the right-handed).
Brain area	Cerebral cortex - left and right temporal lobes.
Organ	Larynx mucosa and/or musculature + bronchial mucosa and/or musculature.
Bio. function	The individual is "lifted away" from an oppressive reality = psychic relief.

Hearing constellation - hearing voices (auditory hallucinations)[5]

Conflict	Hearing conflicts. One hears voices.
Characteristics	Imaginary or real voices from another dimension - both are possible. CM: paranoid schizophrenia. Clairaudience, channeling and composers' constellation.
Brain area/Organ	Cerebral cortex - auditory cortex right and left (lower than pictured!) Inner ear right + left.
Bio. function	Voices, tinnitus warn the individual of similar situations ("alarm system").

Obsessive-constellation - compulsive actions

Characteristics	Compulsiveness, e.g., washing, cleanliness, control, order, touch etc.
Conflict	Fear-disgust conflict + sensory conflict (in the right-handed).
Brain area	Diencephalon left + right sensory and motor cerebral cortex.
Organ	Pancreas - alpha-islet cells, beta-islet cells, skin + musculature.

Anorexia constellation - loss of appetite (anorexia)[5]

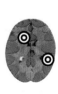

Conflict	Any left-cerebral territorial conflict + territorial-anger conflict (in the right-handed).
Brain area	Cerebral cortex - left + right temporal lobes.
Organ	Any left-cerebral territorial SBS + ectodermal stomach mucosa.
Notes	Anorexia begins often after the first menstrual cycle = indication of territorial relationship.

Bulimic constellation - bulimia addiction (bulimia)[5]

Conflict	Fear-disgust conflict + territorial-anger conflict in persistent repair (in the right-handed).
Brain area	Diencephalon left + cerebral cortex - right temporal lobe.
Organ	Pancreas - alpha-islet cells + ectodermal stomach mucosa.
Note	Cravings from hypoglycemia, nausea through repair phase crisis of the stomach mucosa.

Loss of intellectual capacity - dementia, Alzheimer's disease

Characteristics	Extreme forgetfulness, learning difficulties (e.g., with students).
Conflict	Chronic-active or recurring separation conflicts (see p. 271f). In my experience: little self-love. The longing for love. Having lost contact with one's own feelings and the joy of life.
Label	Sensory constellation.
Examples	➜ *Loss of life partner after many years = separation conflict.* ➜ *Someone has to go to a nursing home. Everything that was dear to them is suddenly gone.*
Brain area	Cerebral cortex - sensory-cortex left + right (image: sensory legs).

E C T O

−+

---

5   See Dr. Hamer, Charts p. 110

Conflict-active	Limitation of short-term memory, loss of cognitive abilities, problems with simple tasks such as making shopping lists.
Organ	Most likely only a manifestation of the brain, the skin does not have to be affected.
Bio. function	Forgetting the separations so the individual no longer has to suffer.
Therapy	Determine the conflict and conditioning and, if possible, resolve in real life. Coconut oil 1 tbsp/day.

Further possible causes for dementia

- **Constellation of the brainstem:** Here, spatial and temporal disorientation are paramount. The person cannot find his way around his own room, no longer recognizes people or objects, thinks he is somewhere else or for instance is living at another time in another place. (See p. 313.)
- **No longer being part of life,** has no tasks and goals anymore (everything is done by others, e.g., nursing home). One loses curiosity and interest in life.

- **Chronic malnutrition** due to industrial foods or poisoning through food additives/pesticides such as glutamate, aspartame, glyphosate, preservatives, citric acid, food coloring, aluminum, fluorine etc.
- **Chronic poisoning through medication** (e.g., psychotropic drugs, blood thinners, blood pressure medication), vaccinations.
- **Chronic exposure to electro-smog** (see below).

FINAL REFLECTIONS

The 5 Biological Laws of Nature and relationships

In our daily practice, we see that a large part of biological conflicts involve, directly or indirectly, problems between men and women. This leads us to conclude that if there were more harmony in our relationships and marriages, many of our conflicts wouldn't even arise in the first place. There is certainly no panacea. However, if we learn to understand the fundamental differences between men and women and learn to adapt ourselves to this reality, it will be easier. Family therapist, John Gray has written a much-to-be-recommended book, *Men Are from Mars, Women Are from Venus*, which every new couple should read.

The 5 Biological Laws of Nature and sport

As a former competitive athlete, I see sport through different eyes: Sport is only good for you if you do it for the joy of movement. Competitive thinking is damaging, because it is bound to lead to conflicts. This applies both for children and older athletes. Whether or not competition is controversial is only of secondary importance if one's inner attitude has been formed by false ambition.

However, and without a doubt, sport in moderation is good for us for so many reasons, including: having fun, promoting team spirit, improving energy flow, compensating for the lack of movement in our civilized (sedentary) lives, working off stress (breaking down sugar), connecting with nature and for our own bodies (grounding), strengthening self worth, etc. My friend, Adi Sandner, has been studying the 2nd Biological Law for years: He discovered that the so-called "training effect" also represents the two-phase process: The stress of training represents the sympathicotonic first phase. In the training pauses, the parasympathicotonic second phase repairs and strengthens the body. This rhythm leads to increased performance (overcompensation and sore muscles when you overdo it).

The 5 Biological Laws of Nature and radiation

Radioactive radiation

This is a poison that damages molecules and cells. At high doses, it "burns" the body. Lower doses have the effect that many body cells must be exchanged or replaced during the repair phase. When blood or bone marrow cells are destroyed, the body responds by increasing the rate of cell reproduction. We then find many unripe, enlarged blood cells in the blood, which can lead to a CM diagnosis of leukemia, which is principally a repair measure (see p. 135f).

Electromagnetic radiation (cell phones, electricity, radio waves)

In recent decades, the earth's natural electromagnetic information field has been superimposed with countless technologically produced electromagnetic fields. The negative effects of this "wave chaos" on man, animal, and plants, are being deliberately played down by the mass media. Added to that is radiation inside and outside the house, for example from Wi-Fi (WLAN) routers, clock-radios, TVs in the bedroom, microwave ovens, fluorescent lights, LED lamps, cordless telephones and other devices, transmitters, military communications, atmospheric projects like HAARP (High Frequency Active Auroral Research Program) and EISCAT (European Incoherent Scatter Scientific Association) and others. (These are very powerful transmitting sites in Alaska and Norway, respectively. This is an attempt to influence the ionosphere. Both projects have been linked to earthquakes and weather abnormalities). Such electro-smog "poisoning" that we are all exposed to - some more, some less - falls outside the scope of the 5 Biological Laws of Nature. What this means is that often, illness is not caused by the psyche, but by radioactive contamination. Hartmut Müller has proven that it would be possible to forgo mobile communications: By coupling into Earth's natural energy field he was able to transmit information and energy without friction loss and without artificial fields (See www.global-scaling-institute.de).

Earth rays and water veins

Are earth rays as powerful and water veins as harmful as some people say? Are they not part of Mother Earth?

The fact is: every geographic location has certain characteristics and effects on living organisms. Some places suit some people but not others. It is known, for example that ants, bees and cats, "look for" earth energies, while dogs, pigs, and horses, avoid them. Human beings are also said to avoid them. Along with earth rays, there are also grid networks like the Curry and Hartmann grids. Also, there are places that are "haunted" (e.g., old dungeons) or "holy" (e.g., Lourdes) based on their history. There is really a lot more than meets the eye.

One thing is certain: The most dangerous things are the things we are convinced will hurt us. If we address the issues as calmly as possible, then we will get a sense of which places are good for us (e.g., where we sleep well) and which are not.

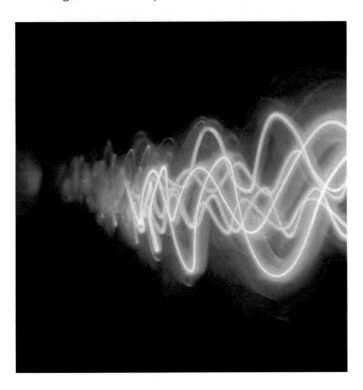

The 5 Biological Laws of Nature and the theory of evolution

Regarding the origin of life, there are two basic theories: The creation theory, which I personally believe in, and the evolution theory. In the 1980s, the evolutionary biologists were sure that they had found the "missing link" (the missing form of life between apes and human beings or, in a broader sense, between all forms of life).

Thirty years later, they have not come a step further. Even worse, between similar species, not a single transitional form has been found, although the search continues uninterrupted.

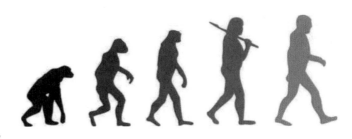

"From the amoeba to Shakespeare" (= macroevolution) is evidently mistaken. The facts (fossils) say clearly that no evolution crosses the borders of the given species and that there are only varying characteristics within a species caused by adaptation (= microevolution).

Undeniably, however, is that we are composed of "building blocks" (programs and special programs) of the animal kingdom, which is attested to by i.e., the different embryonic stages.

To this, Ivita Blömer provides in her book, *Crazy Truths*, extremely valuable information by the clairvoyants Svetlana and Nikolay Levashov: In a fixed order, different animal beings "visit" the embryo. This round starts one month after fertilization when the cells are grown to approximately 5 mm. First, a fish-essence comes and forms fishlike structures (e.g., gill arches). In the second month, an amphibious entity settles in - now amphibious structures are formed (e.g., webbed extremities). In the third month a reptile essence comes and in the fourth month, one of a mammal. Only in the fifth month of development, does the etheric body of a human enter the embryo - the actual incarnation starts. Up to this point, according Blömer, a quality barrier between essence and embryo biomass existed. The human soul must basically wait "on hold" until the foreman (animal entities) have prepared everything.

Biology confirms the chronology: From the sixth month of development, the rudiments, such as the animal-tail, regress. Now the embryo develops, until birth, into the kind of individual, human, etheric body it is going to be. Mrs. Ivita Blömer points out that the birthing process is the easiest and most painless in the sitting, squatting, or kneeling positions (gravity helps).

The conventional supine position today is actually the worst position.

The 5 Biological Laws of Nature and inheritance

In CM, it has been thought that faulty genes are due to certain "illnesses" and that the genetic substance remain unchanged during one's entire life.

This belief is beginning to falter, largely due to the work of the New York cell biologist Bruce Lipton: He has discovered that a human being is determined less by its genes than by its environment. Genes are subject to the influences of the environment and can mutate. Only its basic constituents remain unchanged. His knowledge of the cell membrane has made him a pioneer in the so-called field of epigenetics.

The link, according to Dr. Hamer, is simple. Longer lasting conflicts can, of course, change the genetic substance as can conflict resolution.

In this way, an individual's genes are constantly changing (being modified/updated) to meet life's demands.

Why do we find a preponderance of certain illnesses in certain families?

According to the law of attraction (resonance), like attracts like. Thus, mother and father attract a similar child-soul, which relates to their characters.

> A daughter, whose psychic landscape is akin to her mother's, has genes similar to hers and perceives similar conflicts > the similar perceptions lead to similar SBSs.

Furthermore, from the beginning of pregnancy, the child senses every feeling of its mother (and father) > this basic pattern of thought and feeling is internalized and adopted > it develops into a body much like the parents', just as its immortal soul is similar to the parents'. It is clear that having the same foundation, the new organism will have similar conflicts and illnesses.

However, we are only partly subject to this fate, for in principle, we can leave these limitations behind us at any time.

There are no incurable (hereditary) diseases, but only incurable (rigid) people.

The 5 Biological Laws of Nature and life expectancy

Can we use this knowledge to avoid illnesses and remain healthy?
- Yes, because we have recognized that psychic well-being and harmony is the basis for health. With this in mind, we will pay attention to what is good for us and what is not. We will free ourselves from the compulsions, expectations and norms and, as far as possible, live a self-determined life.
- Yes, if we have recognized which conflicts and conflict triggers are making us ill and make concrete changes accordingly. It is quite simple if we change our lives and no longer produce our own stress.
- Yes, because thanks to our knowledge, we will hardly suffer diagnosis and prognosis shocks and take a detour around damaging therapies such as chemotherapy, radiation, vaccinations and pointless surgeries. Statements like: *"You have a metastases in the liver!"* or *"Enjoy your life while you can,*

because we cannot do anything more for you!" may possibly worry us, but should not send us into a panic.
- No, because nobody among us is completely immune to biological conflicts. The unexpected is simply unexpected. Remaining calm is surely a good attitude in life, but it's hard to remain calm when it comes to our "weak spots," the very things in life, with which we identify ourselves with and hold dear.

For example: If somebody, to whom we have no special relationship dies, we can stay calm.

However, if our own child dies, we can no longer stay calm.

A car lover whose car was stolen cannot remain calm, nor can an athlete who loses a championship title when they were the "favorite."
- The expectations of this "New Medicine" are simply too high in some people. Dr. Hamer claiming a "98% New Medicine chance of survival" was completely illusory and unrealistic in the present system.

I have seen countless people die in CM treatment, but I have also seen many people die, who did everything right when they were sick from my point of view.

The 5 Biological Laws of Nature cannot guarantee survival. Rather, we live and die "within" the 5 Biological Laws of Nature.

Now, we can understand health and sickness in most people, but often, we have no other choice but to "understand" that a human being will die. For instance, when the conflict mass was too great and/or the conflict kept recurring.

Death is not a disorder, it is as much a part of life as birth.

Unfortunately, this is being measured by a double standard: When a single person dies practicing New Medicine, all hell breaks loose: *"He could be alive today, if he hadn't believed that nonsense!"*

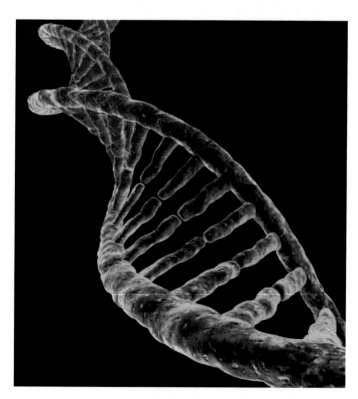

For the thousands that die every hour in CM's care, we hear: *"We did our best but they couldn't be saved!"*
The fact is, we all die one day and we should reflect on the concept that our lifespan, at least from a spiritual point of view, is at least in part, predetermined. When the bell tolls, no medicine will help: not this one, not that one. That's right, nothing will help, for when fate wants us, for whatever reason, our incarnation will come to an end. Of course, we can shorten this span through our own mistakes, e.g., disregarding spiritual, biological and physical laws, recklessness, self-indulgence, destructive thoughts and actions, etc.

The 5 Biological Laws of Nature and spirituality

Let's imagine a person who remains calm, regardless of what happens to them. No dreadful event, be it loss, attack, separation or death can move them. A person full of love, in total harmony with themselves, their environment, united with all, free from dependencies, free from shocks and from illness.
It may sound unrealistic, but we must recognize that there are people, who have come close to this ideal through spiritual development. What I want to say with this is: let's not get carried away. The special biological programs discovered by Dr. Hamer are, if you will, "animal-biological" survival programs.
We need to obey the "laws of the jungle" only if we are tangled up in the perceptions of chunk, attack, defence, fear and territorial conflicts.
However, we are not animals. While it is true that we live in animal bodies, we differ from animals in that each of us has an individual, immortal soul. Unlike plants and animals, we can make mistakes, reflect upon our actions and are capable of self-recognition. With our primitive, animal biology, we navigate amongst conflicts and diseases within the 5 Biological Laws of Nature.
Through spiritual development, that is, by maturation and refinement of character, by loving thoughts and deeds and by dissolving dependencies, our spiritual nature can flourish.
Not overnight, but at least within several incarnations.
By gradually decoupling ourselves from our animal instincts and urges, biological conflicts no longer affect us so strongly.
However, if we are caught in its orbit (conflict), we must solve the conflict at the corresponding biological level. If we speak with admiration today of the exemplary and harmonious life of the Native Americans or other aboriginal cultures, we should not forget that the lives of these peoples were not only biologically natural but also marked by deep spirituality.
When one expands the scope of the 5 Biological Laws of Nature too far, they risk succumbing to a "evolutionary-theory-justified materialism," of believing that "might makes right" in property and territorial thinking.
Such an attitude prevents spiritual development.
As happy as we can consider ourselves in our knowledge of what causes disease, we should not forget about the most important questions in life:

Who am I? What is the meaning of my life? Where do I come from? Where am I going?

The spiritual and energy healers among the readers will forgive me that their methods were glossed over in this book. My intention was to elaborate on health and illness from a psyche-biological view, on the connections between the body and psyche. That things are possible for the creative spirit, which by far exceed our current horizons, is clearly evident to me.
That we have infinitely more to learn is also clear.
One needs only to think about the healing of broken bones within minutes, as practiced by the aborigines or of the countless spiritual healings by the Brazilian, Joao de Deus. Nevertheless, I think that it is good to start with a solid knowledge of biology and from there, embrace the spiritual levels.
I am convinced: The basis of every intentionally healing is the connection with God and the acknowledgement of this connection, for we have always been bound to God since the beginning of time, just as a child is and was always will be bound to its parents.

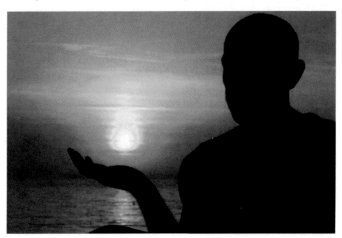

Ethereal beings

A touchy subject, because many might regard this as pure rubbish and not even a pseudoscience.
In my own experience, I have no doubt that behind the material plane, subtle levels and beings exist, which can have a significant impact on our lives and our health.
The senses of children and animals, such as dogs and cats, are often open to these worlds.
Among us "civilized adults," only a few can, while awake, feel or see deceased souls, angels, ghosts, fairies, or gnomes.
One of these is the Swiss architect Anton Styger. According to his descriptions, there is lively activity and a sheer unfathomable variety of different beings in the ethereal world. This all has intense interrelationships to plants, animals, and human beings. Styger has been asked by psychologically and physically disturbed people to take a look at what is going on with them or their houses. While doing so he finds, for example:
• People who are being bothered or occupied by dead relatives.
• Children who can not sleep and are afraid, because deceased former residents move around.
• People who created demons by negative thinking and with which they can't cope anymore.
• Cows who are being mistreated by the deceased and become sick because of it.

- People who are no longer happy on their property, because they have incurred the hatred of earth spirits, etc.

The difficulties with these phenomena are, firstly, being able to recognize what is going on and secondly, taking the right steps. Anton Styger is praying with the persons concerned and addresses the troublemakers directly. He explains the situation to them and then sends them to the light. He always asks his angels and guardian spirits for help.

His reports show how important a loving coexistence and the respectful treatment of all living things is.

I am convinced:

Conflict events, family forces, influences from subtle beings and everything else that happens to us in our lives always „fits in" with our personal destiny.

The law of cause and effect functions like clockwork.

Everything that occurs in our lives only happens for one reason: So that we may learn from it and develop our spirit and soul!

Conclusion

The New Medicine has emerged in these changing times in which we live, because spirit and psyche have once again become centers of our attention. Purely materialistic, reductionist thinking is "running out of steam," for it does not fit into the new era. The time of medical materialism is over.

With the discovery of the 5 Biological Laws of Nature, Dr. Hamer has placed the key to the understanding of health and disease and the key to therapy in our hand.

Nobody needs to wait until "the men in the ivory towers" say, *"Yes, the 5 Biological Laws of Nature are correct!"*

We do not need to wait until all the doctors have switched over. - No, our own health and that of our loved ones are too precious. We can begin to use the 5 Biological Laws of Nature right now.

The rules are simple once they've been understood. We don't need to know all the details - we can look them up as need be. Of course, this knowledge brings with it a responsibility: not letting others literally "die of ignorance." In my experience, one is most successful when one offers help discreetly.

I also learned that some people will never be ready for this information at any time and now I can accept this wholeheartedly. With doctors, one has to speak more directly. After all, it is their duty to keep up with the latest advances in science.

It is tragic, but not surprising, that at the present time, there are no surgeons, specialists nor clinics that work under our criteria. It is also dreadful that children are taken away from their parents if families want to follow this new path. This will probably not change until the 5 Biological Laws of Nature have been officially recognized.

Now, with all of this information swirling around in our heads about conflict analyses, cell growth here and cell degradation there - we shouldn't forget the most beneficial, the most important and easiest principle:

Love heals all wounds.

Let's practice the New Medicine with love, joy, compassion, and gratitude in union with God.

Also, let this biological knowledge resonate with the tidings of spiritual teachers, the spiritual principles, and combine the essence of all religions.

Let's build bridges to other therapeutic approaches - almost all have valuable insights to offer us.

God bless us all.

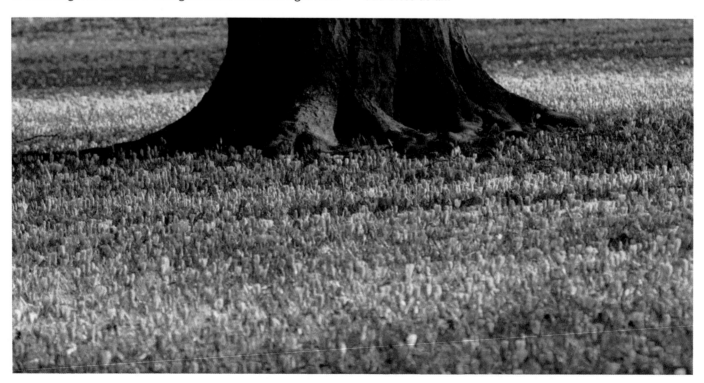

Literature by Dr. med. Mag. theol. Ryke Geerd Hamer

- Scientific Chart of Germanic Medicine®, Amici di Dirk Ediciones dela Nuevo Nedicina, S.L., as of December 2008, ISBN: 978-84-96127-29-9, www.amici-di-dirk.com
- Vermächtnis einer Neuen Medizin, Part 1, Amici di Dirk Verlag, 7th edition, 1999, ISBN: 84-930091-0-5
- Vermächtnis einer Neuen Medizin, Part 2, Amici di Dirk Verlag, 7th edition, 1999, ISBN 84-930091-0-5
- Kurzfassung der Neuen Medizin, Amici di Dirk Verlag, ISBN: 84-930091-8-0
- Celler Dokumentation, Amici di Dirk Verlag, Kologne 1994, ISBN: 3-926755-07-5
- 12 + 1 Hirnnerventabelle der Neuen Medizin, 1st edi-tion, as of July 2004 and 2nd edition, 2009, Amici di Dirk Verlag, ISBN 84-96127-11-7
- Wissenschaftlich-embryologische Zahntabelle der Germanischen Neuen Medizin,® 2009, Amici di Dirk Verlag, ISBN: 978-84-96127-36-4
- Krebs und alle sog. Krankheiten, 2004, Amici di Dirk Verl., ISBN: 84-96127-13-3
- Präsentation der Neuen Medizin, 2005 Amici di Dirk Verlag
- Germanische Neue Medizin® Kurzinformation, 2008, Amici di Dirk Verlag, ISBN: 978-84-96127-31-9
- Brustkrebs - Der häufigste Krebs bei Frauen? Amici di Dirk Verlag, 2010, ISBN: 978-84-96127-47-0 Available from AMICI DI DIRK ® - Deliverie: Germany South: Michaela Welte, Tel.: 07202/7756, e-Mail: michaelawelte@yahoo.de, Austria: Ing. Helmut Pilhar, Tel./Fax: 02638-81236, www.germanische-heilkunde.at

Literature by other authors

- Angela Frauenkron-Hoffmann, Biologisches Dekodieren - So befreien Sie Ihr Kind, Resonaris Verlag, Köln 2013
- Angela Frauenkron-Hoffmann, 1-2-3 Migränefrei, Resonaris Verlag, Köln 2016
- Claudio Trupiano, Danke Doktor Hamer, Secondo Naura s.r.l.,Bagnone, 2010, 3. Auflage, ISBN: 978-88-95713-10-6
- Mirsakarim Norbekov, Eselsweisheit - Der Schlüssel zum Durchblick oder wie Sie Ihre Brille loswerden, Goldmann Verlag, 2. Auflage, 2006
- Marion Kohn, Die fünf geistigen Gesetze der Heilung, Verlag Silberschnur, Güllesheim, 1st edition, 2010
- Karl Dawson & Sasha Allenby, Matrix Reconditioning, Trinity Verlag in the Scorpio Verlag GmbH & Co.KG, Berlin, Munich 2010
- Bert Hellinger, Ordnungen der Liebe, Carl-Auer Verlag Heidelberg, 8th edition, 2007
- Monika Berger-Lenz & Christopher Ray, 100 Tage Herzinfarkt, faktuell, 2009
- Dr. Ralph Bircher, Geheimarchiv der Ernährungslehre, Bircher-Benner Verlag Bad Homburg, 11th edition, 2007
- Böcker/Denk/Heitz, Pathologie, Urban & Fischer, 2004
- Walter & Lao Russel, Radioaktivität Das Todesprinzip in der Natur, Genius Verlag, Bremen, 2006
- Callum Coats, Naturenergien verstehen und nutzen - Viktor Schaubergers geniale Entdeckungen, Omega Verlag, Düsseldorf, 1999
- Harold J. Reilly & Ruth H. Brod, Das Große Edgar-Cayce-Gesundheits - Buch, Bauer Verlag, 9th edition, 1989
- Rainer Körner, BioLogisches Heilwissen, Heilwissen Verlag 2011, www.BioLogisches Heilwissen.de, ISBN: 978-3-9814795-0-8
- Woschnagg, Exel, Mein Befund, Ueberreuter Verlag, 1991
- Heinrich Krämer, Die stille Revolution der Krebs-und AIDS-Medizin, Ehlers 2001
- Michael Leitner "Mythos HIV", Verlag videel, 2005
- Ulrich Abel, ChemoTherapy fortgeschrittener Karzinome, Eine kritische Bestandsaufnahme, 2nd updated edition, Stuttgart, Hippokrates Verlag, 1995
- Richard Willfort, Gesundheit durch Heilkräuter, Rudolf Trauner Verlag, 1986
- Leo Angart, Vergiss deine Brille, Nymphenburger Verlag, 5th edition, 2007
- Kurt Allgeier, Die besseren Pillen, Mosaik Verlag, 2003
- Susanne Fischer-Rizzi, Medizin der Erde, AT Verlag, 2006
- Dr. Gottfried Herztka und Dr. Wighard Strehlow, Große Hildegard-Apotheke, Christiana-Verlag 2007
- Brandon Bays, The Journey - Der Highway zur Seele, Ullstein, Berlin, 2008
- Franz-Peter Mau, EM - Fantastische Erfolge mit Effektiven Mikroorganismen, Goldmann Verlag, 2002.
- Jürgen Schilling, Kau dich gesund, Haug Verlag, 2003
- John Gray, Männer sind anders. Frauen auch (original title: Men Are From Mars, Women From Venus), Goldmann Verlag, Munich, 1992
- Karin Achleitner-Mairhofer, Dem Schicksal auf der Spur, Ennsthaler, 2010
- Johannes F. Mandt, was Gesund macht, Mandt-Verlag, 1st edition, 2009, Bergstraße 48, 53919 Weilerswist, www.mandt-verlag.de, ISBN: 978-3-00-028725-1
- Anton Styger, Erlebnisse mit den Zwischenwelten, volumes 1 and 2, Styger-Verlag Oberägeri, Switzerland, 2008 und 2010

Graphics und photographs

Photos on pp. 6, 7, 13, 18, 22, 26, 30, 32, 33, 39, 43 - 63 from www.fotolia.com.
Photos on pp. 40, 64 pixabay.com.
Graphics and photos on pp. 8, 10, 12, 14-17, 19, 20, 23, 24, 28, 29, 35 by the author.
Franz Geroldinger: 25
Hospital laboratory: 21
Hospital documents: 36
The anatomical graphics on cover and reference section (P. 65 - 307) were drawn by a Viennese illustrator with pencil and colored in by the author.

List of Abbreviations

Adeno-Ca . . . . Glandular or mucosal tissue cancer
Ca . . . . Cancer (from the Latin carcinoma) (p 20ff)
CT . . . . Cerebral CT = Computed tomography (29)
CM . . . . Conventional Medicine
EM . . . . Effective Microorganisms (55)
MMS . . . . Miracle Mineral Supplement of Jim Humble - gentle antibiotic (57)
SBS . . . . Significant Biological Special Program (p 8f)
OP . . . . Surgery
Syndrome . . . . Active kidney collecting tubules SBS + other SBS in healing (p 226ff)

Index

A

Abdominal aorta 141
Abdominal wall 212
Abdominal wall, hernia 215
Abscesses, skin 284
Absence seizures 69
ACE inhibitors, medicine 63
Acetaminophen, medicine 62
Acetylsalicylic acid, aspirin, medicine 62
Achilles tendon, inflammation 305
Achromatopsia, eye 99
Acid-base balance 58
Acne, skin 279
Acoustic neuroma, ear 106
Acromegaly, hypophysis 114
Actinic keratosis, skin 281
Acupressure, acupuncture (massage) .. 61
Addison's disease, adrenal glands 116
Adenoviruses, small intestine 198
Adiposity (obesity)............................... 67
Adnexitis, fallopian tubes 245
Adrenal cortex, hyperfunction 116
Adrenal gland, insufficiency 116
Adrenal gland, stimulating 114
Adrenal glands 116
Adrenal medulla, tumor 118
ADS (ADHD), children 33
Advil, medicines 62
Age warts, seborrheic keratosis, skin . 276
Aggression, constellation 316
Aggressiveness, children 33
AIDS 138
AIDS-Tests 41
Allergic "cold", runny nose 153
Allergic contact, eczema 274
Allergic rhinitis 153
Alopecia areata/totalis, hair 284
Alpha cells, pancreas 224
Alpha-fetoprotein, AFP, laboratory 42
ALS, muscular system 308
Alveolar pulmonary edema 167
Alveoli, lungs 159
Alzheimer's disease 313, 317

Amelanotic melanoma, skin 278
Amends, therapy 52
Amenorrhea, ovaries 242
Amoebic dysentery, small intestine 198
Amylase (alpha-amylase), laboratory .. 40
Amyotrophic lateral sclerosis, ALS 308
Anal fissures 206
Anal mucosa 205
Anemia, red blood cell deficiency 134
Angina tonsillaris 175
Angina, pectoris, heart 124
Ankle or toe joint, inflammation 305
Ankylosing spondylitis, bones 293
Anorectal abscess 205
Anorexia 68, 317
Anosmia, nose 154
Anti-fungal drugs, antimycotics 63
Anti-viral drugs 63
Antibiotics, medicines 63
Antibodies 42
Antihypertensive medications 63
Antimycotics, medicines 63
Antirheumatics, medicines 62
Anus 204
Anxiety neurosis, constellation 316
Aortic aneurysm, blood vessels 141
Aortic arch, blood vessels 145
AP (alkaline phosphatase), laboratory . 39
Apaxiban, medicament 63
Aphthous stomatis, mouth 172
Appendicitis, colon 200
Appendix, ruptured, colon 200
Arrhythmia absoluta, heart 131
Arrhythmia, heart 132
Arteria subclavia dextra 145
Arteriosclerosis, blood vessels 140
Arteriosclerosis in coronary arteries 125, 145
Artery disease, peripherial 140
Arthritis, bones and joints 291
Asbestos pleurisy 170
Asbestosis 168
Ascending aorta 145
Ascites, exsudative, peritoneum 214

Asocial, constellation 314
Aspergillus, small intestine 198
Aspirin, medicines 62
Astigmatism, eye 103
Astramorph, medicines 62
Astrocytoma, brain 74
AT1 antagonists, medicines 63
Athlete's foot 279
Atrial fibrillation, heart 131
Atrial fibrillation, paroxymal, heart 131
Atrioventricular block, heart 126
Attention Deficit Syndrome (ADHD) ... 33
Auditory hallucinations, constellation 317
Auricular perichondritis, ear 107
Autism, constellation 315
Autonomous adenoma, thyroid 119
AV block, atrioventricular block, heart 126
Avinza, medicament 62

B

Bach Flower Remedies 54
Bacteria 18
Bacterial intestinal dysentery 198
Balance, vestibular nerve, ear 106
Balanitis, penis 261
Barrett's esophagus 191
Bartholin's cyst, Bartholinitis 253
Basal cell cancer, basalioma, skin 271
Basal-cell carcinoma, BCC, skin 274
Basalioma, skin 271
Bechterew's disease, bones 293
Bed wetting, enuresis nocturna . 236, 316
BED, pancreas 225
Benign melanocytic nevus 281
Benign, cancer 21
Besnier-Boeck disease, lungs 160
Beta-blocker, medicines 63
Bewilderment 313
Big toe joint, bunion, deformation 306
Bile ducts, cancer 218
Bilharziosis, schistosomiasis 198
Biliary colic, microlithiasis liver 219
Bilirubin, laboratory value 39

Binge eating disorder, BED, pancreas 225
Bioaggressive constellation 316
Biological conflict 11
Bird and swine flu 68
Birth, conditioning 31
Black lung disease 168
Bladder 235
Bladder cancer, adeno-ca 237
Bladder infection, purulent 237
Bladder stones 240
Bladder, inflammation 236
Bladder, inverted papilloma 236
Bladder, irritable, overactive 238
Bleeding diathesis, blood 137
Blepharitis, eye 82
Bloating, intestine 208
Blood 133
Blood in the stool, laboratory value 41
Blood in urine, laboratory value 41
Blood sugar fluctuating, pancreas 225
Blood vessels 139
Blood, laboratory 37
Blood, pressure 65
Blood, sugar 39, 224
Blood, vessel tension 142
Boils, skin 284
Bone fracture 295
Bone marrow fibrosis 290
Bone tumor, marrow tumor 292
Bones 286
Bony labyrinth, ear 110
Borrelia antibodies, laboratory value ... 42
Brain chambers 75
Brain hemorrhage 77, 79
Brain tumor 74
Brain, blood vessels 79
Brain, inflammation 79
Brainstem 16
Branchial arches 178
Branchiogenic cysts 147
Breast 265
Breast cancer 265
Breast gland, adhesions 267
Breastbone pain 299
Breasts, sagging 270
Brittle bone disease 290
Bronchi 158
Bronchi, inflammation, lungs 162
Bronchial asthma 163
Bronchial epithelial cancer 161
Bronchial inflammation, spastic 163
Bronchial tumor 161
Bronchiectasis 162
Bronchitis 162
Bruising, blood 137
Bruxism, teeth 185
Bubonic plague, skin 280
Bulge in the small intestine 195
Bulimia, constellation 317

Bunion, hallus valgus 306
Burnout syndrome 70
Bursitis, inflammation, bones 291, 304

C
C-reactive protein, laboratory value 38
Calcaneal spur, bones 306
Calcifying aortic valve stenosis, heart 129
Calcium, increased parathyroidea 122
Calluses on the feet, skin 276
Campylobacter coli bacteria 198
Campylobacter, laboratory 42
Candida albicans 198
Candidiasis 174, 281
Canker sores, mouth 172
Carbamazepine, medicines 72
Carbohydrate antigen 19/9, 19/9 CA . 42
Carbuncles, skin 284
Carcinoembryonic antigen, CEA 42
Cardia insufficiency, stomach 191
Cardiac insufficiency, heart weakness 132
Carpal tunnel syndrome, bones 299
Cartilage 288
Cartilage of the outer ear 107
Cartilaginous tumor 292
Catalepsy, constellation 316
Cataracts, eye 92
CEA, laboratory value 42
Cecum 200
Cecum, appendix, inflammation 200
Celiac disease, small intestine 197
Cellulite, legs 148
Cellulite, skin 283
Cerebellum 16
Cerebral cortex 17
Cerebral hemorrhage, nervous system 79
Cerebral white matter 17
Cervical cancer 247
Cervical disk herniation 296
Cervical syndrome, bones 295
Cervix Mucosa 247
CF, mucoviscidosis, lungs 165
CFS, Chronic Fatigue Syndrome .. 67, 116
Chalazion, eye 85
Chancroid, ulcus molle, men 262
Chancroid, female 252
Chemotherapy 63
Chest pain 124
Chicken pox, varicella, skin 275
Children 32
Chills phase, repair phase crisis 13
Chlamydia, laboratory value 42
Cholangiocarcinoma, liver 218
Cholecystitis, liver 218
Cholelithiasis, liver 219
Cholera, small intestine 198
Cholesterol, laboratory value 38
Cholinesterase, laboratory value 39
Chondrosarcoma, bones 292

Choroid cancer 94
Choroid plexus papilloma 75
Choroid, Choroiditis eye 94
Chronic eosinophilic leukemia, blood 135
Chronic Fatigue Syndrome, CFS .. 67, 116
Chronic lymphocytic leukemia, blood 135
Chronic obstructive pulmonary disease 168
Ciliary muscle, eye 100
Cirrhotic kidney 234
Claustrophobia, constellation 316
Clavus, skin 281
Cleft lip, jaw or palate 178
Closed-angle glaucoma, eye 97
Clotting tendency, hypercoagulability 138
Clouding of the lenses, cataracts 92
Cod liver oil, remedies 61
Cold, rhinitis, nose 151
Cold abscess, skin 215
Cold lumps 122
Cold stroke, nervous system 77
Cold, purulent 154
Colds, infection 68
Colitis ulcerosa, colon 202
Collateral ligament, bones 305, 306
Collecting tubules, kidneys 230
Coloboma, eye 94
Colon cancer, polyps 201
Colonic diverticula 203
Color blindness, eye 99
Color vision deficiency, eye 99
Compulsive actions, constellation 317
Compulsive stealing, kleptomania 315
Conditioning 24
Condyloma acuminata female 248, 252, 276
Condylomata acuminata, male 261
Conflict 9
Conflict resolution 46
Conflict-active phase 13
Confusion, constellation 313
Conjunctivitis, eye 82
Conn's syndrome, adrenal glands 117
Consciousness, loss of 69
Constellations 313
Constipation 199, 208
Constriction of the foreskin, penis 263
Constriction of the larynx 157
COPD, lungs 168
Cornea, inflammation, keratitis, eye ... 93
Corneal clouding, eye 93
Corns, clavus, skin 281
Coronary arteries, heart 124
Coronary heart attack 125
Coronary veins, heart, lungs 165
Corticotropes, hypophysis 114
Cortisone, medicines 62
Cough coming from the larynx 158
Coumadin, medicines 63
Coumarins, medicines 63
Coxarthrosis, bones 303

Coxsackie virus, small intestine 198
Creatinine, laboratory value 40
Crohn's disease, small intestine 202
Crossed eyes, strabismus 90
Crossed-eye(s), inwardly, esotropia 91
Croup, cough, larynx 158
CRP, laboratory value 38
CRPS, Sudeck's dystrophy, joints 290
Cruciate ligament, knee 305
Cushing's syndrome, adrenal glands . 117
Cystademona, serous, pancreas 226
Cystic fibrosis, eye 84
Cystic fibrosis, lungs 165
Cystic kidney 232
Cytotoxics, medicines 63

D

Dacryoadenitis, eye 84
Dancing eyes 92
Dandruff, hair 284
Daytime blindness, hemeralopia ... 89, 99
DCIS, breast 267
Deafness, ear 108
Dedentition, teeth 184
Dentin, deep cavities, teeth 182
Degenerative joint disease 288
Dementia, constellation 317
Dental calculus, tartar 185
Depression, constellation 314
Depression, general symptoms 70
Dermatomycosis, skin 279, 281
Dermoid cysts, ovaries 242
DES, dry eye syndrome 84
Despondency, constellation 315
Destructive anger, children 33
Diabetes mellitus type 1 222
Diabetes mellitus type 1 or 2 225
Diagnosis 37
Diaphragm 209
Diaphragm cramps 210
Diaphragmatic hernia 212
Diarrhea 199, 207
Diclofenac, medicines 62
Diphtheria, laryngitis 158
Diuretics, medicines 63
Diverticulitis, colon 203
Dizziness, vertigo, ear 112
Down syndrome, trisomy 21 69
Drooping eyelids, ptosis 87
Dry eye syndrome, DES 84
Dry mouth 177
Ductal carcinoma in situ, DCIS, breast 267
Ductal hyperplasia, breast 267
Duodenal bleeding 195
Duodenal ca 194
Duodenal mucosa 195
Duodenal polyps 195
Duodenal ulcer, ulcus duodeni 194
Duodenum 194

Dupuytren's contracture, bones 299
Duramorph, medicines 62
Dust mite allergy, nose 153
Dwarfism, short stature 115

E

Ear 104
Ear canal furuncle, otitis externa 109
Ear polyp 105
Ear, outer, auditory canal 107
Eating disorders, anorexia 68
ECHO virus 198
Eclampsia, pregnancy 249
Ectoderm 15
Ectopic pregnancy, tubal pregnancy .. 246
Ectropium, eye 87
Eczema, skin 271
Effective Microorganisms, EM 59
Efflorescence 271
EFT, Emotional Freedom Techniques ... 55
Carotid, left and right 145
Egyptian ophthalmia 93
Elephantiasis 148
Eliquis, medicines 63
EM, Effective Microorganisms 59
Empyema of the frontal sinus 154
Encephalitis, encephalomeningitis 79
Encopresis, paradoxical diarrhea 207
Endocarditis valvularis, heart 128
Endoderm 15
Endometrial cancer 244
Endometriosis 246
Enteritis, acute 197
Enteroida adeno-ca, eye 94
Entropion, eye 87
Enuresis nocturna, bladder 236
Ependymoma, nervous system 75
Epicondylitis, joints 297
Epidermis, inflammation 271
Epidermomycosis, skin 281
Epilepsy, muscular System 310
Epiphora, eye 88
Epithelial metaplasia, uterus 248
Epulis, teeth 186
Erectile dysfunction, penis 264
Erysipelas, skin 271
Erythema, skin 271
Erythrocyte sedimentation rate 38
Erythrocytes, laboratory value 37
Escherichia coli bacteria, small intestine 198
Esophageal cancer, adeno-ca 187
Esophageal cancer, ulcer-ca 188
Esophageal reflux 191
Esophageal submucosa 187
Esophageal varices 188
Esophagitis 189
Esophagus 187
Esophagus, inflammation 189
Esotropia, eye 91

ESR, laboratory value 38
Ethereal beings 321
Eustachian tubes, inflammation, ear . 106
Euthyroid cyst, thyroidea 121
Euthyroid goiter, thyroidea 121
Evolution 319
Evolution 319
Ewing's sarcoma, bones 292
Exaggeration, constellation 316
Exanthema, skin 271
Exotropia, eye 91
External female sex organs 251
Extremities, enlargement, acromegaly .. 114
Extroversion, constellation 316
Eye 81
Eye muscles, outer 90, 101
Eye socket 296
Eye(s), outwardly crossed 91
Eyelid 82
Eyelid muscles 86
Eyelid tremor 88
Eyelid, inflammation 82
Eyelid, jittering, eyelid tremor 88
Eyelid, outward-turned, ectropium 87

F

Facial nerve 76
Facial nerve, paralysis 76
Fallopian tube cancer 245
Fallopian tubes 244
Family 48
Farsightedness, hyperopia, eye 102
Farsightedness, age related 103
Fatigue, Chronic Fatigue Syndrome, CFS 67
Fatigue fracture, bones 295
Fatigue fracture, pelvic bone 302
Fear of the future, constellation 316
Fecal soiling, rectum 207
Fever blisters, mouth 173
Fibroadenoma, breast 267
Final reflections 318
First worsening 57
Flatulence 208
Floaters, eye 95
Floating constellation 317
Flu infections 68
Fluid retention 230
Fluor genitalis, female 254
Folliculitis, boils, carbuncles, skin 284
Foreign language problems, children .. 34
Foreskin, inflammation 261
Forgiving, therapy 49
Frenulum breve, penis 263
Frigidity 242
Frontal-fear constellation 316
Fronto-occipital constellation 316
Fungal infection, skin 281
Fungal infection, small intestine 198
Fungi, microbes 18

G

G-strophanthin, heart medicines 133
Gallbladder 216
Gallbladder inflammation 218
Gallstones, cholelithiasis 219
Gamma-GT, laboratory value 39
Ganglioglioma, nervous system 74
Gastric mucosa, inflammation 190
Gastric ulcer, stomach 191
Gastritis, stomach 190
Gastroduodenal prolapse 191
Gastroparesis, gastroptosis, stomach . 191
Genital herpes, male 261
Genital warts, condyloma, female 252
Genital warts, condylomata, male 261
Genital warts, condylomata, cervix ... 248
Geographic tongue, mouth 174
Germ cell tumor, teratoma, testicles .. 242
Germ layer 14
Gestosis, late, pregnancy 249
Gigantism, hypersomnia, hypophysis 114
Gingival hyperplasia, teeth 186
Gingivitis, teeth 186
Glaucoma, eye 95
Glaucoma, normal pressure 96
Glioblastoma, nervous system 74
Glomerulonephritis, kidneys 232
Gluten intolerance, celiac disease 197
Goblet cell tumor, lungs 164
Goiter, thyroid 121
Golfer's elbow, bone and joints 297
Gonorrhea, female 254
Gonorrhea, male 260
GOT, laboratory value liver 39
Gout, bones and joints 293
GPT, glutamate pyruvate transaminase 39
Grammar problems, children 33
Grave's disease, thyroid 120
Gray hair 285
Greater omentum, cancer 215
Grinding of the teeth, bruxism 185
Gum proliferations, teeth 186

H

Hair 271
Hair loss, alopecia totalis 284
Hair-cell leukemia 135
Hallucinations, constellation 316
Hamer focus, HF 10
Handedness 12
Hardening of arteries, arteriosclerosis 140
Harelip, mouth 178
Hashimoto's thyroiditis 122
Hay fever, nose 153
HCG, laboratory value 42
Headaches 71
Hearing constellation 317
Hearing impairment, hypacusis 111
Hearing loss, sudden deafness 110

Hearing voices, auditory hallucinations 317
Heart 123
Heart attack 125
Heart muscle, inflammation 128
Heart rhythm disturbances, arrhythmia 132
Heart valve insufficiency, leakage 132
Heart valves 128
Heart valves, inflammation 128
Heart weakness 132
Heartburn, stomach 190
Heavy menstruation 249
Heel spur, bones and joints 306
Hemangioma, infantile hemangioma 140
Hematuria, laboratory value 41
Hemeralopia, eye 89, 99
Hemoglobinuria, laboratory value 41
Hemophilia, blood 137
Hemorrhagic diathesis, blood 137
Hemorrhoids, internal 205
Hemorrhoids, superficial 205
Hepatic coma, liver 220
Hepatic encephalopathy 220
Hepatitis, liver 218
Hepatocellular cancer 216
Herpes labialis, simplex, mouth 173
Herpes zoster, skin 278
Hiatus hernia, abdominal wall 212
Hiccups (singultus), diaphragm 211
High blood pressure 65
Hip joint arthrosis, coxarthrosis 303
Hip pains 302
Hirsuties coronae glandis, penis 261
Histamine intolerance 152
Hives, urticaria, skin 271
Ho'oponopono, therapy 56
Hodgkin's disease, lymphatic system 146
Homeopathy 60
Hordeolum, eye 85
Hormonal and vegetative imbalance . 115
Hormonal contraception, medicines 63
Hospital germs, MRSA 69
Hot lumps, thyroidea 122
Hot stroke, nerve system 78
HPV-induced cell proliferation 252
Human chorionic gonadotropin, HCG 42
Hydrocele, testicles 257
Hydrocephalus, water on the brain 81
Hydronephrosis, kidneys 234
Hypacusis, ear 111
Hyperacidity of the stomach 190
Hyperactivity, children 33
Hyperaldosteronism, adrenal glands . 117
Hypercalcemia, parathyroid 122
Hypercoagulability, blood 138
Hypercortisolism, adrenal glands 117
Hyperfunction of the thyroid 120
Hyperglycemia, pancreas 222, 223
Hyperhidrosis, skin 280
Hyperinsulinanemia, pancreas 224

Hyperkeratosis, skin 276
Hypermenorrhea, uterus 249
Hyperopia, eye 102
Hyperparathyroidism, parathyroidea . 122
Hyperplasia of the endometrium, uterus 244
Hyperplasia of the stomach mucosa . 192
Hypersomnia, hypophysis 114
Hypertension, high blood pressure 65
Hyperthyrosis, thyroidea 120
Hypertonia, high blood pressure 65
Hypertropia, eye 91
Hypoglycemia, pancreas 224
Hypophysis 113
Hyposmia, nose 154
Hypothalamus, tumor 115
Hypothyroidism, thyroidea 120
Hypotonia 66

I

Ibuprofen, medicines 62
Icterus, liver 219
Iga nephropathy, kidneys 232
Ileum, small intestine 196
Ileus, large intestine 202
Immune system 22
Immunoglobulins, (Ig) M, G, A, E, D .. 41
Imperative urinary incontinence 238
Indocin, medicines 62
Indomethacin, medicines 62
Induratio penis plastica, penis 263
Infarction of the heart muscle 126
Infection laboratory value 41
Infertility in women 242
Inflamed bone marrow 291
Influenza 68
Inguinal canal, peritoneum 257
Inguinal hernia, abdominal wall 215
Inheritance 320
Inner ear 109
Inner germ layer 15
Inner labia or vagina, fungal infection . 253
Inner navel, cancer 214
Inoculation, vaccination 64
Insomnia, sleep disorders 66
Intercerebral hemorrhage, nervous system 79
Intermittent claudication, blood vessels 140
Intestinal infarct, small intestine 198
Intestinal obstruction, ileus 202
Intestines, inflammation 202
Intraductal prostatic cancer 260
Intraductal cancer, breast 267
Introversion, constellation 315
Invagination 199
Inverted eyelid, entropion, trichiasis 87
Iris musculature, eye 89
Iris nevus, eye 94
Iris, ciliary body, tumor 94
Iritis, eye 94
Ischium bone, pain 302

J

Jaundice, icterus, gallbladder 219
Jaundice in newborn babies 219
Jaw 181
Jaw cysts 184
Jaw Tumor, odontoma, osteosarcoma 184
Jejunum 196
Jim Humble, MMS 62
Joint body, loose, knee 305
Joints 286
Joints, inflammation 291
Juvenile kyphosis, spine 300

K

Kadian, medicines 62
Kahler's disease, bone marrow tumor 292
Keloid, skin 283
Keratitis, eye 93
Keratoconus, eye 93, 101
Kernicterus, liver, baby 219
Kidney arteries 234
Kidney cavity 229
Kidney collecting tubules 230
Kidney cyst 229
Kidney failure, acute 232
Kidney gravel 234
Kidney laboratory values 40
Kidney poisoning 234
Kidney stones, nephroliths 234
Kidney tumor 229
KIdney-collecting tubules 230
Kidney, sacculated 234
Kidneys 228
Kidneys, ischemic tubulopathy 232
Kleptomania, constellation 315
Klinefelter syndrome, testicles 256
Knee joint, mouse 305
Knee joint, inflammation, arthritis, ... 304
Knee pains 304
Knee, cruciate or collateral ligament . 304
Knee, damaged cartilage 304
Knee, torn meniscus 304

L

Laboratory Values 37
Lack of appetite 68
Lacrimal gland excretory ducts 86
Lacrimal gland, inflammation, tumor .. 84
Lacrimal glands 84
Lactose intolerance, malabsorption ... 197
Large intestine 201
Laryngeal asthma 157
Laryngeal musculature 157
Laryngitis, inflammation 156
Larynx 155
Larynx carcinoma, papilloma 156
Larynx mucosa 156
Lateral or branchiogenous neck cyst . 178
Laws of Nature 9

LCIS, breast 265, 267
Leg veins 143
Leg veins, inflammation 143
Legg-Calve-Perthe's disease, bones .. 303
Legionnaire's disease, lungs 159
Leiomyoma, myoma, uterus 248
Lense, eye 92
Lentigo maligna, skin 281
Leper, term 281
Leprosy, skin 280
Leucopenia, blood 135
Leukemia, blood 135
Leukocytes, blood 38
Leukoplakia, blood 174
Leydig cell tumor, testicles 255
Life expectancy 320
Ligaments 288
Light, hypersensitivity, eye 89
Lip, tumor 172
Lipase, phospholipase, laboratory value 40
Lipedema, skin 283
Lipoma, skin 282
Liver 216
Liver abscess 217
Liver adeno-ca 216
Liver cirrhosis 221
Liver cysts, PLD - polycystic liver disease 221
Liver failure 220
Liver tuberculosis 217
Liver, laboratory value 39
Lobular breast cancer 265
Lobular cancer in situ = LCIS, breast . 267
Lobular carcinoma in situ, breast 265
Local conflict 12
Loss of appetite, anorexia 317
Love 322
Low blood pressure 66
Lower back pain, LBP, ... 300
Lues, skin 262
Lumbar spine or coccyx, pain 300
Lumps, toxic 119
Lung artery, occlusion 165
Lungs 158
Lupus erythematodes, skin 271
Lying, constellation 316
Lyme borreliosis, disease 69
Lymph drainage 61
Lymph node cancer, lymphoma 146
Lymph node inflammation 146
Lymphadenitis, lymphadenopathy 146
Lymphangitis 146
Lymphatic system 145
Lymphedema 148
Lymphoblastic leukemia, blood 135
Lymphoma 146

M

Macular degeneration, eye 97
Macular, eye 97

Malaria, sickle-cell disease, blood 136
Male sterility 264
Malignant 21
Mammary glands, cancer 265
Mania, constellation 314
Massage 60
Mast cell leukemia, blood 135
Mastitis, breast 270
Math problems, children 34
Matrix Reimprinting, therapy 55
MC (molluscum contagiosum), eye 82
Measles, rubella, skin 275
Meckel's diverticulum, small intestine 195
Medial neck cysts 121, 179
Medication 62
Medipren, medicines 62
Meditation, therapy 52
Megalomania, constellation 314
Melanoma of the iris, eye 94
Melanoma on the breast 269
Melanoma, skin 278
Ménière's disease, MD, ear 111
Meningitis, encephalomeningitis 79
Menopausal complaints 243
Menstrual distress, pains 250
Menstruation, absence of, irregular .. 242
Metastases 21
Microbes 18
Micropenis 264
Midbrain 16
Middle ear infection 105
Middle germ layer 15
Migraines, nervous system 71
Miosis, eye 89
Miscarriage, premature birth 250
Mitral valve, heart 129
MMS, Jim Humble 62
Molluscum contagiosum, MC, eye 82
Molluscum contagiosum, MC, skin ... 276
Mononucleosis, lymphatic system 146
Morphine, medicines 62
Motor neuropathy, muscular system . 310
Motrin, medicines 62
Mouth 171
MRSA, hospital germs 69
MS, multiple sclerosis 309
Mucoviscidosis of the salivary glands 177
Multiple myeloma, bones 292
Multiple sclerosis, MS 308
Mumps, throat 179
Muscle fibers, torn 312
Muscle paralysis 308
Muscle spasms 309
Muscle tension, distension, ruptured 312
Muscular system 307
Music therapy 53
Mycoses, small intestine 198
Mydriasis, eye 89
Myelofibrosis, bone 290

Myeloid leukemia, acute, chronic 135
Myocardial infarction, heart 126
Myocarditis, heart 128
Myogelosis, muscular system 312
Myoma, uterus 248
Myopia, eye 100
Myosclerosis, bones 312
Mythomaniac constellation 316
Myxedema, thyroid 120
Myxoma, jaw tumor 184

N
Nail bed infection 280
Nail fungus, tinea 279
Navel 212
Nearsightedness, eye 100
Neck cyst 147
Neck pain, bones 295
Necrosis of the femoral head, bones . 303
Nephroblastoma, kidneys 229
Nephroliths, kidneys 234
Nephrotic syndrome, kidneys 232
Nerve sheath 80
Nerve tumor, neurofibroma 80
Nervous system 71
Neuralgia 72
Neuroblastoma, adrenal glands 118
Neurodermatitis, skin 271
Neurofibroma, nerve tumor 80
Neuropathy, skin 273
New-mesoderm 15
Newborn icterus, liver 219
Night blindness, eye 89
Nodular malignant melanoma 278
Nodules of the pupillary seam 94
Non-Hodgkin's lymphoma 147
Norwalk virus 198
Nose 151
Nose polyps 154
Nosebleeds 137, 155
Nuprin, medicines 62
Nutrition 57
Nympho, and Casanova constellation . 315
Nymphomania, constellation 315
Nystagmus, dancing eyes 92

O
Obesity, overweight 67
Obsessive-constellation 317
Occipital constellation 316
Odontoma, jaw tumor 184
Oil pulling, therapy 61
Old-mesoderm 15
Olfactory epithelium 154
Oligodendroglioma, nervous system ... 74
Omentum majus, ... 215
Omentum, gr. 212
Ontogenetic system 14
Onychomycosis, skin 279

Open leg ulcer, blood vessels 144
Open-angle glaucoma, eye 97
Optical nerve, eye 96
Orange peel syndrome, skin 283
Orofacial cleft, mouth 178
Osteoarthritis, bones 288
Osteoblastoma, bones 292
Osteochondritis dissecans, bones 305
Osteochondroma, bones 292
Osteogenesis imperfecta, bones 290
Osteoma, bones 292
Osteomyelitis, bones 291
Osteomyelosclerosis, bones 290
Osteoporosis, bones 289
Osteosarcoma, bones 184, 292
Otitis externa circumscripta, ear 109
Otitis externa, ear 107
Otitis media, ear 105
Otosclerosis, otospongiosis, ear 110
Otospongiosis, ear 110
Ouabain, medicines, heart 133
Outer germ layer 15
Ovarian abscess 242
Ovarian cysts, cancer 240
Ovaries 240
Overweight, adiposity 67
Oxcarbazepine, medicines 72

P
Paget's disease, bone 290
Paget's disease, breast 267
Pain medications 62
Painting therapy 54
Palatal cancer, adeno-ca, mouth 174
Pancreas 222
Pancreas insufficiency, exogene 227
Pancreas laboratory value 39
Pancreas, inflammation 227, 228
Pancreatic cancer, adeno-ca 226
Pancreatic ductal/intraductal cancer . 227
Pancreatic excretory ducts 227
Pancreatic islet, alpha cells 224
Pancreatitis 227, 228
Papillary adenoma, breast 267
Paracetamol, medicines 62
Paranoia, constellation 316
Parathyroid gland 122
Parathyroid hormone, PTH 122
Paratyphus, small intestine 198
Parkinson's disease, muscular system 311
Parodontitis, teeth 184, 186
Paronychia, nail bed infection 280
Parotid salivary gland ducts 179
Parvovirus 198
Pelvic bone, pain 302
Pelvic organ prolapse, uterus 249
Pemphigus, skin 271
Penile melanoma 262
Penile papules 261

Penis 261
Penis deformation, deviation 263
Pericardial effusion, exsudative 130
Pericardial effusion, transudative 130
Pericardial sac, inflammation 129
Pericarditis, heart 129
Pericardium, heart 129
Periodontal abscess, tooth fistula 186
Peritoneal cancer, mesothelioma 213
Peritoneum 212
Peritonitis, inflammation 213
Pernicious anemia 137
Persistent conflict activity 22
Persistent repair 22
Perspiration, hyperhidrosis, skin 280
Pertussis, lungs 168
Petroleum, medicines 62
Peyronie's disease, penis 263
Pharyngeal polyps 175
Pharyngitis, inflammation 176
Pheochromocytoma, adrenal glands . 118
Phimosis, penis 263
Phlebitis, veins, blood vessels 143
Phlegm, mucus, lungs 164
Pigment nevus, skin 281
Pigmentation disturbances, vitiligo ... 277
PIN, prostate gland 260
Pineal tumor 76
Pinealozytes 76
Pineoblastoma, pineocytoma 76
Pinguecula, eye 83
Pink eye, conjunctivitis 82
Pituitary gland, hypophysis 113
Plantar warts, skin 276
Plasmacytoma, bones 292
PLD, polycystic liver disease 221
Pleura cancer 169
Pleura mesothelioma 169
Pleural adhesions, empyema 170
Pleural effusion, exsudative 170
Pleurisy 170
Pneumoconiosis 168
Pneumocystis pneumonia 159
Pneumonia, lungs 159
Polio, muscular system 308
Polyarthritis of the finger joints 298
Polyarthritis, joints 293
Polycystic liver disease 221
Polycythemia vera, blood 135
Polycythemia, blood 139
Polyneuropathy, skin 273
Polyps, small intestine 196
Posterior vitreous detachment, PVD, eye 95
Posthitis, penis 26
Postmortem constellation 315
Potency disturbances 264
Praying 52
Pre-eclampsia, PE, pregnancy 249
Pregnancy 28

Premature birth, therapy 250
Premenstrual syndrome 250
Prepuce, inflammation, penis 264
Presbyopia, eye 103
Pressure within the eye 95
Procreation 28
Prolactinoma, hypophysis 113
Prolapsed cervical disc 296
Prolapsed disc, lumbar spine 301
Prostate cancer, adeno-ca 258
Prostate gland 258
Prostate-specific antigen, PSA 41
Prostate, enlargement 258
Prostate, laboratory value 41
Prostatic hyperplasia 258
Prostatic intraepithelial neoplasia 260
Protein, albumin, microglobulin 40
Proteinuria, laboratory value 40
PSA, laboratory value 41
PSA, prostate gland 260
Pseudocroup, bronchi 158
Psoriasis, skin 274
Psycho-pharmaceuticals 63
Psychodrama, Moreno, therapy 50
Psychotherapy 54
PTB, pulmonary tuberculosis 159
Pterygium, eye 83
Ptosis, eyelid 87
Pubic bone, pain 302
Pulmonary abscess, tuberculosis 159
Pulmonary embolism 165
Pulmonary emphysema, sarcoidosis .. 160
Pupil constriction, miosis, eye 89
Pupils, unevenly shaped 89
PVD, posterior vitreous detachment ... 95
Pyelectasis, renal pelvis 234
Pyelonephritis, renal pelvis 233

Q
Q & A examples 45
Questions about conditioning 44
Questions about the conflict 43

R
Radiation therapy 63
Radiation, electromagnetic 318
Raynaud syndrome, blood vessels 142
Raynaud's phenomenon, blood vessels 142
Raynaud's phenomenon, nipple, breast 269
Reading problems, children 33
Reconciling, therapy 49
Rectal cancer, adeno-ca, colon 204
Rectal cramps, anus 206
Rectum 204
Recurring conflicts 22
Red-green color blindness, eye 99
Reduced sexual drive 242, 264
Reflux, stomach 191
Regression therapy 55

Reincarnation therapy 55
Relationships, therapy 318
Religiousness, therapy 52
Renal artery stenosis 234
Renal pelvis, inflammation, cancer 233
Renal pelvis, enlargement 234
Repair phase 13
Repair phase crisis 13
Residual urine, bladder 238
Restless activity, mania, constellation 315
Restless legs syndrome 310
Retina, eye 98
Retinal detachment, edema, eye 98
Rhagades, mouth 173
Rheumatic spectrum disorder 293
Rheumatism 293, 294
Rheumatism laboratory value 41
Rhinitis, nose 151
Rhinophyma, blood vessels 141
Rib pain, bones 299
Ring calcification, heart valves 129
Rituals, therapy 51
Rolling of the eyes, zyklotropia 91
Rosacea, blood vessels 141
Rotavirus, small intestine 198
Round back, spine 300
Round liver lesions 216
Rubella, skin 275
Running amok, constellation 316
Runny nose 153
Rupture of the Achilles tendon 306

S
Salivary gland cysts 178
Salivary glands 177
Salpingitis, fallopian tube 245
Satyriasis, constellation 315
SBS, Significant Biological Special Program 11
Scar proliferation, keloid, skin 283
Scarlet fever 173, 277
SCD, sickle-cell anemia 136
SCD, Sudden cardiac death 128
Scheuermann's disease, spine 300
Schistosomiasis, worm disease 198
Sciatica, lumbar spine 300
Sclerosing adenosis, breast glands 267
Scoliosis, spine 300
Seborrheic keratosis, skin 276
Seclusion, autistic constellation 315
Semicircular canals, dizziness, ear 112
Seminoma, testicles 255
Sense of smell, nose 154
Sex drive, increased, constellation 315
Sexual desire, lack of 242
Shiatsu, therapy 61
Shingles (herpes zoster), skin 278
Shock kidney (acute ischemic tubulopathy) 232
Shocked solidification, constellation .. 316
Short frenulum, penis 263

Short stature - dwarfism 115
Short stature, somatotropin deficiency 114
Shortening of the flexor tendons, joint 299
Shortsightedness, eye 100
Shoulder pain 296
Sialadenitis, salivary glands, mouth . 177, 180
Sickle-cell anemia, blood 136
Side stitches, diaphragm 211
Sigmoid colon 203
Sigmoid colon, cancer 203
Significant Biological Special Program . 11
Silicosis, black lung disease 168
Singultus, diaphragm 211
Sinus infection, sinusitis, nose 151
Sinuses, suppuration, nose 154
Sinusitis 151
Sjögren Syndrome, eye 84
Skin 271
Skin cancer, melanoma 278
Skin rash 271
Sleep apnea, diaphragm 210
Sleep disorders 66
Sliding, rocking, walking testicles 256
Slipped vertebrae, spondylolisthesis .. 302
Small cell bronchial cancer 167
Small intestine 194
Small intestine, inflammation 197
Smegma-producing glands 264
Smoking, lungs 168
Social, overly constellation 314
Sodium chlorite, MMS, medicines 62
Somatotropin deficiency, hypophysis 114
Soor vulvitis 253
Sounds in the ear, tinnitus 109
Spastic bronchitis 163
Spasticity, muscular system 310
Spelling problems, children 34
Sphincter spasms, anus 206
Spinal stenosis 302
Spirituality, therapy 321
Spleen 149
Spleen enlargement, splenomegaly .. 150
Splenic abscesses, cysts 150
Splenitis, inflammation 150
Spondylolisthesis, bones 302
Sport 318
Spot baldness, hair loss 284
Squamous cell cancer, skin 271
Stammering, stuttering 157
Stapedius muscle, ear 108
Stapedotomy, ear 111
Staphylococcal pneumonia 159
Stomach 189
Stomach bleeding, colic 193
Stomach polyps, cancer (adeno-ca) .. 192
Stomach ulcer, epithelial cancer 190
Strabismus, eye 90
Stress incontinence, bladder 239
Stretch marks, skin 282

Striae cutis atrophicae 282
Stroke of the optical nerve 96
Stroke, nervous system 77
Stuttering, stammering 157
Styes, hordeolum, eye 85
Subarachnoid hemorrhage, brain 79
Subclavian artery, blood vessels 145
Subconscious mind, therapy 47
Subglottic-stenosing laryngitis 158
Sudden cardiac death, SCD, heart 128
Sudden deafness, ear 110
Sudeck's dystrophy, joints 290
Sun allergy, skin 274
Sunburn, skin 281
Sweat glands, skin 279
Swine flu 68
Synovial membrane, bones and joints 298
Syphilis, lues, male 262

T
Tarry stool 193, 195, 197
Tartar, teeth 185
Tear fluid, eye 84
Tear Gland Ducts, eye 86
Teeth 181
Telangiectatic rosacea, blood vessels . 141
Tenesmus, rectal cramps 206
Tennis elbow, bones and joints 297
Tenosynovitis, bones and joints 298
Teratoma, female 242
Teratoma, male 257
Territory marking constellation 316
Testicles 255
Testicles, rocking, walking 256
Testicular cancer, tumor 255
Testicular hypogonadism 256
Testicular pouch, fluid in 257
Thalamus 115
The clap 254
Theater therapy 50
Thelitis, breast glands 270
Therapy 46
Thinning of the cornea, keratoconus, eye 93
Thinning of the cornea, eye 101
Thoracic spine 300
Throat 171
Thromboembolism, blood vessels 165
Thrombophilia, blood 138
Thrombosis, Thrombophlebitis leg veins 143
Thrombosis tendency, thrombophilia . 138
Thyreotropes, hypophysis 114
Thyroglossal duct cysts 179
Thyroid 118
Thyroid excretory ducts 121
Thyroid stimulating cells, hypophysis 114
Thyroid tumor 119
Thyroid, hyperfunction 120, 122
Thyroid, laboratory value 37
Thyroiditis, inflammation 120

Tinnitus, ear 109
Tongue 172
Tongue, musculature, paralysis 179
Tonsil cancer, adeno-ca 175
Tonsil infections, tonsillitis 175
Tooth enamel 182
Tooth fistula 186
Tooth loss 184
Trachea 158
Trachea, inflammation, tracheitis 163
Tracheal cancer, tracheitis 163
Trachoma, Egyptian ophthalmia, eye .. 93
Transudative pleural effusion 171
Trench mouth, leukoplakia 174
Trichiasis, inverted eyelid 87
Trigeminal neuralgia 72
Trigon Mucosa, bladder 237
Trisomy 21 69
Tromboembolism, intestinal infarct 198
TSH, thyroid stimulating hormone 121
Tubal pregnancy, fallopian tubes 246
Tubo-ovarian abscess, fallopian tubes 245
Tubulopathy, toxic, kidneys 234
Tumor markers, laboratory values 42
Turner syndrome, underdevelopment 241
Two-phased process 13
Tympanic muscle, ear 108
Typhus, small intestine 198

U
Ulcus duodeni, ... 194
Ulcus molle, men 262
Ulcus molle, women 252
Ultraviolet (UV) rays, skin 281
Umbilical hernia, Abdominal wall 215
Unconsciousness (absence seizures) 69
Undersized penis 264
Underweight 68
Undescended testicles 256
Urea, laboratory value 40
Uremia, kidneys 230
Urethra, bladder 235
Uric acid, laboratory value 40
Urinary incontinence, bladder 238
Urinary stones, bladder 240
Urine loss, bladder 239
Urine retention, prostate 260
Urocystitis, bladder 236
Urothelium cancer, bladder 236
Urothelium papilloma 236
Urticaria, skin 271
Uterine adeno-ca 244
Uterine and pelvic organ prolapse 249
Uterine muscles, tumor 248
Uterus 244
Uveal melanoma, eye 94
Uveitis, eye 94

V
Vaccinations 64
Vaginal cramps, vaginismus 251
Vaginal discharge, fluor genitalis 254
Vaginal epithelial cancer 252
Vaginal glands, inflammation 253
Vaginal inflammation, colpitis 252
Vaginal mycosis 253
Vaginal submucosa 253
Vaginal, yeast infection 254
Vaginismus, vaginal cramps 251
Varices, blood vessels 143
Varicose vein, varices 143
Vascular dilation, face 141
Vegetative state, constellation 313
Venous ulcer, open leg ulcer 144
Verrucae, skin 276
Vertigo, ear 112
Vestibular schwannoma 106
Viruses, microbes 18
Visualization, therapy 53
Vitamin B12 deficiency, pernicious anemia 137
Vitiligo, skin 277
Vitreous body, opacity, eye 95
Vocal cord polyps, larynx 157
Volvulus, small intestine 199
Vulva 251
Vulvitis 252

W
Walking testicles 256
Wall-eye (exotropia) 91
Warfarin, medicine 63
Wart-like fat deposits on the eyelid 83
Warts (verrucae), skin 276
Water in the lungs 167
Water on the brain 81
Wedge vertebrae, spine 300
Weeping eyes (epiphora) 88
White blood cell deficiency (leucopenia) 135
Whooping cough (pertussis) 168
Widening of the pupils (mydriasis), eye 89
Wilms' tumor, kidneys 229
Wilms' tumor, nephroblastoma 229
Withdrawn aloofness, constellation .. 317
Worm diseases, small intestine 198

X
Xanthelasma, eye 83
Xerophthalmia, eye 84

Z
Zyklotropia, rolling of the eye 91

Have you ever wondered if diseases could be related to what goes on in our psyches?
Have you searched in vain for answers? Refusing to believe that everything in life just happens for no reason?
If so, then this is the book for you!

Inside, the author presents the groundbreaking discovery of the 5 Biological Laws of Nature. These are the basic laws that govern our organism and they are explained here in easy-to-understand, layman's terms.

The 5 Biological Laws of Nature are a solid foundation for understanding the nature of health and disease.

The comprehensive reference section is organized by organ and describes the roots, meaning, course, and support options for all common diseases.

More than 500 examples and 65 anatomical illustrations make this book not only a handy guide for therapists and medical professionals, but everyone interested in leading a healthy life. Thanks to its simplicity, this book is an ideal resource for every home library.

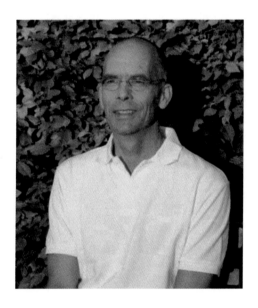

The author, Björn Eybl, was born in 1965 in Austria. After finishing high school, he finished in 8th place at the Los Angeles Olympics in windsurfing.

Rather than becoming a part of his father's commercial business, he opted to become a massage therapist.

Since then, he has worked as a therapist for over 29 years in private practice. He is married and spends his free time with his wife in the mountains.

For the last 15 years, he has worked intensively with Dr. Hamer's discoveries and is committed to liberating humanity from our current medical paradigm through the dissemination of Dr. Hamer's life work.

"Everything must be based on a simple idea.
If we ever discover it, will be so persuasive and wonderful
that we will say to each other:
Of course, it could not be any different. "

John Wheeler, Physicist

Made in the USA
Las Vegas, NV
16 March 2024